Bariatric Surgery Cookbook

A Complete Informative Guide For You To Go Through Before Going For The Surgery With A Meal Plan For You To Follow And 1001 Amazingly Delicious Recipes

By

FAYE ELLEDGE

Table of Contents

Chapter 14-Dips, Dressings and Sauces Recipes 350

Introduction

The battle is genuine. It's a constant battle to lose weight. Knowing what to eat, when to eat it, and how to eat it can be difficult, especially in today's world of fad diets and inconsistent instructions and advice. When you add in the ever-changing trends in the world of exercise, the prospect of reducing weight might be intimidating. However, it is a crucial struggle that must be fought. It's a fight worth fighting.

Obesity is a multifaceted disease with several causes. Genetics, diet, the environment, and even the microorganisms in our gut all have an impact. Obesity continues to rise despite substantial advancements in nutrition science and medicine. In the United States, three-quarters of adults are overweight or obese. Obesity is the leading cause of death in the United States. The entire economic cost of obesity is projected to be $1.72 trillion per year or nearly 9.3% of GDP. Traditional diet and exercise plans can lead to significant weight loss, but keeping the weight off is usually the challenge. No treatment has been found to produce significant, long-term weight loss other than bariatric surgery, especially for those who suffer from extreme obesity.

The object of bariatric surgery is to attain significant weight loss that leads to improved health and quality of life. The number on the scale is an element of the broader goal, but it isn't the end goal. Bariatric surgery is a potent surgical intervention for weight loss that encourages behavioral changes. It necessitates a considerable change in lifestyle.

It's almost like having a full-time job as a bariatric surgery patient. You must consume several small meals throughout the day, stay hydrated by sipping water, take multivitamins, and exercise in between all of this. A significant part of altering one's lifestyle is changing one's food, which is much easier to do with a book like this one.

This is one of the first cookbooks to offer advice and suggestions for both before and after bariatric surgery. Furthermore, the techniques espoused in this book can be used by family members who want to assist their loved ones on their bariatric journey or even apply them to their own life in order to improve their health. The healthy behavior induced by bariatric surgery has been proven in studies to create a halo effect, resulting in weight loss in patients' family members as well.

This book is an essential resource for any bariatric patient. It includes a well-organized, simple-to-follow, comprehensive plan with delectable recipes and nutritious meal plans that are simple to prepare and help you lose weight.

Bariatric surgery can have a dramatic influence on one's health, sometimes practically immediately. The wonderful thing is that small moments of delight and accomplishment continue throughout the wellness journeys of those who have the surgery performed. They relish "non-scale triumphs," such as being able to cross their legs, buy items off the rack, keep active with loved ones, and face life with confidence in both new and old familiar ways. It can be difficult to learn how to care for oneself after surgery, but this book is here to help you through every step, both before and after surgery.

You'll find ideas and advice for dietary and lifestyle changes in the first few chapters, which will help you prepare for surgery and life afterward.

You'll also receive tips on how to handle social occasions, eat out, and breakthrough plateaus. The dishes in this book are simple, tasty, and healthy. Knowing what to eat, as well as how to cook and organize meals for success, can give you confidence. Of course, your wellness journey begins with you, but it's critical that you work closely with your surgical facility for support throughout this particular procedure. There is no such thing as a "one-size-fits-all" solution, so talk to your care team about your specific needs. Throughout this journey, there will undoubtedly be many joys and trials, and as you know, success does not come easily. Begin each day with a new perspective and a commitment to achieving little goals each day. This is an opportunity for a fresh start, a chance to let go of the past and move on with confidence and excitement. Surgery, as well as a major lifestyle change, can be frightening, and you may not have made this decision lightly. Whatever decision you choose, you've just made a huge investment in the remainder of your life. Let's get this party started!

Chapter 1-Bariatric Journey: Surgery Guide

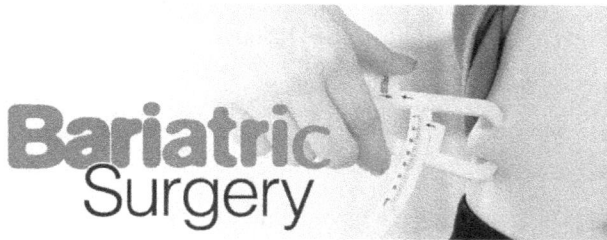

Your initiative

Congratulations on your weight-loss surgery decision!

This is a fresh start, an opportunity to reset your mind, body, and lifestyle. Your decision was most likely the result of a lot of thought and preparation. Even if you have a lot of information regarding the treatment, surgery, and lifestyle adjustments that come with it can be intimidating. Some of your friends and family members may have questioned your decision or advised other, more traditional methods for losing weight and improving your health. However, surgery appeared to be a crucial step toward greater health control, and your medical team concurred.

This book will help you overcome your worries and provide you with the tools you need to accept your new way of life. You'll discover advice on how to prepare for surgery, what to eat afterward, and how to buy for and cook meals in the first few chapters, as well as, perhaps, inspiration for making long-term adjustments to live your healthiest life. The remaining chapters, of course, are jam-packed with delectable dishes that will help you feel your best.

Food that is delicious and healthy

It's difficult to conceive that you'll ever enjoy genuine, chewable food again during the first few weeks after surgery when you're reliant on liquids for nutrition. You might even be questioning whether surgery was the best decision in between sips of protein shakes and hydrating beverages. It's tough to envision how your life and diet will be in a few years, or even a few months, after surgery. However, when you heal and return to normal textures, you'll be able to eat a greater variety of nutritious foods. This book will help you learn new and innovative ways to cook with familiar products using simple kitchen items you probably already have at home as you work toward a better lifestyle. You'll soon be inventing creative ways to employ products that are easily available at your local supermarket, regardless of the season.

A few improvements

You'll discover that little, long-term adjustments have the greatest influence on your life and health as you go. It's easy to compare yourself to others and fear that you won't achieve the same results. But, with hard effort and determination, you can get there one step at a time. Rather than becoming overwhelmed by the distance between where you are and where you want to go, concentrate on what you can do right now. Consider taking the stairs instead of the elevator or getting off the bus a stop early to walk the rest of the way if your goal is to become more active. Consider foregoing the starchy side dish and piling on more vegetables to your plate if you want to make better dietary choices. These minor decisions, like taking a shower or brushing your teeth, will become everyday habits as you practice them.

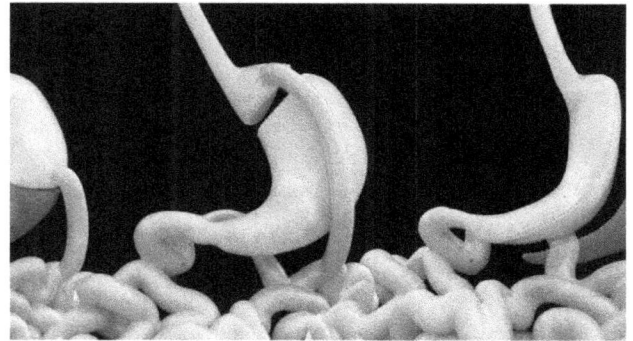

Your surgery your opinion

The Roux-en-Y gastric bypass (RYGB), laparoscopic sleeve gastrectomy (LSG), and the adjustable gastric band are the most popular bariatric operations nowadays (AGB). All bariatric operations aim to curb hunger and promote portion management. Some procedures, on the other hand, work at a far deeper biochemical level. Type 2 diabetes, high blood pressure, sleep apnea, fatty liver, and other comorbidities have all been proven to improve after certain operations. Your surgeon and medical team's knowledge will be required to choose which procedure is best for you. Each surgery has its own set of benefits and drawbacks, but they all assist you in regaining control of your health. Regardless of which procedure you choose, you may feel comfortable that it was the greatest choice for you.

The Roux-En-Y gastric bypass

This treatment is considered the "gold standard" of weight-loss surgery. It is also known as gastric bypass. There are two stages to the procedure: Your surgical team will first divide the small intestine and form a small stomach pouch of about one ounce in capacity. The pouch is then attached directly to the small intestine's lower portion. Food eaten will bypass much of the stomach and the first segment of the small intestine, traveling directly from the stomach pouch to the bottom section of the small intestine.

Advantages

- Reduces stomach capacity and food intake by altering gastrointestinal hormones in a positive way, reducing appetite and increasing satiety.

- Weight loss and maintenance may be aided by changes in energy expenditure.

- If required, reversible

- Possibility of large (60 to 80 percent) long-term excess weight loss with more than 50% weight maintenance

Disadvantages

- Surgical complication rates are higher when compared to gastric sleeve and band treatments.

- Long-term vitamin and mineral deficiency is a high danger.

- The most time spent in the hospital

- Food intolerances and dumping syndrome are very common.

Laparoscopic sleeve gastrectomy

Under the supervision of their surgical teams, sleeve patients will have around 80% of their stomachs removed. The operation works by limiting the amount of food that the stomach can hold at one time, leaving just a small, tubular pouch in the shape of a banana. However, it has the largest impact on gut hormones, which influence hunger, satiety, and blood sugar management.

Advantages

- Limits the amount of food you can eat by limiting the capacity of your stomach.

- Changes gut hormones in a positive way, lowering appetite and increasing satiety.

- When compared to gastric bypass, there are fewer surgical complications.

- When compared to gastric bypass, there is a lower chance of dumping syndrome.

- It does not necessitate the use of a foreign device (such as a gastric band) or the rerouting of the food stream (as in gastric bypass)

- In comparison to gastric bypass, hospital stays are shorter.

- Possibility of large excess weight loss (more than 50%)

Disadvantages

- Long-term vitamin and mineral deficiency is a possibility.

- Acid reflux is a possibility.

- Nonreversible

The adjustable gastric band

An inflatable band is put near the top of the stomach to produce a tiny stomach pouch in gastric band procedures. The pouch can be gradually reduced in size over time by filling the band with saline through a port beneath the abdominal wall. The ease with which food can flow from the tiny pouch into the lower stomach is affected by tightening the band in this way. The pouch is intended to satisfy hunger while also promoting a sense of fullness.

Advantages

- Limits food intake by reducing stomach capacity.

- With no incisions in the stomach wall or intestines, this procedure is completely customizable and reversible.

- Early post-operative surgical complication rates are the lowest.

- Vitamin and mineral shortages are the least likely to occur.

- Hospital stays that are the shortest

- Excess weight loss of 40 to 50 percent is achieved.

Disadvantages

- Slower and less rapid weight loss than gastric bypass and band procedures

- Requires the use of a foreign device that must be kept in the body for an extended period of time

- Complications such as band slippage and erosion are possible.

- Risk of esophageal dilatation in overeating individuals Risk of developing intolerances to particular food textures Requires more regular follow-ups for band adjustment

- The highest re-operation rate.

Friends and family support

The individuals in your life can influence your ability to stick to post-op lifestyle modifications. Involving trustworthy family members in your journey will help them prepare for the changes ahead, as well as understand how you prefer to receive support and encouragement. Making the decision to have surgery is a personal one, and deciding who to inform and how to tell them can be difficult. Naturally, you won't want to share with those who aren't close to you or who might have an unfavorable opinion of you. If and when you decide to tell others, do so with the intention of gaining support and encouragement. Keep your conversations short when discussing with others, but highlight the personal significance of this decision: "You're a very important person to me, and I want you to be a part of this shift in my life," or "I've made a huge decision, and I want to share it with you." If you choose to be transparent about your decision, you may find that you have a large number of fans cheering you on. However, there may be detractors, some of whom may have little understanding of the process or may even be jealous of your weight-loss and health-improvement quest. Rather than allowing their criticisms to discourage you, remember why you chose this path and that you, as well as the outcomes that await you, are worth the effort. Keep in mind that you have no one but yourself to answer to. Follow your own path with your head held high; this is your decision and your adventure.

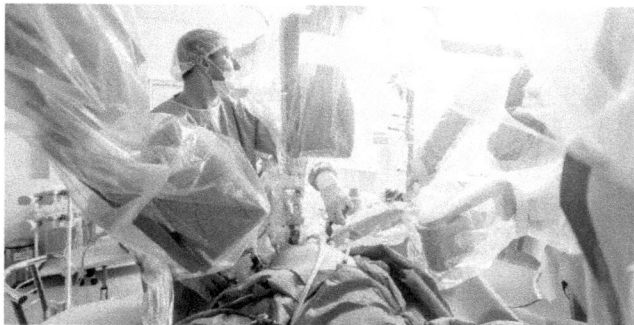

Common misconceptions about surgery

The easy way out is surgery. Surgery is a tool, not a miracle cure. Hard work and dedication will be required to achieve success.

Most patients find that surgery does not help them lose weight; instead, they gain it back. According to research, bariatric patients who underwent surgery lost more weight and maintained their success better than those who lost weight through diet and exercise.

Bariatric surgery is not without risks. The risk of death during the first 30 days after surgery is 0.13 percent, according to statistics from the ASMBS Bariatric Centers of Excellence database. This rate is much lower than that of other major surgical operations such as gallbladder and hip replacement. Furthermore, post-surgery data demonstrates a considerable decrease in mortality rates associated with various weight-related disorders. The death rate associated with diabetes, for example, drops by more than 90%.

Bariatric Surgery

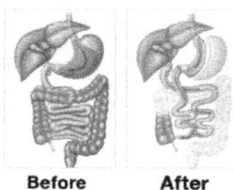

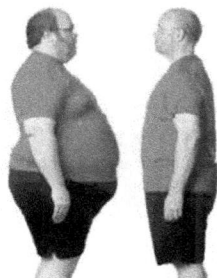

Before   After

Mental preparation

You're ready to move on after attending innumerable seminars, meetings, lectures, and more, and your care team agrees. However, it is totally normal to feel a mixture of excitement and fear as your surgery date approaches.

If your nerves are getting the best of you, try the following ways to relax your mind and body:

- Slowly and deeply, inhale and exhale.

- Listen to a guided meditation or practice mindful meditation techniques.

- Slowly tensing and releasing each muscle group in your body, starting with your toes and working your way up to your jaw, is a good way to practice progressive muscle relaxation.

- Visualize yourself in a place that provides you comfort, joy, and tranquillity using guided imagery techniques.

- Play your favorite relaxing music.

- Talk to a friend or family member about your feelings and thoughts, or write them down in a notebook.

- Get some fresh air by going for a walk.

- Focus on why you're having surgery and the results you are most excited about achieving.

- Additionally, preparing for your hospital stay and the first few weeks after surgery can help put your mind at ease. For your stay, consider packing comfortable clothing, a pillow to hold against your abdomen on the car ride home, protein shakes, chargers for your personal electronics, and any toiletries you may need. Having your post-op supplies ready before your surgery will also help you feel confident and equipped for the journey ahead.

Useful things to have at home when you return from the hospital:

- Measuring cups

- Hydrating fluids

- Protein shakes

- A reusable water bottle

- A blender or blender bottles

- Small bowls and plates

- Small airtight storage containers

- Appetizer spoons and forks

- A mug warmer (to keep small plates warm)

- Recommended vitamin and mineral supplements

- A food scale

- A food journal to track your fluid and protein intake

- An insulated bag or cooler

The day off

The first day of the rest of your life begins on the day of your surgery. You've probably spent months, if not years, getting ready for this. You've learned a lot about your procedure and put in a lot of time understanding and executing post-operative food and lifestyle advice. You've prepared your mind, body, and house for the following steps. If you're having second thoughts about your decision, remember why you made it in the first place. Consider how your life might change six or twelve months after surgery. Have faith in yourself and your capacity to accomplish your objectives. It will not always be easy following surgery, but your hard work and dedication will pay off. You can do it!

Keep the following in mind on the day of your surgery:

- You will most likely be asked to refrain from drinking anything for at least 4 hours before your treatment.

- When you wake up after surgery, you'll probably be advised to drink cautiously. Because your stomach can only hold a limited amount of liquid, drinking 8 ounces of water could take over an hour.

- With gas trapped in your abdomen, you will most likely feel uncomfortable. To relieve some of the pain, get up and walk around as much as possible.

Going home after surgery

You'll probably feel sleepy after surgery when the anesthetic wears off. You may also have nausea, gas sensations, and tenderness near the incision sites in your abdomen. Patients are often advised to start cautiously sipping liquids to check tolerance and support frequent hydration. To ease gas pain and prevent blood clots, your doctor may advise you to start walking. You will likely spend 1 to 3 days in the hospital, depending on your surgery. Many individuals who have pain after surgery worry that it will become their "new normal." Despite the frequent issues that accompany surgery, most people find that their energy and emotions improve over time. Your doctor will likely send you home to recover once you are ambulatory, with control over your pain, ability to urinate, and fluid tolerance. Make sure you and your surgical team go through your post-op instructions before you leave. Discuss your medication needs and when you should begin taking your post-operative vitamin and mineral supplements. Make sure you've planned your post-operative follow-up appointments and that you know who to contact if you have any questions or concerns. If you've made it this far, let me congratulate you on your achievement. You're all set to return home and begin your quest.

Chapter 2~Bariatric Journey: Nutritional Guide

Phases of Diet Before and After Bariatric Surgery

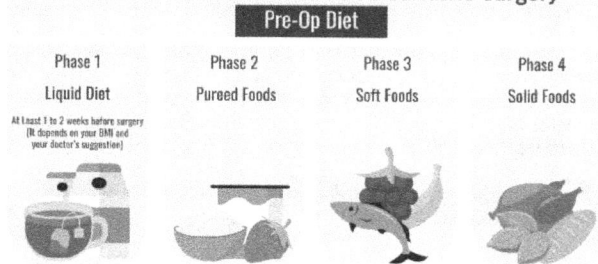

Pre-Op Diet

Phase 1	Phase 2	Phase 3	Phase 4
Liquid Diet	Pureed Foods	Soft Foods	Solid Foods
At Least 1 to 2 weeks before surgery (It depends on your BMI and your doctor's suggestion)			

Surgery is only a minor portion of your weight-loss and health-improvement journey. Your new lifestyle will require effort, time, and devotion, just like learning a new activity or sport. To set yourself up for success, you'll learn what to eat before and after surgery, how to shop wisely, and how to stock your bariatric-friendly kitchen.

The pre-operation diet

Most patients are needed to follow a pre-operative diet in order to lose weight and minimize the amount of fat in and around the liver and abdomen prior to surgery. This will reduce the risk of difficulties during your treatment and help you get used to a new way of eating. Your surgical team will determine your specific pre-op instructions and any required weight-loss goals, but this section provides basic advice for the pre-operative period that will also help you adjust to post-op life.

Pre~op diet recommendations

Pre-operative instructions differ from clinic to clinic and are occasionally patient-specific. Prior to surgery, you will most likely be required to follow a low-calorie, low-carbohydrate, or liquid diet for at least two weeks. Supplements and Protein Shakes Protein smoothies or powders will be used at some stage after bariatric surgery. Protein helps to build and preserve muscular tissue while also encouraging your body to burn fat rather than muscle. Protein shakes are a wonderful meal replacement alternative if you have to follow a liquid diet before surgery. Some commercial protein smoothies are heavy in sugar or have a low protein content per serving. Look for shakes that include at least 20 grams of protein per serving and are low in fat and carbohydrates as a general guideline.

Here are a few recommendations for protein supplements to get you started:

Whey Protein Isolate: Lactose-free, milk-based, complete protein (best tolerated and most absorbable for bariatric patients)

Soy Protein-Plant-based, complete protein

Egg White Protein-Non-milk-based, complete protein

Whey Protein Concentrate: Milk-based, complete protein containing lactose (may cause discomfort for gastric bypass patients with lactose intolerance after surgery) Fat Prior to surgery, you will need to be mindful about the amount and type of fat you consume to gain control over your caloric intake and help you lose weight. Use a food tracking app, and read labels to identify hidden sources of fat.

What to eat

- Almonds
- Avocados
- Canola oil
- Chia seeds
- Fatty fish (like salmon, tuna, and mackerel)
- Flaxseed
- Nut butter, all-natural
- Olives
- Olive oil
- Peanuts
- Seafood
- Walnuts

What to limit

- Animal fats
- Baked goods
- Chips
- Chocolate
- Cream sauces
- Foods high in saturated fat
- Fried foods
- Full-fat dairy products
- High-fat condiments (like mayonnaise)
- High-fat salad dressings
- Stick margarine containing hydrogenated oils
- Tropical oils

Sugar

Sugar is a particularly deceptive element that may be found in practically any prepared dish you buy. Ketchup, yogurt, dried fruit, barbecue and other sauces, fruit juices, spaghetti sauce, flavored coffees, pre-made soups, sports drinks, frozen dinners, protein bars, granola bars, and even some protein shakes are among the items with unexpectedly high sugar content. It can be difficult to eliminate sugar from your diet, but choosing healthier alternatives will aid in weight loss and promote better post-operative habits.

High Carbohydrate-Foods

Reducing carbohydrate intake has been demonstrated to help with weight loss, blood sugar control, and desire management. Giving up carbs, on the other hand, is easier said than done. While going fully carb-free before surgery may not be necessary, it is a good time to make some changes. For example, instead of a bun, try a lettuce-wrapped burger, cauliflower rice instead of white rice, or zucchini noodles instead of pasta noodles.

What to eat

- Dairy products, low-fat
- Nuts
- Seeds
- Vegetables, non-starchy (like asparagus, broccoli, cauliflower, kale, onions, spinach, and zucchini)
- Whole fruits

What to avoid

- Chips
- Corn
- Dried fruit
- Flour, white (as in bread, crackers, pasta, and tortillas)
- Fried foods
- Potatoes
- Rice
- Sweet sauces and dressings

Drinks

Because you won't be able to drink with your meals or ingest substantial amounts of fluid shortly after surgery, staying hydrated may be difficult. Aim for at least 48 to 64 ounces of hydrating fluids every day before surgery. Limit your caffeine intake and avoid high-fat or high-sugar beverages.

What to drink

- Broth, low-sodium
- Sports drinks, sugar-free
- Tea, unsweetened
- Water
- Water, flavored, sugar-free
- Water, infused

What to avoid

- Coffee
- Fruit juices
- Sodas and other carbonated drinks

Habits to Avoid Prior to surgery, you will be asked to quit smoking or using tobacco—both can delay healing and increase your risk for blood clots, pneumonia, and ulcers. You will also be asked to abstain from alcohol for a period of time before and after surgery.

Pre-op favorites

These pre-op staples are simple to prepare, high in protein, and low in carbs. They're also healthy and delicious options for the rest of your life.

Meals

- Denver Egg Muffins with Ham Crust
- Curried Chicken Salad
- Roasted Garden Vegetables
- Soy-Ginger Salmon with Bok Choy
- Sheet Pan Fajitas
- Barbecue Chicken and Portobello Pizzas
- Philly Cheesesteak–Stuffed Bell Peppers

Snacks

- String cheese wrapped in deli turkey
- Tuna salad with celery
- Plain, low-fat Greek yogurt mixed with flavored protein powder
- Protein shake with less than 5 grams of carbohydrates
- Hard-boiled egg with 10 almonds.

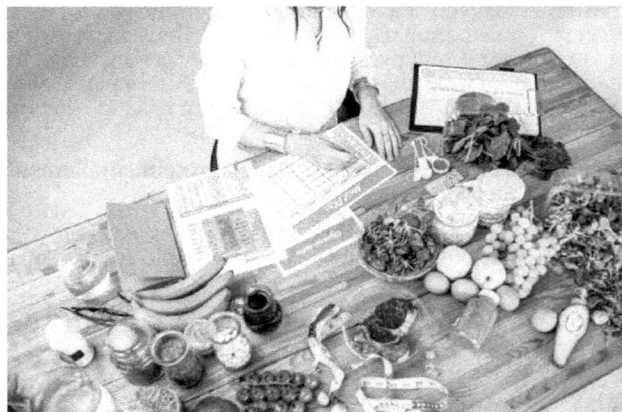

A new relationship with food

Many patients' relationships with food must shift as a result of surgery. You may have eaten while bored, stressed, or upset in the past, but continuing these habits after surgery may jeopardize your long-term success. Consider different strategies to cope with emotional events instead of relying on food for comfort.

Are you feeling lonely? Make a call to a friend.

Bored? Make progress on a project.

Stressed? Take a quick stroll.

Change your focus from what you're eating to what you're doing. Plan an activity instead of going out to dinner to catch up with friends. Food will lose some of its power in your life over time. Much of your success will be determined by your relationship with food, and you must be the leader in that relationship.

Here are some pointers to help you get started:

- If you're feeling down, don't turn to food for comfort. Practicing non-food tactics for controlling your emotions is a good idea.

- Instead of getting a mid-afternoon coffee or pastry "pick-me-up," take a quick stroll during your shift.

- To avoid the temptation of less-healthy options, bring meals and snacks with you when you run errands.

- To avoid impulse purchases, make a list before going grocery shoping.

- Don't be too hard on yourself if you do indulge. At your next meal, try to get back on track.

How to eat?

After surgery, how you eat is almost as essential as what you consume. Patients tolerate food better when they take small bites, chew their meal thoroughly (25 to 30 times), and eat slowly due to anatomical changes associated with bariatric surgery (over the course of 20 to 30 minutes). You should be finished with your dinner in 30 minutes. To avoid filling your pouch with fluid instead of food or causing food to drain out of your stomach too rapidly, you should avoid drinking with meals. You'll have to drink fluids in between meals instead. Due to a decrease in the hunger hormone ghrelin, which is produced predominantly by the stomach, patients report a loss of appetite after surgery. It may feel unusual to eat when you aren't hungry; make a meal schedule or set alarms to remind yourself to eat. To satisfy their protein and nutrient needs, most patients must eat three to six times each day. You can prepare for surgery by incorporating these practices into your daily routine. You might wish to start experimenting with some of the recipes in this book. Choose a few meals and shop ahead of time to try meal planning.

Here are some suggestions for changing your eating habits:

- Smaller dishes and bowls should be used.

- Take little bits of food.

- Chew for at least 25 to 30 seconds.

- Slowly eat.

- A hiccup, sneeze, sigh, burp, or runny nose are all satiety indicators to look out for.

What to eat after the surgery?

Your post-operative diet will begin with liquids, progressing to purées, soft meals, and finally, normal textures. Protein will be your main source of energy during this time of mending.

Your doctor will establish the specific length and requirements of each phase of your rehabilitation, but here are some broad recommendations to consider:

Clear-liquid diet: This stage normally only lasts a couple of days. It enables your healthcare staff to assess your liquid tolerance and assists you in practicing frequent hydration.

Full-liquid diet: This stage is aimed to enhance your fluid consumption and include protein supplements once you have fully tolerated liquids.

Purée diet: It's time to start reintroduction of foods to your body. Your body will be able to acquire more nutrients and return to regular digestion as you begin to recuperate. Pay attention to portion sizes and how much food your stomach can comfortably process.

Soft-foods diet: You may be able to wean yourself off of protein smoothies and powders if you reintroduce more foods with soft textures to your diet. To accomplish your nutritional goals, eat protein-rich foods as often as possible.

General diet: You can reintroduce a range of textures when you've finished your transitional diet. Continue to consume in reasonable portions, prioritizing protein over carbohydrates, and avoiding high-fat and high-carb items.

Post-op diet phases

	PHASE ONE: FULL LIQUIDS	PHASE TWO: PURÉES	PHASE THREE: SOFT FOODS	PHASE FOUR: GENERAL DIET
ADJUSTABLE GASTRIC BAND	Weeks 1 and 2	Week 3	Week 4	Weeks 5 or 6+
LAPAROSCOPIC SLEEVE GASTRECTOMY	Weeks 1 and 2	Week 3	Weeks 4 to 6	Weeks 7 or 8+
ROUX-EN-Y GASTRIC BYPASS	Weeks 1 and 2	Weeks 3 and 4	Weeks 5 to 8	Week 9+

Texture is important

As you can see, the texture is vital and will play a part in your healing at every step.

Fluids and meals that convert to liquid at normal temperature are also considered liquids.

Soft, moist, and smooth purées are required. They shouldn't have any lumps or require chewing.

Soft foods must be chewed and swallowed easily. Chopped, ground, mashed, or puréed are all options. They shouldn't require the use of a knife to cut through.

The texture is not a limiting factor in general diets, although nutrient-dense foods should still be prioritized.

The right liquids

Drinking fluids to stay hydrated will be your first priority after surgery. While this may appear to be straightforward, persistent edema may limit the amount of fluid you may drink at any given time. Throughout the day, take little sips of water. You'll eventually be able to add hydrating fluids like sugar-free sports drinks, broth, and sugar-free juices to your diet. Dehydration is the most prevalent post-surgery consequence, although it is readily avoidable.

Tips for staying hydrated: ~

- Drink a glass of water first thing in the morning.

- Keep a reusable water bottle on you at all times.

- Set a reminder on your phone to remind you to drink.

Enough protein

The most crucial of the three macronutrients to watch following bariatric surgery is protein. At least 60 to 80 grams of protein per day is recommended by the American Society of Metabolic and Bariatric Surgery (ASMBS). You can maintain muscle mass, avoid hair loss, feel invigorated, strengthen your immune system, and remain fuller for longer when you eat enough protein.

If you're having trouble getting enough protein, try the following:

- Protein smoothies, powders, and bars are all good options.

- Protein-rich foods, such as dairy, eggs, meat, fish, and legumes should be included in your meals.

- At all meals and snacks, put protein first.

- Maintain a supply of protein-rich snacks in your purse, desk, exercise bag, or laptop bag, among other places.

Simple and complex carbs

Some carbs are high in calories, fiber, and micronutrients, but not all carbohydrates are the same.

Carbohydrates are divided into two types: simple and complicated.

Complex carbohydrates are strong in fiber, vitamins, and minerals and take a long time to digest. Simple carbs need little energy to digest and should be avoided following surgery. They can not only obstruct weight loss, but they can also put you at risk for dumping syndrome, which is particularly dangerous for gastric bypass patients. You can always go back to the pre-surgery menus. While you may be eating different textures post-surgery, the macronutrient guidelines remain roughly the same.

Fats

Dietary fats, the third macronutrient, are high in energy and maintain cell health by producing key hormones and aiding nutrient absorption. Saturated, unsaturated, and trans fats are the three basic kinds of fats. Saturated fats (like butter or lard) are solid at room temperature and should be consumed in moderation. At room temperature, unsaturated fats are liquid, and they're mostly found in plant-based meals. Essential fatty acids (omega-3s and omega-6s) are unsaturated fats that human systems cannot produce on their own.

Trans fats, on the other hand, are created by humans and should be avoided:

They can increase your risk of heart disease and type 2 diabetes by raising bad cholesterol and lowering good cholesterol. While fat is an important part of our diet, it also has the highest calorie density, with 9 calories per gram. When consuming high-fat foods, remember to eat in moderation. However, be wary of items branded as low- or reduced-fat, as they frequently contain additional sugars to retain flavor quality. If you're unclear what to eat, consult the pre-surgery meal lists, just like you did with carbs.

Supplements

Because you won't be able to eat a lot after surgery, you'll have to rely on supplements to meet your vitamin and mineral requirements. Vitamin B12, iron, thiamine, and calcium deficits are the most common in gastric bypass and sleeve patients. Because gastric band patients are rarely in danger of malabsorption, a daily multivitamin and calcium supplement is usually sufficient. Keep in mind, however, that you should always follow your doctor's specific instructions.

The following are some common supplements that you may require:

Multivitamins with minerals for bariatric patients are available in liquid, chewable, and pill form and must be taken for the rest of their lives.

For bone health and parathyroid function, calcium plus vitamin D is essential. Calcium and any iron you're taking should be separated by at least 2 hours, as they compete for absorption.

For most gastric bypass patients and many sleeve patients, iron is suggested.

Vitamin B12 is helpful for gastric sleeve and bypass patients because it reduces nerve damage and anemia.

Sugar and fried foods

After surgery, you must completely avoid high-sugar and fried foods. Foods heavy in sugar and/or fat can trigger dumping syndrome in gastric bypass and, to a lesser extent, sleeve patients. Stevia, sucralose, erythritol, and monk fruit are all good sugar alternatives.

Early Dumping Syndrome: It can produce nausea, lightheadedness, perspiration, a quick pulse, an overwhelming need to lie down, and diarrhea shortly after eating. It's more prevalent than late dumping syndrome, and it's caused by a quick emptying of the stomach. It'll go away once the food has passed through your system.

Late Dumping Syndrome: Shakiness, sensations of hunger, dizziness, cold chills, bewilderment, and anxiety might occur 1 to 3 hours after eating a meal. It is a type of hypoglycemia that occurs as a result of hormonal changes in your body in reaction to a certain type of food consumed. It will also resolve itself once the offending meal has passed through your system.

What to do at home

You should be able to move around carefully once you return home from surgery, although you may suffer pain or tenderness in your abdominal muscles or near your incision sites. Walk as much as you can to increase your stamina, reduce stomach gas, and prevent blood clots. Your energy levels may fluctuate from one day to the next or even hour to hour. If you have a lot of energy, be sure you're not overworking yourself and that you're getting enough rest. If you're fatigued, check your fluids to make sure you're getting enough protein and staying hydrated. Hunger sensations will most likely be absent, but emotional or sensory cues may cause you to feel hungry in your thoughts. Use books, music, puzzles, a hobby, or friends and family to distract yourself. If you eat or drink too much at once, or if you advance your diet too quickly, you may have nausea, discomfort, or vomiting. When it comes to diet, take small nibbles, eat carefully, and stick to your doctor's post-op diet recommendations. You may realize that your taste preferences have altered when you begin to consume a larger variety of drinks and foods. For the first few weeks after surgery, you may experience both loose stools and constipation. Discuss any persistent issues or concerns with your surgical team. Hair loss is common after surgery and usually begins 3 to 6 months after the procedure. Consume the correct amount of protein, take vitamins as directed, and eat consistently to ensure your body has the nutrition it needs to help your hair regenerate. Following surgery, you may experience a flood of emotions, including second thoughts or regrets. These are natural thoughts that will pass as your rehabilitation develops. If you observe any changes in your mood or if your depression is getting worse, see your doctor or a psychologist right once.

Kitchen

Before and after surgery, your kitchen is one of your most powerful tools. It can help you achieve your objectives while also defending your flaws. How many times have you told yourself, "I didn't intend to eat the ice cream, but it was in the house, and I had a weakness"?

Clean up your cupboards before surgery to keep your kitchen free of temptations. You won't be able to reach for something indulgent if this is the case.

Quick, Healthy Meals

- Rotisserie chicken
- Deli meat and cheese
- Chili
- Tuna or chicken salad
- Yogurt
- Cottage cheese
- Hummus and veggies

- Shrimp and cocktail sauce
- Meatballs and pasta sauce
- Low-carb frozen meals
- Protein bars
- Protein shakes

Kitchen gadgets

You won't need any sophisticated culinary equipment to make the dishes in this book. Knives, stock pots, measuring cups, and sauté pans are typically all that is required. However, there are a few tools that you may find handy. For a fair price, you can find modest selections online or at many big retailers.

Blender: Blend protein drinks and purée sauces, soups, or meats with this blender.

Food processor: Purée or cut foods into tiny pieces with this tool.

Hand or Stand Mixer: For recipes, combine, mix, or knead the ingredients.

Muffin tin or small ramekins: Use to portion single servings.

Slow cooker: Use for making soups, roasts, and casseroles. A 4- or 5-quart size is sufficient for most recipes.

Spiralizer or vegetable peeler: Use for making vegetable noodles, like zucchini noodles.

Stock up pantry

Protein, high fiber carbohydrates, and healthy fats will make up your post-surgery diet. As a result, make sure you have a variety of protein-rich foods on hand, such as meats, low-fat dairy products, eggs, seafood, fish, and legumes. You'll also need a range of nutritious carbs and fats, such as non-starchy vegetables, seeds, nuts, whole fruit, and 100 percent whole grains, to keep your meals balanced.

Avoid

- After surgery, you will need to make every bite count.
- Make sure to avoid the temptation to buy:
- Foods with empty calories (pastries, sweets, pretzels, chips, rice cakes, and popcorn)
- Foods with doughy or sticky textures (bread, rice, and pasta)
- Foods high in fat or sugar (high-fat dairy products, desserts, sausages, butter, and some frozen or packaged foods)
- Sugary, highly caffeinated, or alcoholic beverages

Toss

When clearing out your cupboards, remember that it's fine to throw any food that doesn't fit your new diet. You do not have to consume all of the food in your kitchen simply because you bought it. If you don't want to waste food, give it to a friend or donate it to a local food bank.

Make sure to toss:

- Baked beans
- Boxed potatoes
- Bread
- Candies
- Cereals
- Chips
- Cookies
- Crackers
- Dried fruit
- Frozen desserts
- High-sugar condiments
- High-carb frozen meals
- High-fat soups
- Pasta
- Popcorn
- Rice

Staple foods for your bariatric kitchen

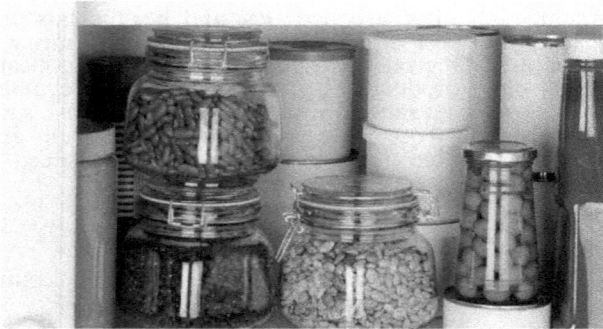

Stock up on these basics to make life simpler or less expensive in your bariatric kitchen:

- Almond flour
- Canned beans (garbanzo, pinto, black)
- Canned tuna, chicken, or salmon
- Dried lentils
- Dried spices and herbs
- Eggs
- Extra-virgin olive oil
- Frozen fruit
- Frozen meat
- Frozen vegetables
- Low-sodium chicken broth
- Nuts and seeds
- Old-fashioned oats
- Plain pasta sauce
- Quinoa
- Reduced-fat dairy products
- Whole wheat flour

Things to consider when living with others

If you live with others, it's a good idea to talk to them about the changes you'll be making before and after surgery. Often, the entire family may improve their health. If you have family members that are hesitant to change, talk to them about how they can support you. Also, keep in mind that not everyone requires dietary changes. Establish boundaries for the first 8 weeks following surgery when

transitioning back to ordinary textures, allow family members to choose goodies that they like but don't, and keep simple meals and snacks on hand for you and your family to avoid being a short-order cook.

Chapter 3-Bariatric Journey: Lifestyle Change

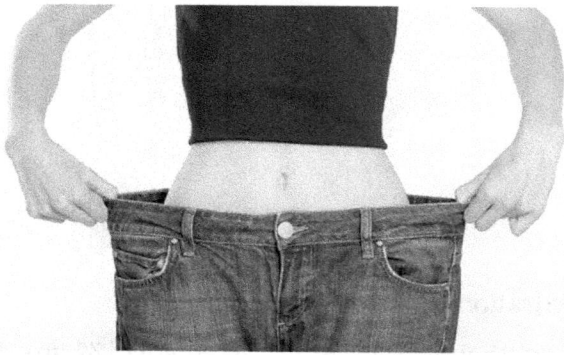

While weight loss begins in the kitchen, it spreads to other areas. Taking control of your lifestyle, understanding how to deal with difficult eating situations, and navigating maintenance mode are all part of setting yourself up for weight-loss success. It may take some time for new habits to take hold, but they will eventually become second nature. Start making modifications before surgery if you can—it will be less overwhelming.

Exercise

While surgery is by far the most drastic step in your weight-loss journey, exercise can help speed things up by increasing muscle mass, lowering stress, and improving general health. Do not be concerned if you did not exercise consistently before surgery.

To build stamina and strengthen the habit, start by including modest activities into your day. Consider stretching, going for a 15-minute walk, utilizing resistance bands, or doing chair exercises. Even modest modifications, such as parking farther away from the grocery store entrance or climbing the stairs, can help you boost your activity level.

If, on the other hand, you used to exercise more frequently before surgery, gradually return to the frequency, length, and intensity you were used to. When patients consume fewer calories during the early stages of recuperation, they often feel a loss of strength and stamina. To avoid harm, be patient when you reintroduce your favorite activities. Low-impact workouts are an excellent choice for the first month after surgery. For the first several weeks, the ideal activity is walking. Simple yoga position stretches, and deep-breathing exercises may also be beneficial.

Later on

The American Heart Association recommends at least 2 hours 30 minutes of moderate-intensity aerobic activity per week, or 1 hour 15 minutes of strong aerobic activity per week (or a combination of both), spread out over the week. Include moderate- to high-intensity muscle-strengthening activity at least two days each week (such as resistance bands or weights). As you gain strength, increase the volume and intensity of your activities. An exercise physiologist or physical therapist can advise you

on where to start if you are unfamiliar with weight-training routines or if you have injuries that limit you from completing particular activities.

Find a companion

A workout companion could be the answer if you're having trouble motivating yourself to exercise. They can motivate you to show up to sessions you were considering skipping, encourage you to work out harder, or simply make your workout more enjoyable. They might even be able to assist you in overcoming the fear of starting a new class or activity.

Journaling

Journaling is one of the most effective strategies to keep on track. You can manage what you can measure! You may have had some experience tracking your food consumption before surgery, but now you may add measurements, fluid intake, bowel movements, energy level, mood, exercise, and more to your list of things to track. Some patients like to write down their plans for the day in their journals, so they know what they'll eat and how much exercise they'll get. You can check your journal throughout the day to make sure you're on track. You can use a pen and paper journal or a phone app like Baritastic or MyFitnessPal to keep track of your calories.

Restaurants

You'll probably find yourself at a restaurant ordering takeout or at a particular social function soon after your surgery. These are supposed to be enjoyable occasions, not stressful ones. If you know where you're going to eat, look over the menu ahead of time. Make a plan for what you'll eat before you arrive so you're not tempted by other options when you're hungry. There's no need to order an entrée for your dinner; instead, go over the appetizer and side-dish menus to put together your own protein- and veggie-rich meal. You'll be in command with a little strategy and practice.

Here are some dining-out suggestions:

- When dining out, avoid trying unfamiliar foods or textures for the first time. If you're not sure what to get, go for softer textures because they'll be more bearable.

- Fried foods, doughy or sticky carbohydrates, cream sauces, sugary drinks, and desserts should all be avoided.

- It's perfectly acceptable to be fussy; most restaurants are accustomed to customers requesting substitutes or alterations to their dishes. Ask if they can substitute vegetables for starch, put your dressing or sauce on the side, or give you a half quantity instead of a full meal.

- If you're eating with others, see if they'd like to share a meal or store your leftovers for the next day.

Friend's house

Eating at a friend's house can be more challenging than eating at a restaurant because you not only have fewer options, but you also know the cook. Imagine showing up to a dinner gathering and seeing that your friend has prepared a delicious pasta dish, steak, and garlic toast. This may have been possible before surgery, but what about now?

Here are some suggestions to make things easier:

- Before you go, call your acquaintance and inquire about the food.

- To contribute to the meal, offer to bring a side dish that satisfies your diet rules.

- Alternatively, 1 to 2 hours before your arrival, have a balanced lunch.

Holidays

The holidays are a time for revelry, which usually entails food and booze. They can be enticing and nostalgic at the same time. Consider arriving at a holiday gathering and being greeted with a glass of champagne from a dear friend. Following that, you'll find a vast buffet with all of your favorite meats, sides, and desserts. What are your options if you've had surgery to cope with this situation?

Here are a few recommendations:

- Before an event, eat a protein-rich meal or snack.

- To prevent eating "simply because it's there," move away from any appetizers or buffet tables.

- Bring a dish that you can eat and share as a side dish.

- Before you take a plate from a buffet, have a look around. Aim for a small protein, vegetables, and a small piece of a carb you can't live without if required.

- If you don't want others to question why you're not drinking, ask for a cocktail glass filled with water, a splash of juice, and a lime wedge.

Snacking

The majority of bariatric patients cannot achieve their protein and calorie requirements in three meals. Instead, they are encouraged to take snacks in between meals, resulting in four to six times per day of eating. Make sure to include a source of protein in your snack. When you're on the run and need a healthy alternative, bring nonperishable products like protein bars, nuts, jerky, and seeds with you.

Here are some other snack ideas:

- Apple slices with peanut butter

- Deli meat and cheese

- Hard-boiled eggs

- Hummus and vegetables

- Low-fat cottage cheese

- Low-fat Greek yogurt and berries

- Low-fat string cheese and almonds

- Protein bars Protein shakes

- Tuna or chicken salad wrapped in lettuce

- Turkey jerky and sliced apple

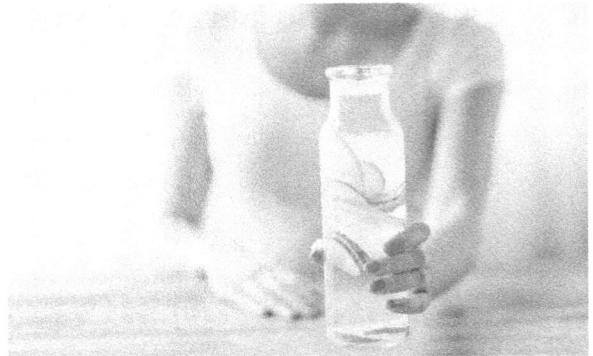

Hydration tips

As a bariatric patient, you must prioritize hydration throughout your life, not just in the first few weeks after surgery. Beyond your initial recovery, adequate fluid consumption will aid weight loss, minimize constipation, and boost your energy levels. Maintain the habits you acquired in the weeks following your operation. Start your day with a glass of water and keep a reusable water bottle with you at all times.

Alcohol

If you drank alcoholic beverages on occasion before surgery, you might be wondering if you can do so again post-surgical. Yes, but only in moderation and with some tweaks is the quick response. Drinking should be avoided for 3 to 12 months after surgery. Because of your altered metabolism, if you start drinking again, your blood alcohol level may peak higher and faster. Furthermore, eating less food causes faster absorption of nutrients into the bloodstream. It just takes one drink for many post-operative patients to reach the threshold of intoxication, therefore never drink and drive. Individuals with a history of addiction are also more likely to develop transference addiction, which occurs when patients shift their food addiction to other addictive behaviors. Shopping, sex, gambling, drugs, and alcohol are examples of these activities. If you see any behavioral changes in yourself, you should see a doctor.

Cocktail hour

If you do decide to consume alcohol, avoid doing so while eating, and choose low-sugar, low-calorie options like white or red wines, vodka blended with light cranberry juice, or whiskey on the rocks. Avoid sugary mixers and fizzy beverages. It's also worth noting that just because you're at happy hour doesn't mean you have to drink. Take advantage of the social side of the event and catch up with friends. Choose iced tea or coffee, water with a lime wedge, or sugar-free juice if you want a drink in your hands but don't want alcohol.

Additional tips

Alcoholic beverages can dehydrate you, so drink plenty of water while you're drinking them.

Before you come, eat a snack or drink some water.

Look for protein-rich alternatives such as hummus and veggies, shrimp with cocktail sauce, steak bits, steamed edamame, or mini-sliders without the buns if you plan to eat.

Maintenance

Many patients may attain a weight they want to keep between 6 and 24 months after surgery. Patients who have gastric band, sleeve, or bypass surgery lose 40 to 80 percent of their excess weight on average, with gastric bypass patients losing the most. This timetable will be influenced by a variety of factors, including the patient's initial weight, food habits, degree of activity, and so on. The length of time it takes you to lose weight is determined by your food and lifestyle choices, as well as your health history and genetics. Weight loss necessitates a calorie deficit and a rather rigorous dietary plan, whereas weight maintenance allows for a little more leeway. Patients must, however, continue to make healthy choices on a daily basis to avoid regaining weight, focusing on protein-rich options and avoiding foods heavy in sugar and fat.

Changes you may notice

Many obesity-related problems have been demonstrated to be improved or resolved by bariatric surgery. Patients also report good long-term outcomes such as decreased appetite, improved portion control, higher energy, decreased joint pain, improved sleep quality, decreased use of drugs for linked disorders (such as diabetes), and increased self-esteem.

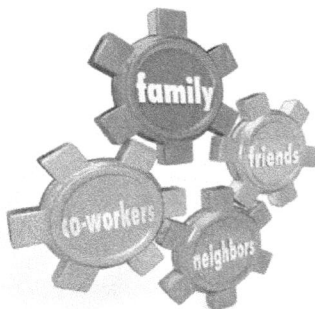

Support systems

Your support system is one of the most important aspects of successful weight loss and maintenance. Family and friends, as well as coworkers, medical professionals, and peers from a bariatric surgery support group, may be included. The amount of help you require will most likely change over time. According to research, those who regularly attend follow-up consultations and support groups have a better chance of losing weight and keeping it off.

Food rules for maintenance

Surgery, as you may know, is merely a tool. Maintaining your accomplishments necessitates a lifelong commitment to a healthy way of living. If you return to unhealthy habits like nibbling, drinking high-calorie beverages, eating high-sugar and high-fat foods, and cutting back on exercise, it's simple to gain weight. In comparison to the first few months after surgery, you may realize that you can eat greater portions or tolerate more variety of food as your body adjusts. The band may be required for patients with adjustable gastric bands to ensure portion control and dietary tolerance. Patients who have had gastric bypass surgery may notice a reduction in dumping syndrome and the resolution of food intolerances, making it simpler to eat more.

Don't be alarmed; these adjustments are rather typical. They should not, however, affect how you follow basic nutrition requirements.

Protein will always be a priority. Aim for protein at every meal and snack to fulfill your daily goals while also staying full and satisfied for longer. Furthermore, protein should come first at meals, followed by produce, and then complete grains. Aim for 60 to 80 grams of protein per day or as directed by your doctor.

Make healthy choices. There will be holidays and special occasions, but what you do on a daily basis is more essential than what you occasionally do. Lean proteins, fruits, vegetables, seeds, nuts, and whole grains should all be included in your diet. There's no need to be harsh on yourself if you have a bad day; instead, focus on getting back on track the next day.

Stay hydrated. To stay hydrated, use low-calorie, low-sugar beverages. Calories are easier to drink than to consume. Liquid calories from sugar, fat, and alcohol should be avoided.

Take your supplements as instructed. Vitamins and minerals should be consumed for the rest of one's life. What you require, though, may alter with time. Make an appointment with your doctor for follow-up care.

Exercise regularly. Exercise is an important part of weight-loss and weight-maintenance wellbeing. To keep involved, increase the length, intensity, and frequency of your workouts as you are able, or try new activities.

Staying on track

Here are some guidelines to help you make good dietary and other decisions as you move forward:

- Make a meal and snack schedule.
- Pay attention to the labels.
- Portion control is important.
- Keep track of what you eat.
- Make protein a priority in your diet.
- Avoid high-sugar and high-fat foods and beverages.
- Drink plenty of water in between meals.
- Take small nibbles, chew thoroughly, and savor your food carefully.
- Take the supplements that are suggested.
- Find new methods to stay active.
- Every night, try to get at least 6 to 8 hours of sleep.
- Make use of stress-relieving practices.
- For continued support, contact your bariatric clinic.

Enjoy yourself

You now have all of the resources you need to achieve your weight-loss objectives right at your fingertips. Take it easy and enjoy the journey; you've got this. And, in between the hard effort, remember to congratulate yourself on your accomplishments, whether they are weight-related or not. You are deserving of it. Now it's time to go to the kitchen! The recipes that follow offer step-by-step directions as well as nutritional data.

~Meal Plan

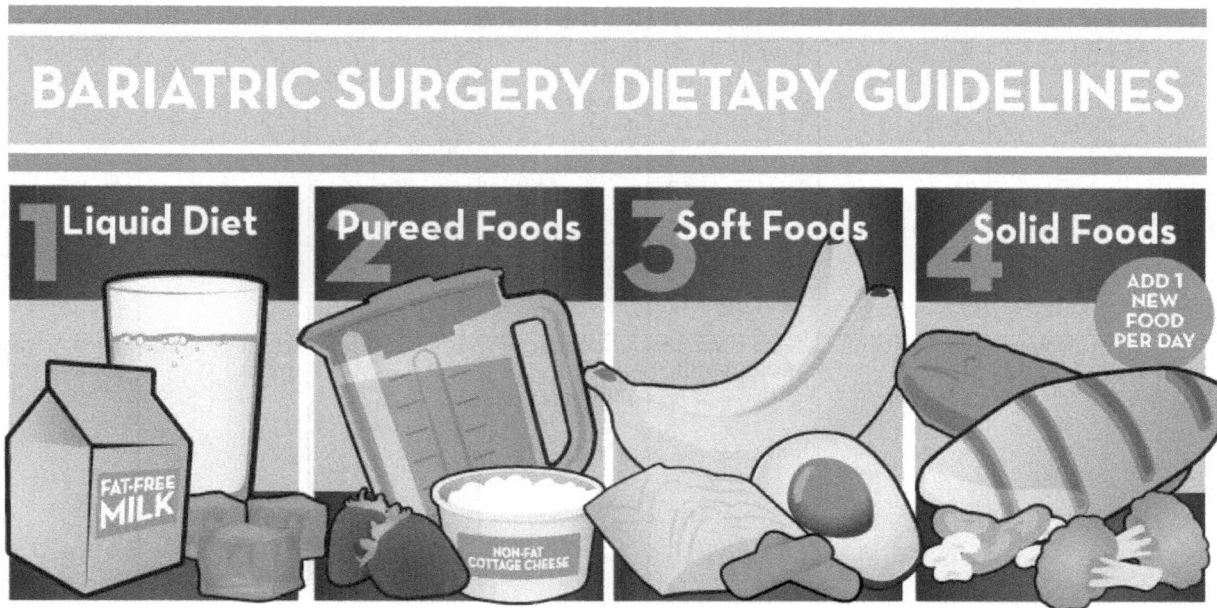

For optimum healing, a transitional diet is required for the first eight weeks after surgery. Keep in mind that you may not have a full grasp of the capacity of your new pouch when eating. If you're having trouble progressing to the next step of your diet, go back to the previous level for a few days.

The physician will make recommendations to assist you in transitioning more smoothly from one phase of the plan to the next.

Liquids (Week 1 and 2)

You'll start with a full-liquid diet after surgery. Liquid textures require less effort to digest, allowing your stomach to heal properly. Keeping hydrated is the most important goal at this point, but you'll also be using protein drinks to meet your protein targets for recovery. You'll find a number of recipes to help you get through this phase in the chapter titled beverages. Check with your medical staff for precise instructions.

DAYS/ MEALS	Monday	Tuesday	Wednesday	Thursday	Friday	Saturday	Sunday
BREAK- -FAST	Peanut butter and chocolate protein shake	Banana Cream Protein Shake	Vanilla Bean Protein Shake	Berry-Mango Breakfast Shake	Peanut butter and Chocolate protein Shake	Banana Cream pie smoothie	Vanilla Bean Protein Shake
SNACK	High protein milk	Bone broth	Zero waste protein milk	Chocolate orange pudding	Bone broth	High protein milk	Zero waste protein milk
LUNCH	Banana Cream Protein shake	Berry Bliss Protein Shake	Protein-packed peanut Buttercup shake	Classic Vegetable soup	Chocolate-mint Protein shake	Vanilla Bean Protein Shake	Pina colada Protein shake
SNACK	Bone broth	Strawberry Lime Ginger Punch	High protein milk	Protein hot chocolate	Zero waste protein milk	Cool-as-a-cucumber water	High protein milk
DINNER	Classic Vegetable soup	Chocolate-Raspberry Truffle Protein shake	Berry Bliss Protein Shake	Banana Cream pie smoothie	Green Machine Protein Shake	Protein-packed peanut Buttercup shake	Classic Vegetable Soup

Pureed Foods (Week 3 and 4)

You can start transitioning to a purée diet after 1 to 2 weeks of tolerating liquids. Foods should be the consistency of a smooth paste at this point, with no solid parts or chunks. Soft meats with sauce, fruits, cooked vegetables, low-fat dairy products, eggs, low-fiber hot cereals, lentils, and low-fat soups are all good purée candidates. A competent blender or food processor can purée most of them.

Because of the limited capacity of your stomach, you should limit your meals to 2 to 3 ounces (4 to 8 tablespoons) at a time. To meet your protein goals, try adding unflavored protein powder or fat-free powdered milk to your dishes, or stick to protein smoothies (at least 60 grams per day).

It's critical to stay hydrated while you transition from liquids to purées, drinking 48 ounces of fluids per day, including protein shakes. Also, don't drink with your meal; wait at least 30 minutes after you've finished eating before drinking.

You can start doing low-impact workouts to increase strength and flexibility now that your body is recovering. You can also start walking greater distances or at a faster pace.

DAYS/ MEALS	Monday	Tuesday	Wednesday	Thursday	Friday	Saturday	Sunday
BREAK- -FAST	Perfectly soft scrambled eggs	Overnight Oatmeal	Banana Brulee Yogurt Parfait	Vanilla Probiotic Shake	Sweet Maple Protein Oatmeal	Strawberry- Banana Protein Smoothie	Protein- Packed Peanut Buttercup Shake
SNACK	Pumpkin Spice Latte Protein Shake	High Protein milk	Strawberry Protein Shake	Smoothie Bowl	Zero waste protein milk	Summer Rhubarb Cooler	High Protein milk
LUNCH	Lemon- Dijon Tuna salad	Classic Turkey chili	Curried chicken salad	Mom's turkey meatloaf	Homestyle refried beans	Southwest Deviled eggs	Split pea soup
SNACK	High Protein milk	Protein hot chocolate	Zero waste protein milk	Pumpkin Spice Latte Protein Shake	Smart Banana Blender	High Protein milk	Lemon Pie Protein Shake

DINNER	Italian Ricotta Bake	Old Fashioned Salmon Soup	Mom's turkey meatloaf	Classic Turkey Chili	Tuna salad	Veggie-Quinoa Soup	Turkish Soup

Soft Foods (Week 5 to 8)

A soft-food diet gives you more texture, but you must still be able to cut through your food with a fork. Small, delicate, and easy-to-chew food pieces are ideal. Make sure you only try one or two new items at a time as you move to a soft-food diet. Ground lean meat or poultry, eggs, flaky fish, cottage cheese, yogurt, soft cheese, soft fresh or canned fruits (without seeds or skin), hot cereal, beans, cooked vegetables (without skin), and lentils are some options for this period.

To reach your daily protein goal of 60 to 80 grams, you'll probably eat at least three meals and 1 to 2 protein-rich snacks or drinks. 13 to 12 cups of food should be served at each meal.

Continue to abstain from drinking while eating. To hydrate, wait 30 minutes after a meal.

DAYS/ MEALS	Monday	Tuesday	Wednesday	Thursday	Friday	Saturday	Sunday
BREAK--FAST	Breakfast Pizza	Slow Cooker Cinnamon Oatmeal	Farmers Market Scramble	Denver Egg Muffins with Ham Crust	Slow-cooked Peppers Frittata	Spicy Deviled Eggs	Protein Pancakes
SNACK	Any beverage from the list	Any beverage from the list	Any beverage from the list	Any beverage from the list	Any beverage from the list	Any beverage from the list	Any beverage from the list
LUNCH	Mahi-Mahi with Mango-Avocado Salsa	Classic Slow Cooker Pulled Pork	Slow-cooker Chicken Tikka Masala	Chicken Casserole	Blackened Salmon with Avocado Cream	Slow-cooker pork chili	Special Fish Pie

SNACK	Any beverage from the list	Any beverage from the list	Any beverage from the list	Any beverage from the list	Any beverage from the list	Any beverage from the list	Any beverage from the list
DINNER	Broiled tuna and tomato	Black-Eyed Dill Tuna	Chicken piccata	Salmon Patties	Boneless Chicken Cutlets	Oven-baked Chicken Tenders	White Bean Chicken Chili

General Diet (Week 9 -Throughout Life)

You will no longer have texture constraints when you are ready to transition to a more general diet. Make prudent eating choices, prioritize protein-rich foods and avoid empty calories. Make sure to introduce only one or two new meals at a time, just like you did when transitioning from liquids to purées and purées to soft foods. Certain foods can make you feel sick, cause pain, or make you vomit. Bread, dry meats, fibrous veggies, and sugary or fatty foods are common causes, and you should continue to avoid them.

Stick to three meals and one to two snacks per day, keeping portion limits in mind. Most patients can eventually handle roughly 12 to 1 cup of food. Maintain a daily fluid intake of 48 ounces and a protein intake of 60 grams, as on a soft foods diet. Make sure you're getting enough exercise and taking your supplements.

DAYS/ MEALS	Monday	Tuesday	Wednesday	Thursday	Friday	Saturday	Sunday
BREAK- -FAST	Apple Oatmeal with Cinnamon	Broccoli Egg and Cheese Bake	Denver Egg Muffins with Ham Crust	Awesome Egg Salad Sandwich	Breakfast Pizza	Greek Bowl	Banana-Amarnath Porridge
SNACK	Any beverage from the list	Any beverage from the list	Any beverage from the list	Any beverage from the list	Any beverage from the list	Any beverage from the list	Any beverage from the list

LUNCH	Braised Chicken and Mushrooms	Crab salad	Classic Slow Cooker Chicken	Thai Chicken Coconut Curry	New England Chicken	Tuna salad	Halibut with Creamy Parmesan-Dill Sauce
SNACK	Cajun Onion Rings	Asian Cabbage Slaw	Pesto Crackers	Homestyle refried Beans	Baked Tofu Bites	Spiced Maple Nuts	Baked sweet potato fries with basil pesto
DINNER	Lemon-Pepper Chicken Bake	Roasted Leg Lamb	Broccoli Cheddar Bake	Greek Chop-Chop Salad	Sloppy Joes	Curry Salmon with Mustard	Mushroom and Barley salad

Chapter 5~Breakfast Recipes

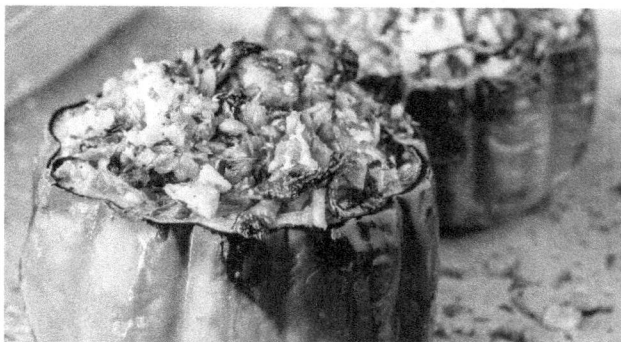

Acorn Squash ~ Stuffed with Cheese

Preparation time- 10 minutes| Cook time-35 minutes| Servings-4 |Difficulty-Moderate

Nutritional value- Calories-298| Fat-16g |Carbohydrates-2.8g| Protein-20.9g

Ingredients

- One pound of ground turkey breast (extra-lean)
- Three acorn squash
- One can (8 ounces) tomato sauce
- One cup of fresh mushrooms
- One cup of chopped onion
- One cup of diced celery
- One teaspoon of garlic powder
- One teaspoon of Basil
- One teaspoon of Oregano
- One teaspoon of Black pepper
- One teaspoon of salt
- Shredded cheddar cheese (reduced-fat)

Instructions

- Program the oven temperature to 350°F. Slice the squash in half and remove the seeds.
- Arrange the squash, cut side down, in a dish, and microwave high for 20 minutes. Brown the turkey in a skillet and add the onion and celery.
- Sauté for two to three minutes. Blend in the mushrooms and add the sauce and seasonings. Divide into quarters and spoon into the squash.
- Cover and bake for 15 minutes. Garnish with the cheese and bake until the cheese has melted.

Almond Chia Porridge

Preparation time-10 minutes |Cook time-30 minutes |Servings-2 |Difficulty-Easy

Nutritional value: ~Calories-150|Proteins-4g| Fat-8g|Carbohydrates-18g

Ingredients

- Three cups of organic almond milk
- 1/3 cup of chia seeds, dried
- One teaspoon of vanilla extract
- One tablespoon of honey
- A quarter teaspoon of ground cardamom

Instructions

- Pour almond milk into the saucepan and bring it to a boil.
- Then chill the almond milk to room temperature (or appx. For 10-15 minutes).
- Add vanilla extract, honey, and ground cardamom. Stir well.
- After this, add chia seeds and stir again.
- Close the lid and let chia seeds soak the liquid for 20-25 minutes.
- Transfer the cooked porridge into the serving ramekins.

Apple Oatmeal with Cinnamon

Preparation time- 5 minutes| Cook time-10 minutes| Servings-1 |Difficulty-Easy

Nutritional value- Calories-108| Fat-2.4g |Carbohydrates-12g| Protein-9g

Ingredients

- One fresh green apple
- One teaspoon of lemon juice
- ¾ cup of skim milk
- Half cup of oats
- Half teaspoon of cinnamon

Instructions

- Cut the apple into cubes, then place it in a bowl. Drizzle the lemon juice over the cubed apple, then set aside.
- Pour skim milk into a saucepan and bring it to a boil. Once it is boiled, add the oats and apple, then bring the mixture to a simmer.
- Transfer everything to a serving bowl, and sprinkle cinnamon on top. Serve and enjoy!

Artichoke Omelet

Preparation time-5 minutes |Cook time-10 minutes |Servings-2 |Difficulty-Easy

Nutritional value: ~Calories-231|Proteins-14.9g| Fat-15g|Carbohydrates-4g

Ingredients

- Four eggs, beaten
- One tomato, chopped
- Half cup of artichoke hearts, chopped
- Four ounces of goat cheese, crumbled
- One tablespoon of olive oil

Instructions

- Mix up eggs, chopped artichokes, goat cheese, and tomato. Then brush the baking mold with olive oil and pour the mixture inside.
- Bake the omelet for 10 minutes at 365 degrees F. Serve.

Asparagi All'uovo

Preparation time-10 minutes | Cook time-15 minutes | Servings-4 | Difficulty-Easy

Nutritional value: ~310 Calories | Fat-25g | Protein-16g | Carbohydrates-4g

Ingredients

- One pound of asparagus
- One clove garlic, crushed
- A quarter cup of olive oil
- Salt and ground black pepper, to taste
- Half cup of grated Parmesan cheese
- Eight eggs

Instructions

- Preheat the oven to broil.
- Break the asparagus tips off where they typically break. In a microwave-safe baking dish or a glass pie plate, place the asparagus spears. Cover with a couple of teaspoons of water.
- Microwave for four minutes on high.
- Mash the cloves of garlic into the olive oil while the asparagus is cooking.
- Drain the asparagus when it's done.
- Asparagus should be divided among the four dishes. If not, a rectangle glass baking dish will be required.
- In the baking dish, arrange the asparagus in four groups.
- Drizzle garlic oil over each serving of asparagus.
- Season with a pinch of salt and pepper, then divide the cheese among the four plates. Place the asparagus underneath the broiler at a distance of 4 inches (10 cm) from the heat source.
- Allow for five minutes of broiling.

- Fry the eggs to your taste while the asparagus is broiling. To cook them all at once, use your largest pan, or divide them between two skillets.
- Remove the asparagus from the grill when the Parmesan is faintly browned.
- Remove the asparagus from the grill when the Parmesan is faintly browned.
- Carefully transfer each serving to a plate with a large spatula.
- Serve 2 fried eggs on top of each asparagus portion.

Avocado Egg Scramble

Preparation time-8 minutes | Cook time-15 minutes | Servings-2 | Difficulty-Easy

Nutritional value: ~Calories-236 | Proteins-8.6g | Fat-20g | Carbohydrates-7.4g

Ingredients

- Two eggs, beaten
- One white onion, diced
- One tablespoon of avocado oil
- One avocado, finely chopped
- Half teaspoon of chili flakes
- One ounce of Cheddar cheese, shredded
- Half teaspoon of salt
- One tablespoon of fresh parsley

Instructions

- Pour avocado oil into the skillet and bring it to a boil.
- Then add diced onion and roast it until it is light brown.
- Meanwhile, mix up together chili flakes, beaten eggs, and salt.
- Pour the egg mixture over the cooked onion and cook the mixture for 1 minute over medium heat.
- After this, scramble the eggs well with the help of the fork or spatula. Cook the eggs until they are solid but soft.
- After this, add chopped avocado and shredded cheese.
- Stir the scrambled well and transfer in the serving plates.
- Sprinkle the meal with fresh parsley.

Avocado Toast

Preparation time-10 minutes | Cook time-0 minutes | Servings-2 | Difficulty-Easy

Nutritional value: ~Calories-282 | Proteins-6g | Fat-18g | Carbohydrates-35g

Ingredients

- One tablespoon of goat cheese, crumbled
- One avocado, peeled, pitted, and mashed
- A pinch of salt and black pepper
- Two whole wheat bread slices, toasted
- Half teaspoon of lime juice
- One persimmon, thinly sliced
- One fennel bulb, thinly sliced
- Two teaspoons of honey
- Two tablespoons of pomegranate seeds

Instructions

- In a container, mix the avocado flesh with salt, pepper, lime juice, and the cheese and whisk.
- Spread this onto toasted bread slices, top each piece with the remaining ingredients and serve for breakfast.

Awesome Egg Salad Sandwich

Preparation time-5 minutes |Cook time-0 minutes |Serving-2 |Difficulty- Easy

Nutritional value: ~ Calories-164| Fat-6g| Protein-13.4g| Carbohydrates-14g

Ingredients

- Two whole hard-boiled eggs
- Two hard-boiled eggs, whites only
- Two teaspoons of nonfat mayonnaise
- A quarter teaspoon of Dijon mustard
- One teaspoon of finely chopped chives
- Half teaspoon of celery seed
- Two whole-grain English muffin halves, toasted

Instructions

- In a small bowl, crush the hard-boiled eggs and egg whites with a fork. Add the mayonnaise, mustard, chives, and celery seed and mix to combine.
- Top each muffin half with half of the egg salad and serve.

Backward pizza

Preparation time-10 minutes |Cook time-20 minutes|Servings-6 |Difficulty-Easy

Nutritional value: ~262 Calories| Fat-22g|Protein-14g|Carbohydrates-3g

Ingredients

- One clove of garlic
- Three tablespoons of olive oil

- 1/3 cup of no-sugar-added pizza sauce
- One and a half teaspoons of dried oregano
- Half teaspoon of red pepper flakes (optional)
- A quarter cup of grated Parmesan cheese

Instructions

- Preheat oven to 375°F.
- Line a jelly roll tin with non-stick foil.
- Spread the mozzarella evenly over the foil, all the way to the corners.
- Bake for 5 minutes, turn the pan to help it cook evenly, and give it another 5 to 7 minutes—you want the cheese golden brown all over.
- While the cheese is baking, crush the garlic into a little cup and cover with the olive oil, stirring once.
- Put your pizza sauce in a microwavable dish, and give it 1 minute to warm.
- When your cheese is an even, golden layer, pull it out of the oven. Drizzle the garlicky oil all over it, spreading with a brush or the back of a spoon.
- Sprinkle with oregano and red pepper flakes if using.
- Spread the pizza sauce over the oil, and sprinkle the Parmesan over that. Cut into 6 big rectangles to serve.

Bacon, Tomato, Lettuce, and Cream Cheese Sandwich

Preparation time-5 minutes |Cook time-0 minutes |Serving-1 |Difficulty- Easy

Nutritional value: ~ Calories-186| Fat-6.5g| Protein-12g| Carbohydrates-23g

Ingredients

- Two slices of diet whole grain bread, toasted
- One ounce of nonfat cream cheese
- Two strips reduced-sodium, reduced-fat turkey bacon or veggie bacon
- Two 2-inches thick slices of tomato
- Two red or green leaf lettuce leaves stems removed
- Fresh cracked black pepper (optional)

Instructions

- On each slice of bread, evenly spread the cream cheese. Place the bacon strips in a cross from corner to corner on one slice.
- Layer the tomato, the pepper (if using), then the lettuce leaves, and top with the remaining slice of bread.
- Spear each half of the sandwich with a toothpick, cut in half, and serve.

Baked Eggs with Parsley

Preparation time-15 minutes | Cook time-20 minutes | Servings-2 | Difficulty-Easy

Nutritional value: ~Calories-167 | Proteins-4g | Fat-12g | Carbohydrates-11g

Ingredients

- One green bell pepper, chopped

- Two tablespoons olive oil

- One yellow onion, chopped

- One teaspoon of sweet paprika

- Three tomatoes, chopped

- Three eggs

- A quarter cup of parsley, chopped

Instructions

- Warm a pan with the oil over medium heat, add all ingredients except eggs and roast them for 5 minutes.

- Stir the vegetables well and crack the eggs.

- Transfer the pan with eggs in the preheated to 360°F oven and bake them for 15 minutes.

Baked Ham and Cheese Sandwich

Preparation time-5 minutes | Cook time-5 minutes | Serving~1 | Difficulty- Easy

Nutritional value: ~ Calories-266 | Fat-8g | Protein-24g | Carbohydrates-26g

Ingredients

- Two slices of fresh diet whole-grain bread

- Two teaspoons of nonfat mayonnaise

- Half teaspoon of Dijon mustard

- Two ounces of reduced-sodium, reduced-fat sliced ham

- Two sis-inch (6.25-cm) thick slices of tomato

- One slice (1 ounce) reduced-fat Swiss cheese

Instructions

- Preheat the oven to 350°F.

- On one slice of bread, spread the mayonnaise and spread the mustard on the other. Place the ham on one slice, then the tomato slices, then the cheese. Top with the remaining slice of bread and place on a sheet pan.

- Bake the sandwich for about 2 minutes, until the bread is nicely toasted and the cheese is melted. Cut in half and serve warm.

Baked Oatmeal with Cinnamon

Preparation time-10 minutes | Cook time-25 minutes | Servings-2 | Difficulty-Easy

Nutritional value: ~Calories-151 | Proteins-5g | Fat-4g | Carbohydrates-24g

Ingredients

- One cup of oatmeal

- 1/3 cup of milk

- One pear, chopped

- One teaspoon of vanilla extract

- One tablespoon of Splenda

- One teaspoon of butter

- Half teaspoon of ground cinnamon

- One egg, beaten

Instructions

- The big bowl mixes up together oatmeal, milk, egg, vanilla extract, Splenda, and ground cinnamon.

- Melt butter and add it to the oatmeal mixture.

- Then add chopped pear and stir it well.

- Transfer the oatmeal mixture to the casserole mold and flatten gently. Cover it with foil and secure the edges.

- Bake the oatmeal for 25 minutes at 350 degrees F.

Baked Tofu in Cup

Preparation time- 5 minutes | Cook time-25 minutes | Servings-4 | Difficulty-Easy

Nutritional value- Calories-298 | Fat-16g | Carbohydrates-2.8g | Protein-20.9g

Ingredients

- One lb. of tofu

- Half cup of diced tomatoes

- One cup of chopped kale

- Half cup of ground chicken

- Two organic eggs

- Two teaspoons of minced garlic

- Half teaspoon of pepper

Instructions

- Preheat an oven to 350°F and prepare 8 muffin cups. Coat with cooking spray then set aside.

- Place the tofu in a food processor, then add eggs and ground chicken to the food processor. Season with pepper and minced garlic. Blend until smooth.

- Transfer the tofu mixture to a bowl, then stir diced tomatoes and chopped kale into the bowl. Mix until just combined.

- Fill each muffin cup with the tofu mixture, then bake for approximately 25 minutes.

- Once the tofu is set and lightly golden, remove it from the oven and let them cool. Take the tofu from the cups and arrange it on a serving dish. Serve and enjoy!

Banana Berry

Preparation time- 5 minutes| Cook time-0 minutes| Servings-1 |Difficulty-Easy

Nutritional value- Calories-140| Fat-0g |Carbohydrates-29g| Protein-8g

Ingredients

- A quarter cup of blueberries, fresh or frozen
- A quarter cup of ice
- 1/8 teaspoon of vanilla extract
- A quarter cup of sliced banana
- A quarter cup of raspberries, fresh or frozen
- Two tablespoons of non-fat dry powdered milk
- One packet of sugar substitute, or to taste
- Half cup of non-fat milk

Instructions

- Mix the non-fat milk and powdered milk well and leave it on for 2 to 3 minutes.
- Now, put all the rest of the ingredients in a food blender and run it until a smooth consistency is reached.

Banana Brûlée Yogurt Parfait

Preparation time- 5 minutes| Cook time-2 minutes| Servings-1 |Difficulty-Easy

Nutritional value- Calories-168| Fat-0g |Carbohydrates-20g| Protein-24g

Ingredients

- Dash ground cinnamon
- One cup of non-fat plain Greek yogurt
- One teaspoon of brown sugar
- A quarter cup of banana slices
- Nonstick cooking spray

Instructions

- Spray a skillet and put it over medium flame.
- Put the banana slices in the hot skillet and top with some brown sugar. Then cook for a few minutes. Move everything frequently. Take off from the stove.
- Add yogurt to a bowl, then pour the banana mixture on top. Dust it with cinnamon. Serve and enjoy.

Banana Oats

Preparation time-10 minutes |Cook time-0 minutes |Servings-2 |Difficulty-Easy

Nutritional value: ~Calories-312|Proteins-8g| Fat-18g|Carbohydrates-35g

Ingredients

- One banana, peeled and sliced
- ¾ cup of almond milk
- Half cup of cold-brewed coffee
- Two dates pitted
- Two tablespoons of/ cocoa powder
- One cup of rolled oats
- One and a half tablespoons of chia seeds

Instructions

- In a blender, combine the banana with the milk and the rest of the ingredients, pulse, divide into bowls, and serve breakfast.

Banana-Amaranth Porridge

Preparation time-10 minutes |Cook time-10 minutes |Servings-4 |Difficulty-Easy

Nutritional value: ~Calories-271|Proteins-8g| Fat-6g|Carbohydrates-47g

Ingredients

- Two and a half cups of unsweetened almond milk
- One cup of amaranth
- Two sliced bananas
- Dash of cinnamon

Instructions

- Mix the amaranth, milk, and bananas in your pressure cooker or a deep pan.

- Close the lid.

- Cook on high pressure/heat for about 5 minutes.

- When time is up, wait for the pressure to come down on its own.

- When all the pressure is gone, you can serve the porridge with cinnamon.

Banana-Buckwheat Porridge

Preparation time-10 minutes ·|Cook time-10 minutes |Servings-4 |Difficulty-Easy

Nutritional value: ~Calories-240|Proteins-6g| Fat-4g|Carbohydrates-46g

Ingredients

- Three cups of almond (or rice) milk

- One cup of buckwheat groats

- One sliced banana

- A quarter cup of raisins

- One teaspoon of cinnamon

- Half teaspoon of pure vanilla extract

Instructions

- Rinse off the buckwheat and put it right in the pressure cooker or a deep pan with a lid.

- Pour in the milk, and add the rest of the ingredients.

- Close the lid.

- Cook for 6 minutes on high pressure/heat.

- When time is up, wait 20 minutes or so for the pressure to go all the way down.

- Open the lid and stir well. Add more milk if it's too thick for you.

- Serve!

Bell Pepper Frittata

Preparation time-10 minutes |Cook time-15 minutes |Servings-2 |Difficulty-Easy

Nutritional value: ~Calories-105|Proteins-6g| Fat-8g|Carbohydrates-4g

Ingredients

- One cup of red bell pepper, chopped

- One tablespoon of olive oil, melted

- One tomato, sliced

- Four eggs, beaten

- A quarter teaspoon of ground black pepper

- A quarter teaspoon of salt

Instructions

- Brush the baking pan with melted olive oil. Then add all the remaining ingredients, mix gently and transfer in the preheated to 365 degrees F oven.

- Cook the frittata for 15 minutes.

Berry Oats

Preparation time-5 minutes |Cook time-0 minutes |Servings-2 |Difficulty-Easy

Nutritional value: ~Calories-382|Proteins-8g| Fat-21g|Carbohydrates-31g

Ingredients

- Half cup of rolled oats

- One cup of almond milk

- A quarter cup of chia seeds

- A pinch of cinnamon powder

- Two teaspoons of honey

- One cup of berries, pureed

- One tablespoon of yogurt

Instructions

- In a bowl, combine the oats with the milk and the ingredients except for the yogurt.

- Toss, divide into bowls, top with the yogurt, and serve cold for breakfast.

Best Scrambled Eggs

Preparation time- 5 minutes| Cook time-15 minutes| Servings-2 |Difficulty-Easy

Nutritional value- Calories-87| Fat-6g |Carbohydrates-1g| Protein-7g

Ingredients

- One tablespoon of low-fat milk

- Freshly ground black pepper

- Half teaspoon of dried thyme

- Two large eggs

- Nonstick cooking spray

Instructions

- Spray a skillet with some cooking spray and put it over medium heat.

- Whisk the eggs lightly. Then mix in the thyme and milk.

- Put the egg mixture in the skillet lower the heat to medium. For 10 to 15 minutes, keep moving the eggs slowly but continuously with a spatula or until they're cooked properly.

- Sprinkle with black pepper and serve.

Black bean and avocado breakfast burrito with lime cream

Preparation time-5 minutes |Cook time-0 minutes |Serving-3 |Difficulty- Easy

Nutritional value: ~ Calories-124| Fat-9g| Protein-4g| Carbohydrates-8g

Ingredients

For Burrito

- One egg plus one egg white

- One tablespoon of shredded white cheddar or provolone cheese

- One tablespoon of chopped fresh cilantro or parsley

- Two teaspoons of your favorite salsa

- One tablespoon of canned black beans drained and rinsed

- Two teaspoons of freshly scooped avocado

- One low-carb, high-fiber whole wheat tortilla wrap

- One tablespoon of lime cream

For Lime Cream

- A quarter cup of light sour cream or 0% fat-free Greek Yogurt

- Zest and juice of half lime

- A quarter teaspoon o salt

Instructions

- In a small skillet sprayed with nonstick spray, scramble the egg and egg white on medium heat. Season with a little salt. When eggs are almost done, add in cheese and parsley or cilantro.

- Place eggs on the tortilla. On top of eggs, add salsa, then beans, avocado, and lime cream. Roll up "burrito style" and enjoy immediately!

For Lime Cream

- In a small bowl, whisk all ingredients. Salt to taste. Use as a dip or as a condiment for soups and stews. Store in the refrigerator.

Black Bean plus sweet Potato Hash

Preparation time- 5 minutes| Cook time-10 minutes| Servings-4 |Difficulty-Easy

Nutritional value- Calories-133| Fat-1g |Carbohydrates-28g| Protein-5g

Ingredients

- Two cups of peeled, chopped sweet potatoes

- One cup of chopped onion

- One cup of cooked and drained black beans

- One minced garlic clove

- ⅓ cup of vegetable broth

- A quarter cup of chopped scallions

- Two teaspoons of hot chili powder

Instructions

- Prepare your vegetables.

- In a deep saucepan with a lid, saute and cook the chopped onion for 2-3 minutes, stirring, so it doesn't burn.

- Add the garlic and stir until fragrant.

- Add the sweet potatoes and chili powder, and stir.

- Pour in the broth and give one last stir before locking the lid.

- Cook on high pressure for 3 minutes.

- When time is up, quick-release the pressure carefully.

- Add the black beans and scallions, and stir to heat everything up.

- Season with salt and more chili powder if desired.

Blueberry Muffins

Preparation time-15 minutes| Cook time-25 minutes| Servings-12 |Difficulty-Easy

Nutritional value- Calories-133| Fat-1.8g |Carbohydrates-22g| Protein-2.3g

Ingredients

- One and 3 /4 cups of all-purpose flour

- Half teaspoon of baking soda

- Half cup of sugar

- Half teaspoon of baking powder

- A quarter teaspoon of kosher salt

- A quarter teaspoon of ground cinnamon

- Three teaspoons of egg replacer, such as Ener-G

- A quarter cup of warm water

- Half cup of nondairy vanilla yogurt

- A quarter cup of grapeseed oil

- Two tablespoons of nondairy milk

- One teaspoon of lemon zest

- One teaspoon of freshly squeezed lemon juice

- One and a quarter cup of roughly chopped fresh or frozen blueberries

Instructions

- Preheat the oven to 350°F (180°C). Lightly coat the cups of a 12-cup muffin tin with nonstick baking spray.

- In a medium bowl, whisk together baking soda, all-purpose flour, kosher salt, sugar, baking powder, and cinnamon.

- In a small bowl, whisk egg replacer with warm water until well blended. Whisk in vanilla nondairy yogurt, grapeseed oil, nondairy milk, lemon zest, and lemon juice.

- Quickly stir wet ingredients into flour mixture until ingredients are just combined, taking care not to overmix. Fold in blueberries.

- Using an ice-cream scoop or a large spoon, evenly divide batter among muffin cups. The batter will be thick, like biscuit dough.

- Bake on the bottom rack of the oven for 22 to 25 minutes or until muffins spring back when lightly pressed in the center. Cool in the pan for 5 minutes before turning out on a wire rack to cool. Serve warm or at room temperature.

Blueberry-Almond Overnight Oats

Preparation time-5 minutes | Cook time-2 minutes |Serving-4 |Difficulty- Easy

Nutritional value: ~ Calories-225| Fat-8g| Protein-9g| Carbohydrates-30g

Ingredients

- One and a half cups of old-fashioned rolled oats

- Two cups of unsweetened vanilla almond milk

- One teaspoon of vanilla extract

- Two tablespoons of flaxseed meal

- A quarter teaspoon of ground cinnamon

- A quarter teaspoon of salt Sugar substitute for added sweetness (optional)

- Half cup of low-fat, plain Greek yogurt

- One cup of blueberries

- A quarter cup of sliced almonds for topping

Instructions

- In a medium bowl, combine the oats, milk, vanilla, flaxseed, cinnamon, salt, and up to one tablespoon of your preferred sugar substitute (if using).

- Divide the oat mixture among 4 jars or serving cups.

- Layer Two tablespoons of Greek yogurt over each cup of oats, and cover.

Place the blueberries in a microwave-safe bowl, cover them, and heat for 1½ to 2 minutes, or until they burst to form a sauce.

Top each yogurt with about 2 ounces of blueberries, and finish with sliced almonds.

Refrigerate overnight or for at least 2 hours.

Eat cold or warm slightly in the microwave for 20 to 30 seconds.

Braunschweiger omelet

Preparation time-10 minutes |Cook time-8 minutes |Servings-1 |Difficulty-Easy

Nutritional value: ~443 Calories| Fat-39g|Protein-19g|Carbohydrates-4g

Ingredients

- One tablespoon of butter

- Two eggs, beaten

- Two ounces of braunschweiger (liverwurst), mashed a bit with a fork

- A quarter medium ripe tomato, sliced

- Mayonnaise (optional)

Instructions

- Make your omelet, spoon the mashed braunschweiger over half of your omelet and top with the tomato slices.

- If you'd like to gild the lily, a dollop of mayonnaise is good on top of this.

Breakfast burritos

Preparation time-10 minutes |Cook time-10 minutes |Servings-2 |Difficulty-Easy

Nutritional value: ~113 Calories| Fat-1.8g|Protein-2.3g|Carbohydrates-22g

Ingredients

- Two tablespoons of olive oil

- Half small red onion, thinly sliced (A quarter cup)

- Two cups of sliced button mushrooms

- One teaspoon of crumbled dried sage

- Half teaspoon of kosher salt

- Half teaspoon of freshly ground black pepper

- One cup of cooked black beans

- Two (10-in.) whole-wheat tortillas

- One large tomato, diced (one cup)

- One medium Hass avocado halved, seeded, and sliced

- A quarter cup of prepared salsa

Instructions

- Heat olive oil in a medium sautés pan over medium-high heat. Cook, stirring once or twice, for 2 to 3 minutes with button mushrooms and red onion.

- Cook for 2 minutes more after adding the kosher salt, sage, and black pepper.

- Cook, stirring a few times and pressing to break up the beans and brown them a little, for approximately 5 minutes, turning a few times and pushing to break them up and brown them a little. Remove the pan from the heat and set it aside.

- Place half of the mushroom filling in the center of each tortilla, then divide the avocado, tomato, and salsa among the burritos. Fold the two short ends in first, then fold one long end inside to form a burrito.

Breakfast Egg Muffin

Preparation time-10 minutes | Cook time-20 minutes | Servings-6 | Difficulty-Easy

Nutritional value- Calories-120 | Fat-13g | Carbohydrates-1g | Protein-16g

Ingredients

- Six eggs

- Cooking spray

- ⅓ cup of cooked turkey bacon

- ⅓ cup of shredded cheddar cheese

- Half cup of frozen chopped spinach

Instructions

- Preheat the oven to 375 degrees Fahrenheit.

- Coat 6 muffin cups with cooking spray or line with paper cups.

- In a large mixing bowl, crack eggs and whisk until smooth, about 1 minute.

- To the egg mixture, add bacon, cheese and spinach. Combine well.

- Evenly distribute egg mixture among muffin cups.

- Bake for 16-18 minutes, or until the eggs are firm to the touch.

- Remove from oven and tin, and serve immediately.

Breakfast Pizza

Preparation time-15 minutes | Cook time-5 minutes | Serving-1 | Difficulty- Easy

Nutritional value: ~ Calories-189 | Fat-6g | Protein-23g | Carbohydrates-9g

Ingredients

- Four large egg whites (or a half cup of liquid egg whites)

- Nonstick cooking spray

- Half teaspoon of Italian seasoning

- A quarter teaspoon of garlic powder

- A quarter cup of pizza sauce

- A quarter cup of shredded mozzarella cheese

- One tablespoon of chopped fresh basil (optional)

Instructions

- In a small bowl, whisk together the egg whites.

- Over medium-low heat, lightly spray an 8-inch sauté pan with cooking spray. Pour the egg whites into the pan.

- Allow the egg whites to cook for 1 to 2 minutes.

- Using a rubber spatula, gently lift the edges of the egg and tilt the pan, allowing the unset white to run underneath and start to cook. Repeat until no liquid remains.

- Sprinkle with Italian seasoning and garlic powder once the egg is almost cooked through, top with the sauce and cheese. Cook for another minute until the cheese has melted.

- Slide the pizza onto a plate and serve immediately, topping with fresh basil (if desired).

Breakfast Scramble

Preparation time-10 minutes | Cook time-10 minutes | Serving-2 | Difficulty- Easy

Nutritional value: ~ Calories-113 | Fat-5.7g | Protein-6.2g | Carbohydrates-19g

Ingredients

- Two tablespoons of olive oil

- Half cup of silken tofu

- Half small red onion, thinly sliced (A quarter cup)

- One tablespoon of nutritional yeast

- Two cups of sliced button mushrooms

- One teaspoon of crumbled dried sage

- Half teaspoon of kosher salt

- Half teaspoon of freshly ground black pepper

- One cup of cooked black beans

- Two (10-in.; 25cm) whole-wheat tortillas

- One large tomato, diced (one cup)

- One medium Hass avocado halved, seeded, and sliced

- A quarter cup of plant-based sour cream

- A handful of chopped cilantro

- Chopped fruits and vegetables of your choice

- A quarter cup of prepared salsa

Instructions

- Heat olive oil in a medium sautés pan over medium-high heat. Cook, stirring once or twice, for 2 to 3 minutes with button mushrooms and red onion.

- Cook for 2 minutes more after adding the kosher salt, sage, and black pepper.

- Cook, stirring a few times and pressing to break up the beans and brown them a little, for approximately 5 minutes, turning a few times and pushing to break them up and brown them a little.

- Toss half a cup of crumbled silken tofu and one tablespoon of nutritional yeast into the pan with black beans. Remove the pan from the heat and set it aside.

- Place half of the mushroom filling in the center of each tortilla, then divide the avocado, tomato, and salsa among the burritos.

- Add plant-based sour cream, chopped cilantro, or chopped fresh fruits or veggies to your burrito.

- Fold the two short ends in first, then fold one long end inside to form a breakfast scramble.

Breakfast Toast

Preparation time-10 minutes |Cook time-20 minutes |Servings-2 |Difficulty-Easy

Nutritional value: ~Calories-153 | Proteins-6.2g | Fat-5.7g | Carbohydrates-19.2g

Ingredients

- Two eggs, beaten

- Half cup of yogurt

- One banana, mashed

- Half teaspoon of ground cinnamon

- Six whole-grain bread slices

- One tablespoon of olive oil

Instructions

- In the mixing bowl, mix up eggs, cream, and ground cinnamon, add mashed banana.

- Coat the bread in the egg mixture. Then heat olive oil.

- Put the coated bread in the hot olive oil and roast for 3 minutes per side until light brown.

Breakfast Tofu Scramble

Preparation time-5 minutes |Cook time-5 minutes |Serving-4 |Difficulty- Easy

Nutritional value: ~ Calories-139 | Fat-5g | Protein-12g | Carbohydrates-15g

Ingredients

- One block of extra-firm, crumbled tofu

- One cup of cherry tomatoes

- One onion

- One diced potato

- One diced apple

- A quarter cup of veggie broth

- Two minced garlic cloves

- One teaspoon of dry dill

- Half teaspoon of ground turmeric

- Salt and pepper to taste

Instructions

- Sauté and dry-cook the garlic and onion until the onion begins to soften in a deep saucepan with a lid.

- Add a bit of water if it starts to stick.

- Pour broth and add the rest of the ingredients.

- Close the lid.

- Cook on high pressure for 4 minutes.

- Stir, season to taste, and enjoy!

Breakfast Tostadas

Preparation time-15 minutes |Cook time-6 minutes |Servings-2 |Difficulty-Easy

Nutritional value: ~Calories-246 | Proteins-13.7g | Fat-11.1g | Carbohydrates-24.5g

Ingredients

- Half white onion, diced

- One tomato, chopped

- One cucumber, chopped

- One tablespoon of fresh cilantro, chopped

- Half jalapeno pepper, chopped

- One tablespoon of lime juice

- Six corn tortillas

- One tablespoon of canola oil

- Two ounces of Cheddar cheese, shredded

- Half cup of white beans, canned, drained

- Six eggs

- Half teaspoon of butter

- Half teaspoon of Sea salt

Instructions

- For Pico de Gallo, in the salad bowl, combine diced white onion, tomato, cucumber, fresh cilantro, and jalapeno pepper.

- Then add lime juice and a half tablespoon of canola oil. Mix up the mixture well. Pico de Gallo is cooked.

- After this, preheat the oven to 390 degrees F.

- Line the tray with baking paper.

- Arrange the corn tortillas on the baking paper and brush with the remaining canola oil from both sides.

- Bake the tortillas for 10 minutes or wait until they start to be crunchy.

- Chill the cooked crunchy tortillas well.

- Meanwhile, toss the butter in the skillet.

- Crack the eggs in the melted butter and sprinkle them with sea salt.

- Fry the eggs until the egg whites become white (cooked). Approximately 3-5 minutes over medium heat.

- After this, mash the beans until you get a puree texture.

- Spread the bean puree on the corn tortillas.

- Add fried eggs.

- Then top the eggs with Pico de Gallo and shredded Cheddar cheese.

Broccoli and cheese frittata

Preparation time-10 minutes |Cook time-37 minutes |Servings-2 |Difficulty-Moderate

Nutritional value: ~Calories-121|Proteins-12g| Fat-8g|Carbohydrates-5g

Ingredients

- One cup of broccoli florets

- One tablespoon of extra-virgin olive oil

- Half cup of finely chopped onion

- Half cup of chopped red bell pepper

- Two cloves of fresh garlic, minced

- One cup of shredded mozzarella cheese

- Dash of crushed red hot pepper flakes

- One cup of egg substitute or One cup of egg whites, or two large eggs

- Olive oil spray

Instructions

- Steam broccoli until crispy tender and remove from heat. In a large skillet over medium-high heat, heat olive oil and sauté onion, bell pepper, and garlic until vegetables are soft (about 5 minutes).

- Add broccoli and cook about 2 minutes longer. Transfer vegetable mixture to a bowl, then add mozzarella cheese and hot pepper flakes. If using whole eggs, beat in a separate bowl until blended. Stir eggs into vegetable mixture and pour into a round cake pan lightly sprayed with olive oil spray.

- Bake in 325 degrees F oven until eggs are set, about 30 minutes.

- Serve hot or at room temperature.

Broccoli Casserole

Preparation time- 5 minutes| Cook time-20 minutes| Servings-12 |Difficulty-Easy

Nutritional value- Calories-298| Fat-16g |Carbohydrates-2.8g| Protein-20.9g

Ingredients

Four cups of cut-up broccoli

Sleeve Ritz crackers

Two cups of cheddar cheese

Instructions

Add the casserole ingredients into a Pyrex dish with the crumbled crackers on top.

Bake long enough to melt the cheese at 375°F.

Broccoli~Cheddar Puree

Preparation time- 5 minutes| Cook time-15 minutes| Servings-4 |Difficulty-Easy

Nutritional value- Calories-78| Fat-3g |Carbohydrates-7g| Protein-8g

Ingredients

- ⅓ cup of part-skim shredded Cheddar cheese

- ⅔ cup of low-fat cottage cheese

- Two cups of diced broccoli florets

Instructions

- Fill a medium saucepan with a few inches of water. Then place a steam basket. Put broccoli florets in it and boil the water. Close the lid and steam the broccoli until it softens. Turn off the heat.

- Throw the Cheddar cheese, cottage cheese, and softened broccoli into a food processor. Enjoy.

- Refrigerate the leftovers for up to 5 days.

Broccoli Egg and Cheese Bake

Preparation time~10 minutes |Cook time-One hour 30 minutes |Serving~8 |Difficulty-Hard

Nutritional value: ~Calories~114| Fat~5g| Protein~12g| Carbohydrates~6g

Ingredients

- Four ounces of light margarine

- Six tablespoons of flour

- Ten ounces of frozen, chopped broccoli (thawed)

- A dash of black pepper

- One 4-ounce jar chopped pimento (optional)

- Six large eggs

- Half pound of low-fat cheddar cheese

- Two pounds of non-fat cottage cheese

- One teaspoon of salt

- Dash paprika (optional)

- Half cup of sliced mushrooms, fresh or canned (optional)

Instructions

- Preheat the oven to 350 degrees Fahrenheit.
- Combine all ingredients in a mixing bowl.
- Using cooking spray, coat a 2-quart casserole dish.
- Bake for 90 minutes with the combined ingredients in the prepared pan.
- Serve immediately.

Broiled Fish Fillet

Preparation time- 5 minutes| Cook time-12 minutes| Servings-2 |Difficulty-Easy

Nutritional value- Calories-298| Fat-16g |Carbohydrates-2.8g| Protein-20.9g

Ingredients

- Two cod fish fillets
- 1/8 teaspoon of curry powder
- Two teaspoons of butter
- A quarter teaspoon of paprika
- 1/8 teaspoon of pepper
- 1/8 teaspoon of salt

Instructions

- Preheat the broiler. Spray broiler pan with cooking spray and set aside. In a small bowl, mix together paprika, curry powder, pepper, and salt.
- Coat fish fillet with paprika mixture and place on broiler pan. Broil fish for 10-12 minutes. Top with butter and serve.

Buffalo wing omelet

Preparation time-5 minutes |Cook time-5 minutes |Servings-1 |Difficulty-Easy

Nutritional value: ~384 Calories| Fat-34g|Protein-17g|Carbohydrates-2g

Ingredients

- One and a half teaspoons of bacon grease
- Two eggs, beaten
- Three tablespoons of crumbled blue cheese
- One tablespoon of butter
- One tablespoon of hot sauce (preferably Frank's Red Hot, or Tabasco or Louisiana brand)

Instructions

- Make your omelet using the bacon grease for the fat. Fill with the blue cheese.

- While your omelet is covered on low heat, melt the cheese, melt the butter with the Tabasco sauce in a small saucepan or nuke for a minute in a custard cup.
- Stir them together well.
- When your omelet's done, fold and plate, and then top with the sauce and eat.

California omelet

Preparation time-10 minutes |Cook time-10 minutes |Servings-1 |Difficulty-Easy

Nutritional value: ~545 Calories| Fat-47g|Protein-26g|Carbohydrates-5g

Ingredients

- One tablespoon of olive oil
- Two eggs, beaten
- Two ounces of Monterey Jack cheese, shredded
- A quarter avocado, sliced
- A quarter cup of alfalfa sprouts

Instructions

- Make your omelet, place the Monterey Jack over half of your omelet when you're ready to add the filling.
- Cover, turn the heat to low and cook until the cheese is melted (2 to 3 minutes).
- Arrange the avocado and sprouts over the cheese, and follow the directions to finish making the omelet.

Cauliflower Fritters

Preparation time-10 minutes |Cook time-10 minutes |Servings-2 |Difficulty-Easy

Nutritional value: ~Calories-167|Proteins-9g| Fat-12g|Carbohydrates-8g

Ingredients

- One cup of cauliflower, shredded
- One egg, beaten
- One tablespoon of wheat flour, whole grain
- One ounce of Parmesan, grated
- Half teaspoon of ground black pepper
- One tablespoon of canola oil

Instructions

- In the mixing bowl, mix up together shredded cauliflower and egg.
- Add wheat flour, grated Parmesan, and ground black pepper.
- Stir the mixture with the help of the fork until it is homogenous and smooth.
- Pour canola oil into the skillet and bring it to a boil.

- Make the fritters from the cauliflower mixture with the fingertips' help, or use a spoon and transfer in the hot oil.
- Roast the fritters for 4 minutes from each side over medium-low heat.

Chai-Spiced Oatmeal with Mango

Preparation time-10 minutes |Cook time-10 minutes |Servings-2 |Difficulty-Easy

Nutritional value: ~Calories-236|Proteins-6g| Fat-4g|Carbohydrates-44g

Ingredients

- Three cups of water
- One cup of steel-cut oats
- Half teaspoon of vanilla
- Dash of cinnamon
- Dash of ginger
- Dash of cloves
- Dash of cardamom
- Dash of salt
- Half mango, cut into pieces

Instructions

- Mix water and oats in a deep saucepan with a lid.
- Close the lid.
- Cook for 5 minutes on high flame.
- Turn off the flame and let it rest.
- Open the lid and stir well.
- Season and taste.
- Divide into even servings and add chopped mango.

Cheesy Slow Cooker Egg Casserole

Preparation time-15 minutes |Cook time-4 to 8 hours |Serving-8 |Difficulty- Hard

Nutritional value: ~Calories-348| Fat-17g| Protein-27g| Carbohydrates-24g

Ingredients

- One pound of fresh Italian chicken sausage

Nonstick cooking spray

- One (30-ounce) bag of frozen hash browns
- One medium red bell pepper, seeded and diced
- Half medium onion, diced
- One (4-ounce) can mild diced green chiles

- One and a half cups of low-fat shredded Cheddar cheese, divided into three ½- cup servings
- Twelve large eggs
- One cup of low-fat milk
- Half teaspoon of salt
- Half teaspoon of freshly ground black pepper

Instructions

- Remove the casings from the sausage, and discard.
- In a large skillet over medium heat, brown the meat, breaking it into smaller pieces as it cooks, about 7 minutes, or until no longer pink.
- Spray a 5-quart slow cooker with nonstick cooking spray, and layer half of the frozen hash browns, cooked sausage, pepper, onion, and chiles, plus half a cup of cheese. Repeat with the remaining hash browns, sausage, pepper, onion, and chiles, plus another half cup of cheese.
- In a large bowl, whisk the eggs, milk, salt, and pepper.
- Pour the egg mixture over the potato-sausage layers, and top with the remaining half cup of cheese.
- Cook on high for 4 hours or on low for 8 hours, and serve.

Chicken Cheesesteak Wrap

Preparation time- 5 minutes| Cook time-10 minutes| Servings-1 |Difficulty-Easy

Nutritional value- Calories-298| Fat-16g |Carbohydrates-2.8g| Protein-20.9g

Ingredients

- Two teaspoons of sliced pickled hot chili peppers
- One whole wheat flour tortilla
- A quarter lb. of boneless skinless chicken breast
- One wedge of Swiss cheese spread
- Half cup of sliced mushrooms
- A quarter cup of sliced green pepper
- A quarter cup of chopped onion

Instructions

- Put chicken on cutting board and pound to ¼-inch thickness. Slice into strips. Spray the skillet with a nonstick cooking spray, or you can brush it with a very little amount of oil as an alternative.
- Place the onion and the chicken cooking until the chicken is done. Mix in mushrooms and green peppers. Cook until mushrooms and pepper are soft.
- Put the tortilla between two damp paper towels. Microwave 20 seconds. Put the tortilla on a plate and put Swiss cheese in a strip down the middle.

- Top with mushrooms, onions, peppers, and chicken. Add pickled chili peppers. Fold sides over the middle. Serve and enjoy.

Chili Garlic Salmon

Preparation time-7 minutes| Cook time-5 minutes| Servings-3 |Difficulty-Easy

Nutritional value- Calories-194| Fat-4g |Carbohydrates-23g| Protein-20g

Ingredients

- One lb. of salmon fillet, cut into three pieces
- One teaspoon of red chili powder
- One garlic clove, minced
- One teaspoon of ground cumin
- Pepper
- Salt

Instructions

- Pour one and a half cups of water into the instant pot and place the trivet into the pot.
- In a small bowl, mix together chili powder, garlic, cumin, pepper, and salt. Rub salmon pieces with spice mixture and place on top of the trivet. Seal the instant pot with a lid and cook on steam mode for 2 minutes.
- Once done, release pressure using the quick-release method and then open the lid. Serve and enjoy.

Cinnamon Flax-and-Almond Breakfast Cakes

Preparation time- 5 minutes| Cook time-20 minutes| Servings-4 |Difficulty-Easy

Nutritional value- Calories-117| Fat-8g |Carbohydrates-7g| Protein-7g

Ingredients

- Nonstick cooking spray
- A quarter teaspoon of stevia
- Two large eggs
- One teaspoon of vanilla extract
- One teaspoon of ground cinnamon
- Two teaspoons of brown sugar
- Four tablespoons of unsweetened almond milk
- Four tablespoons of almond flour
- Four tablespoons of flax meal

Instructions

- Combine almond flour, stevia, eggs, cinnamon, brown sugar, flax meal, almond milk, and vanilla extract. Then beat it fast to make it thick.
- Spray a skillet and put it over medium flame.

- Pour one tablespoon of batter to make each cake. Let them cook until they're golden. You'll see bubbles emerging on the surface of the cakes.
- Continue with all the batter. Serve warm on a plate and enjoy.

Cinnamon spice pancakes

Preparation time-10 minutes |Cook time-10 minutes |Servings-2 |Difficulty-Easy

Nutritional value: ~Calories-98|Proteins-9g| Fat-7g|Carbohydrates-12g

Ingredients

- A quarter cup plus Two tablespoons of coconut flour
- Half teaspoon of baking soda
- A quarter teaspoon of ground nutmeg
- One teaspoon of ground cinnamon
- Four large eggs, beaten
- Half cup of full-fat, canned coconut milk
- One teaspoon of lemon juice
- Two teaspoons of honey
- Two tablespoons of unsalted butter, ghee, or coconut oil, for cooking
- Melted butter or ghee, for serving

Instructions

- In a large mixing basin, sift together the baking soda, coconut flour, nutmeg, and cinnamon. In a mixing bowl, combine the eggs, lemon juice, coconut milk, and honey. Whisk until the mixture is completely smooth.
- In a medium skillet over medium heat, melt the fat. Pour For each pancake, pour a quarter cup of batter into the hot pan, leaving room for it to spread. Cook for 2 minutes on one side, then flip and cook for another 2 minutes on the other side.
- Place the cooked pancakes on a platter and cover with plastic wrap to keep warm while you finish the remainder of the pancakes.
- Serve with melted butter on top.

Cinnamon-Spice Overnight Cereal

Preparation time- 5 minutes| Cook time-0 minutes| Servings-1 |Difficulty-Easy

Nutritional value- Calories-336| Fat-17g |Carbohydrates-26g| Protein-27g

Ingredients

- Three tablespoons of almond flour
- A quarter teaspoon of stevia
- One teaspoon of ground cinnamon

- One tablespoon of chia seeds

- Two tablespoons of quick oats

- Four tablespoons of unsweetened almond milk

- ¾ cup of non-fat plain Greek yogurt

Instructions

- In a pint-size canning jar, thoroughly mix oats, cinnamon, almond milk, stevia, chia seeds, almond flour, and yogurt.

- Tightly close the jar and refrigerate it. Let it sit for the whole night.

- Take out a half cup of if only you're eating. Enjoy cold or microwave it for half a minute. You will need to check it every 10 seconds if it's only one serving you're heating up to prevent overcooking.

Classic Turkey, Cranberry, and Cream Cheese Sandwich

Preparation time-15 minutes |Cook time-0 minutes |Serving-1 |Difficulty- Easy

Nutritional value: ~ Calories-214| Fat-5g| Protein-17g| Carbohydrates-27g

Ingredients

- Two slices diet whole grain bread, toasted

- One teaspoon of nonfat mayonnaise

- Two teaspoons of reduced-fat cream cheese

- Two tablespoons of cranberry sauce

- Two ounces of sliced turkey meat, no skin or fat

- One leaf green or red leaf lettuce

Instructions

- On one slice of the bread, spread the mayonnaise, and spread the cream cheese on the other.

- On top of the cream cheese, spread the cranberry sauce.

- Place the turkey on top of the cranberry sauce and the lettuce on top of the turkey. Top with the remaining slice of toast and cut in half.

Club Omelet

Preparation time-10 minutes |Cook time-8 minutes |Servings-1 |Difficulty-Easy

Nutritional value: ~383 Calories| Fat-28g|Protein-29g|Carbohydrates-5g

Ingredients

- Two slices of bacon

- Two ounces of sliced turkey breast

- Half small tomato

- One scallion

- Two eggs

- One tablespoon of mayonnaise

Instructions

- Cook and drain your bacon.

- Cut the turkey into small squares, and slice the tomato and scallion.

- Beat the eggs, and make your omelet, using a couple of spoonfuls of the bacon grease.

- Add just the bacon and turkey before covering. Once it's cooked to your liking, sprinkle the tomato and scallion over the meat, spread the mayonnaise on the other side, fold, and serve.

Cocoa Oatmeal

Preparation time-10 minutes |Cook time-15 minutes |Servings-2 |Difficulty-Easy

Nutritional value: ~Calories-230|Proteins-5g| Fat-11g|Carbohydrates-28g

Ingredients

- One and a half cups of oatmeal

- One tablespoon of cocoa powder

- Half cup of heavy cream

- A quarter cup of water

- One teaspoon of vanilla extract

- One tablespoon of butter

- Two tablespoons of Splenda

Instructions

- Mix up together oatmeal with cocoa powder and Splenda.

- Transfer the mixture to the saucepan.

- Add vanilla extract, water, and heavy cream. Stir it gently with the help of the spatula.

- Close the lid and cook it for 10-15 minutes over medium-low heat.

- Remove the cooked cocoa oatmeal from the heat and add butter. Stir it well.

Coconut flax bread

Preparation time-10 minutes |Cook time-One hour 20 minutes|Servings-20 slices |Difficulty-Hard

Nutritional value: ~111 Calories| Fat-9g|Protein-4g|Carbohydrates-5g

Ingredients

- Four cups of shredded coconut meat

- 3/4 cup of flaxseed meal

- One tablespoon of xanthan or guar

- One teaspoon of erythritol

- One and a half teaspoons of baking soda

- Half teaspoon of salt

- Half cup of water

- Two tablespoons of cider vinegar

- Four eggs

Instructions

- Preheat the oven to 350 degrees Fahrenheit.

- Grease a typical loaf pan, not a super-large one. Using nonstick aluminum foil or baking paper, line the pan.

- Combine the flaxseed meal, coconut, xanthan gum, baking soda, erythritol, and salt in a food processor fitted with the S-blade.

- Run the machine until all of the ingredients are finely ground. Scrape down the sides of the processor and run it again.

- While that's going on, combine the water and vinegar in a glass measuring cup. Place this near the food processor.

- Add the eggs one at a time through the feed tube while the food processor is running.

- Finally, through the feed tube, pour the water-and-vinegar combination in. Just another 30 seconds or so of running.

- Scoop or transfer the batter into the loaf pan that has been prepared. Preheat oven to 350°F and bake for 1 hour and 15 minutes. Allow cooling on a wire rack.

- This is an excellent slicer. Refrigerate this or, better yet, slice it and freeze it as soon as it's cool.

Coconut-Almond Breakfast Cakes

Preparation time- 5 minutes| Cook time-20 minutes| Servings-4 |Difficulty-Easy

Nutritional value- Calories-209| Fat-17g |Carbohydrates-7g| Protein-9g

Ingredients

- One teaspoon of baking powder

- A quarter teaspoon of salt

- Half teaspoon of stevia

- One teaspoon of ground cinnamon

- Two large eggs

- Half cup of unsweetened coconut milk

- One cup of almond flour

- Two teaspoons of vanilla extract

- Nonstick cooking spray

Instructions

- Spray a skillet and put it over medium flame.

- In a medium bowl, mix the coconut milk eggs, salt, cinnamon, stevia, baking powder, vanilla extract, almond flour, and whisk them swiftly.

- Pour two tablespoons of batter to make each cake. Then leave them for a while as they cook.

- Continue with all the batter. Make sure that cakes are at minimum 1 inch away from each other when making multiples in the same skillet.

- Serve warm on a plate with your favorite topping and enjoy.

Coconut-Almond Risotto

Preparation time-10 minutes| Cook time-20 minutes| Servings-4 |Difficulty-Easy

Nutritional value- Calories-337| Fat-7g |Carbohydrates-66g| Protein-6g

Ingredients

- Two cups of vanilla almond milk

- One cup of coconut milk

- One cup of Arborio rice

- ⅓ cup of sugar

- Two teaspoons of pure vanilla

- A quarter cup of sliced almonds and coconut flakes

Instructions

- Pour the milk into a deep-bottomed saucepan with a lid.

- Stir until it boils.

- Add the rice and stir before closing the lid.

- Cook for 5 minutes on high pressure.

- Turn off the flame and wait 10 minutes.

- Add the sugar and vanilla.

- Divide up oats and top with almonds and coconut.

Confetti frittata

Preparation time-10 minutes |Cook time-30 minutes|Servings-4 |Difficulty-Moderate

Nutritional value: ~279 Calories| Fat-22g|Protein-16g|Carbohydrates-4g

Ingredients

- Four ounces of bulk pork sausage

- A quarter cup of diced green bell pepper

- A quarter cup of diced red bell pepper

- A quarter cup of diced sweet red onion

- A quarter cup of grated Parmesan cheese

- One teaspoon of original flavor Mrs. Dash

- Eight eggs, beaten

Instructions

- Preheat the oven to broil.

- Brown and crumble the sausage in a large, ovenproof skillet over medium heat.

- Add the onions and peppers to the skillet as the fat begins to render.

- Sauté the sausage and vegetables until the sausage is no longer pink.

- In the bottom of the skillet, spread the mixture into an equal layer.

- In a medium bowl, whisk together the eggs, Parmesan cheese, and seasonings, then pour over the sausage and vegetables in the skillet.

- Reduce to a low heat setting and cover the skillet. (If your skillet doesn't come with a lid, cover it with foil.)

- Cook until the eggs are mostly set in the frittata. This could take up to 25 or 30 minutes, but the size of your skillet will influence how quickly it cooks, so keep an eye on it.

- When the frittata has all set except for the very top, place it under the broiler for about 5 minutes or until the top is brown. Serve wedges cut into wedges.

Cranberry~Walnut Quinoa

Preparation time~10 minutes| Cook time~10 minutes| Servings~4 |Difficulty~Easy

Nutritional value- Calories~661 | Fat~29g |Carbohydrates~82g| Protein~13g

Ingredients

- Two cups of water

- Two cups of dried cranberries

- One cup of quinoa

- One cup of chopped walnuts

- One cup of sunflower seeds

- Half tablespoon of cinnamon

Instructions

- Rinse quinoa.
- Put quinoa, water, and salt in a deep-bottomed saucepan with a lid.
- Lock the lid.
- Cook for 10 minutes on high pressure.
- Turn off the flame.
- When the pressure is gone, open the lid.
- Mix in the dried cranberries, nuts, seeds, sweeteners, and cinnamon.
- Serve and enjoy!

Creamy Oatmeal with Figs

Preparation time-10 minutes |Cook time-20 minutes |Servings-2 |Difficulty-Easy

Nutritional value: ~Calories-222 |Proteins-7g | Fat-6g |Carbohydrates-35g

Ingredients

- Two cups of oatmeal
- One and a half cups of milk
- One tablespoon of butter
- Three figs, chopped
- One tablespoon of honey

Instructions

- Pour milk into the saucepan.
- Add oatmeal and close the lid. Cook the oatmeal for 15 minutes over medium-low heat.
- Then add chopped figs and honey.
- Add butter and mix up the oatmeal well.
- Cook it for 5 minutes more. Close the lid and let the cooked breakfast rest for 10 minutes before serving.

Creamy Pumpkin Mousse

Preparation time- 5 minutes| Cook time-0 minutes| Servings-4 |Difficulty-Easy

Nutritional value- Calories-149| Fat-4.4g |Carbohydrates-28g| Protein-2g

Ingredients

- One can of pumpkin, 15-ounce
- One teaspoon of cinnamon
- Two cups of sugar-free whipped topping (Cool Whip)
- Half cup of skim milk
- One package of fat-free vanilla pudding 4-ounce

- Allspice, clove, ginger, nutmeg and Splenda to taste

Instructions

- Combine all ingredients in a mixing bowl.
- Whip until smooth and creamy.

Cumin and cauliflower frittata

Preparation time-5 minutes |Cook time-30 minutes |Servings-2 |Difficulty-Easy

Nutritional value: ~Calories-131 |Proteins-16g | Fat-7g |Carbohydrates-9g

Ingredients

- One medium head cauliflower
- Two tablespoons of unsalted butter, ghee, or coconut oil
- Two teaspoons of minced garlic
- One cup of cherry tomatoes halved
- Fine sea salt and ground pepper
- Two tablespoons of chopped fresh cilantro
- Two teaspoons of ground cumin
- Four large eggs

Instructions

- Preheat the oven to 350°F.
- Core the cauliflower and cut it into small florets; discard the core.
- Place the cauliflower in the top of a steamer pot with a few inches of water in the bottom. Steam the cauliflower over medium heat for about 10 minutes until it is slightly soft but still firm.
- Melt the fat in a large oven-safe skillet over medium heat. Sauté the garlic for 1 minute in the butter.
- Add the tomatoes to the skillet and sauté for 2 to 3 minutes, until softened. Add a pinch of salt and pepper, the cilantro, and the cumin to the pan and stir to combine.
- Add the drained cauliflower to the skillet and season with a pinch of salt and pepper. Sauté the cauliflower and tomato mixture for two more minutes to allow the flavors to meld.
- In a bowl, beat the eggs with a pinch of salt and pepper. Pour the beaten eggs into the skillet, evenly covering the vegetables, and cook for 1 minute without stirring.
- Put the skillet in the oven and bake for 7 to 10 minutes, until the eggs are cooked through.
- Turn the oven to broil to brown the top of the eggs for 1 minute.
- Remove the skillet from the oven and slice the frittata into wedges. Serve and enjoy.

Delicious Breakfast Bowl

Preparation time-5 minutes |Cook time-20 minutes | Servings-1 | Difficulty-Easy

Nutritional value: ~Calories-131 | Proteins~16g | Fat~7g | Carbohydrates~9g

Ingredients

- Four ounces of ground beef
- One chopped yellow onion
- Eight sliced mushrooms
- Salt and black pepper as per taste
- Two whisked eggs
- One tablespoon of coconut oil
- Half a teaspoon of teaspoon smoked paprika
- One avocado, pitted, peeled and chopped
- Twelve pitted and sliced black olives

Instructions

- Heat a saucepan over medium heat with the coconut oil, add the onions, mushrooms, pepper and salt, stir and cook for five minutes.
- Add the beef and paprika, stir, cook and transfer to a bowl for 10 minutes.
- Over medium heat, heat the pan again, add the eggs, some pepper and salt and scramble.
- Put the beef mix back in the pan and stir.
- Add the olives and avocado, stir, and cook over medium heat for a minute
- Transfer and serve in a bowl.

Delicious Eggs and Sausages

Preparation time-10 minute |Cook time-35 minutes | Servings-6 | Difficulty- Moderate

Nutritional value-Calories-192 | | Carbohydrates-0.5g | Protein~11.8g   Fat-4.5g

Ingredients

- Five tablespoons of ghee
- Twelve eggs
- Salt and black pepper as per taste
- One of torn spinach
- Twelve slices of ham
- Two chopped sausages
- One chopped yellow onion
- One chopped red bell pepper

Instructions

- Heat a saucepan over medium heat with one tablespoon of ghee, add the onion and sausages, stir and cook for five minutes.
- Add the bell pepper, pepper and salt, stir and cook for an additional three minutes and place in a bowl.
- Melt and divide the rest of the ghee into one-two cupcake mold.
- In each cupcake mold, add a slice of ham, divide each spinach and then the sausage mix.
- Break an egg on top, place everything in the oven and bake for 20 minutes at 425 ° Fahrenheit.
- Before serving, leave your cupcakes to cool down a bit.

Delicious Poached Eggs

Preparation time-10 minute| Cook time-35 minutes | Servings-4 | Difficulty- Moderate

Nutritional value-Calories-151 | | Carbohydrates-0.4g | Protein-8.8g   Fat-2.5g

Ingredients

- Three minced garlic cloves
- One tablespoon of ghee
- One chopped white onion
- One chopped Serrano pepper
- Salt and black pepper to the taste
- One chopped red bell pepper
- Three chopped tomatoes
- One teaspoon of paprika
- One teaspoon of cumin
- A quarter teaspoon of chili powder
- One tablespoon of chopped cilantro
- Six eggs

Instructions

- Heat the pan over medium heat with the ghee, add the onion, stir and cook and stir for ten minutes.
- Add the garlic and Serrano pepper, stir and cook over medium heat for a minute.
- Add red bell pepper and cook for 10 minutes, stirring and cooking.
- Add the tomatoes, pepper, salt, chili powder, paprika and cumin, stir and cook for 10 minutes.
- In the pan, crack the eggs, season them with pepper and salt, cover the pan and cook for another 6 minutes.
- In the end, sprinkle with cilantro and serve.

Dense Oatmeal Cake

Preparation time- 5 minutes| Cook time-40 minutes| Servings-4 |Difficulty-Moderate

Nutritional value- Calories-298| Fat-16g |Carbohydrates-2.8g| Protein-20.9g

Ingredients

- ¾ teaspoon of baking powder
- One cup of rolled oats
- Half cup of low-fat buttermilk
- Two organic eggs
- Four tablespoons of applesauce
- Two teaspoons of brown sugar
- One teaspoon of cinnamon

Instructions

- Preheat an oven to 325°F and line a small baking pan with parchment paper. Set aside.
- Combine the rolled oats with baking powder, brown sugar, and cinnamon. Stir well.
- In another bowl, crack the eggs and add the applesauce and buttermilk. Whisk until incorporated. Pour the liquid mixture over the dry mixture, then whisk until combined. Transfer the mixture to the prepared baking pan. Spread evenly.
- Bake the cake for approximately 40 minutes or until a skewer that is inserted into the cake, comes out clean. Remove from the oven, then let the cake cool for a few minutes.
- Take the cake out from the pan, then cut it into slices. Serve and enjoy.

Denver Egg Muffins with Ham Crust

Preparation time-15 minutes |Cook time-30 minutes |Serving-12 |Difficulty- Moderate

Nutritional value: ~ Calories-99| Fat-6g| Protein-8g| Carbohydrates-1g

Ingredients

- Nonstick cooking spray
- Twelve slices of deli ham
- One teaspoon of extra-virgin olive oil
- Half onion, diced
- Half green pepper, minced
- Ten large eggs
- A quarter cup of low-fat milk
- Half cup of Cheddar cheese

Instructions

- Preheat the oven to 350°F.

- Grease a 12-compartment muffin tin with cooking spray.
- Line each cup with a ham slice, pushing it down to fit tightly against the edge of the well.
- In a small skillet over medium heat, heat the oil. Add the onion and green pepper, and sauté for 3 minutes, or until soft. Remove from the heat, and drain any liquid from the pan.
- In a large bowl, whisk the eggs and milk. Add the cheese and cooked vegetables, and whisk again.
- Ladle A quarter cup of the egg mixture into each cup. If there is any leftover, divide evenly among the cups.
- Bake for 20 to 25 minutes, or just until the eggs are firm and no longer runny, and serve.

Egg Chilada

Preparation time- 5 minutes| Cook time-5 minutes| Servings-1 |Difficulty-Easy

Nutritional value- Calories-171| Fat-8g |Carbohydrates-3g| Protein-23g

Ingredients

- One egg
- One egg white only
- Black pepper
- Salt to taste
- One tablespoon of shredded, Mexican blend cheese
- A one-ounce protein of choice (tofu, ground beef or chicken)
- Two tablespoons of plain Greek yogurt (fat-free)
- Two tablespoons of salsa

Instructions

- In a small bowl, scramble the egg yolk and white.
- Coat a skillet or griddle with nonstick cooking spray and place over medium heat.
- Pour the scrambled eggs into the heated pan and spread them out into a roughly circular shape.
- Allow a minute or two for the eggs to set on their own.
- While the eggs are set, season with a pinch of black pepper and salt.
- Slip right a spatula underneath the eggs and flip (don't be alarmed if some egg drips off at this point).
- Cook eggs on the other side for approximately two minutes longer or until fully cooked and transfer to a serving dish.
- Create a filling strip for your egg-enchilada by combining 1-ounce protein of your choice and Mexican cheese.
- Roll the egg "pancake" into an enchilada shape.

- Garnish with salsa and sour cream.

Egg White "Pizza"

Preparation time- 5 minutes| Cook time-5 minutes| Servings-4 |Difficulty-Easy

Nutritional value- Calories-181| Fat-9g |Carbohydrates-14g| Protein-12g

Ingredients

- One cup of sliced tomato One large tomato)
- Half cup of shredded mozzarella cheese
- Nonstick cooking spray (optional)
- A quarter teaspoon of salt
- Half teaspoon of garlic powder
- Half teaspoon of Italian seasoning
- Twelve large egg whites One and a half cups of egg whites)
- One tablespoon of extra-virgin olive oil

Instructions

- Heat oil over medium heat.
- Whisk the egg whites with garlic powder, some seasoning and salt.
- Put the mixture in the skillet and close it. Then cook until the egg whites begin bubbling on top. Now lift at the corners to prevent egg whites from sticking to the skillet. If they still stick, lift the egg whites and spray the skillet with cooking spray.
- Now sprinkle with mozzarella and arrange tomato slices on top. Close and cook till the cheese melts.

Eggplant Pesto Mini Pizza

Preparation time- 5 minutes| Cook time-45 minutes| Servings-4 |Difficulty-Easy

Nutritional value- Calories-298| Fat-16g |Carbohydrates-2.8g| Protein-20.9g

Ingredients

- One chopped bell tomato
- One chopped Eggplant
- One sliced red onion
- 1/8 teaspoon of salt
- Three cloves of garlic
- Pinch of oregano
- A quarter cup Extra-virgin olive oil
- A quarter cup Pesto sauce
- A quarter cup Humus

- A quarter cup Vegan Parmesan cheese
- Sandwich thins — Arnold Oro-wheat used
- Pepper flakes (Optional)

Instructions

- Set the oven to 400°F.
- If desired, chop the vegetables and combine the oil, pepper, salt, oregano, and pepper flakes.
- Arrange on a baking tin and toast for approximately 30 to 45 minutes or until they are done the way you like them.
- Toast the buns, spread the hummus on them, and add the veggies and pesto sauce. Sprinkle with the vegan cheese and enjoy.

Eggs Baked in Avocados

Preparation time- 5 minutes| Cook time-30 minutes| Servings-4 |Difficulty-Easy

Nutritional value- Calories-181| Fat-9g |Carbohydrates-14g| Protein-12g

Ingredients

- Two avocados, cut in halves and pitted
- Four eggs
- Salt and black pepper to the taste
- One tablespoon of chopped chives

Instructions

- Scoop some of the avocado halves with some flesh and assemble them in a baking dish.
- In each avocado, crack an egg, season with pepper and salt, place them at 425 degrees F in the oven and bake for 20 minutes.
- In the end, sprinkle the chives and serve them for breakfast.

Eggs florentine

Preparation time-5 minutes |Cook time-10 minutes |Servings-2 |Difficulty-Easy

Nutritional value: ~Calories-191|Proteins-19g| Fat-12g|Carbohydrates-9g

Ingredients

- Two tablespoons of apple cider vinegar
- Two tablespoons of unsalted butter, ghee, or coconut oil
- Four cups of tightly packed fresh spinach
- A quarter cup of chopped fresh basil
- fine sea salt and ground black pepper
- Two large tomatoes, sliced into eight rounds

Four large eggs

- Hollandaise Sauce, for serving

- One teaspoon of paprika for garnish

Instructions

- Combine three cups of water and the vinegar in a saucepan and bring to a rolling boil over medium heat.

- Meanwhile, prepare the spinach: In a sauté pan, melt the butter over medium heat. Add the spinach and basil with a pinch of salt and pepper and sauté until wilted. Transfer the spinach mixture to a bowl and cover to keep warm. (Do not clean the pan; you'll use it momentarily.)

- Return the pan to medium heat and add the tomato slices. Sprinkle with salt and pepper and cook for 1 minute on each side, or until slightly browned. Set the tomatoes aside.

- Crack one egg into a small bowl, then gently drop it into the saucepan with the boiling water. Repeat until all the eggs are in the water. Cook for 1 to 2 minutes until the whites are firm and opaque and the yolks are slightly firm but still runny.

- Place two tomato slices on each plate and top with the spinach. Remove the eggs one by one with a slotted spoon and tap over a dry, clean cloth to remove the excess water. Place one egg on top of each spinach and tomato base.

- Top the eggs with the hollandaise sauce and paprika. Season with a pinch of salt and pepper, serve and enjoy.

Eggs with Zucchini Noodles

Preparation time-10 minutes |Cook time-12 minutes |Servings-2 |Difficulty-Easy

Nutritional value: ~Calories-279|Proteins-15g| Fat-22g|Carbohydrates-11g

Ingredients

- Two tablespoons of extra-virgin olive oil

- Two zucchinis, cut with a spiralizer

- Two eggs

- Salt and black pepper to the taste

- A pinch of red pepper flakes

- Cooking spray

- One tablespoon of basil, chopped

Instructions

- In a bowl, combine the zucchini noodles with salt, pepper, and olive oil and toss well.

- Grease a baking sheet using cooking spray and divide the zucchini noodles into two nests on it.

- Crash an egg on top of each nest, sprinkle salt, pepper, and pepper flakes on topmost, then bake at 350 degrees F for 11 minutes.

- Divide the mix between plates, sprinkle the basil on top, and serve.

Farmers' Market Scramble

Preparation time-10 minutes |Cook time-20 minutes |Serving-4 |Difficulty- Easy

Nutritional value: ~ Calories-386| Fat-25g| Protein-35g| Carbohydrates-4g

Ingredients

- Eight large eggs

- A quarter cup of low-fat milk

- Four ounces of sharp Cheddar cheese, plus more for topping

- Half teaspoon of extra-virgin olive oil

- Half cup of mushrooms, sliced

- Half pound of extra-lean turkey breakfast sausage

- One cup of firmly packed baby spinach

- One medium ripe tomato, seeded and diced

Instructions

- In a large bowl, whisk together the milk, eggs, and cheese.

- In a pan over medium heat, heat the oil. Add the mushrooms, and sauté for 2 to 3 minutes, or until soft. Transfer to a plate.

- Add the turkey sausage to the skillet. Using a rubber spatula, break the sausage into smaller pieces and cook until browned and no longer pink, 5 to 8 minutes.

- Reduce heat to medium-low, and add the egg mixture to the skillet with the sausage. Gently push the eggs around the pan, cooking halfway through before adding the spinach and tomato.

- Continue cooking until the eggs are fluffy and the spinach has wilted.

- Return the mushrooms to the skillet and gently mix until combined.

- Top with cheese, divide among four plates and serve.

Feta and Asparagus Delight

Preparation time-1 minutes |Cook time-35 minutes |Serving-2 |Difficulty- Easy

Nutritional value: ~ Calories-386| Fat-25g| Protein-35g| Carbohydrates-4g

Ingredients

- Twelve asparagus spears

- One tablespoon of olive oil

- Two chopped green onions

- One minced garlic clove

- Six eggs

- Salt and black pepper to the taste

- Half cup of feta cheese

Instructions

- Heat a pan over medium heat with some water, add asparagus, stir for eight minutes, drain well, chop two spears and reserve the remainder.

- Over medium heat, heat a pan with the oil, add the garlic, onions and chopped asparagus, stir and cook for five minutes.

- Add salt, pepper and eggs, stir, cover and cook for five minutes.

- On top of your frittata, arrange the whole asparagus, sprinkle with cheese, place in the oven at 350 ° F and bake for nine minutes.

- Divide and serve between plates.

Fried mush

Preparation time-10 minutes |Cook time-30 minutes|Servings-4 |Difficulty-Moderate

Nutritional value: ~232 Calories| Fat-21g|Protein-9g|Carbohydrates-2g

Ingredients

- Four eggs

- Half cup of ricotta cheese

- A quarter cup of heavy cream

- Thirty-six drops of liquid stevia

- Half teaspoon of ground cinnamon

- A quarter teaspoon of ground nutmeg

- Six drops of corn flavoring (optional)

- One teaspoon of oil

Instructions

- Preheat oven to 350°F.Coat an 8-inch (20 cm) square baking dish with non-stick cooking spray.

- Simply put everything but the oil in a mixing bowl. Whisk together, and pour into the prepared baking dish.

- Bake for 25 minutes, or until a knife inserted in the center comes out clean. Pull it out of the oven and let it cool for a few minutes.

- Put your large, heavy skillet over medium heat, and add the oil. Cut the mush into 4 squares, and fry until they're golden on both sides. Serve with Cinnamon "Sugar".

Fried sweet potato omelet

Preparation time-5 minutes |Cook time-10 minutes |Servings-2 |Difficulty-Moderate

Nutritional value: ~Calories-132|Proteins-12g| Fat-7g|Carbohydrates-23g

Ingredients

- One tablespoon of unsalted butter, ghee, or coconut oil

- Some Sweet Potato Fries

- Four large eggs, beaten

- Fine sea salt and ground black pepper

- A quarter cup of chopped fresh cilantro for garnish

Instructions

- Melt the fat in a large skillet over medium heat.

- Add the sweet potato fries to the skillet and pour the eggs on top. Season the egg mixture liberally with salt and pepper.

- Lift the edges of the omelet with a spatula and tilt the pan slightly to let the uncooked egg run underneath the omelet and cook on the bottom of the pan. Continue this process until the omelet is fully cooked, 8 to 10 minutes.

- Sprinkle the cilantro on top of the omelet and slide it onto a plate.

- Serve and enjoy.

Garlic Shrimp

Preparation time-10 minutes| Cook time-50 minutes| Servings-8 |Difficulty-Hard

Nutritional value- Calories-298| Fat-16g |Carbohydrates-2.8g| Protein-20.9g

Ingredients

- Two lbs. large shrimp, peeled and deveined

- Two tablespoons of parsley, minced

- A quarter teaspoon of chili flakes, crushed

- One teaspoon of paprika

- Six garlic cloves, sliced

- 3/4 cup of olive oil

- A quarter teaspoon of pepper

- One teaspoon of kosher salt

Instructions

- Add all ingredients except shrimp and parsley into the crockpot and stir well. Cover and cook on high for 30 minutes. Add shrimp and stir well.

- Cover and cook on high for 20 minutes. Garnish with parsley and serve.

Greek Bowl

Preparation time-10 minutes |Cook time-7 minutes |Servings-2 |Difficulty-Easy

Nutritional value: ~Calories-253|Proteins-16.5g| Fat-11g|Carbohydrates-22.5g

Ingredients

- A quarter cup of Greek yogurt

- Six eggs

- A quarter teaspoon of ground black pepper

- Half teaspoon of salt

- One tablespoon of avocado oil

- Half cup of cherry tomatoes, chopped

- Half cup of quinoa, cooked

- Half cup of fresh cilantro, chopped

Half red onion, sliced

Instructions

- Boil the eggs in the water within 7 minutes. Then cool them in the cold water and peel.

- Chop the eggs roughly and put them in the salad bowl.

- Add Greek yogurt, ground black pepper, salt, avocado oil, tomatoes, quinoa, cilantro, and red onion.

- Shake the mixture well. Serve.

Greek cheese, spinach, and olive omelet

Preparation time-7 minutes | Cook time-6 minutes | Servings-1 | Difficulty-Easy

Nutritional value: ~457 Calories | Fat-40g | Protein-4g | Carbohydrates-4g

Ingredients

- One tablespoon of olive oil

- Two eggs, beaten

- Two tablespoons of crumbled feta cheese

- Two tablespoons of shredded kasseri cheese

- Half cup of chopped fresh spinach or baby spinach leaves

- Four kalamata olives, pitted and chopped

Instructions

- Make your omelet using olive oil for the fat.

- Layer in the cheeses, then the spinach, with the chopped olives on top. Let it cook till the cheese is hot and the spinach just starts to wilt a bit.

Ground Beef and Spinach Scramble

Preparation time-5 minutes | Cook time-20 minutes | Serving-1 | Difficulty- Easy

Nutritional value: ~ Calories-141 | Fat-7.9g | Protein-17.4g | Carbohydrates-0.8g

Ingredients

- One teaspoon of light butter

- A quarter cup of lean, browned ground beef

- 1/3 cup of chopped fresh spinach leaves, stems removed

- A quarter cup of liquid egg substitute

- One tablespoon of shredded Parmesan cheese

Instructions

- In an omelet pan over medium heat, melt the butter, swirling the pan to coat evenly. Add the ground beef and saute for 4 to 5 minutes, until warmed through.

- Add the spinach and continue cooking until the spinach is completely wilted. Add the egg substitute, stirring gently but constantly with a heat-resistant rubber spatula, scraping the bottom of the pan to keep the eggs moving to avoid browning.

- When the eggs are almost finished, add the cheese and turn off the heat. Gently fold the cheese into the eggs, turning over with the rubber spatula.

- When the cheese becomes soft but not dissolved, turn the scramble onto a plate.

Ham and zucchini frittata

Preparation time-10 minutes | Cook time-15 minutes | Servings-2 | Difficulty-Easy

Nutritional value: ~Calories-140 | Proteins-14g | Fat-8g | Carbohydrates-0g

Ingredients

- One tablespoon of olive oil

- Half medium white onion, chopped

- One clove of fresh garlic, minced

- One medium zucchini, halved lengthwise, cut to 1/4 inch thick slices

- One cup of diced low-sodium ham

- One and a half cups of liquid eggs

- A quarter cup of low-fat milk

- One teaspoon of dry Italian seasoning mix plus more to sprinkle

- Salt and freshly ground pepper to taste

- Two Italian plum tomatoes, sliced

- One cup of shredded, part-skim milk mozzarella cheese

Instructions

- Preheat oven to broil. In an oven-safe skillet, heat olive oil over medium heat. Add onion, garlic, and zucchini, sauté till soft.

- Reduce heat to medium-low, add ham, and cook for about 2 minutes. In a bowl, combine liquid eggs, milk, Italian seasoning mix, and salt and pepper to taste.

- Pour mixture into skillet with ham and cook unstirred for about 5 minutes or until eggs begin to set. Arrange tomato slices on top of the egg mixture and sprinkle with mozzarella cheese.

- Place skillet about 6 inches under the broiler and broil for about 4–5 minutes until eggs set and cheese is lightly browned.

- Sprinkle top of the frittata with a dash of Italian seasoning mix and serve.

Ham Muffins

Preparation time-10 minutes |Cook time-15 minutes |Servings-2 |Difficulty-Easy

Nutritional value: ~Calories-109|Proteins-9.3g| Fat-6.7g|Carbohydrates-9.3g

Ingredients

- Four ham slices

- Two eggs whisked

- 1/3 cup of spinach, chopped

- A quarter cup of feta cheese, crumbled

- Half cup of roasted red peppers, chopped

- A pinch of salt and black pepper

- One and a half tablespoons of basil pesto

- Cooking spray

Instructions

- Grease a muffin tin using the cooking spray and line each muffin mold with one and ½ ham slices.

- Divide the peppers and the rest of the ingredients except the eggs, pesto, salt, and pepper into the ham cups.

- In a container, blend the eggs with the pesto, salt, and pepper, whisk and pour over the peppers mix.

Bake the muffins in the oven at 400F for 15 minutes and serve for breakfast.

Harvest Vegetable Chicken Bone Broth

Preparation time- 5 minutes| Cook time-5-8 hours| Servings-8 |Difficulty-Hard

Nutritional value- Calories-171| Fat-6g |Carbohydrates-6g| Protein-19g

Ingredients

- Two bay leaves

- One teaspoon of salt

- Twelve to sixteen cups of water

- One (5- to 7-pound) whole chicken

- Four large carrots, peeled and chopped

- One medium yellow onion, sliced

- Two cups of diced celery

- Nonstick cooking spray

Instructions

- Oil a shallow roasting pan with some nonstick cooking spray.

- Place the celery, onion, carrot, and whole chicken in the pan. Let it roast for 1.5 hours (20 minutes per lb. of chicken), or just when the reads 165°F.

- Now, take the pan out and remove the meat from the bones. Then put it aside.

- Put the veggies with the carcass and in a pot. Now pour water to submerge the carcass and veggies fully. Add salt and bay leaves, and then boil them.

- Let it cook for 4 hours over medium heat. Stir a couple of times every hour.

- Remove the bones and veggies and enjoy the warm broth.

High-protein Cottage Cheese Pancakes

Preparation time-10 minutes| Cook time-7 minutes| Servings-4 |Difficulty-Easy

Nutritional value- Calories-152| Fat-7g |Carbohydrates-10g| Protein-13g

Ingredients

- 1/3 cup of all-purpose flour

- Half teaspoon of baking soda

- One cup of low-fat cottage cheese

- Half tablespoon of canola oil

- Three eggs, lightly beaten

Instructions

- In a small bowl, whisk together flour and baking soda.

- In a large mixing bowl, combine the remaining ingredients.

- Stir the flour mixture into the cottage cheese mixture until just combined.

- Coat a large skillet with cooking spray and heat over medium heat.

- Spoon 1/3-cup portions of batter into skillet and cook until surface bubbles appear.

- Cook until brown on the other side.

- Drizzle with calorie-free syrup.

Hummus toast

Preparation time-10 minutes |Cook time-0 minutes |Servings-2 |Difficulty-Easy

Nutritional value: ~Calories-300|Proteins-10g| Fat-8g|Carbohydrates-7g

Ingredients

- Hummus Whole-grain bread seeded

- One tablespoon of Sprouts

- Sliced avocado

- Black sesame seeds

- Two tablespoons of Za'atar spice

- One cup of Roasted chickpeas

Topping option

- One teaspoon of Sunflower seeds

- One teaspoon of Pumpkin seeds

- One teaspoon of Hemp seeds

- One teaspoon of Sesame seeds

Instructions

Spread hummus using a knife over toast and top with any of the topping options given in ingredients and serve.

Insta-quiche

Preparation time-10 minutes |Cook time-15 minutes|Servings-4 |Difficulty-Easy

Nutritional value: ~438 Calories| Fat-34g|Protein-28g|Carbohydrates-4g

Ingredients

- Eight slices of bacon

- Five eggs

- A quarter cup of heavy cream

- A quarter cup of carb-reduced milk or sugar-free almond milk

- One tablespoon of dry vermouth

- Half teaspoon of salt

- A quarter teaspoon of ground black pepper

- A pinch of ground nutmeg

- One tablespoon of butter

- Eight ounces of shredded Swiss cheese

Instructions

- Place a 10-inch (25 cm) non-stick skillet over medium heat. Let it heat.

- Lay the bacon on a microwave bacon rack or in a microwavable baking dish. Stick it in the microwave on high for 8 to 9 minutes. (The length of time will depend a bit on your microwave.)

- In a medium mixing bowl, whisk together the eggs, cream, carb-reduced milk, vermouth, salt, pepper, and nutmeg.

- Put your butter in your now-hot skillet and swirl it around as it melts to coat the bottom. Now pour in your egg mixture.

- Use a spatula—preferably one for non-stick skillets—to gently stir the eggs around, pulling back the part that's setting and letting the liquid egg run underneath. It won't work like an omelet, where it sets up firm enough that you can lift the whole edge.

- Just scramble them gently until they're about half-set, half-liquid.

- Spread the eggs out evenly in the skillet and sprinkle the shredded cheese over the top. Cover the skillet and turn the burner to low. (If you have an electric stove, you'll need to shift your pan to a low burner.)

- Turn on the broiler and set the rack 4 inches (10 cm) below it.

- When the bacon is done, take it out, drain it, and let it cool for just a minute or two. Then crumble it, or easier, you can use your kitchen shears to snip it into bits. Uncover your Insta-Quiche and sprinkle the bacon bits evenly over the top.

- Now slide the whole thing under the broiler for just a minute until you're sure the top is set, then cut into wedges and Serve.

Italian-Style Scramble

Preparation time- 5 minutes| Cook time-5 minutes| Servings-4 |Difficulty-Easy

Nutritional value- Calories-241| Fat-16g |Carbohydrates-6g| Protein-21g

Ingredients

- A quarter teaspoon of salt

- One cup of shredded mozzarella cheese

- One teaspoon of garlic powder

- One teaspoon of Italian seasoning

- One cup of canned diced tomatoes, drained

- Eight large eggs

- Nonstick cooking spray

Instructions

- Warm the oil.

- Whisk the eggs with mozzarella, Italian seasoning tomato, cheese, salt, and garlic powder. Whisk until it's well-mixed.

- Put the beaten eggs in the skillet and cook for 2 to 4 minutes, moving several times until the eggs are well-cooked.

- Serve hot and enjoy.

Keto Breakfast Mix

Preparation time-10 minutes| Cook time-0 minutes| Servings-2 |Difficulty-Easy

Nutritional value- Calories-241| Fat-16g |Carbohydrates-6g| Protein-21g

Ingredients

- Five tablespoons of unsweetened coconut flakes

- Seven tablespoons of Hemp seeds

- Five tablespoons of Ground Flaxseed

- Two tablespoons of ground Sesame

- Two tablespoons of unsweetened cocoa, dark

- Two tablespoons of Psyllium husk

Instructions

- Grind the sesame and the flaxseed. Ensure that you only grind the sesame seeds for a short time.

- In a jar, mix all the ingredients and shake them well.

- Keep refrigerated until ready for consumption.

- Serve softened with black coffee or still water and, if you want to increase your fat intake, add coconut oil. It also combines well with cream or with cheese from mascarpone.

Keto Fall Pumpkin Spiced French Toast

Preparation time- 5 minutes| Cook time-15 minutes| Servings-2 |Difficulty-Easy

Nutritional value- Calories-241| Fat-16g |Carbohydrates-6g| Protein-21g

Ingredients

- Four slices of Pumpkin Bread

- One large Egg

- Two tablespoons of cream

- Half teaspoon of Vanilla Extract

- 1/8 teaspoon of Orange Extract

- A quarter teaspoon of Pumpkin Pie Spice

- Two tablespoons of butter

Instructions

- Cook the pumpkin, butter, milk and spices over a medium-low flame.

- Add two cups of solid coffee and blend together until bubbling.

- Remove from the stove, apply cream and stevia, and then whisk together with an electric mixer.

- Top with whipped cream and serve.

Keto Frittata

Preparation time- 5 minutes| Cook time-55 minutes | Servings-4 |Difficulty-Hard

Nutritional value- Calories-241| Fat-16g |Carbohydrates-6g| Protein-21g

Ingredients

- Nine ounces of spinach
- Twelve eggs
- One ounce of pepperoni
- One teaspoon of minced garlic
- Salt and black pepper to the taste
- Five ounces of shredded mozzarella
- Half cup of grated parmesan
- Half cup of ricotta cheese
- Four tablespoons of olive oil
- A pinch of nutmeg

Instructions

- Squeeze out the spinach liquid and put it in a bowl.
- Mix the eggs with the salt, nutmeg, pepper, and garlic in another bowl and whisk well.
- Add the spinach, ricotta and parmesan and whisk well.
- Pour this into a saucepan, sprinkle on top with mozzarella and pepperoni, place in the oven and bake for 45 minutes at 375 ° Fahrenheit.
- Leave the frittata for a few minutes to cool down before serving.

Lemon Mug Cake

Preparation time- 5 minutes| Cook time-5 minutes| Servings-1 |Difficulty-Easy

Nutritional value- Calories-298| Fat-16g |Carbohydrates-2.8g| Protein-20.9g

Ingredients

- One organic egg
- A quarter cup of skim milk
- Two tablespoons of applesauce
- One and a half tablespoons of avocado oil
- Half teaspoon of grated lemon zest
- Half tablespoon of lemon juice
- Two tablespoons of whole grains flour
- One scoop of protein powder

Instructions

- Crack the eggs and place them in a measuring cup. Pour skim milk, applesauce, lemon juice, and avocado oil into the cup, then mix until incorporated.
- In a microwave-safe mug, put protein powder, flour, and grated lemon zest, then mix well. Pour the liquid mixture into the dry mixture, then stir until smooth and incorporated.
- Place the mug in the microwave, then microwave for 2 minutes. Check the doneness of the cake by inserting a skewer into the cake. When it comes out clean, it means that the cake is completely cooked. Microwave for another 30 seconds if it is necessary.
- Remove the mug cake out from the microwave, then let it cool. Serve and enjoy.

Lentil Vegetarian Loaf

Preparation time-10 minutes| Cook time-1 hour 30 minutes| Servings-10 |Difficulty-Hard

Nutritional value- Calories-298| Fat-16g |Carbohydrates-2.8g| Protein-20.9g

Ingredients

- Half cup of rinsed dried lentils
- One medium yellow onion
- Half cup of cooked brown rice

Two tablespoons of canola/olive oil

- Half cup of ketchup
- One can of tomato paste (6 ounces)
- One teaspoon of Marjoram
- One teaspoon of Garlic powder
- One teaspoon of Sage
- Half cup of quartered cherry tomatoes
- ¾ cup of tomato/pasta sauce
- Salt as per taste
- More ketchup as per taste

Instructions

- Preheat the oven to 350°F. Rinse and cook the lentils in 3 to 4 cups of water for approximately 30 minutes. Drain and slightly mash the lentils. Peel and chop the onions. Cook in the oil until golden.
- Combine the onions, lentils, tomato paste, rice, tomatoes, sauce, and spices into a large pot. Mix well.
- Press the mixture into a well-greased baking dish with a half cup of ketchup over the top. Bake for one hour.

Make-Ahead Breakfast Burritos

Preparation time-15 minutes |Cook time-20 minutes |Serving-8 |Difficulty- Moderate

Nutritional value: ~Calories-264| Fat-12g| Protein-21g| Carbohydrates-24g

Ingredients

- Twelve large eggs
- A quarter cup of low-fat milk
- One teaspoon of extra-virgin olive oil
- Half medium yellow onion, diced
- One medium green bell pepper, seeded and diced
- One cup of canned black beans drained and rinsed
- Eight (7- to 8-inch) whole wheat tortillas
- Half cup of shredded Cheddar cheese
- Eight ounces of salsa

Instructions

- In a large bowl, whisk together the eggs and milk.
- In a large skillet over medium heat, heat the oil. Add the onion, bell pepper, and black beans. Sauté until the onion is translucent, about 5 minutes, and transfer to a plate.
- Pour the egg mixture into the skillet and gently stir until the eggs are fluffy and firm. Remove from the heat.
- Divide the eggs and onion mixture evenly among the tortillas, and top with the cheese and salsa.
- With both sides of the first tortilla tucked in, roll tightly to close. Repeat with the remaining tortillas.
- Serve immediately, or freeze for up to 3 months. If freezing, wrap the burritos in paper towels and cover them tightly with aluminum foil for storage.

Mango Tropical Salsa

Preparation time- 5 minutes| Cook time-15 minutes| Servings-4 |Difficulty-Easy

Nutritional value- Calories-298| Fat-16g |Carbohydrates-2.8g| Protein-20.9g

Ingredients

- Two ripe mangoes
- Half cup of chopped onion
- Two tablespoons of cilantro
- Three tablespoons of lemon juice
- A quarter cup of diced tomatoes
- A pinch of salt
- A pinch of pepper

Instructions

- Peel the mangoes, then cut them into small cubes. Place the cubed mangoes in a salad bowl.
- Add chopped onion, cilantro, and diced tomatoes. Sprinkle salt and pepper over the ingredients. Drizzle lemon juice on top. Toss to combine.

- Cover the bowl with the lid, then chill the mango mixture in the fridge. Serve and enjoy.

Meat Cups and Creamy Topping

Preparation time-10 minutes| Cook time-40 minutes| Servings-4 |Difficulty-Easy

Nutritional value- Calories-298| Fat-16g |Carbohydrates-2.8g| Protein-20.9g

Ingredients

- One lb. of ground turkey
- ¾ cup of grated zucchini
- Two tablespoons of chopped onion
- Half cup of whole-wheat crumbs
- Three tablespoons of ketchup
- Half lb. of potatoes
- Two teaspoons of minced garlic
- One and a half tablespoons of non-fat sour cream
- One and a half tablespoons of low sodium chicken broth
- Two tablespoons of skim milk
- Half teaspoon of pepper
- One and a half tablespoons of thyme

Instructions

- Peel and cut the potatoes, then place them in a steamer. Steam the potatoes for approximately 15 minutes or until the potatoes are tender. Meanwhile, preheat an oven to 350°F and coat 8 small muffin cups with cooking spray. Set aside.
- Place the ground turkey in a food processor, then add grated zucchini, chopped onion, wholewheat crumbs, and ketchup to the food processor. Process until smooth.
- Fill the prepared muffin cups with the turkey mixture, then arrange them on a baking sheet.
- Bake the turkey cups for approximately 20 minutes or until the meat cups are cooked through. Remove the turkey cups from the oven, then let them cool for a few minutes. While waiting for the turkey cups, take the potatoes from the steamer, then place them in a bowl.
- Using a potato masher, mash the potatoes until smooth. Add the minced garlic and non-fat sour cream, then pour skim milk and low-sodium chicken broth over the mashed potatoes. Season with pepper and thyme. Mix until combined.
- Take the turkey cups out from the cups, then arrange them on a serving dish. Top each turkey cup with mashed potatoes, then serve. Enjoy!

Meaty Breakfast Omelet

Preparation time- 5 minutes| Cook time- 15 minutes| Servings-2 |Difficulty-Easy

Nutritional value- Calories-228|Fat-11.1g |Carbohydrates-0.4g| Protein-17.9g

Ingredients

- Three big whisked eggs
- One spoonful of heavy cream
- Salt and onions
- One-inch uncooked, sliced bacon
- Two tablespoons of sausage for cooking crumbled
- A quarter cup of ham

Instructions

- Whisk the eggs together in a small bowl of heavy cream, salt, and pepper.
- Cook the bacon over medium to high heat in a small skillet.
- Spoon it out into a mug until the bacon is crisp.
- Cook the sausage in the saucepan until browned, then add to the dish.
- Steam the pan up with the bacon fat and sausage.
- Put in the whisked shells, and simmer until the egg's bottom begins to set.
- To scatter the egg, tilt the saucepan, and cook until almost finished.
- Sprinkle the bacon, egg ham, and spread over half the omelet.
- Cook the omelet until the eggs are firm, and then serve soft.

Mini Frittatas

Preparation time-5 minutes |Cook time-15 minutes |Servings-2 |Difficulty-Easy

Nutritional value: ~Calories-56|Proteins-5g| Fat-3g|Carbohydrates-4g

Ingredients

- One yellow onion, chopped
- One cup of parmesan, grated
- One yellow bell pepper, chopped
- One red bell pepper, chopped
- One zucchini, chopped
- Salt and black pepper to the taste
- Eight eggs whisked
- A drizzle of olive oil

- Two tablespoons of chives, chopped

Instructions

- Heat a pan with the oil over medium-high heat, add the onion, the zucchini, and the rest of the ingredients except the eggs and chives, and sauté for 5 minutes, often stirring.
- Divide this mix on the bottom of a muffin pan, pour the egg mixture on top, sprinkle salt, pepper, and the chives, and bake at 350 degrees F for 10 minutes.
- Serve the mini frittatas for breakfast right away.

Mixed vegetable frittata

Preparation time-10 minutes |Cook time-25 minutes |Servings-2 |Difficulty-Easy

Nutritional value: ~Calories-170|Proteins-17g| Fat-1g|Carbohydrates-7g

Ingredients

- Five large fresh asparagus spears
- One and a half cups of egg substitute or one and a half cups of egg whites or six whole eggs
- 3/4 cup of low-fat cottage cheese
- Two teaspoons of spicy brown mustard
- A quarter teaspoon of crushed dried tarragon
- A quarter teaspoon of marjoram
- Salt and freshly ground pepper to taste
- Half teaspoon of extra-virgin olive oil
- One cup of sliced fresh mushrooms
- Half cup of diced onion
- A quarter cup of chopped seeded tomato for garnish

Instructions

- Boil asparagus for 8–10 minutes until crispy tender. Drain. Cut all but three spears into 1-inch pieces. Set aside. In a bowl, mix together eggs, cottage cheese, mustard, tarragon, marjoram, and salt and pepper. Set aside.
- Heat olive oil in a large oven-safe skillet, and sauté mushrooms and onion until tender. Stir in asparagus pieces, pour egg mixture over the top, and cook an additional 5 minutes over low heat until it bubbles and begins to set.
- Arrange the remaining three uncut asparagus spears on top of the mixture. Place skillet in oven and bake uncovered at 400 degrees for 10 minutes or until frittata sets.
- Remove from heat. Sprinkle with tomato and serve.

Monterey jack and avocado omelet

Preparation time-2 minutes |Cook time-5 minutes |Servings-1 |Difficulty-Easy

Nutritional value: ~372 Calories| Fat-32g|Protein-19g|Carbohydrates-7g

Ingredients

- Two eggs, beaten
- Two teaspoons of butter
- One ounce of Monterey Jack, pepper Jack, or Cheddar cheese, sliced or shredded
- Half avocado, sliced

Instructions

- Just make a regular omelet.
- Add the cheese, turn the burner to low, cover, and let the cheese melt. Add the avocado just before folding.

Monterey scramble

Preparation time-10 minutes |Cook time-8 minutes|Servings-2 |Difficulty-Easy

Nutritional value: ~449 Calories| Fat-36g|Protein-26g|Carbohydrates-5g

Ingredients

- Two canned artichoke hearts
- Two scallions
- One ounce of Monterey Jack cheese
- Three eggs
- One teaspoon of pesto sauce
- One tablespoon of butter

Instructions

- Thinly slice your artichoke hearts, slice your scallions, shred your cheese and have them standing by.
- Scramble up your eggs with the pesto until it is completely blended in.
- Give your medium skillet a squirt of non-stick cooking spray, and put it over medium-high heat. Add the butter and let it melt.
- Throw your veggies in the skillet, and pour the eggs in on top of them. Scramble it all together until the eggs are set almost to your liking.
- Scatter the cheese over the top, cover the skillet, turn off the burner, let the residual heat melt the cheese and finish cooking the eggs.

Morning Oats

Preparation time-5 minutes |Cook time-0 minutes |Servings-2 |Difficulty-Easy

Nutritional value: ~Calories-196|Proteins-7g| Fat-11.6g|Carbohydrates-16.5g

Ingredients

- One ounce of pecans, chopped

- A quarter cup of oats
- Half cup of plain yogurt
- One date, chopped
- Half teaspoon of vanilla extract

Instructions

- Mix up all the ingredients and leave for 5 minutes.
- Then transfer the meal to the serving bowls.

Multigrain apple and nut pancakes

Preparation time-10 minutes |Cook time-30 minutes |Servings-2 |Difficulty-Moderate

Nutritional value: ~Calories-87|Proteins-3g| Fat-2g|Carbohydrates-15g

Ingredients

- 3⁄4 cup of multigrain pancake flour
- Half cup plus Two tablespoons of skim milk
- One tablespoon of canola oil
- Half medium sweet apple, cored, peeled, and diced
- 1⁄8 cup of chopped walnuts
- Canola oil cooking spray
- Fat-free sour cream or sugar-free or low-sugar fruit jams as garnish (optional)
- Sugar-free syrup

Instructions

- In a mixing bowl, combine pancake flour, milk, and canola oil. Using a wire whisk, mix

- ingredients until smooth. Add apple and walnuts and stir to combine all ingredients. Spray griddle with cooking spray and heat over medium heat.

- Drop a few droplets of water onto the heated griddle. If droplets are bead, then the griddle is hot enough. Pour about one tablespoon of batter per pancake onto the griddle.

- Cook pancake until it begins to bubble up and edges turn brown, then flip over and continue cooking until the other side is golden brown.

- Remove cooked pancakes to a warmed platter or hold in a low-heat oven (175 degrees) while preparing other pancakes.

- Repeat this process until all the batter is gone. Serve with a dollop of fat-free sour cream, low-sugar fruit jam, or your favorite sugar-free syrup, if desired.

Multigrain nutty blueberry pancakes

Preparation time-10 minutes |Cook time-30 minutes |Servings-2 |Difficulty-Moderate

Nutritional value: ~Calories-85 |Proteins-3g| Fat-1g |Carbohydrates-15g

Ingredients

- 3/4 cup multigrain pancake flour
- Half cup plus Two tablespoons of skim milk
- One tablespoon of canola oil
- A quarter cup of blueberries (either fresh or frozen)
- 1/8 cup of chopped walnuts
- Canola oil cooking spray
- Fat-free sour cream or sugar-free or low-sugar fruit jams as garnish (optional)
- Sugar-free syrup

Instructions

- In a mixing bowl, combine pancake flour, milk, and canola oil. Using a wire whisk, mix ingredients until smooth.

- Add blueberries and walnuts and stir to combine all ingredients.

- Spray griddle with cooking spray and heat over medium heat. Drop a few droplets of water onto the heated griddle.

- If droplets are bead, then the griddle is hot enough. Pour about one tablespoon of batter per pancake onto the griddle.

- Cook pancake until it begins to bubble up and edges turn brown, then flip over and continue cooking until the other side is golden brown.

- Remove cooked pancakes to a warmed platter or hold in a low-heat oven (175 degrees) while preparing other pancakes. Repeat this process until all the batter is gone.

- Serve with a dollop of fat-free sour cream, low-sugar fruit jam, or your favorite sugar-free syrup, if desired.

No Flour Pumpkin Bread

Preparation time- 5 minutes| Cook time-30 minutes| Servings-4 |Difficulty-Easy

Nutritional value- Calories-298| Fat-16g |Carbohydrates-2.8g| Protein-20.9g

Ingredients

- One cup of quick-cooking oats
- One cup of pumpkin puree
- Three tablespoons of applesauce
- One organic egg
- Half teaspoon of baking soda
- ¾ teaspoon of cinnamon

Instructions

- Preheat an oven to 350°F and line a loaf pan with parchment paper. Set aside.

- Place the pumpkin puree and oats in a blender, then add egg, baking soda, applesauce, and cinnamon to the bowl. Using an electric mixer, mix the ingredients until smooth and combined.

- Transfer the batter to the prepared loaf pan, then spread evenly.

- Bake the pumpkin bread for approximately 30 minutes, or until the top of the bread is lightly golden. Insert a toothpick into the bread, and if it comes out clean, it means that the bread is completely done.

- Remove the bread from the oven and let it cool for a few minutes. Take the pumpkin bread out of the loaf pan and cut it into slices.

- Arrange the sliced bread on a serving dish, then serve. Enjoy!

Nutty granola

Preparation time-5 minutes |Cook time-25 minutes |Servings-10 |Difficulty-Easy

Nutritional value: ~113 Calories| Fat-1.8g |Protein-23g |Carbohydrates-22g

Ingredients

- Four cups of rolled oats (not instant)
- Two tablespoons of lightly packed brown sugar
- One teaspoon of ground cinnamon
- Half teaspoon of kosher salt
- Half cup of grapeseed oil
- Half cup of maple syrup
- Half cup of chopped pecans, walnuts, or your favorite nut
- Half cup of raisins
- A quarter cup of roasted, salted, shelled pumpkin seeds (pepitas)

Instructions

- Preheat the oven to 300 degrees Fahrenheit (150 degrees Celsius).
- Combine cinnamon, brown sugar, rolled oats, and kosher salt in a large mixing bowl.
- Whisk together maple syrup and grapeseed oil in a small basin, then pour over oat mixture. Fold the ingredients together with a big spatula until well combined.
- Spread the granola out on a big baking sheet and toast it for 20 to 25 minutes, stirring twice, until golden brown.
- Allow cooling completely in a clean basin, stirring in raisins, pecans, and pumpkin seeds.
- For up to a week, store in a firmly sealed glass jar.

Onion and Cheese Egg Muffins

Preparation time- 5 minutes| Cook time-25 minutes| Servings-4 |Difficulty-Easy

Nutritional value- Calories-298| Fat-16g |Carbohydrates-2.8g| Protein-20.9g

Ingredients

- Eight organic eggs
- Three tablespoons of coconut flour
- Half teaspoon of olive oil
- A quarter cup of chopped onion
- A quarter cup of grated skim Mozzarella cheese

Instructions

- Preheat an oven to 400°F and coat 4 muffin tins with cooking oil.
- Crack the eggs into your bowl. Add the coconut flour to the eggs, then whisk until the flour is completely

dissolved. Set aside.

- Over medium heat, preheat a skillet, then pour olive oil into it. Once it is hot, stir in the chopped onion and sauté until aromatic. Remove from heat.
- Add the onion to the egg mixture, then stir well. Divide the egg mixture into the prepared muffin cups, then sprinkle grated skim Mozzarella cheese on top.
- Bake the egg muffins for approximately 20 minutes or until the egg is set. Once it is done, take the egg muffins out from the oven.
- Let them cool for a few minutes. Arrange the egg muffins on a serving dish. Enjoy!

Orange blossom pancakes

Preparation time-10 minutes |Cook time-10 minutes |Servings-2 |Difficulty-Easy

Nutritional value: ~Calories-98|Proteins-9g| Fat-7g|Carbohydrates-12g

Ingredients

- Two tablespoons of coconut flour
- Half teaspoon of baking soda
- A quarter teaspoon of ground nutmeg
- Two tablespoons of cashew meal or blanched almond flour
- Four large eggs
- 3/4 cup of full-fat, canned coconut milk
- Two teaspoons of orange blossom water or grated orange zest
- Half teaspoon of apple cider vinegar
- Two teaspoons of honey (optional)
- Two tablespoons of unsalted butter, ghee, or coconut oil
- Sliced fruit of choice, for serving

Instructions

- Sift the coconut flour, baking soda, and nutmeg into a large bowl. Add the cashew meal and whisk to combine.
- In another bowl, whisk together the eggs, coconut milk, orange blossom water, vinegar, and honey, if using. Add the wet mixture to the dry and whisk until smooth.
- Melt the fat in a large skillet over medium heat. Pour about A quarter cup of the batter per pancake into the hot pan, leaving room for it to spread. Cook each pancake for 2 minutes, then flip it over and cook for two more minutes on the opposite side.
- Transfer the cooked pancakes to a plate and cover to

keep warm while you cook the rest of the pancakes.

- Top with sliced fruit and enjoy.

Orange Mango Popsicles

Preparation time-10 minutes | Cook time-0 minutes | Servings-4 | Difficulty-Easy

Nutritional value- Calories-118 | Fat-1g | Carbohydrates-13g | Protein-9g

Ingredients

- Two ripe bananas
- Two ripe mangoes
- One and a half cups of unsweetened orange juice

Instructions

- Peel the bananas then cut them into slices. Place in a blender.
- Peel the mangoes, then cut them into cubes, then also place them in the blender. Pour the orange juice over the fruits, then blend until incorporated.
- Pour the mixture into 4 popsicle molds, then freeze. Enjoy cold.

Overnight Oatmeal

Preparation time-10 minutes | Cook time-0 minutes | Servings-2 | Difficulty-Easy

Nutritional value-Calories- 203 | Carbohydrates- 36.9g | Protein- 5.9g | Fat- 4.4g

Ingredients

- Two teaspoons of honey
- One cup of unsweetened almond milk
- One cup of rolled oats, gluten-free
- A quarter cup of fresh blueberries
- Half teaspoon of ground cinnamon

Instructions

- In a wide mixing bowl, combine all ingredients (except blueberries) and stir well.
- Refrigerate the bowl overnight, covered.
- Serve with blueberries on top in the morning.

Parmesan Omelet

Preparation time-5 minutes | Cook time-10 minutes | Servings-2 | Difficulty-Easy

Nutritional value: ~Calories-148 | Proteins-10.6g | Fat-11.5g | Carbohydrates-1.4g

Ingredients

- One tablespoon of cream cheese
- Two eggs, beaten
- A quarter teaspoon of paprika
- Half teaspoon of dried oregano
- A quarter teaspoon of dried dill
- One ounce of Parmesan, grated
- One teaspoon of coconut oil

Instructions

- Mix up together cream cheese with eggs, dried oregano, and dill.
- Put coconut oil in the frypan and heat it until it coats all the skillet.
- Then pour the egg mixture into the skillet and flatten it.
- Add grated Parmesan and close the lid.
- Cook the omelet for 10 minutes over low heat.
- Then transfer the cooked omelet to the serving plate and sprinkle with paprika.

Parmesan-rosemary eggs

Preparation time-10 minutes | Cook time-8 minutes | Servings-2 | Difficulty-Easy

Nutritional value: ~448 Calories | Fat-36g | Protein-26g | Carbohydrates-4g

Ingredients

- Six eggs
- Half cup of grated Parmesan cheese
- A quarter cup of heavy cream
- One teaspoon of ground rosemary
- One clove of garlic, crushed
- One tablespoon of butter

Instructions

- Whisk together the eggs, cheese, cream, rosemary, and garlic. Put a large skillet over medium-high heat (if it isn't non-stick, give it a shot of non-stick cooking spray first).
- When the pan is hot, add the butter, give the egg mixture one last stir to make sure the cheese hasn't settled to the bottom, then pour the egg mixture into the skillet.
- Scramble until the eggs are set, and serve.

PB and J Overnight No-Oats Cereal

Preparation time-5 minutes | Cook time-2 minutes | Servings-2 | Difficulty-Easy

Nutritional value- Calories-232 | Fat-13g | Carbohydrates-14g | Protein-19g

Ingredients

- A quarter cup of diced fresh or frozen strawberries

- A quarter teaspoon of stevia

- One tablespoon of unsweetened peanut butter powder

- One tablespoon of chia seeds

- Six tablespoons of almond flour

- One cup of non-fat plain Greek yogurt

Instructions

- Combine the almond flour, stevia, chia seeds, peanut butter powder, and yogurt in a canning jar. Put it aside.

- Over medium heat, put a small skillet and put strawberries in it. Then cook them until the strawberries become slimy and soft. Keep medium heat.

- Now, put the strawberries in the jar and incorporate them with the remaining ingredients. Tightly shut the jar and refrigerate it. Leave it in the fridge for the whole night.

- Take out a half cup of if only you're eating. Enjoy cold or microwave it for half a minute.

Pear Oats with Walnuts

Preparation time-10 minutes| Cook time-10 minutes| Servings-4 |Difficulty-Easy

Nutritional value- Calories-288| Fat-13g |Carbohydrates-39g| Protein-5g

Ingredients

- Two cups of almond milk

- Two cups of peeled and cut pears

- One cup of rolled oats

- Half cup of chopped walnuts

- A quarter cup of sugar

- One tablespoon of melted coconut oil

- A quarter teaspoon of salt

- Dash of cinnamon

Instructions

- Mix everything except the walnuts and cinnamon in an oven-safe bowl.

- Preheat the oven to 350 degrees Fahrenheit.

- Put the bowl in the oven.

- Set the timer for 10 minutes.

- When time is up, carefully remove the bowl, divide into 4 servings, and season with salt and cinnamon.

Perfect protein pancakes

Preparation time-10 minutes |Cook time-8 minutes|Servings-30 pancakes |Difficulty-Easy

Nutritional value: ~45 Calories| Fat-3g|Protein-5g|Carbohydrates-1g

Ingredients

- Four eggs

- One cup of ricotta cheese

- Half cup of vanilla whey protein powder

- One teaspoon of baking powder

- A quarter teaspoon of salt

- Two tablespoons of butter

Instructions

- Coat a heavy skillet or griddle with non-stick cooking spray and place it over medium heat.

- In a mixing bowl, whisk together the eggs and ricotta until quite smooth. Whisk in the protein powder, baking powder, and salt, only mixing until well combined.

- Melt one tablespoon of the butter on the hot skillet or griddle, and drop batter onto it by the tablespoonful.

- When the bubbles on the surface of the pancakes are breaking and leaving little holes around the edges, flip them and cook the other side.

- Add the rest of the butter to cook the rest of the batter.

- Serve these with Maple Butter or Cinnamon "Sugar".

Perfectly Soft Scrambled Eggs

Preparation time-5 minutes |Cook time-10 minutes |Serving-1 |Difficulty- Easy

Nutritional value: ~Calories-176| Fat-11g| Protein-15g| Carbohydrates-2g

Ingredients

- Two large eggs

- Two tablespoons of low-fat milk

- One tablespoon of shredded cheese of your choice

- Salt

- Freshly ground black pepper

Instructions

- In a small bowl, whisk together the eggs and milk.

- Heat a small skillet over low heat.

- Pour the egg mixture into the pan, add the cheese, and gently stir with a rubber spatula, scraping the sides of the pan as needed while it cooks. Season with salt and pepper to taste.

- Cook for roughly 8 to 12 minutes until the eggs form soft and fluffy small curds. The eggs should not brown.

- Transfer to a plate, and enjoy.

Pork rind waffles
Preparation time-15 minutes | Cook time-20 minutes | Servings-12 waffles | Difficulty-Easy

Nutritional value: ~103 Calories | Fat-5g | Protein-12g | Carbohydrates-2g

Ingredients

- Three and a half ounces of plain pork rinds or skins
- A quarter cup of erythritol
- A quarter cup of vanilla whey protein powder
- A quarter cup of almond meal
- Half teaspoon of baking powder
- A quarter teaspoon of ground cinnamon
- Five eggs
- One and a half cups of water

Instructions

- Plugin your waffle iron. You want it hot when the batter is ready.
- Run the pork rinds through your food processor until they're powdered. Dump the pork rind crumbs into a mixing bowl.
- Add the erythritol, protein powder, almond meal, baking powder, and cinnamon. Use a whisk to stir everything together well.
- Separate the eggs, put the whites into a deep, narrow mixing bowl and put the yolks in with the pork rind mixture.
- Since the tiniest speck of yolk will keep your egg whites from whipping, do yourself a favor and separate each one into a custard cup first.
- Whisk the egg yolks and the water into the pork rind mixture. Let this sit while you do the next step.
- Using an electric mixer, whip the egg whites until they stand in stiff peaks.
- With a rubber scraper, gently fold the egg whites into the pork rind mixture, adding one-quarter of the whites and incorporating them well before adding another quarter, and so on.
- Bake the batter according to the instructions that come with your waffle iron.
- Serve immediately, with butter and Cinnamon "Sugar" or Maple Butter.
- To freeze, cool on paper towels to absorb moisture, then put in resealable plastic bags with the towels still between them.
- Reheat in the toaster or toaster oven rather than the microwave, so your waffles will be crisp.

Protein Pancakes

Preparation time-5 minutes | Cook time-5 minutes | Serving-6 | Difficulty- Easy

Nutritional value: ~Calories-89 | Fat-3g | Protein-8g | Carbohydrates-6g

Ingredients

- One cup of low-fat cottage cheese
- ⅓ cup of flour
- Three large eggs
- ⅛ teaspoon of baking powder
- Nonstick cooking spray
- Low-fat Greek yogurt, fresh berries, nut butter, or low-sugar syrup, for serving

Instructions

- In a blender, combine the cottage cheese, flour, eggs, and baking powder, and blend until smooth.
- Heat a small skillet over medium-low heat. Spray with nonstick cooking spray.
- Pour A quarter cup of the pancake mixture onto the skillet. When the pancake begins to bubble, flip.
- Cook until golden brown on both sides, about 2 to 3 minutes per side.
- Repeat with the remaining pancake batter.
- Serve with Greek yogurt, fresh berries, nut butter, or low-sugar syrup.

Protein-packed Pesto

Preparation time- 5 minutes | Cook time-0 minutes | Servings-4 | Difficulty-Easy

Nutritional value- Calories-77 | Fat-5g | Carbohydrates-4g | Protein-6g

Ingredients

- One package of frozen chopped spinach, 10-ounce (thawed & well-drained)
- Half cup of water
- 1/3 cup of 1 % cottage cheese
- One tablespoon of olive oil
- Two tablespoons of grated parmesan cheese
- Two cloves of garlic, minced
- 1/3 cup of fresh basil or two tablespoons of dried basil – fresh preferred

Instructions

- In a blender or food processor, combine all ingredients.
- Process or blend until smooth.
- Spoon a half cup of the mixture over the chicken or fish.

Pumpkin and Black Bean Soup

Preparation time-15 minutes| Cook time-30 minutes| Servings-6 |Difficulty-Moderate

Nutritional value- Calories-290| Fat-6g |Carbohydrates-46g| Protein-15g

Ingredients

- Two cans black beans, 15-ounce (rinsed and drained)
- Two tablespoons of olive oil
- Four garlic cloves, minced
- One medium onion, chopped
- One teaspoon of chili powder
- One tablespoon of ground cumin
- Half teaspoon of black pepper
- Two cups of beef broth
- One cup of canned diced tomatoes
- One can of pumpkin puree, 16-ounce

Instructions

- Sauté garlic, onions, cumin, pepper and chili powder in oil in a soup kettle over medium heat until soft.
- Combine tomatoes, broth, black beans and pumpkin in a large mixing bowl.
- Simmer, uncovered, for approximately 25 minutes, occasionally stirring until soup reaches a thick consistency.
- Serve immediately or puree with an immersion blender until smooth.

Pumpkin Oatmeal

Preparation time-10 minutes| Cook time-2 minutes| Servings-2|Difficulty-Easy

Nutritional value-Calories- 223| Carbohydrates- 28.7g| Protein- 29.9g| Fat- 4.6g

Ingredients

- 1/3 cup of pumpkin puree
- Two cups of hot water
- 1/3 cup of gluten-free rolled oats
- One teaspoon of cinnamon
- Two tablespoons of chia seeds
- One teaspoon of ground ginger
- Two scoops of vanilla vegan unsweetened protein powder
- A quarter teaspoon of ground nutmeg
- One tablespoon of maple syrup

Instructions

- Add pumpkin puree, water, chia seeds, oats, and spices in a microwave-safe bowl and stir well.
- Microwave for around 2 minutes on high.
- Take the oatmeal bowl out of the microwave and whisk in the protein powder as well as maple syrup. Serve it.

Pumpkin Spice Muffins

Preparation time-10 minutes |Cook time-25 minutes |Serving-12 |Difficulty- Easy

Nutritional value: ~Calories-107| Fat-5g| Protein-3g| Carbohydrates-13g

Ingredients

- One and a half cups of whole wheat flour
- Two teaspoons of pumpkin pie spice
- One teaspoon of baking soda
- Half teaspoon of salt
- Four tablespoons of butter softened
- ⅔ cup of erythritol
- Two tablespoons of maple syrup
- One teaspoon of vanilla extract
- Two large eggs

Instructions

- Preheat the oven to 350°F. Line the muffin tin with liners.
- In a large bowl, mix the baking soda, salt, pumpkin pie spice, and flour.
- In another large bowl, using a hand mixer, mix the butter, maple syrup, erythritol, and vanilla until smooth. Add 1 egg at a time, beating until mixed.
- Add the dry flour mixture to the wet ingredients in small amounts, mixing between each addition.
- Divide the batter evenly among the 12 muffin cups. Bake for about 25 minutes, or until a toothpick inserted into the center comes out clean. Cool completely on a wire rack, then store in a resealable bag or air-tight container.

Pumpkin Spice Oatmeal with Brown Sugar Topping

Preparation time-10 minutes |Cook time-10 minutes |Serving-6 |Difficulty- Easy

Nutritional value: ~Calories-207| Fat-4g| Protein-4g| Carbohydrates-38g

Ingredients

- Four and a half cups of water
- One and a half cups of steel-cut oats
- One and a half cups of pumpkin puree

- Two teaspoons of cinnamon

- One teaspoon of vanilla

- One teaspoon of allspice

- Half cup of brown sugar

- A quarter cup of chopped pecans

- One tablespoon of cinnamon

Instructions

- Pour one cup of water into a deep-bottomed saucepan.

- Add everything from the first ingredient list (including the rest of the water) into an oven-safe bowl and set it in the steamer basket.

- Lower the basket into the saucepan and lock the lid.

- Cook on high pressure for 3 minutes.

- Turn off the flame.

- Mix the topping ingredients in a small bowl.

- When you serve, sprinkle on top. If necessary, add a little almond milk to the oats.

Pureed Beef Stew

Preparation time-25 minutes| Cook time-7-8 hours | Servings-30 |Difficulty-Hard

Nutritional value- Calories-38| Fat-2g |Carbohydrates-0.8g| Protein-1.2g

Ingredients

- Oil or cooking spray

- One can tomato sauce with garlic, oregano and basil, 8 ounces

- One pound of beef stew meat (small pieces)

- One can lower-sodium beef broth, 14 ounces

- Four cups of freshly cut vegetables (potatoes, celery, carrots and onions-One cup of each)

- A quarter teaspoon of salt

- One cup of low-sodium beef broth or water (optional)

Instructions

- Using oil or cooking spray, coat the inside of a four-quart slow cooker.

- In a slow cooker, combine all ingredients.

- Cook on low for 8 hours or high for 4 hours, or until the meat and the vegetables are tender.

- Allow cooling slightly after cooking before pureeing. Add about one cup of the mixture (meat, vegetables, and broth) at a time to the blender or food processor.

- Puree until desired consistency is achieved, aiming for a consistency somewhere between a smooth liquid and pudding. As needed, add additional water or broth.

- Puree the remaining stew and refrigerate for 3-4 days or freeze for later use.

Pureed Egg Salad

Preparation time-10 minutes| Cook time-10 minutes| Servings-4 |Difficulty-Easy

Nutritional value- Calories-97| Fat-4g |Carbohydrates-5g| Protein-13g

Ingredients

- Four hard-boiled eggs

- Two tablespoons of plain Greek-style yogurt

- Salt and pepper to taste

- Two tablespoons of low-fat mayonnaise

Instructions

- Slice the hard-boiled eggs.

- In a blender or food processor, combine the egg slices.

- Blend or chop eggs until no large pieces remain.

- In a separate bowl, whisk together Greek yogurt, seasonings and mayonnaise.

- Puree the egg salad until smooth.

Pureed Mushroom Chicken

Preparation time- 5 minutes| Cook time-20 minutes| Servings-4 |Difficulty-Easy

Nutritional value- Calories-90| Fat-5g |Carbohydrates-5g| Protein-9g

Ingredients

- One tablespoon of olive oil

- Salt and pepper to taste

- One medium-sized chicken breast (skinless, boneless)

- Small pinch of paprika to taste

- Half cup of mushroom soup cream (low sodium)

Instructions

- Preheat the oven to 425 degrees Fahrenheit.

- Line a baking sheet with foil. Coat chicken breast with olive oil and season with salt and pepper to taste.

- Bake for 10-12 minutes, or until the internal temperature of the chicken attains 166 degrees.

- Remove the chicken from the oven and set it aside to cool. Transfer to a cutting board and chop into 1/2-inch bits.

- Fill a blender or food processor halfway with a half cup of warmed cream of mushroom soup.

- Blend in the cut chicken until smooth. Add additional soup as necessary to achieve the desired consistency.

- Season with a pinch of paprika or season to taste.

Quinoa and Eggs Pan

Preparation time-10 minutes |Cook time-25 minutes |Servings-2 |Difficulty-Easy

Nutritional value: ~Calories-304|Proteins-17.8g| Fat-14g|Carbohydrates-27.5g

Ingredients

- Two bacon slices, cooked and crumbled

- A drizzle of olive oil

- One small red onion, chopped

- One red bell pepper, chopped

- One sweet potato, grated

- One green bell pepper, chopped

- Two garlic cloves, minced

- Half cup of white mushrooms, sliced

- A quarter cup of quinoa

- Half cup of chicken stock

- Two eggs, fried

- Salt and black pepper to the taste

Instructions

- Heat a pan with the oil over medium-low heat, add the onion, garlic, bell peppers, sweet potato, and mushrooms, toss and sauté for 5 minutes.

- Add the quinoa, toss and cook for one more minute.

- Add the stock, salt, and pepper. Stir and cook for 15 minutes.

- Divide the mix between plates, top each serving with a fried egg, sprinkle some salt, pepper, crumbled bacon, and serve breakfast.

Quinoa and raisins porridge

Preparation time-10 minutes |Cook time-35 minutes |Servings-2 |Difficulty-Moderate

Nutritional value: ~Calories-557|Proteins-15g| Fat-14g|Carbohydrates-91g

Ingredients

- Two cups of almond milk

- One cup of quinoa rinsed through a fine-mesh sieve under cold water

- Half teaspoon of ground cinnamon

- 1/8 teaspoon of ground nutmeg

- 1/8 teaspoon of ground ginger

- Dash of salt (optional)

- Two tablespoons of pure maple syrup

- Half teaspoon of pure vanilla extract

- Two tablespoons of raisins

- A quarter cup of chopped nuts (such as pecans, walnuts, or almonds)

Instructions

- In a saucepan over medium heat, gently heat almond milk, occasionally stirring until it begins to bubble.

- Reduce heat to a simmer and add in quinoa, cinnamon, nutmeg, ginger, and salt. Cook uncovered, occasionally stirring until quinoa is tender and begins to thicken (about 20–25 minutes).

- Remove from heat, add maple syrup, vanilla extract, and raisins.

- Top with a sprinkling of nuts and serve.

Quinoa Muffins

Preparation time-10 minutes |Cook time-30 minutes |Servings-2 |Difficulty-Moderate

Nutritional value: ~Calories-123|Proteins-7.5g| Fat-5.6g|Carbohydrates-10.8g

Ingredients

- Half cup of quinoa, cooked

- Two eggs whisked

- Salt and black pepper to the taste

- Half cup of Swiss cheese, grated

- One small yellow onion, chopped

- Half cup of white mushrooms, sliced

- A quarter cup of sun-dried tomatoes, chopped

Instructions

- In a bowl, combine the eggs with salt, pepper, and the rest of the ingredients and whisk well.

- Divide this into a silicone muffin pan, bake at 350 degrees F for 30 minutes, and serve breakfast

Quinoa Stuffed Pepper Skillet

Preparation time-13 minutes| Cook time-25 minutes| Servings-12 |Difficulty-Easy

Nutritional value- Calories-167| Fat-7g |Carbohydrates-3g| Protein-30g

Ingredients

- One tablespoon of olive oil or similar cooking oil

- One cup of diced yellow onion

- Three garlic cloves

- One pound of 90% lean ground beef

- One red pepper, diced

- One green pepper, diced

- One tablespoon of tomato paste

- 14 ounces of diced fire-roasted tomatoes

- One cup of dry quinoa (rinsed)

- One cup of beef broth, reduced-sodium

- One cup of water

- One and a half teaspoons of dry basil

- One teaspoon of dry oregano

- Half teaspoon of fennel seeds

- A quarter teaspoon of salt

- 1/8 teaspoon of pepper

- One cup of low-fat shredded cheese

Instructions

- Preheat a large skillet over moderately high heat.

- To the pan, add oil and diced onions. Sauté for approximately 2-3 minutes, or until translucent.

- Add garlic and sauté for 30 seconds longer.

- Add ground beef to the pan and stir to break it up. Cook for approximately 3-4 minutes, or until no longer pink.

- Stir in the diced green & red peppers, quinoa, tomato paste, beef broth, fire-roasted tomato, dried basil, fennel seeds, water, dried oregano, salt and pepper to taste. Combine all ingredients in a mixing bowl until well combined.

- Bring to a boil, covered. Reduce to low heat and continue simmering for 15 minutes.

- Once the quinoa is cooked, sprinkle one cup of shredded cheese on top and cover.

- Continue cooking for an additional 2 minutes, or until the cheese is melted, and serve.

Quork

Preparation time-10 minutes |Cook time-55 minutes|Servings-8 |Difficulty-Hard

Nutritional value: ~237 Calories| Fat-19g|Protein-15g|Carbohydrates-0g

Ingredients

- Seven ounces of plain pork rinds or skins

- Half cup of butter

- Half teaspoon of liquid stevia (English toffee)

- A quarter teaspoon of corn flavoring (optional)

- One cup of erythritol

Instructions

- Preheat oven to 275°F (130°C). While it's heating, break your pork rinds up into bits about the size of cold cereal.

- When the oven is hot, put the butter in your biggest roasting pan and put it in the oven to melt.

- When the butter is melted, pull the pan out of the oven. Add the liquid stevia, and corn flavoring is used. Stir them into the butter.

- Add the pork rinds to the pan, and, using a pancake turner, stir them into the butter until they're all evenly coated.

- Sprinkle the erythritol over the pork rinds a quarter cup at a time, stirring each addition well before adding more.

- When all the erythritol is worked in, slide the pan back into the oven. Toast the pork rinds for 40 minutes, stirring everything very well with a pancake-turner every 10 minutes.

- At the end of 40 minutes, remove from the oven and let your Quork cool in the pan before storing it in an airtight container.

Raspberry-Lemon Gluten-Free Muffins

Preparation time-15 minutes |Cook time-25 minutes |Serving-12 |Difficulty- Moderate

Nutritional value: ~Calories-160| Fat-11g| Protein-7g| Carbohydrates-11g

Ingredients

- Two cups of almond flour

- Half teaspoon of baking soda

- Half teaspoon of baking powder

- ⅛ teaspoon of salt

- Three large eggs

- One (6-ounce) container of low-fat, plain Greek yogurt

- Zest of one lemon

- ⅓ cup of freshly squeezed lemon juice

- Three tablespoons of raw honey

- One teaspoon of vanilla extract

- One cup of fresh raspberries

Instructions

- Preheat the oven to 350°F. Place paper muffin liners in a 12- cup muffin pan.

- In a medium bowl, mix the almond flour, baking powder, baking soda, and salt.

- In a separate large bowl, whisk the 3 eggs. Add the yogurt, lemon zest, lemon juice, honey, and vanilla. Mix until smooth.

- Gently mix the dry ingredients into the wet ingredients.

- Fold the raspberries into the batter, trying not to break the berries.

- Using a ⅓ cup measuring cup, scoop the batter into the muffin pan cups. The batter should be even with the top of the muffin liners.

- Bake for 20 to 25 minutes, or until a toothpick inserted into the center of the muffin comes out clean.

- Carefully remove the muffins from the pan and let cool on a wire rack, then store in a resealable bag or airtight container.

Refried Bean Bowl

Preparation time-10 minutes| Cook time-5 minutes| Servings-8 |Difficulty-Easy

Nutritional value- Calories-50| Fat-0g |Carbohydrates-0.8g| Protein-2.9g

Ingredients

- One cup of vegetable broth

- One can of pinto beans, drained and rinsed

- A quarter teaspoon of cumin

- A quarter teaspoon of onion powder

- A quarter teaspoon of chili powder

- A quarter teaspoon of (tsp) garlic powder

- One teaspoon of fat-free sour cream or a pinch of low-fat cheese (Optional)

Instructions

- Use olive oil to spray a sauté pan.

- In a sauté pan, add rinsed and drained pinto beans and cook for 1-2 minutes.

- Add broth, cumin, garlic powder, onion powder and chili powder to the sauté pan.

- Bring the pinto beans to a slow boil in a small saucepan. Continue to cook (about 3-5 minutes) at low heat until the broth has been reduced by half.

- Scatter pinches of freshly chopped cilantro evenly across the pan.

- Allow 5-10 minutes for cooling before transferring the contents of the pan to a blender or food processor and blending until smooth.

- As desired, garnish with the optional toppings listed above.

- Tip: When purchasing packaged foods, opt for low-sodium options. When canned goods, such as the canned beans in this recipe, are not available, rinse them to cut down on sodium.

Refried Black Beans

Preparation time-10 minutes| Cook time-5 minutes| Servings-4 |Difficulty-Easy

Nutritional value- Calories-121| Fat-1g |Carbohydrates-20g| Protein-7g

Ingredients

- One teaspoon of extra-virgin olive oil

- One (15-ounce) can of black beans

- One tablespoon of freshly squeezed lime juice

- A quarter teaspoon of cayenne pepper

- One teaspoon of garlic

- Half teaspoon of ground cumin

- Half teaspoon of dried oregano

- One teaspoon of smoked paprika

Instructions

- Heat olive oil and throw in garlic in a small pot over medium-low heat. Mix for 1 minute. Now cook the beans until warm for 5 minutes. Then, turn the heat off. Incorporate the cayenne, cumin, paprika, lime juice, oregano and mix well.

- Use a blender to puree the beans, or you can mash them with a masher.

Roasted Cauliflower Garlic

Preparation time-5 minutes| Cook time-20 minutes| Servings-4 |Difficulty-Easy

Nutritional value- Calories-298| Fat-16g |Carbohydrates-2.8g| Protein-20.9g

Ingredients

- Three tablespoons of avocado oil

- Two teaspoons of garlic powder

- Half teaspoon of pepper

- Two cups of cauliflower florets

- Half teaspoon of salt

Instructions

- Line a baking sheet with parchment paper and preheat an oven to 425 °F. Set aside.

- Place the cauliflower florets in a bowl, then drizzle avocado oil over them. Sprinkle the pepper, salt, and garlic, then toss to combine.

- Spread the cauliflower florets on the prepared baking sheet, then roast for approximately 15-20 minutes or until the cauliflower florets are tender.

- Once it is done, remove it from the oven, then transfer it to a serving dish. Serve and enjoy.

Roasted Chickpeas

Preparation time-5 minutes| Cook time-45 minutes| Servings-4 |Difficulty-Moderate

Nutritional value- Calories-188| Fat-9g |Carbohydrates-18g| Protein-9g

Ingredients

- Half teaspoon of garlic powder
- Half teaspoon of salt
- One cup of chickpeas
- One teaspoon of olive oil
- A quarter teaspoon of cumin

Instructions

- Preheat an oven to 350°F and line a baking sheet with parchment paper.
- Place the chickpeas in a bowl, then drizzle olive oil over the chickpeas. Season with garlic powder, cumin, and salt. Toss to combine.
- Spread the seasoned chickpeas on the prepared baking sheet, then roast on the top rack of the oven for approximately 40 minutes.
- Once it is done, remove it from the oven, then transfer it to a serving dish. Serve and enjoy!

Rodeo eggs

Preparation time-10 minutes |Cook time-15 minutes|Servings-1 |Difficulty-Easy

Nutritional value: ~438 Calories| Fat-34g|Protein-29g|Carbohydrates-3g

Ingredients

- Four slices of bacon, chopped into 1-inch pieces
- Four thin slices onion—round slices through the equator
- Four eggs
- Four thin slices of Cheddar cheese

Instructions

- Begin frying the bacon in a heavy skillet over medium heat. When some fat has cooked out of it, push it aside and put the onion slices in, too.
- Fry the onion on each side, turning carefully to keep the slices together until it starts to look translucent. Remove the onion from the skillet and set it aside.
- Continue frying the bacon until it's crisp. Pour off most of the grease and distribute the bacon bits evenly over the bottom of the skillet.
- Break in the eggs and fry for a minute or two until the bottoms are set, but the tops are still soft. (If you like your yolks hard, break them with a fork; if you like them soft, leave them unbroken.)

- Place a slice of onion over each yolk, then cover the onion with a slice of cheese. Add a teaspoon of water to the skillet, cover, and cook for 2 to 3 minutes, or until the cheese is thoroughly melted.
- Cut into 4 separate pieces with the edge of a spatula, and serve.

Rosemary cheese crackers

Preparation time-10 minutes |Cook time-25 minutes|Servings-50 crackers |Difficulty-Easy

Nutritional value: ~42 Calories| Fat-3g|Protein-3g|Carbohydrates-1g

Ingredients

- One cup of sunflower seed kernels
- Half cup of rice protein powder
- Half teaspoon of xanthan or guar
- Half teaspoon of baking powder
- Half teaspoon of salt, plus more for sprinkling
- Two tablespoons of butter, at room temperature
- One and a half tablespoons of minced fresh rosemary
- One cup of shredded sharp Cheddar cheese
- Half cup of shredded Parmesan cheese
- One egg white
- Three tablespoons of water

Instructions

- Preheat oven to 350°F.
- Put the sunflower seeds, rice protein powder, xanthan or guar, baking powder, and salt in your food processor, and run till the sunflower seeds are ground up to the texture of cornmeal or finer.
- With the processor running, add the butter and the rosemary. Then work in the cheeses in 3 or 4 additions.
- With the processor still running, add the egg white, then the water. When you have a soft dough, turn off the processor.
- Line a cookie sheet with baking parchment. Make a ball of half the dough, and put it on the parchment, then put another sheet of parchment over it.
- Use your rolling pin to roll the dough out into as thin and even a sheet as you can. Carefully peel off the top sheet of parchment.
- Use a straight, thin-bladed knife to score the dough into crackers. Sprinkle them lightly with salt.
- Bake for 20 to 25 minutes, or until golden. Score again before removing from the parchment.

Salted caramel–cinnamon pancakes

Preparation time-15 minutes |Cook time-20 minutes|Servings-3 |Difficulty-Easy

Nutritional value: ~508 Calories| Fat-42g|Protein-29g|Carbohydrates-3g

Ingredients

- Three and a half ounces of plain pork rinds or skins

- One teaspoon of ground cinnamon

- Half teaspoon of baking powder

- Four eggs

- Half cup of heavy cream

- A quarter teaspoon of liquid stevia (English toffee), or more to taste

- Water, as needed

- Three tablespoons of butter, plus more for serving

- Three tablespoons of caramel sugar-free coffee flavoring syrup

Instructions

- Run the pork rinds through your food processor till you have fine crumbs. Dump them in a mixing bowl.

- Add the cinnamon and baking powder, and stir them into the crumbs.

- In a separate bowl, whisk together the eggs, cream, and stevia. Pour this into the crumbs, and whisk till everything's evenly wet.

- Let this mixture sit for 5 minutes or so. This would be a good time to put your frying pan or griddle over medium heat; you'll want it hot when the batter is ready.

- Come back to your batter. It will have been thick to start with and will have thickened even more on standing, becoming downright gloppy. Thin it with water to a consistency you like.

- Melt half of the butter in your skillet or on the griddle, and start frying your pancakes like you would any pancakes.

- Let them get nicely browned on the first side before flipping and cooking the other. The rest of the butter is for the second round, of course.

- Serve with more butter and a sprinkle of Cinnamon sugar.

Savory Beef Bone Broth

Preparation time-5 minutes| Cook time-5 to 8 hours| Servings-4 |Difficulty-Hard

Nutritional value- Calories-138| Fat-8g |Carbohydrates-2g| Protein-13g

Ingredients

- One tablespoon of garlic

- Two bay leaves

- One pound of stew beef

- One teaspoon of salt

- Three pounds of beef bones

- Twelve cups of water

- One cup of peeled, diced carrot

- One cup of diced celery

- One medium yellow onion, chopped

- Nonstick cooking spray

Instructions

- Preheat the oven to 400°F. Cover the roasting pan with cooking spray and put it aside.

- Place celery, carrot, and onion in the pan evenly. Put the stew beef and beef bones on top. Roast it all for about 40 minutes, moving and turning everything throughout the cooking time.

- Now, take it out of the oven and put the meat, bones, and vegetables into a container. Add salt, bay leaves, water, and garlic and boil it.

- Lower the flame and let it sit for a minimum of 4 hours. Keep moving everything a few times every hour.

- Then, remove the bones, meat, and vegetables out of the pot. Serve hot.

Scrambled Eggs

Preparation time-10 minutes |Cook time-10 minutes |Servings-2 |Difficulty-Easy

Nutritional value: ~Calories-249|Proteins-13.4g| Fat-17g|Carbohydrates-13.3g

Ingredients

- One yellow bell pepper, chopped

- Eight cherry tomatoes, cubed

- Two spring onions, chopped

- One tablespoon of olive oil One tablespoon of caper, drained

- Two tablespoons of black olives, pitted and sliced

- Four eggs

- A pinch of salt and black pepper

- A quarter teaspoon of oregano, dried

- One tablespoon of parsley, chopped

Instructions

- Heat a pan with the oil over medium-high heat, add the bell pepper and spring onions and sauté for 3 minutes.

- Add the tomatoes, capers, and olives and sauté for 2 minutes more.

- Crack the eggs into the pan, then add salt, pepper, and oregano, and scramble for 5 minutes more.

- Divide the scramble between plates, sprinkle the parsley on top, and serve.

Scrambled Tofu Veggie

Preparation time- 5 minutes| Cook time-10 minutes| Servings-4 |Difficulty-Easy

Nutritional value- Calories-298| Fat-16g |Carbohydrates-2.8g| Protein-20.9g

Ingredients

- Three cups of diced tofu

- Two organic eggs

- One cup of chopped kale

- Half cup of diced tomatoes

- Two teaspoons of olive oil

- One and a half teaspoons of garlic powder

- Half teaspoon of pepper

Instructions

- Crack the eggs into a bowl. Mix until incorporated. Preheat a skillet over medium heat. Pour olive oil into it.

- Pour the beaten eggs into the skillet. Add the diced tofu to it.

- Quickly stir the egg and tofu until scramble forms. Add chopped kale and diced tomatoes, then season with garlic powder and pepper. Mix until the vegetables are wilted. Remove the scrambled tofu from the heat.

- Transfer to a serving dish. Serve and enjoy warm.

Shakshuka Egg Bake

Preparation time-10 minutes |Cook time-30 minutes |Serving-4 |Difficulty- Moderate

Nutritional value: ~Calories-144| Fat-9g| Protein-9g| Carbohydrates-7g

Ingredients

- One teaspoon of extra-virgin olive oil

- Half onion, minced

- One garlic clove, minced

- Half teaspoon of smoked paprika

- Half teaspoon of ground cumin

- One (15-ounce) can of diced tomatoes

- Two ounces of feta cheese, crumbled

- Four large eggs

Instructions

- Preheat the oven to 350°F.

- In a medium skillet over medium heat, heat the oil. Add the onions and garlic, and sauté until translucent, about 5 minutes. Add the paprika and cumin, and cook a minute longer.

- Stir in the tomatoes until well combined. Simmer until some of their liquid has evaporated and the mixture begins to thicken to form a sauce, 5 to 10 minutes.

- Divide the sauce evenly among 4 ramekins, and repeat with the cheese, sprinkling evenly across.

- Using a spoon, create wells in the tomato sauce and crack an egg over each, being careful to keep the yolk intact.

- Bake in the ramekins for 15 minutes, until the yolk, is done to you like a hard-cooked yolk, and serve. (If you do not have ramekins, crack the eggs into spoon-made wells in the pan and let cook for 5 to 10 minutes, or per your preference.)

Sheet Pan Eggs with Veggies and Parmesan

Preparation time- 5 minutes| Cook time- 15 minutes| Servings-6 |Difficulty-Easy

Nutritional value- Calories-298| Fat-16g |Carbohydrates-2.8g| Protein-20.9g

Ingredients

- Twelve large eggs whisked

- Salt and pepper

- One small red pepper dipped

- One small yellow onion, diced

- One cup of dipped mushrooms

- One cup of dipped zucchini

- One cup of freshly ground parmesan cheese

Instructions

- Preheat the oven to 350 ° F and sprinkle cooking spray on a rimmed baking dish.

- In a cup, whisk the eggs with salt and pepper until sparkling.

- Bring the peppers, tomatoes, mushrooms, and zucchini together until well mixed.

- Pour the mixture onto the baking sheet and scatter over a layer of evenness.

- Sprinkle with parmesan and bake until the egg is firm for 12 to 15 minutes.

- Let it cool off a bit, then cut into squares to eat.

Silky Cheese with Cinnamon

Preparation time- 5 minutes| Cook time-30 minutes| Servings-4 |Difficulty-Easy

Nutritional value- Calories-298 | | Carbohydrates-2.8g | Protein-20.9g | Fat-16g

Ingredients

- ¾ cup of water
- One package sugar-free Jell-O
- ¾ cup of non-fat yogurt
- One cup of non-fat cream cheese
- One tablespoon of cinnamon

Instructions

- Pour the water into a pot, then add sugar-free Jell-O to the pot. Bring to a boil and vigorously stir until the gelatin is completely dissolved in the water.
- Once it is boiled, remove it from the heat and let it warm for a few minutes.
- Meanwhile, place non-fat cream cheese in a mixing bowl. Using an electric mixer, whisk until softened. Add non-fat yogurt to the mixing bowl, then whisk until fluffy and smooth.
- When the gelatin mixture is warm, slowly pour into the cream cheese and yogurt mixture. Whisk until smooth and incorporated. This may take time.
- Pour the mixture into 4 pudding cups or 8 small pudding cups, then sprinkle cinnamon on top.
- Let them cool, then chill in the fridge until set. Serve and enjoy.

Slow Cooker Cinnamon Oatmeal

Preparation time- 5 minutes | Cook time-10 minutes | Servings-10 | Difficulty-Easy

Nutritional value- Calories-136 | Fat-2g | Carbohydrates-23g | Protein-6g

Ingredients

- One teaspoon of ground nutmeg
- Two teaspoons of ground cinnamon
- Two cups of steel-cut oats
- Eight cups of water
- A quarter cup of pumpkin puree
- ⅛ cup of chopped pecans, walnuts, or almonds
- Half apple, pear, peach, or banana, peeled and sliced
- Half cup of fresh or frozen berries

Instructions

- Gently mix your oats, nutmeg, cinnamon, and water in the slow cooker. Close the cover and cook for 7 to 8 hours on low heat.
- Select any of the flavor add-ins and mix them in. Enjoy warm.

Slow-Cooked Peppers Frittata

Preparation time-15 minutes | Cook time-3 hours | Servings-2 to 4 | Difficulty-Easy

Nutritional value: ~Calories-256 | Proteins-16.4g | Fat-19g | Carbohydrates-5g

Ingredients

- Half cup of almond milk
- Eight eggs whisked
- Salt and black pepper to the taste
- One teaspoon of oregano, dried
- One and a half cups of roasted peppers, chopped
- Half cup of red onion, chopped
- Four cups of baby arugula
- One cup of goat cheese, crumbled
- Cooking spray

Instructions

- In a bowl, combine the eggs with salt, pepper, and oregano and whisk.
- Grease your slow cooker with the cooking spray, arrange the peppers and the remaining ingredients, and pour the egg mixture over them.
- Close the lid on, then set and cook on low for 3 hours.
- Divide the frittata between plates and serve.

Smoked salmon and goat cheese scramble

Preparation time-10 minutes | Cook time-8 minutes | Servings-3 | Difficulty-Easy

Nutritional value: ~407 Calories | Fat-31g | Protein-27g | Carbohydrates-5g

Ingredients

- Four eggs
- Half cup of heavy cream
- One teaspoon of dried dill weed
- Four scallions
- Four ounces of chèvre (goat cheese)
- Four ounces of moist smoked salmon
- Two tablespoons of butter

Instructions

- Combine the eggs, cream, and dill in a mixing bowl. Thinly slice the scallions, including the crisp green part.
- Cut the chèvre into little hunks with a texture comparable to cream cheese. Shred the smoked salmon coarsely.

- Melt the butter in a large (ideally nonstick) skillet over medium-high heat. (If your skillet's surface isn't nonstick, spray it with nonstick cooking spray before adding the butter.)

- When the butter has melted, toss in the scallions and cook for a minute.

- Add the egg mixture and cook, constantly stirring, for 60 to 90 seconds, or until the eggs are halfway set. Add the smoked salmon and chèvre, and heat, constantly stirring, until the eggs are set.

Smooth White Beans with Lemon

Preparation time-5 minutes| Cook time-10 minutes| Servings-1 |Difficulty-Easy

Nutritional value- Calories-298| Fat-16g |Carbohydrates-2.8g| Protein-20.9g

Ingredients

- One cup of cooked white beans

- Half teaspoon of minced garlic

- One teaspoon of olive oil

- ¾ tablespoon of lemon juice

- A quarter teaspoon of pepper

- A pinch of salt

- One tablespoon of diced celeries

Instructions

- Preheat a skillet over medium heat. Pour olive oil into the skillet. Once it is hot, stir in minced garlic. Sauté until aromatic and lightly golden.

- Next, add the cooked beans to the skillet, then season with salt and pepper. Mix well.

- Transfer the seasoned beans to a bowl. Using a potato masher, mash the beans until smooth. Drizzle lemon juice over the mashed beans, then add diced celery to the mashed beans.

- Mix until combined. Serve and enjoy!

Southwest Scramble

Preparation time- 5 minutes| Cook time-10 minutes| Servings-4 |Difficulty-Easy

Nutritional value- Calories-266| Fat-21g |Carbohydrates-6g| Protein-14g

Ingredients

- Half cup of sliced avocado

- Dash ground black pepper (optional)

- Half cup of canned diced tomatoes, drained

- A quarter teaspoon of salt

- Half cup of diced bell pepper

- Half cup of diced red or yellow onion

- Eight large eggs

- Eight teaspoons of extra-virgin olive oil

Instructions

- Over medium-high heat, warm the oil.

- Whisk the eggs to make them fluffy and put them aside.

- Throw in the pepper and onion and sauté them. Keep moving them gently until the onion is translucent.

- Incorporate the eggs and cook until they're well-cooked. Throw the tomatoes on top and cook for another minute to two.

- Season with pepper and salt. Garnish the eggs with avocado slices.

Southwest quinoa with corn and black beans

Preparation time-5 minutes |Cook time-20 minutes |Serving-3 |Difficulty- Easy

Nutritional value: ~ Calories-124| Fat-9g| Protein-4g| Carbohydrates-8g

Ingredients

- One small onion, chopped

- One cup of chopped fresh ripe tomatoes

- Two cups of chicken or vegetable broth

- One teaspoon of ground cumin

- One cup of dry quinoa

- Three teaspoons of sliced green onions

- One cup of canned black beans drained and rinsed

- A quarter cup of fresh cilantro, chopped

- One cup of frozen corn kernels

- Half teaspoon of kosher salt

Instructions

- Spray a medium-sized saucepan with nonstick cooking spray.

- Over medium-high, cook onion until translucent. Turn heat to high and add broth. Bring to a boil.

- Add quinoa, cover, and reduce heat to simmer for 20 minutes.

- Add the rest of the ingredients and continue cooking just until warm. Salt to taste. Serve warm or chilled!

Soy Yogurt

Preparation time-Midnight |Cook time-0 minutes |Servings-2 |Difficulty-Easy

Nutritional value: ~Calories-55|Proteins-4g| Fat-2g|Carbohydrates-5g

Ingredients

- Two quarts of soy milk

- One packet of vegan yogurt culture

Instructions

- Mix milk and yogurt culture together.

- Pour into a container.

- Close the lid.

- Store in a dry place.

- After 12 to 13 hours, take out the yogurt.

- Put the lids on the containers and store them in the fridge for at least 6 hours.

- The yogurt will be very tangy, so sweeten with vanilla, sugar, jam, fruit, and so on!

Spanish omelet

Preparation time-10 minutes |Cook time-30 minutes |Servings-2 |Difficulty-Easy

Nutritional value: ~Calories-125 |Proteins-10g| Fat-1g |Carbohydrates-6g

Ingredients

- One tablespoon of extra-virgin olive oil

- Two whole scallions, coarsely chopped

- Two cloves fresh garlic, thinly sliced

- Half green bell pepper, seeded and thinly sliced

- Half red bell pepper, seeded and thinly sliced

- Half medium zucchini, diced

- Two ripe tomatoes, peeled and cut into wedges

- Salt and freshly ground pepper to taste

- A quarter teaspoon of cayenne pepper

- 3⁄4 teaspoon of ground cumin

- Half teaspoon of ground coriander

- Half teaspoon of ground cinnamon

- Two tablespoons of chopped fresh parsley

- One cup of egg substitute or one cup of egg whites, or Four large eggs

- A quarter-pound of crumbled fresh, low-fat goat cheese

Instructions

- Heat two tablespoons of olive oil in an oven-safe skillet and gently sauté scallions and garlic for about 5 minutes until they begin to soften. Add the green and red bell peppers, zucchini, and tomatoes. Raise the heat slightly and continue sautéing another 5–10 minutes until the vegetables have softened and most of the juice is absorbed. Add salt and pepper to taste. Set aside at room temperature.

- In a large bowl, combine the herbs with the eggs and mix with a fork just enough to break up the yolks. Lift the vegetables out of the skillet with a slotted spoon and combine with eggs.

- Return the skillet to medium heat, adding more olive oil if necessary. When the olive oil is hot, add the eggs and vegetable mixture and cook for 2–3 minutes, lifting the edges with a spatula to allow uncooked eggs to run undercooked ones.

- Crumble goat cheese over the top of the omelet and transfer the skillet to a 400-degree oven to finish cooking for about 15–20 minutes or until the omelet is set and the cheese is melted.

Spicy Deviled Eggs

Preparation time-10 minutes |Cook time-0 minutes |Serving-3 |Difficulty- Easy

Nutritional value: ~Calories-131 | Fat-8.7g| Protein-10g| Carbohydrates-1g

Ingredients

- Two tablespoons of creamy horseradish sauce or Greek yogurt

- A quarter teaspoon of spicy mustard

- Dash of black pepper and paprika

- Six hard-boiled eggs

- Half teaspoon of dill

- 1/8 teaspoon of salt

Instructions

- Cut the eggs in half lengthwise after peeling them.

- Set aside the whites and place three yolks in a mixing dish. Save the remaining three yolks for another recipe.

- Using creamy horseradish sauce or Greek yogurt, dill, mustard, and salt, mash the yolks.

- Fill egg white halves with filling by spooning or piping.

- Season with salt, pepper, and paprika.

Spinach and olive scramble

Preparation time-10 minutes |Cook time-15 minutes |Servings-2 |Difficulty-Easy

Nutritional value: ~Calories-187 |Proteins-26g| Fat-9g |Carbohydrates-12g

Ingredients

- Six ounces of ground meat of choice

- A quarter teaspoon fine sea salt

- A quarter teaspoon of ground black pepper

- One cup of cherry tomatoes halved

- Four tightly packed cups of spinach

- A quarter cup of sliced black olives

- Four large eggs, beaten

- One avocado, sliced, for serving

- Two tablespoons of chopped fresh cilantro for garnish

- A quarter cup of crumbled feta for garnish (optional)

Instructions

- Heat a skillet over medium heat and add the ground meat. Season the meat with salt and pepper and cook until browned, about 6 minutes, stirring to break up the meat as it cooks.

- Add the tomatoes and spinach to the meat in the skillet and cook for 2 minutes, or until the spinach is wilted.

- Add the olives and eggs to the skillet and keep stirring until the eggs are cooked for 2 to 3 more minutes.

- Top with the avocado, cilantro, and feta, if desired.

Spinach Frittata

Preparation time-15 minutes |Cook time-20 minutes |Servings-2 |Difficulty-Easy

Nutritional value-Calories-145|Proteins-9.6g| Fat-11g|Carbohydrates-3g

Ingredients

- A quarter cup of kalamata olives, pitted and chopped

- Four eggs, beaten

- One cup of spinach, chopped

- Half tablespoon of olive oil

- A quarter teaspoon of chili flakes

- One ounce of feta crumbled

- A quarter cup of plain yogurt

Instructions

Brush the pan with olive oil. After this, mix up all the remaining ingredients in the mixing bowl, and pour them into the pan.

Bake the frittata for 20 minutes at 355°F. Serve.

Spinach Mushroom Quiche

Preparation time-10 minutes| Cook time-40 minutes| Servings-4 |Difficulty-Easy

Nutritional value- Calories-298| Fat-16g |Carbohydrates-2.8g| Protein-20.9g

Ingredients

- Six organic eggs

- Half cup of skim milk

- A quarter cup of grated Parmesan cheese

- Three cups of chopped spinach

- Half cup of chopped mushroom

- Two teaspoons of garlic powder

- Half teaspoon of pepper

Instructions:

- Preheat an oven to 400°F and coat a disposable aluminum pan with cooking spray.

- Place the chopped spinach and mushroom in the bottom of the disposable aluminum pan, then spread evenly. Set aside.

- Crack the eggs and place them in a bowl. Pour skim milk in the bowl, then season with garlic powder. Mix well.

- Pour the egg mixture over the spinach and mushroom, and sprinkle grated mozzarella cheese on top. Bake the spinach and mushroom quiche for about 40 minutes or until the egg mixture is set.

- When the quiche is done, take it out of the oven. Let the quiche cool for a few minutes and cut into wedges. Serve and enjoy.

Spinach Scramble

Preparation time-5 minutes| Cook time-11 minutes| Servings-2 |Difficulty-Easy

Nutritional value-Calories- 169 |Carbohydrates- 1.2g| Protein- 11.5g| Fat- 13.5g

Ingredients

- Two teaspoons of olive oil

- Four eggs

- One cup of chopped fresh spinach.

- Salt to taste

- One tablespoon of water

- Black pepper to taste (freshly ground)

Instructions

- In a mixing bowl, whisk together the turmeric, eggs, red pepper flakes, black pepper, salt, and water until foamy.

- Heat the oil in a skillet over moderate heat.

- Add in the egg mixture until it is well mixed. Lower the heat to low and continue to cook for another 1-2 minutes.

- Add the spinach and cook, constantly stirring for 3-4 minutes. Take the pan off the fire and serve right now.

Strawberry muffins

Preparation time-15 minutes| Cook time-25 minutes| Servings-12 |Difficulty-Easy

Nutritional value-Calories- 113 |Carbohydrates-22g| Protein-2.3g| Fat- 1.8g

Ingredients

- One and 3 /4 cups of all-purpose flour
- Half cup of sugar
- Half teaspoon of baking powder
- Half teaspoon of baking soda
- A quarter teaspoon of kosher salt
- A quarter teaspoon of ground nutmeg
- Three teaspoons of egg replacer, such as Ener-G
- A quarter cup of warm water
- Half cup of nondairy vanilla yogurt
- A quarter cup of grapeseed oil
- Two tablespoons of nondairy milk
- One teaspoon of lemon zest
- One teaspoon of freshly squeezed lemon juice
- One and a quarter cups of roughly chopped fresh or frozen strawberries

Instructions

- Preheat the oven to 350°F (180°C). Lightly coat the cups of a 12-cup muffin tin with nonstick baking spray.
- In a medium bowl, whisk together sugar, kosher salt, all-purpose flour, baking powder, baking soda, and nutmeg.
- In a small bowl, whisk egg replacer with warm water until well blended. Whisk in vanilla nondairy yogurt, grapeseed oil, nondairy milk, lemon zest, and lemon juice.
- Quickly stir wet ingredients into flour mixture until ingredients are just combined, taking care not to overmix. Fold in strawberries.
- Using an ice-cream scoop or a large spoon, evenly divide batter among muffin cups. The batter will be thick, like biscuit dough.
- Bake on the bottom rack of the oven for 22 to 25 minutes or until muffins spring back when lightly pressed in the center. Cool in the pan for 5 minutes before turning out on a wire rack to cool. Serve warm or at room temperature.

Strawberry Sorbet with Ricotta Cheese

Preparation time-5 minutes| Cook time-20 minutes| Servings-4 |Difficulty-Easy

Nutritional value- Calories-298| Fat-16g |Carbohydrates-2.8g| Protein-20.9g

Ingredients

- Three cups of frozen strawberries
- ¾ cup of skim ricotta
- One tablespoon of lemon juice

Instructions

- Place the strawberries in a food processor, then add skim ricotta to the food processor. Drizzle lemon juice over the strawberries then processes until smooth.
- Transfer the strawberry mixture to a container and spread evenly. Store the strawberry sorbet in the freezer and scoop it out when you want to eat.
- Enjoy cold!

Stuffed French Toast

Preparation time- 5 minutes| Cook time-10 minutes| Servings-1 |Difficulty-Easy

Nutritional value- Calories-227| Fat-5g |Carbohydrates-26g| Protein-25g

Ingredients

- Reduced calorie bread, 4 slices (34 calories per slice)
- Cooking spray
- Two packets of sugar substitute
- Dash of Salt
- A quarter teaspoon of pumpkin pie spice
- Three egg whites
- Half cup of ricotta cheese (fat-free)
- Dash of vanilla

Instructions

- Evenly divide the ricotta between 2 slices of bread.
- Sprinkle one sugar substitute packet onto each slice of bread.
- Top with remaining bread to form two sandwiches.
- Separate the egg whites.
- Stir in a 1/4 teaspoon pumpkin pie spice, a pinch of salt and a dash of vanilla extract to egg whites.
- Dip sandwiches in egg whites and fry in a small amount of cooking spray in a nonstick skillet.
- Both sides are brown.

Stuffed Tomatoes

Preparation time-10 minutes |Cook time-15 minutes |Servings-2 |Difficulty-Easy

Nutritional value: ~Calories-276|Proteins-13.7g| Fat-20g|Carbohydrates-13g

Ingredients

- Two tablespoons of olive oil
- Four tomatoes, insides scooped
- A quarter cup of almond milk

- Four eggs

- A quarter cup of parmesan, grated

- Salt and black pepper to the taste

- Two tablespoons of rosemary, chopped

Instructions

- Grease a pan with the oil and arrange the tomatoes inside.

- Crack an egg in each tomato, divide the milk and the rest of the ingredients, introduce the pan inside the oven, then bake at 375 degrees F for 15 minutes.

- Serve for breakfast right away.

Sun-Dried Tomatoes Oatmeal

Preparation time-10 minutes |Cook time-25 minutes |Servings-2 |Difficulty-Easy

Nutritional value: ~Calories-170|Proteins-2g| Fat-12g|Carbohydrates-6g

Ingredients

- Three cups of water

- One cup of almond milk

- One tablespoon of olive oil

- One cup of steel-cut oats

- A quarter cup of sun-dried tomatoes, chopped

- A pinch of red pepper flakes

Instructions

- In a pot, mix the water with the milk, bring to a boil over medium heat.

- Meanwhile, heat a pan with the oil over medium-high heat, add the oats, cook them for about 2 minutes, and transfer m to the pan with the milk.

- Stir the oats, add the tomatoes and simmer over medium heat for 23 minutes.

- Divide the mix into bowls, sprinkle the red pepper flakes on top, and serve for breakfast.

Sweet Maple Protein Oatmeal

Preparation time-5 minutes |Cook time-15 minutes |Serving-2 |Difficulty- Easy

Nutritional value: ~Calories-297| Fat-6g| Protein-22g| Carbohydrates-39g

Ingredients

- Two cups of low-fat milk

- One pinch of salt

- One cup of old-fashioned rolled oats

- One scoop (¼ cup) unflavored protein powder

- A quarter teaspoon of maple extract

- One teaspoon of brown sugar substitute

Instructions

- In a small saucepan over medium heat, heat the milk and salt until boiling.

- Add the oats, and cook for 10 minutes.

- Remove from the heat and cool to 140°F, using a liquid, meat, or candy thermometer to check the temperature.

- Mix in the unflavored protein powder and flavorings, stirring well until powder has dissolved, and serve.

Sweet Potato Pancakes

Preparation time-5 minutes| Cook time-25 minutes| Servings-4 |Difficulty-Easy

Nutritional value- Calories-298| Fat-16g |Carbohydrates-2.8g| Protein-20.9g

Ingredients

- One lb. of sweet potatoes

- Two organic eggs

- Three tablespoons of whole-wheat flour

- Half teaspoon of pepper garlic powder

- Three tablespoons of canola oil

Instructions

- Preheat a steamer over medium heat, then place peeled sweet potatoes in it. Steam until tender.

- Once the sweet potatoes are tender, remove them from the steamer.

- Using a potato masher, mash until smooth. Place the mashed sweet potatoes in a bowl, then add eggs and flour to the bowl. Season with pepper and garlic powder, then mix well.

- Shape the sweet potato mixture into thin patties, then set aside.

- Preheat a saucepan over medium heat, then pour canola oil into it. Place the shaped sweet potato in the saucepan. Cook until lightly golden. Flip the sweet potato pancakes and cook again until both sides are lightly golden.

- Repeat with the rest of the batter. Once they are done, arrange the sweet potato pancakes on a serving dish, then serve. Enjoy!

Swiss chard and garlic frittata

Preparation time-5 minutes |Cook time-20 minutes |Servings-2 |Difficulty-Easy

Nutritional value: ~Calories-121|Proteins-12g| Fat-8g|Carbohydrates-5g

Ingredients

- One bunch of Swiss chard
- Two tablespoons of unsalted butter, ghee, or coconut oil, plus more for greasing the dish
- Half cup of diced white onion
- One teaspoon of minced garlic
- Fine sea salt and ground black pepper
- One teaspoon of paprika
- Four large eggs

Instructions

- Preheat the oven to 350°F and grease a 2-quart baking dish.
- Separate the leaves of the Swiss chard from the stems. Discard the stems or save them for another use.
- Cut the leaves into bite-sized pieces and wash them very well, making sure there is no leftover grit.
- Heat a few inches of water in a steamer pot over medium-high heat. Steam the Swiss chard for 5 minutes, then remove the steamer from the heat. When it's cool enough to handle, squeeze the excess water out of the Swiss chard and set it aside.
- In a sauté pan, melt the fat over medium heat. Add the onion and cook until soft, about 3 minutes. Add the garlic, a pinch of salt and pepper, and the paprika and sauté the mixture for 1 minute more.
- Add the steamed Swiss chard to the sauté pan and sauté for 2 minutes or until wilted.
- Beat the eggs in a bowl and season them with a pinch of salt and pepper.
- Transfer the Swiss chard mixture to the prepared baking dish. Pour the eggs over the mixture, making sure they cover the chard evenly.
- Put the baking dish in the oven and cook for 8 to 10 minutes until the eggs are firm. Slice and serve.

Tofu Scramble

Preparation time-7 minutes| Cook time-20 minutes| Servings-10 |Difficulty-Easy

Nutritional value- Calories-75| Fat-6g |Carbohydrates-4g| Protein-6g

Ingredients

- One small onion
- One tablespoon of olive oil
- Three cloves of garlic
- Half teaspoon of turmeric
- One cup of frozen chopped baby spinach, thawed
- A quarter cup of reduced-fat cheese
- Salt and pepper to taste

- Two to three Roma tomatoes
- One pound of extra-firm tofu
- One teaspoon of smoked paprika
- One teaspoon of cumin

Instructions

- Finely dice the onion and tomato, followed by the garlic.
- Sauté onion in olive oil in a large skillet over medium-high heat for 7-8 minutes.
- In the meantime, drain some of the excess liquid from the tofu, slice it into 1-inch slices, place it in a medium bowl, and crumble it with a fork.
- Cook garlic in the pan for 30 seconds. Stir in tofu crumbles and tomato.
- Reduce to medium heat and cook for approximately 10 minutes, stirring occasionally.
- In a small bowl, combine the cumin, paprika, and turmeric.
- Stir in 1-2 tbsp water until combined. Season the pan with seasonings. Stir thoroughly.
- Stir in spinach and cook for an additional 3 minutes, or until all vegetables are tender.
- Garnish with cheese and season with salt and pepper to taste.

Tomato and Fresh Basil Scramble

Preparation time-5 minutes |Cook time-10 minutes |Serving-1 |Difficulty- Easy

Nutritional value: ~ Calories-98| Fat-5g| Protein-9g| Carbohydrates-2g

Ingredients

- One teaspoon of light butter
- Two tablespoons of chopped tomato
- One and a half teaspoons of chopped fresh basil leaves
- A quarter cup of liquid egg substitute
- One tablespoon of shredded Parmesan cheese

Instructions

- In an omelet pan over medium heat, melt the butter, swirling the pan to coat evenly. Add the tomato and continue cooking for 4 to 5 minutes, until soft.
- Add the basil and egg substitute, stirring gently but constantly with a heat-resistant rubber spatula, scraping the bottom of the pan to keep the eggs moving to avoid browning.
- When the eggs are almost finished, add the cheese and turn off the heat. Gently fold the cheese into the eggs, turning over with the spatula.

- When the cheese becomes soft but not dissolved, turn the scramble onto a plate.

Tomato Bruschetta

Preparation time- 5 minutes| Cook time-20 minutes| Servings- 12 |Difficulty-Easy

Nutritional value- Calories-298| Fat-16g |Carbohydrates-2.8g| Protein-20.9g

Ingredients

- Half finely chopped small red onion
- Eight medium coarsely chopped and drained tomatoes
- Two to three crushed garlic cloves
- Six to eight leaves of finely chopped fresh basil
- Two tablespoons of balsamic vinegar
- Four tablespoons of extra virgin olive oil
- One crusty loaf of bread

Instructions

- Mix the onions, tomatoes, garlic, and basil in a big bowl, taking care not to crush or break the tomatoes up too much. Balsamic vinegar and extra virgin olive oil should be added. As needed, add salt and pepper. For at least an hour, cover and relax. This will make it easier to soak and mix the flavors.
- Slice the baguette loaf into 12 thick slices diagonally and lightly toast them until both sides are light brown. On the warm bread slices, serve the mixture.
- Take out from the frozen half an hour before serving if you like the mix at room temperature.

Turkey, Zucchini, and Tomato Hash

Preparation time-5 minutes| Cook time-15 minutes| Servings-4 |Difficulty-Easy

Nutritional value- Calories-110| Fat-4g |Carbohydrates-6g| Protein-12g

Ingredients

- Half cup of diced onion
- A quarter teaspoon of salt
- One cup of canned tomatoes, drained
- Two cups of zucchini cut into ½-inch dice
- Eight ounces of lean ground turkey
- One tablespoon of extra-virgin olive oil

Instructions

- Over medium-high heat, warm the oil. Now in the hot skillet, put the turkey and cook until it's browned. Move to a bowl.
- Place the tomato, onion, and zucchini in the skillet and cook until the zucchini turns soft and the onion becomes translucent. Sprinkle some salt and mix.

- Mix the turkey with veggies and enjoy.

Unpotato tortilla

Preparation time-10 minutes |Cook time-20 minutes|Servings-6 |Difficulty-Easy

Nutritional value: ~139 Calories| Fat-11g|Protein-6g|Carbohydrates-1g

Ingredients

- A quarter head cauliflower
- One medium turnip
- One medium onion, sliced thin
- Three tablespoons of olive oil, divided
- Six eggs
- Salt and ground black pepper, to taste
- Chopped fresh parsley (optional)

Instructions

- Reduce the heat to low and preheat the broiler.
- Cauliflower should be thinly sliced, including the stem, and turnips should be peeled and thinly sliced.
- Put them in a microwave-safe casserole dish with a lid, add a few tablespoons of water, and cook for 6 to 7 minutes on high.
- Meanwhile, start sautéing the onion in two tablespoons of olive oil in an 8- to 9-inch (20- to 23-cm) pan—a non-stick skillet is preferred, but not required—in an 8- to 9-inch (20- to 23-cm) skillet. Give your skillet a nice squirt of non-stick cooking spray if it isn't already non-stick.
- Use a medium heat setting.
- Pull the vegetables out of the microwave when it beeps, drain them, and toss them in the skillet with the onion. Continue to sauté everything, adding a little extra oil if things start to stick, for approximately 10 to 15 minutes, or until the veggies are golden around the edges.
- Reduce the heat to low and arrange the vegetables in an equal layer on the skillet's bottom.
- Combine the eggs, salt, and pepper in a mixing bowl, and pour over the vegetables. Cook for 5–7 minutes on low, raising the edges regularly to allow raw egg to run underneath.
- When everything is ready except the top, place the skillet under a low broiler for 4 to 5 minutes, or until the tortilla is brown on top. (Wrap your skillet in foil first if it doesn't have a flameproof handle.) To serve, cut into wedges. It's good to include a little minced parsley on top, but it's not required.

Vanilla Melon Pudding

Preparation time-5 minutes| Cook time-15 minutes| Servings-4 |Difficulty-Easy

Nutritional value- Calories-298| |Carbohydrates-2.8g| Protein-20.9g Fat-16g

Ingredients

- One and a half cups of melon puree
- Two packages of sugar-free Jell-O
- A quarter cup of protein powder
- Two cups of skim milk
- Half cup of fresh raspberries

Instructions

- Combine the sugar-free Jell-O with skim milk, then pour into a pot. Bring to boil and stir until the Jell-O is completely dissolved.
- Once the milk and Jell-O mixture is boiling, add the protein powder and melon puree. Mix well. Remove from heat.
- Pour the mixture into 8 small pudding cups, then garnish each pudding with fresh raspberries.
- Chill the puddings in the refrigerator, then let them set. Serve and enjoy the cold.

Vanilla Pancakes

Preparation time-15 minutes |Cook time-5 minutes |Servings-2 |Difficulty-Easy

Nutritional value: ~Calories-202|Proteins-12g| Fat-4g|Carbohydrates-29.4g

Ingredients

- Six ounces plain yogurt
- Half cup of whole-grain flour
- One egg, beaten
- One teaspoon of vanilla extract
- One teaspoon of baking powder

Instructions

- Heat non-stick skillet well. Meanwhile, mix up all the ingredients.
- Pour the mixture into the skillet in the shape of the pancakes. Cook them for 1 minute per side. Serve.

Veggie Bowls

Preparation time-15 minutes |Cook time-5 minutes |Servings-2 |Difficulty-Easy

Nutritional value: ~Calories-321|Proteins-11g| Fat-20g|Carbohydrates-24g

Ingredients

- One tablespoon of olive oil

- One pound of asparagus, trimmed and roughly chopped
- Three cups of kale, shredded
- Three cups of Brussels sprouts, shredded
- Half cup of hummus
- One avocado, peeled, pitted, and sliced
- Four eggs, soft boiled, peeled and sliced

For the dressing

- Two tablespoons of lemon juice
- One garlic clove, minced
- Two teaspoons of Dijon mustard
- Two tablespoons of olive oil
- Salt and black pepper to the taste

Instructions

- Heat a pan with two tablespoons of oil over medium-high heat, add the asparagus and sauté for 5 minutes, often stirring.
- In a bowl, combine the other two tablespoons of oil with the lemon juice, garlic, mustard, salt, and pepper and whisk well.
- In a salad bowl, combine the asparagus with the kale, sprouts, hummus, avocado, and eggs and toss gently.
- Add the dressing, toss, and serve for breakfast.

Whole-wheat banana pecan pancakes

Preparation time-15 minutes |Cook time-15 minutes |Servings-4 |Difficulty-Easy

Nutritional value: ~Calories-113|Proteins-2.3g| Fat-1.8g|Carbohydrates-22g

Ingredients

- One and a quarter cups of soy milk or coconut milk beverage, plus a quarter cup if needed
- One tablespoon of flax meal (ground flaxseeds)
- One teaspoon of apple cider vinegar
- One large ripe banana, peeled and mashed well
- One tablespoon of brown sugar
- One tablespoon of maple syrup, plus more for serving (optional)
- One teaspoon of vanilla extract
- One cup of white whole-wheat flour or whole-wheat pastry flour
- 1 /3 cup of buckwheat flour
- Two teaspoons of baking powder
- Half teaspoon of kosher salt

- Half teaspoon of ground cinnamon

- A quarter teaspoon of ground nutmeg

- Half cup of finely chopped toasted pecans

- One cup of fresh mixed raspberries, blueberries, and/or strawberries (optional)

Instructions

- In a small saucepan over medium-high heat, warm a quarter cup of soy milk.

- Place flax meal in a small bowl, add warm milk, stir well, and set aside.

- In a small bowl, whisk apple cider vinegar into remaining soy milk and set aside to thicken and curdle.

- In another small bowl, mash banana with brown sugar, maple syrup, and vanilla extract. Whisk in flax mixture, followed by curdled soy milk, and blend well.

- Heat a cast-iron griddle or frying pan over medium heat until a drop of water sizzles and evaporates immediately.

- Meanwhile, in a medium bowl, whisk together white whole-wheat flour, buckwheat flour, baking powder, kosher salt, cinnamon, and nutmeg. Stir in wet ingredients until just combined, and quickly fold in chopped pecans. Stir in more soy milk as needed to make a thick batter, the consistency of a heavy, pound cake batter.

- Lightly oil or butter the griddle, and drop three tablespoon-size scoops of batter into the pan, spreading with a small spatula if necessary. Cook for 2 minutes without disturbing or until bubbles form on the surface of the pancakes, carefully flip over pancakes, and cook for one and a half more minutes. Grease the pan a little between each batch, as these pancakes will want to stick to the pan otherwise.

- Serve hot with mixed fruit (if using) and more maple syrup (if using). The success of this recipe depends on using nondairy milk that will curdle. Choose a soy or coconut milk beverage, as both will thicken and sour nicely when the apple cider vinegar is introduced.

Wisconsin Scrambler with Aged Cheddar Cheese

Preparation time-10 minutes| Cook time-10 minutes| Servings-2-4 |Difficulty-Easy

Nutritional value- Calories-169| Fat-11g |Carbohydrates-2g| Protein-15g

Ingredients

- Three ounces of extra-sharp Wisconsin Cheddar cheese, shredded

- Half teaspoon of garlic powder

- Six large eggs, beaten

- A quarter cup of fat-free milk

- Half teaspoon of onion powder

- Eight ounces of extra-lean turkey sausage

- Nonstick cooking spray

Instructions

- Spray a skillet with some cooking spray and put it over medium-high heat. Throw in some of the turkey sausages to brown. Then cut it into small chunks and let it cook for around 7 minutes or until it's properly cooked.

- Now, beat the milk and eggs and add garlic and onion powders.

- Place beaten eggs in the skillet. Lower the heat to low and mix slowly for around 5 minutes or until the eggs are cooked properly.

- Serve with some cheese on top.

Yogurt with Dates

Preparation time-10 minutes |Cook time-0 minutes |Servings-2 |Difficulty-Easy

Nutritional value: -Calories-215|Proteins-8.7g| Fat-11.5g|Carbohydrates-18.5g

Ingredients

- Five dates, pitted, chopped

- Two cups of plain yogurt

- Half teaspoon of vanilla extract

- Four pecans, chopped

Instructions

- Mix up all the ingredients in the blender and blend until smooth.

- Pour it into the serving cups.

Zucchini Muffins with Broccoli

Preparation time- 5 minutes| Cook time-55 minutes| Servings-4 |Difficulty-Hard

Nutritional value- Calories-298| Fat-16g |Carbohydrates-2.8g| Protein-20.9g

Ingredients

- One and a quarter cups of grated zucchini

- Eight broccoli florets

- One and a quarter cups of oats

- One medium ripe banana

- Two organic eggs

- A quarter cup of applesauce

- One teaspoon of baking powder

- One teaspoon of cinnamon

Instructions

- Preheat an oven to 350°F and prepare 8 muffin cups. Coat with cooking spray then set aside. Place the oats in a food processor, then process until they become a flour-like consistency. Set aside.

- Peel the banana, then mash until smooth. Crack the eggs, then pour them over the mashed banana. Add applesauce, grated zucchini, and cinnamon. Mix until incorporated. Combine the oat flour with baking powder.

- Mix with the liquid mixture. Fill each muffin cup with the batter, then put a broccoli floret in each muffin. Bake the muffins for approximately 40 minutes or until the top of the muffins are lightly golden.

- Insert a skewer into the muffins, and when it comes out clean, it means that the muffins are completely cooked. Remove the muffins from the oven, then let them cool for a few minutes.

- Arrange on a serving dish.

Chapter 6-Lunch Recipes

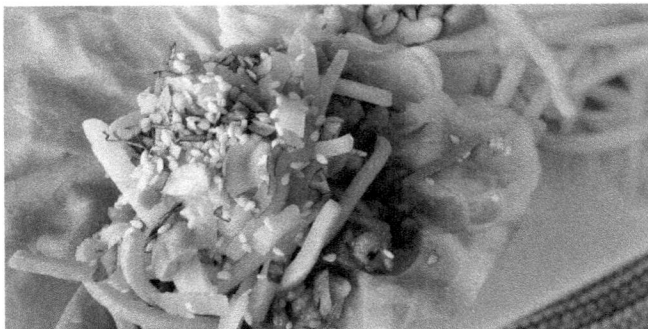

Asian Chicken Lettuce Wraps

Preparation time-10 minutes |Cook time-0 minutes |Serving-4 |Difficulty- Easy

Nutritional value: ~Calories-155| Fat-4g| Protein-16g| Carbohydrates-11g

Ingredients

- One can (8 ounces) water chestnuts, drained and minced
- Two tablespoons of hoisin sauce
- Two teaspoons of low-sodium soy sauce
- Two packets of sugar substitute (such as Splenda)
- One cup of minced onion
- One teaspoon of minced ginger
- One teaspoon of toasted sesame oil
- One whole green onion, chopped
- One can (8 ounces) bamboo shoots, drained and minced
- Three tablespoons of sherry cooking wine
- One tablespoon of unsalted peanut butter
- Two teaspoons of hot pepper sauce, such as Sriracha
- One tablespoon of minced garlic
- Half pound of ground chicken breast
- A quarter teaspoon of salt
- Eight small leaves of butter lettuce
- One small cucumber, seeded and sliced into 1" strips

Instructions

- Mix the bamboo shoots, sherry, water chestnuts, hot-pepper sauce, hoisin sauce, soy sauce, peanut butter, and sugar substitute in a medium mixing bowl. Mix thoroughly. Remove from the heat.
- Set a large nonstick skillet over medium heat, sprayed with cooking spray.

- Cook, occasionally stirring, for 4 minutes, or until the onions are aromatic and softened.
- Cook for another minute after adding the garlic.
- Add the ginger, ground chicken, and salt to the pan and raise the heat to medium-high.
- Cook for 3 to 4 minutes, breaking up the chicken with a spatula or wooden spoon until no longer pink.
- Mix in the bamboo shoots and water chestnuts.
- Cook for 2 minutes, or until thoroughly heated.
- Add the toasted sesame oil and mix well.
- Turn off the heat in the pan.
- To serve, spoon half of the chicken mixture onto each of the eight lettuce leaves.
- Cucumber and green onion are diced and served on top. Serve right away.

Asian Pork Tenderloin

Preparation time-10 minutes |Cook time-40 minutes or 6 hours |Serving-8 |Difficulty- Moderate to hard

Nutritional value: ~Calories-256| Fat-9g| Protein-34g| Carbohydrates-9g

Ingredients

- 1/3 cup of brown sugar
- Two tablespoons of lemon juice
- One tablespoon of dry mustard
- One and a half teaspoons of pepper
- Two pounds of pork tenderloin
- 1/3 cup of light soy sauce
- Two tablespoons of Worcestershire sauce
- Two tablespoons of rice vinegar
- One tablespoon of ginger
- Four garlic cloves or prepared minced

Instructions

- In a freezer-safe bag, combine all of the ingredients.
- Place the tenderloin in a freezer bag and coat it with the marinade.
- Place in refrigerator overnight or freeze for later use.
- Preheat oven to 375°F and bake for 30-40 minutes, or prepare in a slow cooker on low for 4 to 6 hours.

Avocado, Cream Cheese, and Bacon Sandwich

Preparation time-15 minutes |Cook time-0 minutes |Serving-1 |Difficulty- Easy

Nutritional value: ~ Calories-223| Fat-10g| Protein-14g| Carbohydrates-24g

Ingredients

- One ounce of nonfat cream cheese
- Two slices of toasted diet wheat bread
- Two slices of low-sodium turkey bacon, or veggie bacon strips, precooked
- Half ripe avocado, cut into thin slices

Instructions

- Spread the cream cheese equally on each slice of bread.
- Break or cut the bacon strips in half, then distribute them on one slice.
- Next, layer the avocado slices on top of the bacon and top with the other slice of bread. Cut diagonally and serve.

Balsamic-glazed chicken and peppers

Preparation time-10 minutes |Cook time-30 minutes|Servings-4 |Difficulty-Easy

Nutritional value: Calories-221| Fat-11g|Protein-26g|Carbohydrates-7g

Ingredients

- One pound of boneless, skinless chicken breast
- Half green bell pepper
- Half red bell pepper
- One small onion
- Two cloves of garlic, crushed
- Two tablespoons of olive oil
- Two tablespoons of balsamic vinegar
- One teaspoon of Italian seasoning

Instructions

- Cut your chicken into Half-inch (1 cm) cubes. Cut your peppers into strips, cut them thinly lengthwise, then once crosswise.
- Cut your onion in half vertically, and slice vertically. Mince your garlic and have it standing ready, too.
- Put your large, heavy skillet over medium-high heat. Add the olive oil, and let it get hot.
- Now throw in the chicken, peppers, and onions, and stir-fry them until all the pink is gone from the chicken and the vegetables are starting to soften a bit.
- Add the garlic, balsamic vinegar, and Italian seasoning; stir everything up. Let the whole thing cook, often stirring, until the vinegar has reduced and become a bit syrupy, then serve.

Banh mi Burgers

Preparation time-10 minutes |Cook time-35 minutes|Servings-3 |Difficulty-Easy

Nutritional value: Calories-597 | Fat-32g|Protein-19g|Carbohydrates-7g

Ingredients

- Five scallions, divided
- A quarter cup of fresh basil leaves
- One pound of ground pork
- One tablespoon of fish sauce (nam pla or nuoc mam)
- One tablespoon of chili garlic sauce (sometimes called sambal oelek)
- One tablespoon of Splenda, or the equivalent in liquid Splenda
- Two teaspoons of chopped garlic
- One teaspoon of salt
- One teaspoon of ground black pepper
- 1/3 cup of mayonnaise
- One tablespoon of chili garlic sauce

Instructions

- Preheat an electric tabletop grill. If you can choose temperature settings on yours, use 350°F.
- Cut the root and any limp greens off the scallions, whack them into a few pieces, and throw three of them into your food processor with the S-blade in place. (Reserve the other two.) Throw in the basil, too. Pulse until they're finely chopped together.
- Now add the pork, fish sauce, chili garlic sauce, Splenda, garlic, salt, and pepper to the processor and run it until everything is well blended.
- Form the pork mixture into 3 patties and put them on the grill. Set a timer for 6 to 8 minutes.
- Quickly wash out your food processor and reassemble with the S-blade in place. Put the remaining 2 scallions in there and pulse to chop. Now add the mayonnaise and chili sauce and run to blend.
- When the burgers are done, serve with the sauce.

Barbecue Chicken and Portobello Pizzas

Preparation time-15 minutes |Cook time-30 minutes |Serving-6 |Difficulty- Easy

Nutritional value: Calories-181| Fat-9g| Protein-12g| Carbohydrates-14g

Ingredients

- One tablespoon of extra-virgin olive oil
- One garlic clove, minced
- Six large (4- to 5-inch) portobello mushrooms, stems removed
- Half red onion, diced
- ¾ cup of low-sugar barbecue sauce

- One chicken breast, baked and diced

- Four ounces of feta or goat cheese

- ⅔ cup of mozzarella or Monterey Jack cheese

- A quarter cup of roughly chopped fresh cilantro

Instructions

- Arrange the oven shelf to the middle rack. Preheat the oven to 400°F.

- In a small bowl, combine the oil and garlic. Brush the bottoms of each mushroom with the garlic oil mixture, and place each mushroom, oil-side down (stem-side down) on a baking sheet. Bake for 15 minutes.

- Meanwhile, in a small skillet over medium-low heat, sauté the red onion until browned and soft, about 20 minutes. Set aside.

- Drain off any liquid from the mushroom caps, and return to the baking sheet stem-side up. Fill each mushroom cap with Two tablespoons of barbecue sauce. Top with the chicken, red onion, and cheese. Bake until the cheese has melted and is a light golden brown, 5 to 8 minutes.

- Remove from the oven, sprinkle with the cilantro, and serve.

Beef and bacon rice with pine nuts

Preparation time-10 minutes |Cook time-22 minutes|Servings-5 |Difficulty-Easy

Nutritional value: Calories-192 | Fat-6g|Protein-14g|Carbohydrates-4g

Ingredients

- Half head cauliflower

- Four strips bacon

- Half medium onion, chopped

- Two tablespoons of tomato sauce

- One tablespoon of beef bouillon concentrate

- Two tablespoons of toasted pine nuts

- Two tablespoons of chopped fresh parsley

Instructions

- Turn your cauliflower into Cauli-Rice according to the instructions.

- While that's cooking, cut the bacon into little pieces—kitchen shears are good for this—and start the little bacon bits frying in a heavy skillet over medium-high heat. When a little grease has cooked out of the bacon, throw the onion into the skillet.

- Cook until the onion is translucent and the bacon is browned and getting crisp.

- By now, the cauliflower should be done. Drain it and throw it in the skillet with the bacon and onion.

- Add the tomato sauce and beef bouillon concentrate, and stir the whole thing up to combine everything—

you can add a couple of tablespoons (28 ml) of water, if you like, to help the liquid flavorings spread.

- Stir in the pine nuts and parsley (you can just snip it right into the skillet with clean kitchen shears), and serve.

Beef and Broccoli Stir-Fry

Preparation time-1 hour 10 minutes |Cook time-20 minutes |Serving-4 |Difficulty- Easy

Nutritional value: Calories-296| Fat-17g| Protein-27g| Carbohydrates-11g

Ingredients

- One pound of flat iron steak

- One tablespoon of cornstarch

- Half cup of soy sauce

- A quarter cup of oyster sauce

- Half cup of beef broth

- One tablespoon of minced fresh ginger

- 2 garlic cloves, minced

- 5 cups broccoli florets

- One tablespoon of coconut oil

- Cauliflower rice (optional)

Instructions

- Thinly slice the flat iron steak against the grain.

- In a large, resealable bag, toss the meat with the cornstarch. Add the soy sauce, oyster sauce, beef broth, ginger, and garlic. Chill for 1 hour.

- In a large pot, blanch the broccoli for 2 minutes in boiling water, then transfer to an ice bath.

- In a large wok or skillet over medium-high heat, heat the oil. Add the beef (reserve remaining marinade), and stir-fry until brown, 1 to 3 minutes. Transfer to a plate.

- Add the blanched broccoli to the wok or skillet, and stir-fry until crisp but tender, about 3 minutes. Add the remaining marinade, and cook for 2 minutes more.

- Return the beef to the pan with the broccoli, and warm through.

- Serve with cauliflower rice (if desired).

Beef stroganoff

Preparation time-10 minutes |Cook time-8 to 10 hours|Servings-8 |Difficulty-Hard

Nutritional value: Calories-369 | Fat-17g|Protein-44g|Carbohydrates-5g

Ingredients

- Three pounds of beef stew meat in 1-inch (2.5 cm) cubes

- Three tablespoons of olive oil

- Two cups of sliced celery

- Four cloves of garlic

- One teaspoon of salt or Vege-Sal

- A quarter teaspoon of ground cinnamon

- A quarter teaspoon of ground cloves

- A quarter teaspoon of ground black pepper

- 1/8 teaspoon of ground allspice

- 1/8 teaspoon of ground nutmeg

- One can (Fourteen and a half ounces) of diced tomatoes

- Half cup of dry red wine

Instructions

- Put the beef in your slow cooker. Put the onion on top, then dump in the mushrooms, liquid and all.

- Mix the beef broth with the Worcestershire sauce, bouillon concentrate, and paprika, and pour over everything.

- Cover and cook on low for 8 to 10 hours.

- When ready to serve, cut the cream cheese into cubes and stir into the mixture in the slow cooker until melted.

- Stir in the sour cream, and serve.

Blackened Salmon with Avocado Cream

Preparation time-10 minutes | Cook time-10 minutes | Serving-4 | Difficulty- Easy

Nutritional value: Calories-356 | Fat-24g | Protein-35g | Carbohydrates-2g

Ingredients

- Four (6-ounce) salmon fillets, bones removed

- One tablespoon of butter, melted

- Two tablespoons of blackened seasoning

- One tablespoon of extra-virgin olive oil

- Half cup of Avocado Cream

Instructions

- Pat, the salmon, fillets dry on both sides with paper towels.

- Brush the butter over the fleshy side of the salmon fillets.

- Pour the seasoning onto a plate, and press the flesh side of each salmon fillet into the seasoning, coating evenly.

- In a large skillet over medium heat, heat the olive oil. Add the salmon, skin-side up, and cook until blackened, 3 to 4 minutes. Flip the fillets and continue to cook to your liking, 5 to 7 minutes, depending on

the thickness of the fillets, or to an internal temperature of 125 to 145°F. Once done, the fish should flake easily with a fork.

- Transfer to individual plates, and serve with the avocado cream.

Bleu burger

Preparation time-10 minutes | Cook time-14 minutes | Servings-1 | Difficulty-Easy

Nutritional value: Calories-511 | Fat-40g | Protein-34g | Carbohydrates-1g

Ingredients

- Six ounces of ground chuck in a patty

- One tablespoon of crumbled blue cheese

- One teaspoon of finely minced sweet red onion

Instructions

- Cook the burger by your preferred method. When it's almost done to your liking, top with the blue cheese and let it melt.

- Remove from the heat, put on a plate, and top with the onion.

Bok Choy Stir Fry

Preparation time-5 minutes | Cook time-15 minutes | Servings-2 | Difficulty-Easy

Nutritional value: Calories-187 | Fat-9g | Protein-12g | Carbohydrates-12g

Ingredients

- Two minced garlic cloves

- Two cups of chopped bok choy

- Two chopped bacon slices

- Salt and black pepper to the taste

- A drizzle of avocado oil

Instructions

- Heat a pan over medium heat with the oil, add the bacon, stir and brown until crunchy, move to paper towels and drain the oil.

- Return the saucepan to medium heat, stir in the garlic and bok choy, and cook for 4 minutes.

- Stir in salt, pepper and bacon, stir, cook for another 1 minute, divide among plates and serve.

Bourbon-maple glazed pork chops

Preparation time-10 minutes | Cook time-25 minutes | Servings-2 | Difficulty-Easy

Nutritional value: Calories-225 | Fat-12g | Protein-22g | Carbohydrates-2g

Ingredients

- One tablespoon of olive oil

- Twelve ounces of pork loin chops (2 thin-cut chops)
- A quarter cup of minced onion
- One clove of garlic, crushed
- A quarter cup of chicken broth
- One and a half tablespoons of erythritol
- One tablespoon of bourbon
- Five drops of maple extract

Instructions

- Coat your large, heavy skillet with non-stick cooking spray, and put it over medium-high heat. Add the oil, and swirl it around to coat the bottom of the skillet.
- When the whole thing is hot, throw in your chops, and brown them on both sides, about 5 minutes per side.
- Remove the chops from the skillet, and turn the heat down to medium-low. Add the onion and garlic, and sauté in the residual fat for a minute.
- Add the broth, erythritol, bourbon, and maple extract. Stir this around with your spatula, scraping up all the yummy brown bits stuck to the skillet.
- Throw the chops back into the skillet. Turn the heat down to low, and set a timer for 3 minutes.
- When it goes off, flip the chops, and set the timer for another 3 minutes. By this time, the liquid should have cooked down and become syrupy.
- Put the chops on serving plates, scrape the glaze with the bits of onion and garlic over them, then serve.

Braised Chicken with Mushrooms

Preparation time-10 minutes | Cook time-50 minutes | Serving-4 | Difficulty-Hard

Nutritional value: Calories-327 | Fat-12g | Protein-39g | Carbohydrates-20g

Ingredients

- A quarter cup of all-purpose (plain) flour
- Half teaspoon of freshly ground black pepper
- One and a half tablespoons of olive oil or canola oil
- Two skinless, bone-in chicken breast halves, each cut in half crosswise (should be 4 pieces total)
- Two skinless, bone-in chicken thighs
- Two skinless chicken legs
- One shallot, chopped
- One pound of small white button mushrooms brushed clean
- Half pound of peeled pearl onions
- 3/4 cup of low-sodium vegetable stock, chicken stock or broth

- Half cup of port or dry red wine
- Two tablespoons of balsamic vinegar
- Two tablespoons of chopped fresh thyme, plus sprigs for garnish
- A quarter teaspoon of salt

Instructions

- Combine the flour and 1/4 teaspoon of pepper in a small bowl. Using the seasoned flour, dredge the chicken pieces.
- Heat the oil in a big, heavy pot or Dutch oven over medium-high heat. Cook, flipping once until the chicken is browned on all sides, about 5 minutes total. Place on a serving dish.
- Add the shallot to the pan and cook for 1 minute or until softened. Sauté the mushrooms for 3 to 4 minutes, or until gently browned. Stir in the onions and cook for 2 to 3 minutes, or until they start to brown.
- Deglaze the pan by whisking in the stock and wine and scraping out any browned pieces with a wooden spoon. Bring the chicken pieces back to a boil in the pan. Cover, reduce the heat to low, and cook, occasionally stirring, for 45 to 50 minutes, or until the chicken and veggies are cooked. Combine the vinegar, chopped thyme, 1 teaspoon salt, and the remaining 1/4 teaspoon pepper in a mixing bowl.
- To serve, divide the vegetables into shallow individual bowls that have been warmed. Top with 2 pieces of chicken, 1 light meat, 1 dark meat. Serve with thyme sprigs as a garnish.

Broiled Grouper with Teriyaki Sauce

Preparation time-10 minutes | Cook time-15 minutes | Serving-2 | Difficulty- Easy

Nutritional value: Calories-114 | Fat-1g | Protein-22g | Carbohydrates-2g

Ingredients

- One tablespoon of reduced-sodium teriyaki sauce
- Half teaspoon of minced garlic
- Two grouper fillets, each 4 ounces
- Two lemon wedges
- A quarter teaspoon of Italian seasoning

Instructions

- Whisk together the teriyaki sauce and garlic in a small bowl.
- Using cooking spray, lightly coat a baking pan. Fill the pan with grouper fillets. Brush both sides of the fillets with the teriyaki marinade. To marinate the fish, cover and refrigerate for at least 15 minutes.
- Preheat the oven to broil (grill). Place the rack four inches away from the heat source.

- Broil (grill) the salmon for 5 to 10 minutes, or until it is opaque throughout when examined with the tip of a knife. Remove the broiler from the oven.

- Sprinkle each fillet with Italian seasoning after squeezing 1 lemon slice over it. Serve right away.

Buffalo Blue Cheese Chicken Wedges

Preparation time-5 minutes | Cook time-35 minutes | Servings-2 | Difficulty-Easy

Nutritional value: Calories-271 | Fat-12g | Protein-26g | Carbohydrates-11g

Ingredients

- One head of lettuce

- Bleu cheese dressing

- Two tablespoons of crumbled blue cheese

- Four strips of bacon

- Two boneless chicken breasts

- 3/4 cup of any buffalo sauce

Instructions

- Boil a big pot of salted water.

- Add two chicken breasts to the water and simmer for 30 minutes, or until the internal temperature of the chicken reaches 180 ºC.

- Let the chicken rest for 10 minutes to cool.

- Take apart the chicken into strips using a fork.

- Cook and cool bacon strips, crumble reserve,

- Merge the scrapped chicken and buffalo sauce over medium heat, then mix until warm.

- Break the lettuce into wedges and apply the appropriate amount of blue cheese dressing to it.

- Add crumbles of blue cheese.

- Add the chicken-pulled buffalo.

- Cover with more crumbles of blue cheese and fried crumbled bacon.

- Serve.

Burger scramble Florentine

Preparation time-10 minutes | Cook time-20 minutes | Servings-6 | Difficulty-Easy

Nutritional value: Calories~544 | Fat-46g | Protein-27g | Carbohydrates-8g

Ingredients

- One and a half pounds lean ground beef

- Half cup of finely diced onion

- One package of (10 ounces) frozen chopped spinach, thawed and drained

- Eight ounces of cream cheese softened

- Half cup of heavy cream

- Half cup of shredded Parmesan cheese

- Salt and ground black pepper, to taste

Instructions

- Preheat oven to 350°F.

- In a large ovenproof skillet, brown the ground beef and onion.

- Add the spinach and cook through until the meat is done. Add the cream cheese, heavy cream, Parmesan, and salt and pepper to taste. Mix well, then spread evenly in the skillet.

- Bake, uncovered, for 20 minutes or until bubbly and browned on top.

Cauli-bacon dish

Preparation time-10 minutes | Cook time-15 minutes | Servings-5 | Difficulty-Easy

Nutritional value: Calories-161 | Fat-4g | Protein-2g | Carbohydrates-3g

Ingredients

- Four slices of bacon

- Half head cauliflower

- Half green bell pepper

- Half medium onion

- A quarter cup of sliced stuffed olives

Instructions

- Chop the bacon into small bits and start it frying in a large, heavy skillet over medium-high heat. (Give the skillet a squirt of non-stick cooking spray first.)

- Chop the cauliflower into Half-inch (1 cm) bits. Chop up the stem, too; no need to waste it.

- Put the chopped cauliflower in a microwavable casserole dish with a lid—or a microwave steamer if you have one—add a couple of tablespoons (28 ml) of water, cover, and microwave for 8 minutes on high.

- Give the bacon a stir, then go back to the chopping board. Dice the pepper and onion. By now, some fat has cooked out of the bacon, and it is starting to brown around the edges. Add the pepper and onion to the skillet.

- Sauté until the onion is translucent and the pepper is starting to get soft.

- By then, the cauliflower should be done. Add it to the skillet without draining and stir—the extra little bit of water is going to help dissolve the yummy bacon flavor from the bottom of the skillet and carry it through the dish.

- Stir in the olives, let the whole thing cook another minute while stirring, then serve.

Cauliflower Bread Garlic sticks

Preparation time-10 minutes |Cook time-40 minutes|Servings-2 |Difficulty-Moderate

Nutritional value: Calories-211| Fat-9g|Protein-12g|Carbohydrates-15g

Ingredients

- Two +

Instructions

- Preheat the oven to 350° F.

- Sauté the red pepper flakes and garlic for nearly three minutes and transfer to a bowl of cooked cauliflower. Melt the butter in a small skillet over low heat.

- Mix the Italian seasoning and salt together.

- Afterward, refrigerate for 10 minutes.

- Add the mozzarella cheese and egg to the cauliflower mixture until slightly cooled.

- A creamy paste in a thin layer lined with parchment paper on a thinly oiled 9-9 baking dish.

- Bake for thirty minutes.

- Remove from the oven and finish with a little more parmesan and mozzarella cheese.

- Put them back in the oven and cook for an extra 8 minutes.

- Remove from the oven and slice into sticks of the appropriate duration.

Chicken breasts stuffed with artichokes and garlic cheese

Preparation time-10 minutes |Cook time-35 minutes|Servings-4 |Difficulty-Easy

Nutritional value: Calories-298 | Fat-12g|Protein-41g|Carbohydrates-2g

Ingredients

- Four boneless, skinless chicken breasts, total one and a half pounds

- One jar (6 ounces) marinated artichoke hearts, drained

- Three ounces of Boursin cheese (or similar spreadable garlic-herb cheese)

- A quarter teaspoon of ground black pepper

- Half tablespoon of butter

Instructions

- Preheat oven to 375°F.

- One by one, place each chicken breast in a big, heavy resealable plastic bag, and seal it, pressing out the air as you go.

- Then use any heavy, blunt implement that's handy to pound the chicken till it's ¼ inch (6 mm) thick all across. Repeat with all your chicken breasts.

- Throw your drained artichoke hearts and your cheese in your food processor, with the S-blade in place. Add the pepper, too. Pulse until the artichokes are chopped fine but not puréed.

- Spread one-quarter of the cheese mixture on each breast, and roll up jelly-roll fashion. Hold closed with toothpicks.

- Coat your large, heavy skillet with non-stick cooking spray, and put it over medium-high heat.

- When it's hot, add the butter, and swirl it around to cover the bottom of the skillet. Now add your chicken rolls, and sauté till they're lightly golden, about 3 minutes per side.

- If your skillet's handle isn't ovenproof, wrap it in foil. Slide the whole thing into the oven, and let it bake for 15 minutes, or until done through, and serve.

Chicken burgers with basil and sun-dried tomatoes

Preparation time-10 minutes |Cook time-20 minutes|Servings-3 |Difficulty-Easy

Nutritional value: Calories-345| Fat-14g|Protein-47g|Carbohydrates-5g

Ingredients

- One pound of ground chicken

- Two tablespoons of chopped dry-pack sun-dried tomatoes chopped fine

- Two tablespoons of minced onion

- One clove of garlic, minced

- One tablespoon of minced fresh basil (or one teaspoon of dried)

- One teaspoon of minced fresh oregano (or a quarter teaspoon of dried)

- One teaspoon of paprika

- Half teaspoon of salt or Vege-Sal

- A quarter teaspoon of ground black pepper

- A quarter teaspoon of cayenne

Instructions

- Just combine everything in a mixing bowl and use clean hands to mix it all together until it's well blended.

- Form into 3 patties. If you've got a little time, put them on a plate, and chill them for 30 minutes before cooking.

- Pan-broil these in a big, heavy skillet for about 5 to 6 minutes per side.

- Try topping them with mayonnaise with a little lemon juice and chopped basil stirred in.

Chicken Casserole

Preparation time-10 minutes | Cook time-30 minutes | Serving-4 | Difficulty-Moderate

Nutritional value: ~Calories-256 | Fat-8g | Protein-19g | Carbohydrates-27g

Ingredients

- Half cup of whole wheat pasta, uncooked (or one cup of cooked)

- One cup of cubed, cooked skinless chicken breast

- Two cups of frozen mixed vegetables

- One 10.5-ounce can 98% fat-free cream of chicken soup

- One cup of 2% milk reduced-fat shredded cheddar cheese

- Four ounces of canned mushrooms

- 3/4 cup of water

- Pepper, garlic powder and onion powder to taste

Instructions

- Preheat the oven to 350 degrees Fahrenheit.

- Using cooking spray, coat a 9x13 casserole dish.

- Cook pasta and vegetables according to package directions.

- Combine the chicken, soup, milk, half cup of cheese, water, cooked pasta, mushrooms, and veggies in a large mixing bowl.

- To taste, season with pepper, garlic powder, and onion powder.

- Pour the mixture into a greased casserole dish and top with the remaining cheese.

- Bake for 25 to 30 minutes, or until cheese is golden brown and bubbling.

Chicken Fajitas

Preparation time-10 minutes | Cook time-0 minutes | Serving-12 | Difficulty- Easy

Nutritional value: ~Calories-334 | Fat-9g | Protein-34g | Carbohydrates-30g

Ingredients

- One to two cloves of garlic, minced

- Half teaspoon of ground cumin

- One large onion, sliced

- Half a red sweet bell pepper, slivered

- Half cup of salsa

- A quarter cup of lime juice

- One teaspoon of chili powder

- Three pounds of boneless, skinless chicken breasts, cut in 1/4-inch strips

- Half a green sweet bell pepper, slivered

- Twelve whole-wheat 8-inch tortillas

- Half cup of fat-free sour cream

- Half cup of low-fat shredded cheese

Instructions

- In a large mixing bowl, combine the first four ingredients. Stir in the chicken slices until they are evenly covered. 15 minutes of marinating

- Cook chicken for 3 minutes in a pan on the grill or on the stovetop, or until no longer pink.

- Add the onions and peppers and mix well. Cook for 3 to 5 minutes, or until the desired doneness is reached.

- Evenly distribute the mixture among the tortillas.

- Add two tablespoons of salsa, two teaspoons sour cream, and two teaspoons shredded cheese to each tortilla. Serve with a roll-up.

Chicken in creamy horseradish sauce

Preparation time-10 minutes | Cook time-6 hours | Servings-8 | Difficulty-Hard

Nutritional value: Calories-442 | Fat-34g | Protein-30g | Carbohydrates-1g

Ingredients

- Four pounds of cut-up chicken pieces

- One tablespoon of butter

- One tablespoon of olive oil

- 3/4 cup of chicken broth

- One and a half teaspoons of chicken bouillon concentrate

- One tablespoon of prepared horseradish

- Four ounces of cream cheese

- A quarter cup of heavy cream

- Guar or xanthan (optional)

- Salt and ground black pepper, to taste

Instructions

- In your big, heavy skillet, over medium-high heat, brown the chicken in butter and olive oil. Transfer to slow cooker.

- Stir together the chicken broth, bouillon concentrate, and horseradish. Pour over the chicken. Cover the pot, set the slow cooker to low, and let cook for 6 hours.

- When time's up, fish out the chicken and put it on a platter, cut the cream cheese into chunks, and melt it into the sauce, then stir in the heavy cream. Thicken with your guar or xanthan shaker if you think it needs it.

- Season with salt and pepper to taste, and serve.

Chicken in creamy orange sauce

Preparation time-10 minutes | Cook time-6 hours | Servings-8 | Difficulty-Hard

Nutritional value: Calories~384 | Fat-24g | Protein-34g | Carbohydrates-4g

Ingredients

- Four pounds of skinless chicken thighs

- Three tablespoons of oil

- Half cup of white wine vinegar

- Half cup of lemon juice

- Three tablespoons of brandy

- One teaspoon of grated orange zest

- Half teaspoon of orange extract

- A quarter teaspoon of liquid stevia (lemon drop)

- Eight scallions, sliced

- Six ounces of cream cheese

- Salt and ground black pepper, to taste

Instructions

- In your big, heavy skillet, over medium-high heat, brown the chicken in the oil all over. Transfer to your slow cooker.

- Stir together the white wine vinegar, lemon juice, brandy, orange zest, orange extract, and stevia. Pour over the chicken.

- Cover the pot, set the slow cooker to low, and cook for 6 hours.

- When cooking time is up, transfer the chicken to a platter. Add the sliced scallions to the liquid in the pot, then add the cream cheese, cut into chunks, and stir till it's melted.

- Season with salt and pepper. Serve the sauce over the chicken.

Chicken Lettuce Wraps

Preparation time-5 minutes |Cook time-20 minutes |Serving-4 |Difficulty- Easy

Nutritional value: Calories-285| Fat-16g| Protein-22g| Carbohydrates-12g

Ingredients

- One tablespoon of coconut oil
- One pound of ground chicken
- Two tablespoons of low-sodium soy sauce
- A quarter cup of hoisin sauce
- Two tablespoons of unseasoned rice wine vinegar
- One tablespoon of sriracha
- Two teaspoons of freshly grated ginger
- Two garlic cloves, minced
- One (8-ounce) can water chestnuts, drained and diced
- Butter lettuce leaves, for serving

Instructions

- In a large skillet over medium heat, heat the coconut oil. Add the chicken, and cook thoroughly, using a spatula to break into crumbs.
- Add the soy sauce, hoisin sauce, vinegar, and sriracha. Stir to combine, and cook for 5 minutes, or until most of the liquid has been absorbed.
- Add the ginger, garlic, and water chestnuts, and cook for 1 minute.
- Scoop 2 to Three tablespoons of chicken mixture into each lettuce leaf to serve.

Chicken skewers Diavolo

Preparation time-10 minutes |Cook time-35 minutes|Servings-6 |Difficulty-Easy

Nutritional value: Calories-246| Fat-17g|Protein-22g|Carbohydrates-2g

Ingredients

- Two pounds of boneless, skinless chicken thighs
- A quarter cup of olive oil
- A quarter cup of lemon juice
- Two cloves of garlic, minced
- Two tablespoons of red pepper flakes
- Salt and ground black pepper, to taste
- Fresh parsley, for garnish, if desired
- One lemon, cut into six wedges

Instructions

- Cut your chicken into 1-inch (2.5 cm) cubes. Put them in a big resealable plastic bag. Combine the olive oil, lemon juice, garlic, red pepper flakes, and salt and pepper, and pour over the chicken. Seal the bag, pressing out the air as you go.
- Turn to coat, then throw the bag in the fridge, and let the chicken marinate for at least 4 to 5 hours, and all day won't hurt a bit.
- If you're going to use bamboo skewers, put them in water to soak 30 minutes before cooking time.
- When the cooking time comes, preheat your grill pour off the marinade into a dish and reserve.
- Thread the chicken chunks onto 6 skewers. You can now grill them or broil them for about 8 minutes, or until done through (cut into a chunk to see), often basting with the reserved marinade —but stop basting with at least a couple of minutes cooking time to go, to be sure all the raw chicken germs are killed.
- Garnish each skewer with a little minced parsley, if using, and serve with a lemon wedge to squeeze over it.

Classic Slow Cooker Pulled Pork

Preparation time-5 minutes |Cook time-6 hours |Serving-8 |Difficulty- Hard

Nutritional value: Calories-562| Fat-34g| Protein-58g| Carbohydrates-2g

Ingredients

- One onion, peeled and cut into thick rings
- One (4-pound) pork shoulder, trimmed
- One tablespoon of salt
- One teaspoon of freshly ground black pepper
- One teaspoon of garlic powder
- One teaspoon of onion powder
- One tablespoon of paprika
- Two tablespoons of extra-virgin olive oil

Instructions

- Cover the bottom of a 4- to 6-quart slow cooker with the onion slices, and place the pork on top.
- In a small bowl combine the pepper, salt, garlic powder, onion powder, paprika, and olive oil. Rub the mixture over the pork.
- Cook on high for 4 to 6 hours or on low for 7 to 8 hours, or until tender. Discard the excess fat and onions. Shred the pork with two forks, and serve with your favorite sauce.

Cranberry-peach turkey roast

Preparation time-10 minutes |Cook time-7 hours|Servings-8 |Difficulty-Hard

Nutritional value: Calories-255 | Fat-8g|Protein-31g|Carbohydrates-1g

Ingredients

- Three pounds of turkey roast
- Two tablespoons of oil—light olive oil or MCT oil
- One cup of cranberries
- Half cup of chopped onion
- A quarter cup of erythritol
- Three tablespoons of spicy mustard
- A quarter teaspoon of red pepper flakes
- One peach, peeled and chopped

Instructions

- If your turkey roast is like mine (a Butterball), it will be a boneless affair of light and dark meat rolled into an oval roast, enclosed in a net sack. Leave it in the net for cooking, so it doesn't fall apart on you.
- Heat the oil in your big, heavy skillet, and brown the turkey roast on all sides. Transfer it to a slow cooker.
- Put the cranberries, onion, erythritol, mustard, red pepper flakes, and chopped peach in your blender or in your food processor with the S-blade in place. Run it until you have a coarse puree. Pour this over the roast.
- Cover the slow cooker, set it to low, and let it cook for 6 to 7 hours.
- Remove the roast to a platter and stir up the sauce.
- Transfer the sauce to a sauceboat to serve with the turkey. You can remove the net from the turkey before serving if you like, but it's recommended to just use a good sharp knife to slice clear through the netting and let each diner remove his or her own.

Creamy chicken and noodles in a bowl

Preparation time-10 minutes |Cook time-25 minutes|Servings-1 |Difficulty-Easy

Nutritional value: Calories-285 | Fat-22g|Protein-16g|Carbohydrates-5g

Ingredients

- One package (Eight ounces) tofu shirataki, fettuccini width
- A quarter cup of jarred roasted red peppers
- Five kalamata olives
- One scallion
- One tablespoon of minced fresh parsley
- Three tablespoons of chive- and onion cream cheese
- Three ounces of precooked chicken breast strips
- Salt and ground black pepper, to taste

Instructions

- Snip open the packet of shirataki, drain and rinse them, and throw them in a microwavable bowl. Nuke them on high for 2 minutes.
- While that's happening, drain and dice your roasted red peppers.
- When the microwave beeps, drain the shirataki again. Put them back in for another 2 minutes.
- Pit your kalamatas—just squish them with your thumb and pick the pits out—then chop them up. Slice your scallion, including the crisp part of the green, and chop your parsley, too.
- Drain your noodles one last time. Now add the cream cheese and chicken breast strips and nuke the mixture for just 30 more seconds.
- When it comes out, throw in the peppers, olives, scallions, and parsley. Stir it up until the cheese melts, season with salt and pepper to taste, and devour!

Creamy Slow Cooker Chicken

Preparation time-10 minutes |Cook time-5 hours |Serving-6 |Difficulty-Hard

Nutritional value: ~Calories-128| Fat-1.6g| Protein-18.5g| Carbohydrates-3g

Ingredients

- Half cup of chicken stock
- One (0.7-ounce) pack of Italian dressing mix
- One 8-ounce package of mushrooms
- Six boneless and skinless chicken breasts (2 1/2 pounds)
- One cup of plain Greek yogurt or pureed cottage cheese
- One to ¾-ounce of reduced-fat cream of mushroom soup
- Cooking spray

Instructions

- Using frying spray, coat a big skillet. Cook chicken in batches for 2-3 minutes on each side over medium-high heat or until lightly browned. Place the chicken in a 5-quart slow cooker.
- In a skillet, combine the soup, cottage cheese or yogurt, chicken stock, and Italian dressing mix. Cook 2 to 3 minutes over medium heat, stirring regularly until cheese is melted and mixture is smooth.
- Place mushrooms on top of the chicken in the slow cooker. Pour the soup over the mushrooms. Cook for 4 hours on low, covered. Before serving, give it a good stir.
- To prepare ahead of time: Follow the recipe's instructions. Allow it cool completely before transferring to a 13 x 9-inch baking dish. Freeze for up to a month in advance. Refrigerate for 8 to 24 hours to thaw.

- To reheat, wrap firmly in aluminum foil and bake for 45 minutes at 325° F. Remove the top and bake for another 15 minutes, or until well heated.

Easy Chicken Tetrazzini

Preparation time-10 minutes | Cook time-30 minutes | Serving-6 | Difficulty-Moderate

Nutritional value: ~Calories-167 | Fat-3g | Protein-10g | Carbohydrates-25g

Ingredients

- One tablespoon of reduced-calorie margarine
- Half cup of scallions, chopped (about 5 scallions)
- Eight ounces of mushrooms, sliced
- Three tablespoons of all-purpose flour
- A quarter teaspoon of garlic powder
- 1/8 teaspoon of black pepper
- One cup of fat-free chicken broth
- Half cup of fat-free skim milk
- Half pound of cooked, boneless, skinless chicken breasts, cubed
- A quarter cup of canned pimentos, drained and sliced (about equal to a 2 oz. jar)
- Two tablespoons of sherry cooking wine
- Three and a half tablespoons of grated parmesan cheese
- Eight ounces of uncooked spaghetti, broken into thirds and cooked

Instructions

- In a large saucepan over medium-high heat, melt margarine. Cook, occasionally stirring, until the scallions and mushrooms are soft, about 5 minutes.
- In a small mixing bowl, combine flour, broth, garlic powder, pepper, and milk. Mix until everything is well combined.
- Toss the flour mixture into the pot. Cook, stirring regularly until the mixture boils and thickens about 10 minutes.
- Combine the pimentos, chicken, and sherry in a mixing bowl. Cook for about 2 minutes, stirring periodically, until well cooked.
- Toss in the cheese and cook pasta slowly.

Easy Italian beef

Preparation time-10 minutes | Cook time-8 hours | Servings-6 | Difficulty-Hard

Nutritional value: Calories-364 | Fat-28g | Protein-25g | Carbohydrates-1g

Ingredients

- Two pounds of beef chuck
- Two tablespoons of olive oil
- Half cup of beef broth
- One tablespoon of beef bouillon concentrate
- 3/4 teaspoon of lemon pepper
- Half teaspoon of dried oregano
- Half teaspoon of garlic powder
- A quarter teaspoon of onion powder
- Twelve drops of liquid stevia
- Salt and ground black pepper, to taste

Instructions

- Trim the beef of all outside fat. Heat the oil in your big, heavy skillet over medium-high heat, and brown the beef on both sides. Transfer it to your slow cooker.
- In the skillet, mix together everything else but the final salt and pepper, scraping up the nice brown stuff, so it dissolves.
- Pour this over the beef, cover the pot, and set the slow cooker to low. Cook for 6 to 8 hours.
- When cooking time is up, season with salt and pepper to taste.

Egg Roll Bowl

Preparation time-5 minutes | Cook time-20 minutes | Serving-4 | Difficulty- Easy

Nutritional value: Calories-482 | Fat-37g | Protein-28g | Carbohydrates-10g

Ingredients

- Tw0 garlic cloves, minced
- Two teaspoons of freshly grated ginger
- One tablespoon of toasted sesame oil
- One tablespoon of unseasoned rice vinegar
- Two tablespoons of low-sodium soy sauce
- One pound of ground pork
- One (14-ounce) bag coleslaw mix
- Four scallions, chopped

Instructions

- In a small bowl, mix the garlic, ginger, oil, rice vinegar, and soy sauce.
- In a large skillet over medium heat, cook the pork until browned, about 15 minutes. Drain off the excess fat. Add the coleslaw mix, and stir to combine.
- Pour the sauce mixture over the pork mixture and stir, continuing to cook over medium heat until the cabbage is wilted but still a bit crunchy, about 5 minutes.

- Serve with the scallions.

Faux Fried Chicken

Preparation time-10 minutes | Cook time-0 minutes | Serving-3 | Difficulty- Easy

Nutritional value: Calories-210 | Fat-3.5g | Protein-29g | Carbohydrates-17g

Ingredients

- 1/8 teaspoon of paprika
- 1/3 cup of bran cereal
- One tablespoon of dry onion soup mix
- 1/3 cup of reduced-fat buttermilk
- Twelve ounces of raw boneless skinless lean chicken breast tenders (about 10 pieces)
- 1/3 cup of panko breadcrumbs
- Salt, to taste

Instructions

- Combine buttermilk and paprika in a big sealable container or plastic bag and stir thoroughly.
- Coat the bird fully. Refrigerate for at least 1 hour after sealing.
- Preheat the oven to 375 degrees Fahrenheit.
- Spray a large baking sheet with nonstick cooking spray. Remove from the equation.
- Grind cereal to a breadcrumb consistency in a blender or food processor. Fill a large mixing basin halfway with crumbs.
- Combine panko breadcrumbs and onion soup mix in a mixing bowl. Add a dash or two of salt if desired. Make a thorough mix.
- Remove each piece of chicken from the container/bag one at a time, shake it to remove any excess buttermilk, then coat it equally with the crumb mixture and place it flat on the baking sheet.
- Preheat the oven to 350°F and bake for 10 minutes. Cook for an additional 10 minutes, or until the outsides are crispy and the chicken is cooked through, flipping gently (tongs work great!).

Golden triangle chicken kabobs

Preparation time-10 minutes | Cook time-25 minutes | Servings-4 | Difficulty-Easy

Nutritional value: Calories-210 | Fat-3g | Protein-40g | Carbohydrates-3g

Ingredients

- One and a half pounds boneless, skinless chicken thighs
- Two tablespoons of lemon juice
- One tablespoon of lime juice
- One shallot, minced
- Five cloves of garlic, crushed
- One tablespoon of grated fresh ginger root
- Two tablespoons of soy sauce
- Three drops of liquid stevia (plain)
- One teaspoon of ground turmeric

Instructions

- Cut your chicken into 1-inch (2.5 cm) cubes. This is easier if it's somewhat frozen.
- Put your chicken cubes in a resealable plastic bag, then stir together everything else and pour it in. Seal the bag, pressing out the air as you go. Stash the bag in the fridge for at least several hours (24 hours is brilliant).
- If you're going to be using bamboo skewers, you might put them in water to soak now.
- When dinnertime rolls around, preheat your broiler, or fire up your barbecue. Pull the bag out of the fridge, pour off the marinade into a small bowl, and reserve.
- Thread your chicken cubes onto 4 skewers.
- Start your skewers grilling or broiling, giving them about 5 minutes. Baste both sides of your kabobs with that reserved marinade (discard the rest of the marinade to avoid germs), turn them over, and give them another 5 minutes, or till done through.

Grilled Tangy Balsamic Chicken Thighs

Preparation time-1 hour | Cook time-20 minutes | Serving-4 | Difficulty- Easy

Nutritional value: Calories-194 | Fat-11g | Protein-16g | Carbohydrates-10g

Ingredients

- Four boneless, skinless chicken thighs, trimmed
- One tablespoon of extra-virgin olive oil
- A quarter cup of balsamic vinegar
- A quarter cup of freshly squeezed lime juice
- Two tablespoons of brown sugar
- Half tablespoon of chili powder
- Two garlic cloves, minced
- Salt
- Freshly ground black pepper

Instructions

- In a resealable bag, combine the chicken, olive oil, vinegar, lime juice, sugar, chili powder, and garlic, season with salt and pepper to taste, and mix well. Refrigerate and marinate for at least 1 hour or overnight for best results.
- Preheat a grill or a grill pan on the stovetop to medium-high heat. Cook the chicken for 5 to 8

minutes on each side, or until cooked to an internal temperature of at least 165°F, and serve.

Gyro-Style Meatballs

Preparation time-15 minutes |Cook time-15 minutes |Serving-3 |Difficulty- Easy

Nutritional value: Calories-292| Fat-13g| Protein-34g| Carbohydrates-8g

Ingredients

- Nonstick cooking spray
- One pound of ground beef
- A quarter cup of dry Italian bread crumbs
- One large egg
- Two tablespoons of chopped fresh parsley
- One tablespoon of freshly minced garlic
- Half teaspoon of ground cumin
- Half teaspoon of sea salt
- A quarter teaspoon of freshly ground black pepper

Instructions

- Preheat the oven to 425°F. Lightly grease a baking sheet.
- In a large bowl, combine the beef, bread crumbs, egg, parsley, garlic, cumin, salt, and pepper.
- Form the mixture into 1½-inch meatballs, and place them on the prepared baking sheet. Bake for 10 to 15 minutes, or until cooked through and no longer pink inside or until they reach an internal temperature of 160°F, and serve.

Halibut with Creamy Parmesan-Dill Sauce

Preparation time-5 minutes |Cook time-20 minutes |Serving-4 |Difficulty- Easy

Nutritional value: Calories-345| Fat-12g| Protein-52g| Carbohydrates-6g

Ingredients

- Four (6-ounce) fresh halibut fillets (1-inch thick)
- Juice of half lemon
- Salt
- Freshly ground black pepper
- ⅓ cup of low-fat sour cream
- ⅓ cup of low-fat, plain Greek yogurt
- ⅓ cup of Parmesan cheese
- Half teaspoon of garlic powder
- Half teaspoon of dried dill
- Three scallions, finely chopped

Instructions

- Preheat the oven to 400°F.
- Place the halibut fillets in a large baking dish, and add the lemon juice. Season with salt and pepper to taste.
- In a small bowl, mix the sour cream, yogurt, cheese, garlic powder, dill, and scallions. Spread the mixture over the fish.
- Bake for 15 to 20 minutes, or until the internal temperature reaches 145°F, the fish is opaque and flakes easily with a fork, and the cheese is golden, and serve.

Hawaiian Pork Kabobs with Pineapple

Preparation time-30 minutes |Cook time-20 minutes |Serving-4 |Difficulty- Moderate

Nutritional value: Calories-292| Fat-15g| Protein-24g| Carbohydrates-17g

Ingredients

- A quarter cup of low-sodium soy sauce
- Three tablespoons of extra-virgin olive oil, divided
- Two garlic cloves, minced
- Salt
- Freshly ground black pepper
- One pound of pork loin, diced into 1½-inch cubes
- One and a half cups of pineapple chunks
- One white onion, peeled and chopped into 1-inch pieces
- One red bell pepper, trimmed, seeded, and cut into 1-inch pieces
- One yellow pepper, trimmed, seeded, and cut into 1-inch pieces

Instructions

- Prepare 8 to 10 wooden skewers by soaking them in water for 15 minutes to prevent burning. If you are using metal skewers, you can skip this step.
- In a large bowl, whisk the soy sauce, Two tablespoons of olive oil, garlic, and salt and pepper to taste. Add the pork chunks to the bowl, and toss to coat. Cover and chill for at least 15 minutes.
- Carefully thread the skewers with the pork, pineapple, onions, and peppers, repeating until all the ingredients are used.
- Lightly brush the pork and vegetables with the remaining tablespoon of olive oil.
- Heat the grill to high, then reduce to 400°F.
- Place the kabobs on the grill. Cook for 3 to 4 minutes, rotate and repeat until all sides are browned, and the pork is cooked through to 145°F. Serve immediately.

Honey-Mustard Pork Tenderloin with Roasted Green Beans

Preparation time-10 minutes |Cook time-30 minutes |Serving-4 |Difficulty- Moderate

Nutritional value: Calories-313| Fat-9g| Protein-36g| Carbohydrates-26g

Ingredients

- Two tablespoons of whole grain mustard
- Two tablespoons of honey
- Two tablespoons of soy sauce
- Two garlic cloves, minced
- One tablespoon of sriracha
- Salt
- Freshly ground black pepper

- One pound of fresh green beans, trimmed
- One tablespoon of extra-virgin olive oil
- One pound of trimmed pork tenderloin

Instructions

- Preheat the oven to 450°F. Line a baking sheet with aluminum foil.
- In a small bowl, mix the mustard, honey, soy sauce, garlic, and sriracha. Season with salt and pepper to taste.
- Place the green beans on the prepared baking sheet, and toss with the olive oil.
- Place the pork on top of the green beans. Rub half of the sauce on the pork evenly.
- Bake for 15 minutes, then remove from oven. Brush the remaining sauce over the pork. Return the pork to the oven and cook for another 10 to 15 minutes, or until the internal temperature of the pork is between 145 and 150°F and the meat is pale and mostly white with mostly clear juices.
- Remove from the oven and tent the pork with foil. Let rest for 10 to 15 minutes before serving.

Italian Ricotta Bake

Preparation time-5 minutes |Cook time-25 minutes |Serving-6 |Difficulty- Easy

Nutritional value: Calories-132| Fat-8g| Protein-12g| Carbohydrates-4g

Ingredients

- Eight ounces of low-fat ricotta cheese
- Half cup of grated Parmesan cheese
- One large egg, beaten
- One teaspoon of Italian seasoning
- Nonstick cooking spray
- Half cup of low-sugar marinara sauce
- Half cup of low-fat mozzarella cheese

Instructions

- Preheat the oven to 450°F.
- In a medium bowl, mix the ricotta, Parmesan, egg, and Italian seasoning until smooth.
- Spray a 9-by-9-inch baking pan with cooking spray. Spread the ricotta mixture evenly in the pan.
- Top the ricotta mixture with the marinara sauce, then sprinkle with the mozzarella.
- Bake for 20 to 25 minutes, or until the cheese is melted, and serve.

Jakarta steak

Preparation time-10 minutes |Cook time-40 minutes|Servings-6 |Difficulty-Moderate

Nutritional value: Calories~315| Fat~21g|Protein~28g|Carbohydrates~2g

Ingredients

- Two pounds of sirloin steak, trimmed, at least one and a quarter inches (3 cm) thick

- Two tablespoons of soy sauce

- One tablespoon of lime juice

- Two teaspoons of grated fresh ginger root

- One teaspoon of ground turmeric

- One teaspoon of ground black pepper

- Two cloves of garlic, crushed

- Twelve drops of liquid stevia (plain)

Instructions

- Marinate the steak in a shallow, nonreactive container—glass, microwavable plastic, or enamelware. It's easier than finding a resealable plastic bag big enough for your steak. Lay the steak in the container.

- Now mix together everything else, pour it over the steak, and turn the steak once or twice to coat both sides. Stick it in the fridge, and let it marinate for several hours-overnight is brilliant.

- You can grill this on your barbecue grill, or you can broil it. If you want to use charcoal, get it started a good 30 minutes before cooking time.

- Either way, grill or broil it close to the heat, to your desired degree of doneness, basting both sides with the marinade when you turn it.

- Let your steak rest for 5 minutes before carving and serving.

- If you like, you can boil the remaining marinade hard for a few minutes to kill germs, then spoon just a little over each serving.

Joe

Preparation time-10 minutes |Cook time-25 minutes|Servings-6 |Difficulty-Easy

Nutritional value: Calories~406| Fat~29g|Protein~29g|Carbohydrates~5g

Ingredients

- One and a half pounds ground beef

- One package of (10 ounces) frozen chopped spinach, thawed

- One medium onion

- Two cloves of garlic

- Six eggs

- Salt and ground black pepper, to taste

- 1/3 cup of shredded Parmesan cheese

Instructions

- In your large, heavy skillet over medium heat, start browning and crumbling the ground beef. While that's happening, drain the spinach well, chop the onion, and crush the garlic.

- When the ground beef is half done, add the onion and garlic, and cook until the beef is done through. Pour off the extra fat if you like. Now stir the spinach into the beef. Let the whole thing cook for maybe 5 minutes.

- Now, mix up the eggs well with a fork, and stir them into the beef mixture. Continue cooking and stirring over low heat for a couple of minutes until the eggs are set. Season with salt and pepper to taste, and serve topped with Parmesan.

Kalua pig with cabbage

Preparation time-10 minutes |Cook time-16 hours|Servings-8 |Difficulty-Hard

Nutritional value: Calories~384| Fat~27g|Protein~33g|Carbohydrates~1g

Ingredients

- Three pounds of Boston butt pork roast

- Two teaspoons of sea salt

- One tablespoon of liquid smoke flavoring

- One head cabbage

- A quarter medium onion

Instructions

- Take a carving fork, and stab your butt roast viciously all over. Do your best slasher movie imitation. You're making lots of holes to let the smoky flavor in.

- Now sprinkle the salt all over the roast, hitting every bit of the surface, and rub it in a little. Do the same with the smoke flavoring.

- Place your roast, fat-side up, in your slow cooker, cover it, set it to low, and forget about it for a good 7 to 8 hours, minimum.

- Then flip the roast, re-cover, and forget about it for another 7 to 8 hours.

- About one and a half hours before serving time, chop your cabbage fairly coarsely and mince your onion.

- Haul out your pork—it will fall apart and smell like heaven—put it in a big bowl, and shred it with a fork. Scoop out a bit of the liquid from the pot to moisten the meat if it seems to need it. Then keep it somewhere warm (or you can rewarm it later in the microwave).

- Throw the cabbage and onion in the remaining liquid and toss it to coat. Cover the pot, set the slow cooker on high, and let it cook for at least an hour—you want it wilted but still a little crunchy.

- Serve the meat and cabbage together.

Keto Lunch Jambalaya

Preparation time-10 minutes |Cook time-40 minutes|Servings-2 |Difficulty-Moderate

Nutritional value: Calories-239| Fat-12g|Protein-27g|Carbohydrates-8g

Ingredients

- One medium cauliflower
- One coarsely chopped green pepper
- Two stalks of coarsely chopped celery
- One diced small onion
- Two minced cloves of garlic
- Three cubed boneless chicken breasts
- Eight ounces of sliced smoked sausage
- Eight ounces of ham, cubed
- Fourteen and a half ounce can of diced tomatoes, undrained
- Eight ounce can of tomato sauce
- Three teaspoons of Cajun Seasoning
- Salt and pepper according to taste
- Cooking oil

Instructions

- Heat two tablespoons of oil in an 8-quart Dutch oven or skillet.
- On a medium-high flame, sauté the peppers, garlic, chicken, celery, onion and Cajun seasoning until the chicken is almost cooked.
- Add the cauliflower, ham and sausage. Mix thoroughly.
- Add the tomato sauce and tomatoes to the mix. Bring it to a simmer, and then turn it back to low.
- Cover until the cauliflower is moist but not mushy, and cook for around twenty minutes.
- Season with salt and pepper and then serve after removing from heat.

Keto Roasted Pepper and Cauliflower

Preparation time-10 minutes |Cook time-50 minutes|Servings-4 |Difficulty-Moderate

Nutritional value: Calories-223| Fat-12g|Protein-21g|Carbohydrates-15g

Ingredients

- Two halved and de-seeded Red Bell Peppers
- Half head of cauliflower cut into florets
- Two tablespoons of Duck Fat
- Three medium diced green Onions

- Three cups of Chicken Broth
- Half cup Heavy Cream
- Four tablespoons of Duck Fat
- Salt and pepper as per taste
- One teaspoon of Garlic Powder
- One teaspoon of Dried Thyme
- One teaspoon of Smoked Paprika
- A quarter teaspoon of Red Pepper Flakes
- Four oz. Goat Cheese

Instructions

- Preheat the oven to 400 °F
- Clean, de-seed, and half-slice the peppers
- Broil until the flesh is burnt and blackened for about 10-15 minutes.
- Place in a container with a cover to steam when finished cooking cauliflower.
- Sprinkle two tablespoons of melted duck fat, pepper and salt into sliced cauliflower florets.
- Cook for 30-35 minutes in the oven.
- Pick off the skins of the peppers by gently peeling them off.
- Heat Four tablespoons of duck fat in a pot and add the diced green onion.
- To toast, apply seasonings to the plate, then add red pepper, chicken broth, and cauliflower to the skillet.
- For 10-20 minutes, let this boil.
- Bring the mixture to an immersion blender. Make sure that it emulsifies both fats.
- Then apply the cream and combine.
- Serve with some bacon and goats' cheese. Add thyme and green onion to garnish.

Lamb steaks with lemon, olives, and capers

Preparation time-10 minutes |Cook time-30 minutes|Servings-4 |Difficulty-Easy

Nutritional value: Calories-343| Fat-26g|Protein-24g|Carbohydrates-1g

Ingredients

- One and a half pounds leg of lamb in steaks, 3/4 inch (2 cm) thick
- Two teaspoons of olive oil
- One tablespoon of lemon juice
- A quarter cup of chopped kalamata olives
- Two teaspoons of capers

- One clove of garlic

- Salt and ground black pepper, to taste

Instructions

- Coat your large, heavy skillet with non-stick cooking spray and put it over medium-high heat. While it's heating, slash the edges of your lamb steaks to keep them from curling. When the skillet's hot, add the oil and throw in the steaks. You want to sear them on both sides.

- When your steaks are browned on both sides, add the lemon juice, olives, capers, and garlic around and over the steaks.

- Let the whole thing cook another minute or two, but don't overcook—the lamb should still be pink in the middle.

- Season the steaks with salt and pepper, carve them into 4 portions, and serve with all the yummy lemon-caper-olive mixture from the skillet scraped over them.

Lamb, feta, and spinach burgers

Preparation time-10 minutes |Cook time-15 minutes|Servings-6 |Difficulty-Easy

Nutritional value: Calories-352| Fat-28g|Protein-20g|Carbohydrates-5g

Ingredients

- One package of (10 ounces) frozen chopped spinach, thawed and drained

- A quarter cup of minced onion

- One tablespoon of lemon juice

- One teaspoon of dried basil

- A quarter teaspoon of salt or Vege-Sal

- A quarter teaspoon of ground black pepper

- One egg

- One clove of garlic, minced fine

- One and a quarter pounds of ground lamb

- Half cup of crumbled feta cheese

- A quarter cup of chopped sun-dried tomatoes

- Twelve kalamata olives, pitted and chopped

Instructions

- Make sure your spinach is well drained—put in a strainer and then squeeze it with clean hands.

- Transfer it to a big bowl, and add the onion, lemon juice, basil, salt, pepper, egg, and garlic. Stir it all up until it's well blended.

- Now add the lamb, feta, tomatoes, and olives. Use clean hands to mix everything until it's really well combined.

- Make 6 burgers, keeping them at least 1 inch (2.5 cm) thick. Refrigerate them for at least 20 to 30 minutes before cooking.

- Preheat your electric tabletop grill. Slap the burgers on the grill, and give them 6 to 8 minutes, depending on how well done you want them.

- Cook to desired doneness and serve.

Lemon-broiled Orange Roughy

Preparation time-10 minutes |Cook time-0 minutes |Serving-4 |Difficulty- Easy

Nutritional value: Calories-144| Fat-4g| Protein-17g| Carbohydrates-3g

Ingredients

- Three tablespoons of lemon juice

- One tablespoon of Dijon mustard

- One tablespoon of olive oil

- A quarter teaspoon of ground pepper

- Sixteen ounces of orange roughy fillets (4 ounces each)

- Eight medium lemon wedges

Instructions

- Using tin foil, cover the rack of a broiler pan or a baking sheet with cooking spray.

- Stir together the mustard, lemon juice, olive oil, and ground pepper.

- Place the fillets of fish on a rack or baking sheet.

- Brush half of the lemon juice mixture over the fillets, reserving the other half.

- Broil the fish for 5 minutes or until it readily flakes.

- Drizzle the fillets with the reserved lemon juice mixture and season with pepper to taste. Serve with lemon slices on the side.

Lemon Dill Trout

Preparation time-10 minutes |Cook time-20 minutes|Servings-4 |Difficulty-Easy

Nutritional value: Calories-219| Fat-13g|Protein-26g|Carbohydrates-3g

Ingredients

- Two pounds of pan-dressed trout (or other small fish), fresh or frozen

- One and a half teaspoons of salt

- A quarter teaspoon of pepper

- Half cup of butter or margarine

- Two tablespoons of dill weed

- Three tablespoons of lemon juice

Instructions

- Cut fish lengthwise and season its inside with pepper and salt.

- With melted butter and dill weed, prepare a frying pan.

- For about two to three minutes per side, fry the fish flesh side down.

- Remove the fish.

- Add lemon juice to butter and dill to create a sauce.

- Serve the fish and sauce together.

Lemon-herb chicken breast

Preparation time-10 minutes | Cook time-30 minutes | Servings-3 | Difficulty-Easy

Nutritional value: Calories-508 | Fat-40g | Protein-34g | Carbohydrates-5g

Ingredients

- Two cloves of garlic, crushed

- Half cup of olive oil

- One pound of boneless, skinless chicken breast

- Salt and ground black pepper, to taste

- One lemon

- Two tablespoons of water

- A quarter cup of minced fresh basil

- Two tablespoons of minced fresh parsley

Instructions

- Put the garlic in a measuring cup and pour the olive oil over it. Let it sit.

- Give a skillet a squirt of non-stick cooking spray and put it over a high burner.

- Now grab your chicken and a blunt, heavy object and pound your breast out to an even Half-inch (1 cm) thickness. Cut into 3 portions and season with salt and pepper on both sides.

- Pour half of the garlicky olive oil into your now-hot skillet, swirl it around, and throw in your chicken. Cover it with a tilted lid—leave a crack—and let it cook for 3 to 4 minutes.

- Your chicken should be golden on the bottom now; flip it! Re-cover with the tilted lid and give it another 3 to 4 minutes.

- In the meantime, roll your lemon under your palm, pressing down firmly. This will help it render more juice. Slice your lemon in half and flick out the seeds with the tip of a knife.

- When your chicken is golden on both sides, squeeze one of the lemon halves over it. Flip it to coat both sides, turn the burner down to medium-low, and re-cover with that tilted lid. Let it cook until it's done through.

- Plate your chicken and then add the water and the juice of the other lemon half to the skillet.

- Stir it all around with a fork, scraping up the tasty brown bits, and then pour this over the chicken.

- Top with the herbs and a drizzle of the remaining garlic olive oil, and then serve.

Low-fat Turkey Gravy

Preparation time-10 minutes | Cook time-20 minutes | Serving-8 | Difficulty- Easy

Nutritional value: ~Calories-35 | Fat-1g | Protein-2g | Carbohydrates-5g

Ingredients

- Four cups (32 fluid ounces) of unsalted turkey stock, divided

- Two tablespoons of fresh sage, remove from stem and finely chop

- Two tablespoons of fresh thyme, remove from stem and finely chop

- One cup of (8 fluid ounces) skim milk

- A quarter cup of cornstarch

Instructions

- Place the roasting pan on the stovetop over medium heat after the turkey has finished roasting. Stir in two cups turkey stock for 5 minutes, or until the drippings and browned pieces from the bottom dissolve. Over a fat separator cup, place a strainer. Strain the drippings from the pan. To make 4 cups of stock, add enough stock to the drippings.

- If you don't have a fat separator cup, you can extract fat from drippings by freezing the liquid with numerous ice cubes for ten minutes. With a spoon, scrape off the hardened fat and transfer the stock to a saucepan. There should be roughly 4 cups of liquid left. Bring the saucepan to a low simmer on the stovetop over medium heat. Simmer the stock with sage and thyme. Continue to cook until the stock has been reduced by 1/4, or until there are about 3 cups left.

- Fill a small bowl halfway with milk. Stir in the cornstarch until it is equally distributed. Slowly pour the milk mixture into the stock that is simmering, stirring constantly. Bring the sauce to a boil, then keep stirring until the stock thickens and shines for about 3 to 5 minutes.

- Serve the gravy in a warmed gravy boat.

Lunch Stuffed Peppers

Preparation time-10 minutes |Cook time-50 minutes|Servings-4 |Difficulty-Moderate

Nutritional value: Calories-220| Fat-8g|Protein-16g|Carbohydrates-18g

Ingredients

- Four big banana peppers cut into halves lengthwise
- One tablespoon of ghee
- Salt and black pepper to the taste
- Half teaspoon of herbs de Provence
- One pound of chopped sweet sausage
- Three tablespoons of chopped yellow onions
- Some marinara sauce
- A drizzle of olive oil

Instructions

- Season the banana peppers with pepper and salt, drizzle with the oil, rub well and bake for 20 minutes in the oven at 325 ° F.

- Meanwhile, over medium, prepare, heat a skillet, add the pieces of sausage, mix and cook for 5 minutes.

- Combine the onion, herbs, salt, pepper and ghee, mix well and simmer for 5 minutes.

- Take the peppers out of the oven, load them with the sausage mix, place them in a dish that is oven-proof, drizzle them with the marinara sauce, place them back in the oven and bake for another 10 minutes.

- Serve and enjoy.

Lunch Tacos

Preparation time-10 minutes |Cook time-40 minutes|Servings-3 |Difficulty-Moderate

Nutritional value: Calories-223| Fat-10g|Protein-26g|Carbohydrates-7g

Ingredients

- Two cups of grated cheddar cheese
- One small pitted, peeled and chopped avocado
- One cup of cooked favorite taco meat
- Two teaspoons of sriracha sauce
- A quarter cup of chopped tomatoes
- Cooking spray
- Salt and black pepper as per taste

Instructions

- Spray on a lined baking dish with some cooking oil.

- Cover on the baking sheet with cheddar cheese put in the oven at 400 degrees F, and bake for 15 minutes.

- Spread the taco meat over the cheese and cook for a further 10 minutes.

- Meanwhile, combine the avocado with tomatoes, sriracha, salt and pepper in a bowl and swirl.

- Spread this over the layers of taco and cheddar, let the tacos cool down a little, use a pizza slicer to slice and serve for lunch.

Mahi-Mahi with Mango-Avocado Salsa

Preparation time-10 minutes |Cook time-10 minutes |Serving-4 |Difficulty- Easy

Nutritional value: Calories-232| Fat-10g| Protein-28g| Carbohydrates-8g

Ingredients

- Four (4-ounce) mahi-mahi fillets
- Two tablespoons of extra-virgin olive oil
- One tablespoon of ground cumin
- One teaspoon of chili powder
- Half teaspoon of onion powder
- Salt
- Half cup of diced mango
- A quarter cup of diced avocado
- A quarter cup of finely chopped red onion
- ⅓ cup of diced cherry tomatoes
- Two tablespoons of finely chopped fresh cilantro
- Two tablespoons of freshly squeezed lime juice

- One teaspoon of minced jalapeño

Instructions

- Preheat the grill to medium heat. Set the mahi-mahi fillets on a plate, and drizzle with the olive oil. Rub to coat.

- In a small bowl, mix together the cumin, chili powder, onion powder, and salt to taste. Rub the seasonings over each fillet.

- In a small bowl, stir to combine the mango, avocado, onion, tomatoes, cilantro, lime juice, jalapeño, and salt to taste. Refrigerate until serving.

- Place the mahi-mahi on the grill. Cook for 3 to 4 minutes, then gently turn over and cook for 3 to 4 minutes longer, until the fish is opaque and flakes easily with a fork.

- Serve the mahi-mahi with the salsa.

Maple-chipotle glazed pork steaks

Preparation time-10 minutes | Cook time-18 minutes | Servings-4 | Difficulty-Easy

Nutritional value: Calories-412 | Fat-31g | Protein-32g | Carbohydrates-1g

Ingredients

- Two pounds of pork shoulder steaks or pork chops, no more than half an inch (1 cm) thick

- One tablespoon of bacon grease or coconut oil

- A quarter cup of erythritol

- Two teaspoons of spicy brown mustard

- Three chipotle chiles canned in adobo with one and a half teaspoons of the sauce

- Two cloves of garlic, crushed

Six drops of maple extract

Instructions

- Put your large, heavy skillet over medium-high heat and start the pork steaks browning in the bacon grease.

- Throw everything else in your blender or food processor and run until the chipotles and garlic are pulverized.

- When your steaks are browned on both sides, add the glaze to the skillet and flip the steaks to coat on both sides. Cover with a tilted lid and let it cook until the steaks are done through and the glaze has cooked down a little—probably 10 minutes.

- Serve, scraping all the glaze from the skillet over the steaks.

Maple-spice country-style ribs

Preparation time-10 minutes | Cook time-9 hours | Servings-6 | Difficulty-Hard

Nutritional value: Calories-383 | Fat-29g | Protein-27g | Carbohydrates-2g

Ingredients

- Three pounds of country-style pork ribs

- 2/3 cup of erythritol

- A quarter cup of chopped onion

- A quarter cup of chicken broth

- Two tablespoons of (28 ml) soy sauce

- Half teaspoon of ground cinnamon

- Half teaspoon of ground ginger

- Half teaspoon of ground allspice

- A quarter teaspoon of ground black pepper

- 1/8 teaspoon of cayenne

- 1/8 teaspoon of maple extract

- Three cloves of garlic, crushed

Instructions

- Put the country-style ribs in your slow cooker.

- Mix together everything else, and pour over the ribs.

- Cover, and cook on low for 9 hours.

Meatza

Preparation time-10 minutes | Cook time-30 minutes | Servings-6 | Difficulty-Easy

Nutritional value: Calories-527 | Fat-44g | Protein-27g | Carbohydrates-5g

Ingredients

- 3/4 pound of ground beef

- 3/4 pound of Italian sausage

- 1/3 cup of minced onion

- Two teaspoons of Italian seasoning or dried oregano

- One clove of garlic, crushed

- One cup of no-sugar-added pizza sauce

- Three tablespoons of grated Parmesan or Romano cheese (optional)

- Eight ounces of shredded mozzarella cheese

Instructions

- Preheat oven to 350°F.

- In a large bowl, with clean hands, combine the beef and sausage with the onion, Italian seasoning, and garlic. Mix well.

- Pat this out in an even layer in a 9 × 12-inch (23 × 30 cm) baking pan. Bake for 20 minutes.

- When the meat comes out, it will have shrunk a fair amount because of the grease cooking off. Pour off the grease.

- Spread the pizza sauce over the meat. Sprinkle the Parmesan on the sauce, if you like, and then distribute the shredded mozzarella evenly over the top. Set your broiler to high.

- Put your Meatza 4 inches (10 cm) below the broiler.

- Broil for about 5 minutes, or until the cheese is melted and starting to brown.

Mediterranean lamb burgers

Preparation time-10 minutes | Cook time-20 minutes | Servings-3 | Difficulty-Easy

Nutritional value: Calories~578 | Fat-47g | Protein-33g | Carbohydrates-4g

Ingredients

- A quarter medium onion

- Two tablespoons of chopped sun-dried tomatoes

- One pound of ground lamb

- One tablespoon of pesto sauce

- One tablespoon of chopped garlic

Half teaspoon of salt or Vege-Sal

- A quarter teaspoon of ground black pepper

- Two tablespoons of pine nuts

- Three ounces of chèvre (goat cheese)

Instructions

- Preheat your electric tabletop grill to 350°F (180°C).

- Chop your onion, and if your sun-dried tomatoes are in halves rather than prechopped, chop them up, too. Heck, even if they're prechopped, chop them a little more. Throw these things in a mixing bowl.

- Add the ground lamb, pesto, garlic, salt, and pepper. Use clean hands to squish it all together until it's well mixed.

- Form into 3 patties and throw them on the grill. Set a timer for 5 minutes.

- While the burgers are cooking, toast your pine nuts in a dry skillet until they're touched with gold.

- When your burgers are done, plate them, crumble an ounce of chèvre over each one, sprinkle with pine nuts, and then serve.

Middle eastern marinated lamb kabobs

Preparation time-20 minutes | Cook time-20 minutes | Servings-4 | Difficulty-Moderate

Nutritional value: Calories~290 | Fat-20g | Protein-24g | Carbohydrates-5g

Ingredients

- One pound of boneless leg of lamb, cubed

- A quarter cup of olive oil

- A quarter cup of lemon juice

- Four cloves of garlic, minced fine

- One medium onion

- Salt and ground black pepper, to taste

Instructions

- Put your lamb cubes in a big resealable plastic bag. Mix together the olive oil, lemon juice, and garlic and pour over the lamb. Seal the bag, pressing out the air as you go.

- Turn the bag once or twice to coat, and throw it in the fridge for several hours.

- If you plan to use bamboo skewers, put them in water to soak about 30 minutes before cooking time.

- If you want to cook them over charcoal—get your fire going a good 30 minutes before you want to cook.

- When dinner rolls around, cut your onion into chunks, and separate into individual layers. Pull out your lamb cubes, and pour off the marinade into a dish.

- Thread the lamb cubes onto 4 skewers. Alternate your lamb chunks with pieces of onion.

- Keep it compact, with stuff touching, not strung out. When the skewers are full and all the lamb and onion are used up, sprinkle your kabobs with a little salt and pepper.

- Now grill or broil, occasionally basting with the reserved marinade, for 8 to 10 minutes or until done to your liking.

- Stop basting with 3 to 4 minutes to go to make sure any of the raw meat germs in the marinade get killed. Serve 1 skewer per person.

Mom's Turkey Meatloaf

Preparation time-10 minutes | Cook time-1 hour | Serving-4 | Difficulty- Hard

Nutritional value: Calories-258 | Fat-10g | Protein-25g | Carbohydrates-17g

Ingredients

- A quarter cup plus Two tablespoons of ketchup, divided

- Two teaspoons of Worcestershire sauce

- One pound of lean ground turkey

- Half medium onion, minced

- One garlic clove

- Half cup of old-fashioned rolled oats

- One large egg

- One tablespoon of Italian seasoning

- Half teaspoon of salt

- A quarter teaspoon of freshly ground black pepper

- Nonstick cooking spray

Instructions

- Preheat the oven to 350°F.

- In a small bowl, combine Two tablespoons of ketchup and the Worcestershire sauce.

- In a medium bowl, combine the turkey, onion, garlic, oats, egg, the remaining A quarter cup of ketchup, and the Italian seasoning, salt, and pepper. Make sure not to overwork the meat.

- Place the mixture in a greased loaf pan or shape into a loaf and place on a baking pan. Spoon the sauce on top.

- Bake uncovered for 55 to 60 minutes, or until an instant-read thermometer registers 165°F.

- Remove from the oven and allow to sit for 5 minutes before slicing and serving.

Mustard-grilled pork with balsamic onions

Preparation time-10 minutes |Cook time-15 minutes|Servings-4 |Difficulty-Easy

Nutritional value: Calories-369| Fat-29g|Protein-29g|Carbohydrates-4g

Ingredients

- Two tablespoons of brown mustard, divided

- One and a half pounds boneless pork shoulder steaks (4 steaks, about half an inch [1 cm] thick)

- One large red onion, sliced thin

- One and a half tablespoons of olive oil

- One tablespoon of balsamic vinegar

Instructions

- Preheat your electric tabletop grill. Spread two teaspoons of mustard on one side of the pork steaks, flip them, and spread another two teaspoons on the other side. Grill for about 5 minutes, or until done through.

- While that's happening, put your big, heavy skillet over medium-high heat, and start sautéing the onion in the olive oil.

- Forget about tender-crisp—you want your onion soft and turning brown. When good and caramelized, stir in the balsamic vinegar. Set aside.

- By now, your pork is done. Spread the remaining two teaspoons of mustard on the pork (an extra half teaspoon on each piece), divide the balsamic-onions mixture among the steaks, and serve

Mustard-maple glazed pork steak

Preparation time-10 minutes |Cook time-35 minutes|Servings-4 |Difficulty-Easy

Nutritional value: Calories-437 | Fat-32g|Protein-30g|Carbohydrates-1g

Ingredients

- Two pounds of pork shoulder steaks, no more than half an inch (1 cm) thick

- Salt and ground black pepper, to taste

- One tablespoon of olive oil

- A quarter cup of chicken broth or a quarter teaspoon of chicken bouillon concentrate dissolved in a quarter cup of water

- One tablespoon of erythritol

- One tablespoon of spicy brown or Dijon mustard

- Five drops of maple extract

Instructions

- Give your large, heavy skillet a shot of non-stick cooking spray and start it heating over high heat while you season the pork steaks with salt and pepper.

- In a minute or so, add the olive oil, swirl it around to coat the pan, and throw in your steaks.

- Cover them with a tilted lid.

- Mix together everything else and place by the stove.

- After about 5 minutes, flip your pork steaks and let them cook on the other side, again with a tilted lid.

- When your pork steaks are almost done through, transfer them to a plate.

- Pour the mustard-maple mixture into the pan and stir it around, scraping up any tasty brown bits. Let it boil hard until it cooks down by about half.

- Put the steaks back in, flip them to coat, and let the whole thing keep cooking just a minute more until the sauce is the consistency of half-and-half.

- Plate the steaks, pour the sauce over them, and serve.

New England chicken

Preparation time-5 minutes |Cook time-35 minutes |Serving-4 |Difficulty- Easy

Nutritional value: ~ Calories-284| Fat-12g| Protein-24g| Carbohydrates-8g

Ingredients

- Four cups of cubed or shredded cooked boneless, skinless chicken breasts (about 4 chicken breasts)

- Two cans of low-fat cream of chicken soup 1 cup 0% fat Greek yogurt

- Two carrots, grated

- One cup of corn kernels (fresh or frozen)

- Half sweet onion, chopped finely

- Half teaspoon of kosher salt

- One cup of whole-wheat panko breadcrumbs

- Half teaspoon of garlic powder

- Half cup of sliced almonds

Instructions

- Heat oven to 350 F.

- Mix garlic powder into breadcrumbs and set aside.

- In a medium bowl, combine the first seven ingredients until well-mixed. Spray a 9x13 inch pan with nonstick cooking spray. Pour all of the chicken mixtures into the pan. Cover chicken with breadcrumbs.

- Sprinkle almonds on top and bake for 30 minutes, or until bubbly and toasty!

One-Pan Chicken Piccata

Preparation time-15 minutes | Cook time-15 minutes | Serving-4 | Difficulty- Easy

Nutritional value: Calories-227| Fat-15g| Protein-14g| Carbohydrates-13g

Ingredients

- Half cup of flour

- Half teaspoon of salt

- Half teaspoon of freshly ground black pepper

- Two boneless, skinless chicken breasts, butterflied then cut in half

- One to three tablespoons of extra-virgin olive oil, divided

- Half cup of reduced-sodium chicken broth

- A quarter cup of freshly squeezed lemon juice

- Two tablespoons of drained capers

- One tablespoon of unsalted butter

- Freshly chopped parsley for garnish (optional)

Instructions

- In a shallow bowl, mix the flour, salt, and pepper. Dredge the chicken cutlets in the flour mixture, and shake off the excess.

- In a large skillet over medium heat, heat one tablespoon of oil. Add the chicken, cooking in batches if needed to avoid overcrowding and adding more oil as needed. Cook for 2 to 4 minutes on each side, or until the chicken is no longer pink in the center. Transfer to a plate.

- In the same pan, combine the chicken broth, lemon juice, capers, and butter. Whisk until the butter melts and the liquids are well combined, scraping up any brown bits from the pan in the process.

- Return the chicken to the pan, reduce the heat to simmer, and cook for 5 minutes, or until the chicken reaches an internal temperature of 165°F and any juices run clear.

- Transfer the chicken to a rimmed serving platter. Pour the sauce over the chicken, garnish with the parsley (if desired), and serve.

Oven-Baked Chicken Tenders

Preparation time-10 minutes | Cook time-20 minutes | Serving-4 | Difficulty- Easy

Nutritional value: Calories-212| Fat-6g| Protein-32g| Carbohydrates-8g

Ingredients

- Nonstick cooking spray

- Half cup of grated Parmesan cheese

- Half cup of whole wheat panko bread crumbs

- A quarter teaspoon of ground cayenne pepper

- One teaspoon of garlic powder

- Salt

- Freshly ground black pepper

- One pound of skinless chicken breast tenders

- One large egg, beaten

Instructions

- Preheat oven to 400°F.

- Place an oven-safe wire rack on top of a baking sheet, and spray with cooking spray. Set aside. (If you do not have a wire rack, use an aluminum foil– or parchment paper-lined baking sheet.)

- In a small bowl, mix the cheese, bread crumbs, cayenne pepper, garlic powder, and salt and pepper to taste.

- Dip the chicken tenders in the egg, coat with the dry mixture, then transfer to the prepared wire rack/baking sheet. Repeat the process with the remaining chicken.

- Bake for 15 to 20 minutes, depending on the size of the tenders, or until the tenders reach an internal temperature of 165°F.

Pan-broiled steak

Preparation time-10 minutes | Cook time-30 minutes | Servings-4 | Difficulty-Easy

Nutritional value: Calories-403| Fat-33g|Protein-24g|Carbohydrates-0g

Ingredients

- One and a half pounds steak, 1 inch (2.5 cm) thick— preferably rib eye, T-bone, sirloin, or strip

- One tablespoon of bacon grease or olive oil

Instructions

- Put your large, heavy skillet—cast iron is best—over the highest heat and let it get good and hot.

- In the meantime, you can season your steak if you like (Montreal steak seasoning). Instead, you could top the finished steak with salt and pepper.

- When the skillet's hot, add the bacon grease or oil, swirl it around, and then throw in your steak.

- Set a timer for 5 or 6 minutes—your timing will depend on your preferred doneness and how hot your burner gets, but on my stove, 5 minutes per side with a 1-inch (2.5 cm) thick steak comes out medium-rare.

- When the timer goes off, flip the steak and set the timer again. When time is up, let the steak rest on a platter for 5 minutes before devouring.

Pan-Seared Scallops with Garlic-Cream Sauce

Preparation time-5 minutes | Cook time-10 minutes | Serving-4 | Difficulty- Easy

Nutritional value: Calories-242 | Fat-16g | Protein-19g | Carbohydrates-4g

Ingredients

- One pound of scallops, thawed

- Salt

- Freshly ground black pepper

- Two tablespoons of extra-virgin olive oil

- Two tablespoons of unsalted butter

- One tablespoon of minced garlic

- A quarter cup of broth of choice

- Two tablespoons of heavy (whipping) cream

- Two tablespoons of freshly squeezed lemon juice

Instructions

- Dry the scallops with a paper towel. Season with salt and pepper to taste.

- In a large pan or skillet over medium-high heat, heat the olive oil.

- Add the scallops in a single layer without overcrowding the pan (work in batches if needed), and cook until golden brown on one side, about 2 to 3 minutes.

- Gently flip the scallops, and add the butter and garlic to the pan.

- Continue to cook, spooning the butter over the scallops until they are cooked through, 2 to 3 minutes more. The scallops should be opaque and springy, not too firm.

- Transfer the scallops to a rimmed serving dish.

- Add the broth to the pan, and bring to a simmer, scraping up brown bits left behind in the pan. After the broth has been reduced by half, add the cream and allow to simmer until slightly thickened.

- Remove the pan from the heat, and stir in the lemon juice. Pour the sauce over the scallops, and serve immediately.

Pepperoncini beef

Preparation time-10 minutes | Cook time-8 hours | Servings-6 | Difficulty-Hard

Nutritional value: Calories-325 | Fat-24g | Protein-24g | Carbohydrates-3g

Ingredients

- Three pounds of boneless chuck pot roast

- One cup of pepperoncini peppers, with the vinegar they're packed in

- Half medium onion, chopped

- Guar or xanthan

- Salt and ground black pepper, to taste

Instructions

- Put the beef in the slow cooker, pour the pepperoncini on top, and strew the onion over that.

- Put on the lid, set the slow cooker to low, and leave it for 8 hours.

- When it's done, transfer the meat to a platter, and use a slotted spoon for fishing out the peppers and pile them on top of the roast.

- Thicken the juices in the pot just a little with the guar or xanthan, season with salt and pepper to taste, and serve with the roast.

Philly Cheesesteak–Stuffed Bell Peppers

Preparation time-15 minutes |Cook time-35 minutes |Serving-8 |Difficulty- Moderate

Nutritional value: Calories-220| Fat-13g| Protein-18g| Carbohydrates-6g

Ingredients

- Four green bell pepper stems were removed, halved lengthwise, and seeded

- One tablespoon of coconut oil

- One small yellow onion, cut into half-inch strips

- Eight cremini mushrooms, sliced

- Half pound of deli roast beef, sliced into ½- to 1-inch strips

- One garlic clove, minced

- Half teaspoon of paprika

- Half teaspoon of chili powder

- Half teaspoon of dried oregano

- Sixteen thin slices of provolone cheese

Instructions

- Preheat the oven to 350°F. Line a baking sheet with aluminum foil.

- Place the peppers skin-side down on the prepared baking sheet.

- In a large skillet over medium heat, heat the oil. Add the onions, and sauté until golden brown, about 15 minutes. Add the mushrooms, roast beef, garlic, paprika, chili powder, and oregano. Stir fry until the mushrooms are soft, 2 to 3 minutes.

- Place the peppers in the oven to cook for 5 to 10 minutes, or until somewhat softened.

- Gently remove the baking sheet from the oven and carefully line each pepper with 1 slice of provolone cheese.

- Scoop the beef-mushroom mixture into each pepper, and top each with 1 slice of provolone.

- Return the peppers to the oven and bake for another 5 to 7 minutes, or until the peppers are soft and the cheese is melted and golden brown.

Serve immediately.

Poor man's poivrade

Preparation time-10 minutes |Cook time-25 minutes|Servings-1 |Difficulty-Easy

Nutritional value: Calories-587 | Fat-47g|Protein-31g|Carbohydrates-4g

Ingredients

- Six ounces of ground chuck, in a patty half an inch (1 cm) thick

- One tablespoon of coarsely cracked pepper

- One tablespoon of butter

- Two tablespoons of dry white wine or dry sherry

Instructions

- Roll your raw beef patty in the pepper until it's coated all over. Fry the burger in the butter over medium heat until done to your liking.

- Remove the hamburger to a plate.

- Add the wine to the skillet, and stir it around for a minute or two until all the nice brown crusty bits are scraped up.

- Pour this over the hamburger, and serve.

Pork loin with red wine and walnuts

Preparation time-10 minutes |Cook time-40 minutes|Servings-4 |Difficulty-Moderate

Nutritional value: Calories-322 | Fat-21g|Protein-23g|Carbohydrates-4g

Ingredients

- Two tablespoons of butter, divided

- One pound of boneless pork loin, cut into 4 servings

- One small onion, sliced

- Half cup of dry red wine

- Half teaspoon of beef bouillon concentrate

- One clove of garlic, minced

- A quarter cup of chopped walnuts

- A quarter cup of chopped fresh parsley

Instructions

- Coat your large, heavy skillet with non-stick cooking spray, and put it over medium-high heat. When it's hot, add one tablespoon of the butter, swirl it around as it melts, then lay the pork in the skillet. Sauté until it's just golden on both sides.

- Remove the pork from the skillet, but keep it nearby.

- Add half of the remaining butter to the skillet, and let it melt. Add the onion and sauté until it's getting limp. Spread the onion in an even layer in the skillet, and lay the pork on top.

- Mix together the wine, beef bouillon concentrate, and garlic. Pour it over the pork, cover the pan with a tilted lid (leave a 1/4-inch [6 mm] gap for steam to escape), turn the burner to low, and let the whole thing simmer for 20 minutes.

- In the meantime, melt the remaining one and a half teaspoons of butter in a small skillet over medium heat, and stir the walnuts in it for 5 minutes until they smell a little toasty. Remove from the heat and reserve.

- When the timer beeps, add the parsley to the skillet. Let the whole thing simmer for another 5 minutes or so.

- Serve with the pan juices and a tablespoon of walnuts on each serving.

Pork with a camembert sauce

Preparation time-10 minutes | Cook time-30 minutes | Servings-3 | Difficulty-Easy

Nutritional value: Calories-333 | Fat-20g | Protein-32g | Carbohydrates-2g

Ingredients

- One pound of boneless pork loin, cut into three portions, about 3/4 inch (2 cm) thick

- Two ounces of Camembert cheese

- One tablespoon of butter

- Three tablespoons of dry white wine, or better yet, hard cider

- One tablespoon of chopped fresh sage

- 1/3 cup of sour cream

- One and a half teaspoons of Dijon mustard

- Ground black pepper, to taste

Instructions

- One at a time, put the pieces of pork loin in a heavy resealable plastic bag and pound with any handy blunt object until the meat is half an inch (1 cm) thick.

- Using a very sharp, thin-bladed knife, cut the rind off your Camembert as thinly as possible to leave as much of the actual cheese as you can. Cut the cheese into Half-inch (1 cm) chunks and reserve.

- Coat your large, heavy skillet with non-stick cooking spray, and put it over medium-high heat. Add the butter.

- When the butter is melted and the pan is good and hot, swirl the butter around the bottom of the skillet, then lay your pork in it.

- Cook until lightly golden on both sides, but no more—it's easy to dry out boneless pork loin. Put the pork on a plate, and keep it in a warm place.

- Add the wine to the skillet, and stir it around with a spatula, scraping up all the flavorful brown bits.

- Add the sage, and stir again. Turn the heat down to medium-low. Now throw in those chunks of Camembert.

- Use your spatula to stir them around, and cut the chunks into smaller bits until the cheese has completely melted.

- Whisk in the sour cream and mustard, season with pepper to taste, and it's done.

Rib-eye steak with wine sauce

Preparation time-10 minutes | Cook time-35 minutes | Servings-4 | Difficulty-Easy

Nutritional value: Calories-428 | Fat-28g | Protein-35g | Carbohydrates-2g

Ingredients

- One and a half pounds rib-eye steak

- One tablespoon of olive oil

- Two shallots

- Half cup of dry red wine

- Half cup of beef stock or a half teaspoon of beef bouillon concentrate dissolved in a half cup of water

- One tablespoon of balsamic vinegar

- One tablespoon of dried thyme

- One teaspoon of brown or Dijon mustard

- Three tablespoons of butter

- Salt and ground black pepper, to taste

Instructions

- Cook your steak in olive oil as described in Pan-Broiled Steak.

- In the meantime, assemble everything for your wine sauce—chop your shallots and combine the wine, beef stock, vinegar, thyme, and mustard in a measuring cup with a pouring lip. Whisk them together.

- When the timer goes off, flip the steak and set the timer again.

- When your steak is done, put it on a platter and set it in a warm place. Pour the wine mixture into the skillet and stir it around, scraping up the nice brown bits, and let it boil hard.

- Continue boiling your sauce until it's reduced by at least half.

- Melt in the butter, season with salt and pepper, and serve with your steak.

Roman lamb steak

Preparation time-10 minutes |Cook time-15 minutes|Servings-2 |Difficulty-Easy

Nutritional value: Calories-387 | Fat-30g|Protein-26g|Carbohydrates-2g

Ingredients

- 3/4 pound of the leg of lamb steaks, half an inch (1 cm) thick
- Half cup of chopped fresh parsley
- One tablespoon of olive oil
- One tablespoon of lemon juice
- A quarter teaspoon of ground black pepper
- 1/8 teaspoon of salt
- Two anchovy fillets
- One clove of garlic, crushed

Instructions

- Put your lamb steak on a plate. Throw everything else in your food processor with the S-blade in place and pulse to chop the parsley, anchovies, and garlic into a coarse paste.
- Smear half of the resulting mixture on one side of the steak, turn it and smear the rest on the other side. Now let the steak sit for at least half an hour—a couple of hours is great.
- After marinating, preheat your broiler and broil the lamb close to the heat (with the parsley mixture still all over it) for about 6 minutes per side—it should still be pink in the middle—and serve

Sage N Orange Breast of Duck

Preparation time-10 minutes |Cook time-20 minutes|Servings-4 |Difficulty-Easy

Nutritional value: Calories-329| Fat-14g|Protein-26g|Carbohydrates-7g

Ingredients

- Six oz. Duck Breast (~6 oz.)
- Two tablespoons of Butter
- One tablespoon of Heavy Cream
- One tablespoon of Swerve
- Half teaspoon of Orange Extract
- A quarter teaspoon of Sage
- One cup of spinach

Instructions

- Score the duck skin on top of the breast and season with pepper and salt.
- Brown butter in a saucepan over medium-low heat, and swerve.
- Add the extract of sage and orange and cook until it is deep orangey in color.
- Sear duck breasts for a few minutes until nicely crunchy.
- Flip the Breast of the Duck.
- Add the orange and sage butter to the heavy cream and pour it over the duck.
- Cook until finished.
- In the pan that you used to make the sauce, add the spinach and serve with the duck.

Salmon with Caper Sauce

Preparation time-10 minutes |Cook time-30 minutes|Servings-3 |Difficulty-Easy

Nutritional value: Calories-220| Fat-10g|Protein-26g|Carbohydrates-5g

Ingredients

- Three salmon fillets
- Salt and black pepper as per taste
- One tablespoon of olive oil
- One tablespoon of Italian seasoning
- Two tablespoons of capers
- Three tablespoons of lemon juice
- Four minced garlic cloves
- Two tablespoons of ghee

Instructions

- Heat the olive oil pan over medium heat, add the skin of the fish fillets side by side, season with pepper salt and Italian seasoning, cook for two minutes, toss and cook for another two minutes, remove from heat, cover and leave aside for 15 minutes.
- Put the fish on a plate and leave it aside.
- Over medium heat, heat the same pan, add the capers, garlic and lemon juice, stir and cook for two minutes.
- Remove the heat from the pan, add ghee and stir very well.
- Put the fish back in the pan and toss with the sauce to coat.
- Divide and serve on plates.

Sesame ginger salmon

Preparation time-45 minutes |Cook time-20 minutes |Serving-3 |Difficulty- Hard

Nutritional value: - Calories-124| Fat-9g| Protein-4g| Carbohydrates-8g

Ingredients

- A quarter cup of olive oil
- Two tablespoons of soy sauce
- Two tablespoons of rice vinegar
- Two tablespoons of sesame oil
- Two tablespoons of brown sugar
- Two pressed cloves of garlic
- One tablespoon of grated fresh ginger
- One tablespoon of sesame seeds
- Four thinly sliced green onions
- Four salmon filets

For the honey ginger glaze

- Two tablespoons of honey
- One teaspoon of soy sauce
- One teaspoon of sesame oil
- Half teaspoon of Sriracha
- Half teaspoon of grated fresh ginger
- Half teaspoon of sesame seeds

Instructions

- Combine the mixture of honey, soy sauce, sesame oil, cilantro, ginger and some sesame seeds in a small bowl to make the glass.
- In a medium bowl, mix the olive oil, soy sauce, rice vinegar, sesame, brown sugar, garlic, ginger, sesame, and green onion.
- Combine the ginger marinade and salmon file in a gallon-sized ziplock bag or large bowl; turn the bag occasionally and marinate overnight for at least 30 minutes.
- Preheat the oven to 400 ° F. Cover a 9 × 13 baking dish lightly with nonstick spray.
- Place the marine fillets in a marinated baking dish and bake with a fork for about 20 minutes until the fish is easily stirred.
- Serve the salmon with a glass of ginger honey immediately.

Sheet Pan Fajitas

Preparation time-5 minutes |Cook time-25 minutes |Serving-4 |Difficulty- Easy

Nutritional value: Calories-176| Fat-6g| Protein-24g| Carbohydrates-8g

Ingredients

- One pound of chicken breast, cut into strips

- One yellow onion, sliced
- One red bell pepper, sliced
- One yellow bell pepper, sliced
- One tablespoon of extra-virgin olive oil
- Two tablespoons of Taco Seasoning (store-bought or homemade)

Instructions

- Preheat the oven to 350°F.
- In a large bowl, combine the chicken, onion, peppers, oil, and taco seasoning. Mix well to coat evenly.
- Using one or two baking sheets, spread the chicken and veggies out evenly and as flat as possible, trying not to crowd.
- Bake for 20 to 25 minutes, or until the chicken is cooked through and the veggies are soft, stirring halfway through. Serve immediately.

Shrimp Ceviche

Preparation time-10 minutes |Cook time-30 minutes |Serving-4 |Difficulty- Moderate

Nutritional value: Calories-206| Fat-8g| Protein-25g| Carbohydrates-11g

Ingredients

- One pound of cooked jumbo shrimp, peeled, deveined, and diced
- One cup of diced tomatoes
- Half cup of finely chopped red onion
- One jalapeño pepper, seeds and veins removed, minced
- A quarter cup of freshly squeezed lemon juice
- A quarter cup of freshly squeezed lime juice
- Half cup of chopped fresh cilantro
- Salt
- One avocado pitted and diced into half-inch chunks

Instructions

- In a large bowl, mix the shrimp, tomatoes, red onion, and jalapeño.
- Pour in the lemon and lime juice, cilantro, and salt to taste. Gently toss to coat.
- For best flavor, cover and refrigerate for at least 30 minutes.
- Add the avocado right before serving.

Shrimp Scampi with Zucchini Noodles

Preparation time-10 minutes |Cook time-10 minutes |Serving-4 |Difficulty- Easy

Nutritional value: Calories-244 | Fat-12g | Protein-25g | Carbohydrates-9g

Ingredients

- Two tablespoons of extra-virgin olive oil

- One tablespoon of butter

- One tablespoon of minced garlic

- A quarter teaspoon of red pepper flakes

- One pound of peeled and deveined jumbo shrimp, tails removed

- A quarter cup of white wine

- Juice of half lemon

- Four medium zucchinis, cut into noodles using a spiralizer

- Salt

- Freshly ground black pepper

- A quarter cup of fresh parsley

- Freshly grated Parmesan for garnishing

Instructions

- In a large skillet over medium heat, heat the olive oil and butter. Add the garlic and red pepper flakes, and cook for 1 minute, stirring constantly.

- Add the shrimp, and cook until pink, about 3 minutes. Using a slotted spoon, transfer the shrimp to a bowl, leaving the juices in the pan.

- Return the skillet to the heat, and add the wine and lemon juice. Deglaze the pan, using the spoon to scrape up any browned bits from the bottom. Add the zucchini noodles and gently sauté to soften for about 2 minutes.

- Return the shrimp to the pan, and toss to combine. Season with salt and pepper, and serve immediately, garnished with parsley and Parmesan.

Simple Pizza Rolls

Preparation time-10 minutes | Cook time-40 minutes | Servings-6 | Difficulty-Easy

Nutritional value: Calories-217 | Fat-10g | Protein-26g | Carbohydrates-5g

Ingredients

- A quarter cup of chopped mixed red and green bell peppers

- Two cups of shredded mozzarella cheese

- One teaspoon of pizza seasoning

- Two tablespoons of chopped onion

- One chopped tomato

- Salt and black pepper to the taste

- A quarter cup of pizza sauce

- Half cup of crumbled and cooked sausage

Instructions

- On a lined and lightly oiled baking dish, spread mozzarella cheese, sprinkle pizza seasoning on top, put at 400 °F in the oven and bake for 20 minutes.

- Spread the sausage, onion, tomatoes and bell pepper all over and drizzle the tomato sauce at the top. Take the pizza crust out of the oven.

- Place them back in the oven and bake for ten more minutes.

- Take the pizza from the oven, leave it aside for a few minutes, break it into six pieces, roll each slice and eat it for lunch.

Sirloin with Anaheim-lime marinade

Preparation time-10 minutes | Cook time-30 minutes | Servings-4 | Difficulty-Easy

Nutritional value: Calories-415 | Fat-30g | Protein-32g | Carbohydrates-3g

Ingredients

- One and a half pounds sirloin steak, trimmed

- 1/3 cup of lime juice

- Two tablespoons of olive oil

- A quarter teaspoon of ground black pepper

- Half Anaheim chile pepper

- Two cloves of garlic

Instructions

- Put your steak in a shallow, nonreactive pan—glass or stainless steel are good—that just fits it, and pierce it all over with a fork.

- Put everything else in your food processor with the S-blade in place, and run it till the pepper and garlic are pureed.

- Pour the marinade over the steak. Let the whole thing sit for at least half an hour, and an hour or two is great.

- Preheat the broiler or grill. Remove the steak from the marinade, reserving the marinade. Broil or grill your steak, close to high heat, until done to your liking.

- Baste both sides with the marinade when turning the steak over, then quit—you want the heat to kill any germs before your steak is done.

- Let your steak rest for 5 minutes before carving and serving.

Skillet citrus chicken

Preparation time-10 minutes | Cook time-30 minutes | Servings-5 | Difficulty-Easy

Nutritional value: Calories-499 | Fat-36g | Protein-38g | Carbohydrates-4g

Ingredients

- One tablespoon of olive oil

- Three pounds of chicken thighs

- Half cup of chicken broth

- Two tablespoons of low-sugar orange marmalade preserves

- Two tablespoons of lemon juice

- Two tablespoons of lime juice

- Two teaspoons of brown mustard

- Eighteen drops of liquid stevia (lemon drop)

- Two cloves of garlic, crushed

Instructions

- Coat your large, heavy skillet with non-stick cooking spray, and put it over medium-high heat. When it's hot, add the olive oil, then the chicken, skin-side down.

- Sauté until the chicken is lightly golden, then turn bone-side down. Brown for another 5 minutes or so.

- While that's happening, stir together the chicken broth, low-sugar marmalade, lemon juice, lime juice, mustard, stevia, and garlic. When the chicken is browned, pour the broth mixture into the skillet.

- Partially cover the skillet with a "tilted lid" leave a crack of about 1/4 inch (6 mm) to let some steam out. Turn the burner to low, and let the chicken simmer for 20 minutes.

- When the time is up, uncover the chicken and remove it to a platter. Keep it in a warm place while you turn up the burner, and boil down the sauce until it's a little syrupy.

- Pour the sauce over the chicken, and serve.

Slow-cooker Chicken Taco Filling

Preparation time-10 minutes |Cook time-6 to 8 hours |Serving-4 |Difficulty- Easy

Nutritional value: Calories-148| Fat-2.4g| Protein-23g| Carbohydrates-6g

Ingredients

- One pound of boneless, skinless chicken breasts

- One 1.25-ounce) pack of dry taco seasoning mix

- One c(up of chicken broth

Instructions

- In a large mixing bowl, combine the taco seasoning and chicken broth.

- Place the chicken breasts in the slow cooker and set the timer for 6 hours.

- Using a ladle, pour the seasoning and broth mixture over the chicken.

- Cook on a low heat for 6-8 hours, covered. Chicken should be shredded.

- Cook for an additional 30 minutes on low heat to absorb any excess juices.

- Serve as a taco filling, a salad topping, or as a protein source on its own for a complete meal.

Slow-cooker Chicken Tikka Masala

Preparation time-10 minutes |Cook time-4 to 8 hours |Serving-10 |Difficulty- Easy

Nutritional value: Calories-370| Fat-8g| Protein-45g| Carbohydrates-12g

Ingredients

- One large onion, diced

- Two tablespoons of fresh ginger, minced

- One and a half cups of (12 ounces) plain Greek yogurt

- Two tablespoons of Garam masala

- Half tablespoon of paprika

- 3/4 teaspoon of ground black pepper

- Two bay leaves

- Three pounds of boneless, skinless chicken breast

- Four cloves garlic, minced

- One 29-ounce can of tomato puree

- Two tablespoons of olive oil

- One tablespoon of cumin

- 3/4 teaspoon of cinnamon

- Three teaspoons of cayenne pepper

- Chopped cilantro for topping

Instructions

- Place everything up to bay leaves in a large bowl.

- With a spatula, stir to combine and coat chicken well.

- Gently place into a slow cooker, add bay leaves on top.

- Cover and cook for 8 hours on low or 4 hours on high.

- Remove bay leaves, and serve topped with cilantro.

Slow-cooker Salsa Chicken

Preparation time-5 minutes |Cook time-4 hours |Serving-8 |Difficulty- Hard

Nutritional value: Calories-130| Fat-2g| Protein-23g| Carbohydrates-4g

Ingredients

- Four chicken breasts (about 2 pounds total)

- Two cups of your favorite salsa

Instructions

- Place the chicken breasts in a slow cooker, and cover with salsa. Stir around to make sure the chicken is coated.

- Cover and cook on high for 4 hours or on low for 6 to 8 hours.

- Once cooked, shred the chicken in the slow cooker with 2 forks. Stir with the salsa and juices in the crockpot until well mixed, and serve.

Slow-cooker pork chili

Preparation time-10 minutes |Cook time-8 hours|Servings-8 |Difficulty-Hard

Nutritional value: Calories-189| Fat-8g|Protein-3g|Carbohydrates-3g

Ingredients

- One tablespoon of olive oil

- Two and a half pounds of boneless pork loin, cut into 1-inch (2.5 cm) cubes

- One can (Fourteen and a half ounces) diced tomatoes with green chiles

- A quarter cup of chopped onion

- A quarter cup of diced green bell pepper

- One tablespoon of chili powder

- One clove of garlic, crushed

- Sour cream (optional)

- Shredded Monterey Jack cheese (optional)

Instructions

- Heat the olive oil in your big, heavy skillet, and brown the pork cubes all over. Dump them in the slow cooker.

- Stir in the tomatoes, onion, pepper, chili powder, and garlic. Cover and cook on low for 6 to 8 hours.

- Serve with sour cream and shredded Monterey Jack, if you like, but it's darned good as is.

Smothered burgers

Preparation time-10 minutes |Cook time-18 minutes|Servings-4 |Difficulty-Easy

Nutritional value: Calories-508| Fat-41g|Protein-31g|Carbohydrates-2g

Ingredients

- One and a half pounds ground chuck, in 4 patties (6 ounces each)

- Two tablespoons of butter or olive oil

- Half cup of sliced onion

- Half cup of sliced mushrooms

- 1/8 teaspoon of anchovy paste

- One dash of soy sauce

Instructions

- Start cooking your burgers by your preferred method.

- While that's happening, melt the butter in a small, heavy skillet over medium-high heat.

- Add the onion and mushrooms and sauté until the onion is translucent. Stir in the anchovy paste and soy sauce.

- Serve the onion-mushroom mixture over the burgers.

Soy-Ginger Salmon with Bok Choy

Preparation time-20 minutes |Cook time-10 minutes |Serving-4 |Difficulty- Easy

Nutritional value: Calories-247| Fat-12g| Protein-27g| Carbohydrates-8g

Ingredients

- A quarter cup of low-sodium soy sauce

- Two teaspoons of rice vinegar

- One tablespoon of brown sugar

- Two teaspoons of grated ginger

- Two garlic cloves, minced

- Two chopped scallions

- One pound of wild-caught Alaskan salmon fillet, cut into four pieces, bones removed

- Four baby bok choy quartered lengthwise

- Two teaspoons of extra-virgin olive oil

- Salt

- Freshly ground black pepper

Instructions

- In a resealable bag, combine the soy sauce, vinegar, brown sugar, ginger, garlic, and scallions.

- Add the salmon, and mix to coat. Chill for 15 to 30 minutes.

- Preheat the oven to 400°F. Line a baking sheet with aluminum foil.

- Remove the salmon from the bag, reserving any marinade, and place the salmon skin-side down on one side of the baking sheet.

- Place the bok choy on the other side of the baking sheet, drizzle on the olive oil, and toss to coat. Season with salt and pepper to taste.

- Bake for 10 to 12 minutes, or until the internal temperature of the salmon reaches 125 to 145°F and the bok choy is tender.

- Meanwhile, in a small saucepan, heat the reserved marinade to a boil. Simmer on low until thickened and reduced by half, 5 to 10 minutes.

- Transfer the salmon and bok choy to four plates, cover the salmon with the warm marinade and serve.

Spareribs Adobado

Preparation time-10 minutes | Cook time-2 hours 45 minutes | Servings-6 | Difficulty-Hard

Nutritional value: Calories-493 | Fat-43g | Protein-25g | Carbohydrates-2g

Ingredients

- Three cloves of garlic, divided
- Four tablespoons of olive oil, divided
- Three pounds of pork spareribs
- One tablespoon of paprika
- One teaspoon of ground cumin
- One teaspoon of dried oregano
- Half teaspoon of salt or Vege-Sal
- Half teaspoon of ground black pepper
- Half cup of chicken broth

Instructions

- Preheat oven to 325°F.
- Crush two cloves of the garlic, and stir into one tablespoon of the olive oil. Let it sit for 10 minutes.
- Then use clean hands to rub this mixture all over the ribs, coating both sides. Put them in a roasting pan.
- In a small dish, stir together the seasonings. Remove one tablespoon of the mixture to a small bowl and reserve.
- Sprinkle the ribs all over with the seasoning mixture that you didn't reserve in the bowl. Cover all sides.
- Put the ribs in to roast, and set your timer for 25 minutes (a few minutes one way or another won't matter).
- While the ribs are roasting, crush the last clove of garlic and add to the reserved spice mixture with the chicken broth and the remaining three tablespoons of olive oil. Stir to combine. This is your mopping sauce.
- When the timer goes off, baste your ribs with the mopping sauce, turning them over as you do so. Stick them back in the oven, and set the timer for another 20 minutes.
- Repeat for a good one and a half to two hours; you want your ribs sizzling and brown all over and tender when you pierce them with a fork.
- Cut into individual ribs to serve.

Special Fish Pie

Preparation time-10 minutes | Cook time-One hour 20 minutes | Servings-6 | Difficulty-Hard

Nutritional value: Calories-223 | Fat-11g | Protein-29g | Carbohydrates-6g

Ingredients

- One chopped red onion
- Two skinless and medium sliced salmon fillets
- Two skinless and medium sliced mackerel fillets
- Three medium sliced haddock fillets
- Two bay leaves
- A quarter cup and two tablespoons of ghee
- One cauliflower head, florets separated
- Four eggs
- Four cloves
- One cup of whipping cream
- Half cup of water
- A pinch of nutmeg
- One teaspoon of Dijon mustard
- One and a half cups of shredded cheddar cheese
- A handful of chopped parsley
- Salt and black pepper as per taste
- Four tablespoons of chopped chives

Instructions

- In a saucepan, place some water, add some salt, bring to a boil over medium heat, add the eggs, simmer for ten minutes, heat off, drain, cool, peel and break into quarters.
- Place the water in another kettle, bring it to a boil, add the florets of cauliflower, simmer for 10 minutes, rinse, add a quarter of a cup of ghee, add it to the mixer, blend properly, and place it in a bowl.
- Add the cream and half a cup of water to a saucepan, add the fish, toss and cover over medium heat.
- Put to a boil, reduce heat to a minimum, and steam for 10 minutes. Put the cloves, onion, and bay leave.
- Take the heat off, put the fish and set it aside in a baking dish.
- Heat the saucepan with the fish, add the nutmeg, combine and simmer for 5 minutes.
- Remove from the oven, discard the bay leaves and cloves and blend well with one cup of cheddar cheese and two tablespoons of ghee.
- On top of the fish, set the egg quarters in the baking dish.
- Sprinkle with cream and cheese sauce on top of the remaining cheddar cheese, chives and parsley, cover with cauliflower mash, sprinkle with the remaining cheddar cheese, and place in the oven for 30 minutes at 400 ° F.

- Leave the pie until it is about to slice and serve, to cool down a little.

Special Lunch Burgers

Preparation time-10 minutes |Cook time-30 minutes|Servings-8 |Difficulty-Easy

Nutritional value: Calories-243| Fat-4g|Protein-26g|Carbohydrates-13g

Ingredients

- One pound ground brisket
- One pound ground beef
- Salt and black pepper as per taste
- Eight butter slices
- One tablespoon of minced garlic
- One tablespoon of Italian seasoning
- Two tablespoons of mayonnaise
- One tablespoon of ghee
- Two tablespoons of olive oil
- One chopped yellow onion
- One tablespoon of water

Instructions

- Mix the beef, pepper, salt, Italian herbs, mayo and garlic with the brisket in a bowl and stir well.
- Form 8 patties into each one to create a pocket.
- With butter-slices, stuff each burger and seal it.
- Over medium pressure, heat the pan with the oil, add the onions, stir and simmer for 2 minutes.
- Apply the water, swirl and pick them up in the pan corner.
- Put the burgers with the onions in the pan and cook them for ten minutes over moderate flame.
- Flip them over, apply the ghee, and simmer for ten more minutes.
- Break the burgers into buns and place them on top of caramelized onions.

Spinach Dip–Stuffed Chicken

Preparation time-20 minutes |Cook time-40 minutes |Serving-4 |Difficulty- Moderate

Nutritional value: Calories-389| Fat-29g| Protein-32g| Carbohydrates-5g

Ingredients

- Five ounces of frozen chopped spinach, defrosted and drained
- Eight ounces of low-fat cream cheese softened
- A quarter cup of Parmesan cheese
- A quarter cup of shredded mozzarella cheese
- Two garlic cloves, minced
- A quarter teaspoon of salt
- A quarter teaspoon of freshly ground black pepper
- Four boneless chicken breasts
- One tablespoon of extra-virgin olive oil
- Nonstick cooking spray

Instructions

- Preheat the oven to 400°F.
- Place the defrosted spinach in paper towels, and dry off as much water as you can.
- In a medium bowl, mix the spinach, cream cheese, Parmesan, mozzarella, and garlic, and season with salt and pepper.
- Slice your chicken lengthwise to make a pocket, being sure not to cut all the way through.
- Stuff the cream cheese mixture into chicken breasts, and fold to close the pockets. Secure with toothpicks if necessary. Rub with olive oil, and season with salt and pepper.
- Transfer to a greased or parchment paper-lined baking dish. If you have leftover spinach mix, spread it on top of the chicken prior to baking. Cover with aluminum foil and bake for 20 to 40 minutes, depending on thickness, or until the chicken reaches an internal temperature of 165°F and any juices run clear. Serve immediately.

Spinach -Turkey Wraps

Preparation time-15 minutes |Cook time-0 minutes |Serving-4 |Difficulty- Easy

Nutritional value: ~ Calories-184| Fat-6g| Protein-23g| Carbohydrates-21g

Ingredients

- Four ounces of nonfat cream cheese
- Two tablespoons of sliced green onions
- One teaspoon of Dijon mustard
- Four (9-inch, or 22.5-cm) low-carb tortillas
- One and 1/3 cups of fresh spinach, shredded
- Six ounces of thinly sliced roasted turkey breast, skin and fat removed
- A quarter cup of reduced-fat shredded Cheddar or Jack cheese
- Two tablespoons of minced red bell pepper

Instructions

- In a small bowl, combine the cream cheese, green onions, and Dijon mustard.

- Spread the mixture equally onto the tortillas. Next, add in equal portions the spinach, turkey, cheese, and bell pepper.

- Wrap the tortillas tightly around the filling, wrap the rolls in plastic wrap, and refrigerate for at least one hour before serving.

Steak au poivre with brandy cream

Preparation time-10 minutes |Cook time-35 minutes|Servings-2 |Difficulty-Moderate

Nutritional value: Calories-557 | Fat-42g|Protein-32g|Carbohydrates-3g

Ingredients

- Twelve ounces of well-marbled steaks—such as sirloin, T-bone, or rib-eye—Half to 3/4 inch (1 to 2 cm) thick

- Four teaspoons of coarse cracked black pepper, divided

- One tablespoon of butter

- One tablespoon of olive oil

- Two tablespoons of Cognac or other brandy

- Two tablespoons of heavy cream

- Salt, to taste

Instructions

- Place your steak on a plate, and scatter two teaspoons of the pepper evenly over it.

- Using your hands or the back of a spoon, press the pepper firmly into the steak's surface. Turn the steak over, and do the same thing to the other side with the remaining pepper.

- Place a large, heavy skillet over high heat, and add the butter and olive oil. When the skillet is hot, add your steak. For a Half-inch (1 cm) thick steak, four and a half minutes per side is about right; go maybe a minute more for a ¾ inch (2 cm) thick steak.

- When the steak is done on both sides, turn off the burner, pour the Cognac over the steak, and flame it. When the flames die down, remove the steak to a serving platter, and pour the cream into the skillet.

- Stir it around, dis-solving the meat juices and brandy into it.

Season lightly with salt, and pour over the steak.

Stuffed Chicken Breasts

Preparation time-10 minutes |Cook time-0 minutes |Serving-4 |Difficulty- Easy

Nutritional value: Calories-359| Fat-15g| Protein-37g| Carbohydrates-19g

Ingredients

- Three tablespoons of seedless raisins

- Half cup of chopped onion

- Half cup of chopped celery

- A quarter teaspoon of minced garlic

- One bay leaf

- One cup of chopped and peeled apple

- Two tablespoons of chopped water chestnuts

- Four large chicken breast halves, with the bones, removed, each about 6 ounces

- Two tablespoons of olive oil

- One cup of fat-free milk

- One teaspoon of curry powder

- Two tablespoons of all-purpose (plain) flour

- One lemon, cut into 4 wedges

Instructions

- Preheat oven to 425 degrees Fahrenheit. Using cooking spray, lightly coat a baking dish. Place the raisins in a small bowl and cover with warm water. Allow the raisins to swell while you wait.

- Using frying spray, coat a big skillet. Combine the onions, celery, garlic, and bay leaf in a large mixing bowl. Cook for about 5 minutes, or until the onions are transparent. Add the apples after removing the bay leaf. Cook, stirring periodically, for another 2 minutes.

- To remove the extra water from the raisins, drain them and pat them dry using paper towels. Combine the apples and raisins in a mixing bowl. Remove the water chestnuts from the heat and stir them in. Allow cooling.

- Remove the skin from the chicken breasts and loosen it. Between the skin and the breast, place the apple-raisin mixture. Heat the olive oil in a separate skillet over medium heat. Cook for 5 minutes on each side until the chicken breasts are browned.

- Place the chicken breasts in the baking dish that has been prepared. Cover and bake for 15 minutes, or until a meat thermometer reads 165 degrees F. Remove the baking sheet from the oven.

- In a saucepan, cook the milk, curry powder, and flour over low heat while the chicken is roasting. Stir for 5 minutes or until the mixture thickens. Over the chicken breasts, pour the mixture. Return the chicken to the oven and bake for another 10 minutes, covered.

- Place the chicken breasts on individual plates that have been warmed. Serve the chicken with the sauce from the pan and lemon wedges on the side.

Super-easy turkey divan

Preparation time-10 minutes |Cook time-40 minutes|Servings-6 |Difficulty-Moderate

Nutritional value: Calories-614 | Fat-54g|Protein-131g|Carbohydrates-5g

Ingredients

- One pound of frozen broccoli, thawed

- One pound of roasted turkey, sliced

- One cup of grated Parmesan, divided

- One cup of mayonnaise

- One cup of heavy cream

- Two tablespoons of dry vermouth

Instructions

- Preheat oven to 350°F.

- Coat an 8-inch (20 cm) square baking dish with non-stick cooking spray.

- Cover the bottom of the pan with broccoli.

- Cover the broccoli with slices of leftover turkey.

- In a mixing bowl, combine all but two tablespoons of the Parmesan with the mayonnaise, cream, and vermouth.

- Pour over the turkey and broccoli.

- Sprinkle the remaining parmesan on top. Bake until it's getting golden, about a half-hour.

Tandoori chicken

Preparation time-10 minutes |Cook time-1 hour 10 minutes|Servings-6 |Difficulty-Hard

Nutritional value: Calories-387 | Fat-20g|Protein-45g|Carbohydrates-5g

Ingredients

- Five pounds of bone-in chicken thighs without skin

- One and a half cups of plain yogurt

- A quarter cup of olive oil

- Two tablespoons of grated fresh ginger root

- One tablespoon of lemon juice

- Two teaspoons of chili powder

- Two teaspoons of ground turmeric

- One teaspoon of salt or Vege-Sal

- One teaspoon of ground coriander

- Half teaspoon of ground cumin

- Half teaspoon of ground cinnamon

- Half teaspoon of ground cloves

- Four cloves of garlic

- Two bay leaves, whole

Instructions

- Skin the chicken if you didn't buy it that way. Put it in a nonreactive baking pan—glass or enamel are ideal, but stainless steel will do. Don't use aluminum or iron.

- Put everything else in your blender, and run it until you have a smooth sauce.

- Pour the sauce over the chicken, and use tongs to turn each piece to coat. Cover the baking pan with plastic wrap, slide it into the fridge, and let it sit for a minimum of 4 hours; a whole day is ideal.

- Pull your chicken out of the fridge, and let it come to room temperature. Meanwhile, preheat your oven to 350°F.

- When the oven is hot, pull the plastic wrap off the baking pan and slide it in to cook. Roast for 45 minutes to 1 hour, turning the chicken occasionally with your tongs.

Tasty Baked Fish

Preparation   time-10   minutes |Cook   time-30 minutes|Servings-4 |Difficulty-Easy

Nutritional value: Calories-232 | Fat-13g|Protein-27g|Carbohydrates-4g

Ingredients

- One pound of haddock

- Three teaspoons of water

- Two tablespoons of lemon juice

- Salt and black pepper as per taste

- Two tablespoons of mayonnaise

- One teaspoon of dill weed

- Cooking spray

- A pinch of old bay seasoning

Instructions

- With some cooking oil, spray a baking dish.

- Apply the lemon juice, fish and water and toss to cover a little bit.

- Apply salt, pepper, seasoning with old bay and dill weed and mix again.

- Add mayonnaise and spread evenly.

- Place it at 350 ° F in the oven and bake for thirty minutes.

- Split and serve on a plate.

Tasty roasted chicken

Preparation time-10 minutes |Cook time-1 hour 40 minutes|Servings-6 |Difficulty-Hard

Nutritional value: Calories-600| Fat-44g|Protein-48g|Carbohydrates-1g

Ingredients

- One tablespoon of mayonnaise
- One whole chicken
- Salt and ground black pepper
- Paprika
- Onion powder

Instructions

- Preheat oven to 375°F.

- If your chicken was frozen, make sure it's completely thawed—if it's still a bit icy in the middle, run some hot water inside it until it's not icy anymore. Take out the giblets; if you've never cooked a whole chicken before, you'll find them in the body cavity.

- Dry your chicken with paper towels and put it on a plate.

- Scoop your mayonnaise out of the jar and into a small dish, being careful not to contaminate the jar. Using clean hands, give your chicken a nice mayo massage. Rub that chicken all over with the mayonnaise, coating every inch of skin.

- Sprinkle the chicken liberally with salt, pepper, paprika, and onion powder, all four equally, on all sides.

- Put the chicken on a rack in a shallow roasting pan, and put it in the oven.

- Leave the bird there for one and a half hours, or until the juices run clear when you stick a fork in where the thigh joins the body.

- Remove from the oven, and let the chicken sit for 10 to 15 minutes before carving to let the juices settle.

Thai chicken coconut curry

Preparation time-5 minutes | Cook time-20 minutes | Serving-3 | Difficulty- Easy

Nutritional value: ~ Calories-124 | Fat-9g | Protein-4g | Carbohydrates-8g

Ingredients

- Two to three tablespoons of coconut oil
- One large sweet Vidalia or diced small yellow onion
- One pound diced boneless skinless breast of chicken
- Three minced cloves of garlic
- Two to three teaspoons of finely chopped ground ginger
- Two teaspoons of ground coriander
- One 13-ounce can of coconut milk
- One and a half cups of shredded carrots
- One to three tablespoons of Thai red curry paste
- One teaspoon of kosher salt

- Half teaspoon of freshly ground black pepper about
- Three cups of fresh spinach leaves
- One tablespoon of lime juice
- One to three tablespoons of brown sugar
- A quarter cup of finely chopped fresh cilantro rice, quinoa, or naan

Instructions

- Add oil onion and cook over medium-high heat in a large skillet until the onion begins to soften for about 5 minutes; stir occasionally.

- Add the chicken and saute, cook for around 5 minutes or until the chicken is done; to ensure even cooking, flip and stir frequently.

- Add the ginger, garlic, coriander and cook until fragrant or about 1 minute; stir frequently.

- To mix, add coconut milk, carrots, Thai curry paste, salt, pepper and stir. Reduce heat to medium and cook the mixture slowly for around 5 minutes or until the volume of the liquid is preferred and thickened slightly.

- To mix, add spinach, lime juice and whisk. Cook the spinach until it tastes like brown sugar, extra vegetable paste, salt, pepper, etc., for around 1 to 2 minutes.

- Serve evenly slowly. It is best to keep the curry warm and fresh, but keep it airtight for up to 1 week in the fridge.

Thai Red Curry Chicken

Preparation time-10 minutes | Cook time-25 minutes | Serving-4 | Difficulty- Easy

Nutritional value: ~Calories-307 | Fat-16g | Protein-24g | Carbohydrates-19g

Ingredients

- Two tablespoons of extra-virgin olive oil, divided
- One pound of chicken breast, diced into 1-inch cubes
- Two teaspoons of freshly grated ginger
- One garlic clove, minced
- Half large yellow onion, sliced
- One red or green bell pepper, sliced
- Two tablespoons of Thai red curry paste
- One and a half tablespoons of sugar
- One (13.5-ounce) can light coconut milk
- One tablespoon of fish sauce Cauliflower rice (optional)
- Fresh Thai basil leaves for garnish (optional)

Instructions

- In a large skillet over medium heat, heat one tablespoon of oil. Add the chicken, and stir-fry until browned and no longer pink in the middle, 5 to 8 minutes. Transfer to a plate.

- In the same pan over medium heat, heat the remaining tablespoon of oil. Add the ginger, garlic, onion, pepper, and sauté for 2 minutes.

- Add the curry paste, sugar, coconut milk, and fish sauce, and stir well to combine. Simmer, occasionally stirring, for 8 to 10 minutes, until thickened.

- Return the chicken to the pan, adding water to thin if necessary, and reduce to a simmer. Cook for 5 minutes to warm the chicken.

- Plate the curry.

Thanksgiving weekend curry

Preparation time-10 minutes | Cook time-40 minutes | Servings-8 | Difficulty-Moderate

Nutritional value: Calories-349 | Fat-27g | Protein-23g | Carbohydrates-4g

Ingredients

- Three tablespoons of coconut oil

- Two teaspoons of garam masala

- One teaspoon of ground cinnamon

- One teaspoon of ground turmeric

- Half medium onion, chopped

- Two cloves of garlic, crushed

- One tablespoon of grated fresh ginger root

- One teaspoon of cayenne

- One can (14 fluid ounces) of unsweetened coconut milk

- 3/4 cup of chicken broth, or turkey broth, if you have it

- Four cups of diced cooked turkey

- Salt, to taste

Instructions

- In your big, heavy skillet, over medium-low heat, melt the coconut oil. Add the garam masala, cinnamon, turmeric, and stir for a minute or so.

- Add the onion, and sauté until it's translucent.

- Now add the garlic, ginger, and cayenne. Pour in the coconut milk and chicken broth. Stir it up until you've got a creamy sauce.

- Stir in the turkey, and turn the burner to low. Let the whole thing simmer for 15 minutes or so.

- Season with salt to taste and serve in bowls with soup spoons.

Tokyo ginger pork chops

Preparation time-10 minutes |Cook time-20 minutes|Servings-2 |Difficulty-Easy

Nutritional value: Calories-337| Fat-24g|Protein-27g|Carbohydrates-2g

Ingredients

- Twelve ounces of pork chops (2 chops, about 3/4 inch [2 cm] thick)

- Two tablespoons of soy sauce

- Two teaspoons of grated fresh ginger root

- One and a half teaspoons of dry sherry

- One tablespoon of coconut oil

Instructions

- Lay your chops in a shallow nonreactive container—a glass pie plate is great. Mix together the soy sauce, ginger, and sherry, and pour over the chops, turning them once to coat. Let them marinate for 15 to 20 minutes.

- Coat your large, heavy skillet with non-stick cooking spray, and put it over medium-high heat. Let it get good and hot, then add the coconut oil. Swirl it around the bottom of the skillet to cover. Now pick up your chops, let the marinade drip off (reserve the marinade), then throw them in the skillet.

- Brown them a bit on both sides, about 5 minutes each.

- Pour the reserved marinade over the chops, turn the burner down, and let the chops simmer another 5 to 8 minutes, or until done through, then serve, scraping all the pan juices over them.

Tomato-Basil Cod en Papillote

Preparation time-15 minutes |Cook time-15 minutes |Serving-4 |Difficulty- Easy

Nutritional value: Calories-194| Fat-3g| Protein-31g| Carbohydrates-5g

Ingredients

- Two teaspoons of extra-virgin olive oil

- Two garlic cloves, minced

- One shallot, thinly sliced

- A quarter cup of dry white wine

- One tablespoon of freshly squeezed lemon juice

- Four (6-ounce) boneless cod fillets

- Salt

- Freshly ground black pepper

- One pint cherry tomatoes

- Half cup of chopped fresh basil

Instructions

- Preheat the oven to 400°F.

- In a small saucepan over medium heat, heat the oil. Add the garlic and shallot, and sauté until the shallot is softened and the garlic is fragrant for 3 to 5 minutes. Add the white wine and lemon juice, and bring to a gentle simmer. Remove from the heat, and let cool.

- Season the cod fillets with salt and pepper.

- Lay out a 16-inch sheet of parchment paper with a long side facing you. Place one cod fillet in the middle of the paper, and pile with a quarter of the tomatoes and a quarter of the basil.

- Bring the two long ends of the paper together and begin folding in small increments until tightly sealed. Then, roll and tightly crimp the open ends.

- Open the paper back up, as the fold lines have now been established, and pour in ¼ of the lemon-garlic liquid. Refold the paper so that no steam can escape. Repeat with the 3 remaining fillets.

- Transfer the packets to a baking sheet, and bake for 10 to 15 minutes, or until the fish is opaque and flakes easily with a fork (10 minutes for a half-inch fillet, 15 minutes for a one-inch fillet).

- Remove from the oven and allow to rest for 5 minutes before serving.

Turkey Bean Enchilada

Preparation time-5 minutes |Cook time-30 minutes|Servings-4 |Difficulty-Hard

Nutritional value: Calories-387| Fat-20g|Protein-45g|Carbohydrates-5g

Ingredients

- Four medium-sized low-carb or fat-free tortillas

- Two cups of cooked skinless, white turkey meat, cubed

- One cup of taco sauce or canned enchilada sauce, divided

- Half cup of shredded reduced-fat Mexican cheese

- Six medium scallions, green and white parts chopped

- One 15-ounce can of pinto beans, drained and rinsed

Instructions

- Preheat the oven to 350 degrees Fahrenheit (180 degrees Celsius).

- In a large mixing bowl, combine the turkey, onions, beans, and half cup taco or enchilada sauce until well combined.

- Fill each tortilla with a quarter of the turkey-bean mixture.

- Fold in the sides, the top, and the bottom of the tortilla to completely enclose the filling in the tortilla.

- Using a 9x13 inch baking dish, arrange the tortillas so that the seams are facing up.

- The final step is to pour the remaining half cup of sauce and cheese over the enchiladas to finish them off.

- Bake until the cheese is hot and bubbling and the dish is heated through, about 15 minutes (about 20 minutes)

Turkey with mushroom sauce

Preparation time-10 minutes |Cook time-8 hours|Servings-8 |Difficulty-Hard

Nutritional value: Calories-281| Fat-14g|Protein-34g|Carbohydrates-1g

Ingredients

- Three pounds of boneless, skinless turkey breast (in one big hunk, not thin cutlets)

- Two tablespoons of butter

- A quarter cup of chopped fresh parsley

- Two teaspoons of dried tarragon

- Half teaspoon of salt or Vege-Sal

- A quarter teaspoon of ground black pepper

- One cup of sliced fresh mushrooms

- A quarter cup of dry white wine

- One teaspoon of chicken bouillon concentrate

- Guar or xanthan (optional)

Instructions

- In your big skillet, sauté the turkey breast in the butter till it's golden all over. Transfer to the slow cooker.

- Sprinkle the parsley, tarragon, salt, and pepper over the turkey breast. Dump the mushrooms on top. Mix the wine and bouillon concentrate together until the bouillon dissolves, and pour it in as well. Cover the pot, and cook on low for 7 to 8 hours.

- When it's done, fish the turkey out and put it on a platter. Transfer about half of the mushrooms to your blender, and add the liquid from the pot. Blend until mushrooms are puréed.

- Scoop the rest of the mushrooms into the serving dish for the sauce, add the liquid, and thicken further with your guar or xanthan shaker, if needed.

West Coast Crab Cakes

Preparation time-10 minutes |Cook time-25 minutes |Serving-6 |Difficulty- Easy

Nutritional value: Calories-90| Fat-1g| Protein-11g| Carbohydrates-5g

Ingredients

- Nonstick cooking spray

- One large egg, lightly beaten

- One teaspoon of Dijon mustard

- Two tablespoons of low-fat, plain Greek yogurt

- One garlic clove, minced

- Juice of half lemon

- Half teaspoon of ground cayenne

- A few dashes of hot sauce

- Two (7-ounce) cans lump crab meat, drained

- Half cup of whole wheat panko bread crumbs, divided

Instructions

- Preheat the oven to 400°F.

- Spray a baking sheet with nonstick cooking spray.

- In a large mixing bowl, mix the egg, mustard, yogurt, garlic, lemon juice, cayenne, and hot sauce until well combined.

- Gently fold in the crab meat and A quarter cup of bread crumbs.

- Chill the mixture in the refrigerator for 20 minutes.

- Place the remaining A quarter cup of bread crumbs on a plate.

- Using a ⅓ cup measuring cup, scoop the crab mixture from the bowl and gently pack to form into a cake. Transfer to the bread crumb plate by turning the measuring cup upside down and allowing the cake to slide out. Carefully dredge both sides of the cake with crumbs.

- Gently transfer the cake to the baking sheet. Repeat the process with the remaining crab mixture.

- Bake for 10 to 12 minutes, or until the cakes are lightly brown on the bottom. Carefully flip and bake for 10 to 12 more minutes, or until golden and crisp, and serve.

White Sea Bass with Dill Relish

Preparation time-10 minutes |Cook time-0 minutes |Serving-4 |Difficulty- Easy

Nutritional value: Calories-119| Fat-2g| Protein-21g| Carbohydrates-3g

Ingredients

- One teaspoon of pickled baby capers, drained

- One teaspoon of Dijon mustard

- Four white sea bass fillets, each 4 ounces

- One and a half tablespoons of chopped white onion

- One and a half teaspoons of chopped fresh dill

- One teaspoon of lemon juice

- One lemon, cut into quarters

Instructions

- Preheat oven to 375 degrees Fahrenheit.

- Combine the onion, mustard, dill, capers, and lemon juice in a small bowl. Stir everything together thoroughly.

- Each fillet should be placed on a square of aluminum foil. 1 lemon wedge is squeezed over each fillet, and 1/4 of the dill relish is sprinkled over each piece.

- Wrap the aluminum foil around the fish and bake for 10 to 12 minutes, or until the fish is opaque throughout when tested with a tip of a knife. Serve right away.

Yucatán chicken

Preparation time-10 minutes | Cook time-40 minutes | Servings-4 | Difficulty-Moderate

Nutritional value: Calories-389 | Fat-28g | Protein-31g | Carbohydrates-3g

Ingredients

- One tablespoon of ground black pepper

- One tablespoon of ground allspice

- One teaspoon of dried oregano

- Half teaspoon of ground cumin

- One teaspoon of lime juice

- One teaspoon of lemon juice

- Three drops of orange extract

- Two pounds of chicken thighs

Instructions

- Mix together everything but the chicken. Rub this mixture all over your chicken thighs and even up under the skin.

- Refrigerate for several hours.

- When cooking time comes, preheat your broiler, arrange the chicken on your broiler rack, skin-side down, and broil about 6 inches from the heat for 15 minutes or so. Turn, and give it another 10 minutes. Turn again, and give it at least another 5 minutes.

- Now turn a piece skin-side up, and pierce it to the bone. If the juice runs clear, it's done. If it runs pink, you need to give it a little longer.

- You can also cook this on your barbecue grill if you like. Indeed, if you want to take something along to the park or the beach to grill while you're there, do the flavoring step early in the day, marinating the chicken

in a big resealable plastic bag. Then grab the bag of chicken, throw it in your cooler, and go.

- Serve with a big green salad.

Zoodles with Meat Sauce

Preparation time-10 minutes | Cook time-40 minutes | Serving-4 | Difficulty- Moderate

Nutritional value: Calories-410 | Fat-20g | Protein-32g | Carbohydrates-26g

Ingredients

- One pound of ground beef (93%)

- Two tablespoons of extra-virgin olive oil, divided

- One large yellow onion, chopped

- Three garlic cloves, minced

- One tablespoon of tomato paste

- One (24-ounce) jar pasta sauce

- One tablespoon of Italian seasoning

- Four medium zucchinis

- Half cup of shredded Parmesan cheese

Instructions

- In a large saucepan over medium heat, cook the ground beef, breaking it up with the spoon, until browned, 7 to 10 minutes. Drain, and transfer to a plate.

- In the same pan over medium heat, heat one tablespoon of oil. Add the onions and garlic, and sauté until the onions are translucent and the garlic is fragrant for about 5 minutes. Add the tomato paste, and sauté for 1 minute.

- Add the pasta sauce, and stir well to combine. Mix in the Italian seasoning. Simmer for 20 minutes.

- Meanwhile, cut the zucchini noodles to their desired length.

- In a large skillet over medium heat, heat the remaining tablespoon of oil. Add the zucchini, and sauté until soft, 2 to 3 minutes, or to desired texture. Be sure not to overcook the zucchini, as it will end up mushy.

- Plate the zucchini, top with the sauce and Parmesan, and serve.

Zucchini meat loaf Italiano

Preparation time-10 minutes | Cook time- One hour 30 minutes | Servings-5 | Difficulty-Hard

Nutritional value: Calories-521 | Fat-41g | Protein-31g | Carbohydrates-5g

Ingredients

- Two medium zucchinis, chopped—about one and a half cup

- One medium onion, chopped

- Two cloves of garlic, crushed

- Olive oil—a few tablespoons as needed

- One and a half pounds ground chuck

- 3/4 cup of grated Parmesan cheese

- Three tablespoons of olive oil

- Two tablespoons of snipped fresh parsley

- One teaspoon of salt

- Half teaspoon of ground black pepper

- One egg

Instructions

- Preheat the oven to 350°F.

- Sauté the zucchini, onion, and garlic in the olive oil for about 7 to 8 minutes. Let it cool a bit, then put it in a big bowl with the rest of the ingredients.

- Using clean hands, mix thoroughly. This will make a rather soft mixture—you can put it in a big loaf pan if you like or form it on a broiler rack.

- Bake for 75 to 90 minutes, or until the juices run clear, but it's not dried out.

Chapter 7~Dinner Recipes

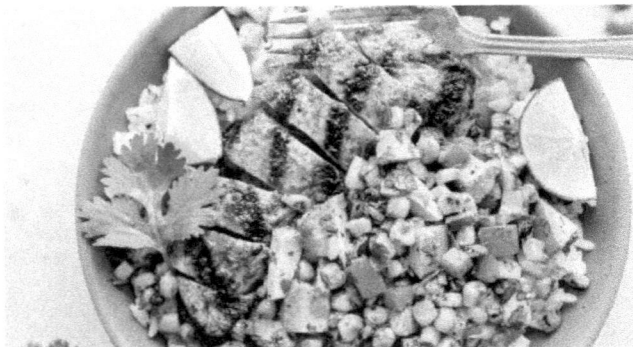

Avocados with Chicken~Corn Salsa

Preparation time~10 minutes| Cook time~10 minutes| Servings~4 |Difficulty~Easy

Nutritional value- Calories~290| Fat~20g |Carbohydrates~19g| Protein~15g

Ingredients

- Two avocados
- One tablespoon of olive oil
- A quarter cup of diced red onion
- A quarter cup of fresh lemon juice
- Half teaspoon of cumin
- Half teaspoon of chili powder
- One clove of garlic, minced
- A quarter cup of chopped fresh cilantro
- Half cup of low-sodium canned black beans
- Half cup of frozen corn, defrosted under cold water
- One cup of ½ -inch pieces of cooked chicken

Instructions

- Mix corn, cilantro, black beans, onion, chicken, cumin, garlic, lemon juice, chili powder, and olive oil.
- Then refrigerate it for 2 hours.
- Cut the avocados in half and seed. Now put avocado halves flat side up and fill each with 1 /2 cup of the chicken-corn salsa.

Baked Cod with Fennel and Kalamata Olives

Preparation time~10 minutes| Cook time~35 minutes|Servings~4 |Difficulty~Easy

Nutritional value- Calories~186| Fat~5g |Carbohydrates~8g| Protein~21g

Ingredients
- Four (4-ounce) cod fillets
- ⅛ cup of freshly squeezed orange juice
- A quarter cup of dry white wine
- Four slices of fresh orange (with rind)
- A quarter cup of Kalamata olives pitted
- One fennel bulb, sliced paper-thin
- Two bay leaves
- Two teaspoons of extra-virgin olive oil
- One teaspoon of freshly ground black pepper

Instructions

- Preheat the oven to 400°F.
- Over medium heat, put on an oven-safe skillet and add some olive oil. Add and cook fennel until softened.
- Add the wine, simmer it and cook for 1 to 2 minutes. Mix in some pepper and orange juice and simmer again for 2 minutes.
- Take it off the heat and place cod over the fennel mixture. Top the fillets with orange slices. Arrange the bay leaves and olives around fish.
- Roast everything until the fish is opaque. Once it flakes easily with a fork, the fish is cooked. It will also reach an inside temperature of 145°F. Serve hot.

Baked Lemon Tilapia

Preparation time~5 minutes| Cook time~22 minutes| Servings~4 |Difficulty~Easy

Nutritional value- Calories~298| Fat~16g |Carbohydrates~2.8g| Protein~20.9g

Ingredients

- Four tilapia fillets
- Two tablespoons of fresh lemon juice
- One teaspoon of garlic, minced
- A quarter cup of olive oil
- Two tablespoons of fresh parsley, chopped
- One lemon zest
- Pepper
- Salt

Instructions

- Preheat the oven to 425°F.
- Spray a baking dish with cooking spray and set it aside. In a small bowl, whisk together olive oil, lemon zest, lemon juice, and garlic. Season fish fillets with pepper and salt and place them in the baking dish.
- Pour olive oil mixture over fish fillets.
- Bake fish fillets in the oven for 10-12 minutes. Garnish with parsley and serve.

Balsamic Roast Chicken

Preparation time-25 minutes| Cook time-30 minutes| Servings-8 |Difficulty-Moderate

Nutritional value- Calories-298| Fat-16g |Carbohydrates-2.8g| Protein-20.9g

Ingredients

- One tablespoon of fresh rosemary (or one teaspoon of dried rosemary)

- One whole chicken, 4 pounds

- Half cup of balsamic vinegar

- One tablespoon of olive oil

- One garlic clove

- 1/8 teaspoon of freshly ground black pepper

- Eight sprigs of fresh rosemary

- One teaspoon of brown sugar

Instructions

- Preheat the oven to 350 degrees Fahrenheit.

- Mince the rosemary and garlic in a small bowl. Separate the skin from the chicken's flesh and rub it with olive oil, followed by the herb mixture. Season with freshly ground black pepper. Two rosemary sprigs should be placed in the cavity of the chicken. Arrange the chicken in a truss.

- Place the chicken in a roasting pan and roast for approximately 20 to 25 minutes per pound, or approximately 1 hour and 20 minutes. The internal temperature of a whole chicken should be at least 165 degrees. Frequently baste with pan juices. When the chicken is browned and the juices run clear, transfer it to a serving platter.

- Combine the brown sugar and balsamic vinegar in a small saucepan. Warm until the brown sugar dissolves, but do not bring to a boil.

- Carve the chicken and skin it. The vinegar mixture should be drizzled over the pieces. Serve immediately garnished with the remaining rosemary sprigs.

Balsamic-Honey Glazed Salmon

Preparation time-2 minutes |Cook time-8 minutes |Servings-2 to 4|Difficulty-Easy

Nutritional value: -Calories-454|Proteins-65g| Fat-17g|Carbohydrates-9.7g

Ingredients

- Half cup of balsamic vinegar

- One tablespoon of honey

- Four (8-ounce) salmon fillets

- Sea salt and freshly ground pepper

- One tablespoon of olive oil

Instructions

- Heat a skillet over medium-high heat. Mix the vinegar and honey in a small bowl.

- Season the salmon fillets with sea salt and freshly ground pepper; brush with the honey-balsamic glaze.

- Add olive oil to the skillet, then sear the salmon fillets, cooking for 3 to 4 minutes on every side until lightly browned and medium-rare in the center.

- Let sit for 5 minutes before serving.

Barbecue Chicken and Portobello Pizzas

Preparation time-15 minutes| Cook time-30 minutes| Servings-6 |Difficulty-Easy

Nutritional value- Calories-181| Fat-9g |Carbohydrates-14g| Protein-12g

Ingredients

- A quarter cup of roughly chopped fresh cilantro

- ⅔ cup of mozzarella or Monterey Jack cheese

- Four ounces of feta or goat cheese

- One chicken breast, baked and diced

- ¾ cup of low-sugar barbecue sauce

- Half red onion, diced

- Six large (4- to 5-inch) portobello mushrooms, stems removed

- One garlic clove, minced

- One tablespoon of extra-virgin olive oil

Instructions

- Preheat the oven to 400°F.

- Mix the garlic and oil. Brush the mushroom bottoms with it. Now put them on a baking sheet with their stem-side down. Bake for 15 minutes.

- Then, sauté the red onion over medium-low heat until browned.

- Discard the mushroom caps juice, and put them back on the baking sheet (this time stem-side up). Fill each one of the caps with Two tablespoons of barbecue sauce. Now put the red onion, cheese, and chicken. Bake again till cheese melts.

- Take it out, garnish with some cilantro, and serve.

BBQ Roasted Salmon

Preparation time-15 minutes| Cook time-15 minutes|Servings-4 |Difficulty-Easy

Nutritional value: Calories-225| Fat-6g |Carbohydrates-7g| Protein-34g

Ingredients

- A quarter cup of pineapple juice

- Two tablespoons of fresh lemon juice

- Four salmon fillets (6 ounces each)
- Two tablespoons of brown sugar
- Four teaspoons of chili powder
- Two teaspoons of grated lemon rind
- 3/4 teaspoon of ground cumin
- Half teaspoon of salt
- A quarter teaspoon of cinnamon

Instructions

- Preheat the oven to 400 degrees Fahrenheit.
- In a Ziploc bag, combine the first three ingredients. Marinate for one hour in the refrigerator, turning occasionally. Take the salmon out of the bag and discard the marinade.
- Combine remaining ingredients in a small bowl and rub over fish.
- Fillets should be placed in a baking dish coated with cooking spray.
- Bake for 12 to 15 minutes, or until the desired degree of doneness is achieved.
- Garnish with a lemon slice.

Beef and Swiss Cheesesteak-Style Lettuce Roll-Up

Preparation time- 5 minutes| Cook time-10 minutes| Servings-4 |Difficulty-Easy

Nutritional value- Calories-227| Fat-15g |Carbohydrates-4g| Protein-20g

Ingredients

- A quarter teaspoon of salt
- Eight thin tomato slices
- Four romaine lettuce leaves
- Half cup of sliced yellow onion
- Four ounces of Swiss cheese (4 slices)
- Eight ounces of stir-fry beef pieces
- One tablespoon of extra-virgin olive oil

Instructions

- Warm-up oil over medium heat. Cook the beef, onion, and salt until the onion becomes translucent.
- Lower the heat and put Swiss cheese on top. Close the lid and cook for one minute to melt the cheese. Take out the onion and beef and arrange them in the middle of the lettuce wraps.
- Top with tomato slices and serve the sandwiches.

Black Bean and Brown Rice Casserole

Preparation time-15minutes| Cook time-25 minutes| Servings-8 |Difficulty-Easy

Nutritional value- Calories-267| Fat-6g |Carbohydrates-22g| Protein-32g

Ingredients

- One cup of vegetable broth
- 1/3 cup of brown rice
- 1 medium thinly sliced zucchini
- 1/3 cup of diced onion
- One tablespoon of olive oil
- Half teaspoon of cumin
- One 15-ounce can of black beans, drained
- Half cup of sliced mushrooms
- 1/3 cup of carrots, shredded
- Two cups of low-fat shredded Swiss cheese
- A quarter teaspoon of cayenne pepper
- One 4-ounce can dice green chilies
- One pound of cooked boneless chicken breast (skinless, chopped into small pieces)

Instructions

- In a saucepan, combine the vegetable broth and rice bring to a boil. Reduce to low heat, cover, and continue cooking for 46 minutes, or until tender rice.
- Preheat the oven to 350 degrees Fahrenheit.
- Coat a large casserole dish lightly with nonstick cooking spray.
- In a skillet over medium heat, heat olive oil and cook onion until tender.
- Combine mushrooms, chicken, zucchini, and seasonings in a large mixing bowl.
- Continue cooking and stirring until the zucchini is lightly browned and the chicken is heated through.
- Combine onion, cooked rice, zucchini, chicken, carrots, beans, mushrooms, chilies, and one cup of Swiss cheese in a large mixing bowl.
- Transfer to a prepared casserole dish and scatter the remaining one cup of Swiss cheese on top.
- Cover casserole loosely with foil and bake in preheated oven for 30 minutes.
- Remove the cover and bake for an additional 10 minutes, or until lightly browned.

Black Bean-Salmon Stir-Fry

Preparation time-5 minutes |Cook time-20 minutes |Servings-2 to 4|Difficulty-Easy

Nutritional value: Calories-330|Proteins-27g| Fat-19g|Carbohydrates-11.8g

Ingredients

- Two teaspoons of cornstarch
- Two tablespoons of rice vinegar
- Two tablespoons of sauce black bean garlic
- Twelve ounces of mung bean sprouts
- One tablespoon of canola oil
- One tablespoon of rice wine
- One lb of salmon
- One pinch of red pepper
- One cup of diced scallions
- A quarter cup of water

Instructions

- Mix all the ingredients except salmon and set aside. The sauce is ready.
- Cook salmon in heated oil for three minutes from each side.
- Add the sauce to salmon and cook for a minute.
- Mix in scallions and beans and cook for five minutes.

Black-Eyed Dill Tuna

Preparation time-15 minutes| Cook time-0 minutes|Servings-4 |Difficulty-Easy

Nutritional value- Calories-150| Fat-8g |Carbohydrates-7g| Protein-15g

Ingredients

- Two teaspoons of chopped fresh dill
- One and a half tablespoons of olive oil
- Two tablespoons of lemon juice
- A quarter cup of finely chopped onion
- Two hard-boiled eggs, chopped fine
- One 6-ounce can water-packed chunk light tuna, drained and flaked
- One medium red pepper, finely diced
- One 15-ounce can of black-eyed peas, drained and rinsed

Instructions

- Just put all of the ingredients in a medium bowl and mix well.

Boneless chicken cutlets

Preparation time-10 minutes |Cook time-15 minutes |Servings-2 to 4 |Difficulty-Easy

Nutritional value: Calories-375|Proteins-30g| Fat-18g|Carbohydrates-10g

Ingredients

- 3/4 cup of all-purpose flour
- Half cup of liquid eggs
- Half cup of unseasoned bread crumbs
- A quarter cup of freshly grated Parmesan cheese
- One tablespoon of mustard powder
- Four (4-ounce) skinless, boneless chicken cutlets
- Four tablespoons of olive oil
- Salt and freshly ground pepper to taste
- Lemon wedges

Instructions

Set out three shallow bowls.

- Place flour in one bowl, eggs in the second bowl, and mix together the bread crumbs, Parmesan cheese, and mustard powder in the third bowl.
- Dredge cutlets with flour, gently shaking cutlets to remove the excess. Then dip chicken into the eggs, coating both sides; again, allow cutlets to drip off any excess egg back into the bowl.
- Finally, coat cutlets with bread crumb mixture. Heat olive oil in a large cast-iron skillet over medium-high heat. Cook cutlets (about 4 minutes on each side) until golden brown and cooked through. Juices should run clear.
- Place cooked chicken on a paper towel-lined plate to absorb any excess oil. Season with salt and pepper to taste and serve with wedges of lemon.

Braised Chicken with Roasted Bell Peppers

Preparation time-30 minutes |Cook time-One hour 15 minutes |Servings-2 to 4|Difficulty-Hard

Nutritional value: Calories-490|Proteins-24g| Fat-28g|Carbohydrates-12g

Ingredients

- Two tablespoons of extra-virgin olive oil
- Three pounds of bone-in chicken, breast and thighs, skin removed
- One and a half teaspoons of kosher salt, divided
- A quarter teaspoon of freshly ground black pepper
- One onion, julienned
- Six garlic cloves, sliced
- One cup of white wine
- Two pounds of tomatoes, chopped
- A quarter teaspoon of red pepper flakes

- Three bell peppers (any colors you like) or two jars of roasted red peppers, drained

- 1/3 cup of fresh parsley, chopped

- One tablespoon of lemon juice

Instructions

- Warm the olive oil in an oven or pot over medium-high heat. Season the chicken with ¾ teaspoon of salt and pepper.

- Add partial chicken to the pot and brown for about 2 minutes on each side. Handover to a plate, and repeat with the remaining half of the chicken.

- Lower the heat to medium and add the onion.

- The next step is to sauté for about 5 minutes. You need to put the garlic and sauté for 30 seconds.

- Add the wine, raise the heat to medium-high, and bring to a boil to deglaze the pot, rubbing up any brown bits on the bottom. Reduce the liquid by half, about 5 to 7 minutes. Add the tomatoes, red pepper flakes, and the remaining ¾ teaspoon of salt and mix well. Add the chicken back to the pot, cover, reduce the heat to low, and simmer for 40 minutes, rotating the chicken halfway through the cooking time.

- While the chicken cooks, prepare the roasted bell peppers.

- Chop the bell peppers into 1-inch pieces and set them aside.

- Once the chicken is cooked through, transfer it to a plate.

- Upsurge the heat to high and bring the mixture to a boil. Reduce by half, about 10 minutes.

- When the chicken is cool enough to grip, remove the meat from the bone, and return it to the pot with the bell peppers. Simmer 5 minutes to heat through. Stir in the parsley and lemon juice.

Broccoli and Garlic Shrimp Stir-Fry

Preparation time-10 minutes| Cook time-25 minutes|Servings-4 |Difficulty-Easy

Nutritional value: Calories-235| Fat-4g |Carbohydrates-10g| Protein-35g

Ingredients

- Half cup of water

- A quarter teaspoon of salt

- One teaspoon of garlic powder

- Two cups of chopped broccoli florets

- One medium bell pepper, diced

- One cup of diced yellow onion

- One tablespoon of extra-virgin olive oil

- Two pounds raw shrimp, deveined

Instructions

- Boil water in a large pot. Add the shrimp once the water is boiling. Now lower the heat to medium and cook for 5 more minutes. Take it off the stove, drain the hot water, and add cold water. Add the shrimp to the cold water for about 5 minutes.

- Drain the cold water, and then peel the shrimp.

- Oil a large skillet and put it over medium-high heat. Add bell peppers and onion. Cook until the pepper is mildly softened and the onion is translucent.

- Add half a cup of water, garlic powder, broccoli, and salt. Cook the broccoli for 5 to 7 minutes.

- Introduce the cooked shrimp and frequently stir for 2 to 3 minutes until everything is well-mixed. Serve hot.

Broccoli Cheddar Bake

Preparation time-15 minutes| Cook time-48 minutes| Servings-6 |Difficulty-Moderate

Nutritional value- Calories-173| Fat-9g |Carbohydrates-8g| Protein-15g

Ingredients

- Half cup of finely chopped onion

- Four cups of chopped fresh broccoli

- One and a half cups of egg substitute

- Half teaspoon of ground black pepper

- One cup of shredded cheddar cheese

- Two tablespoons of water

- One cup of fat-free milk

Instructions

- Preheat the oven to 350 degrees Fahrenheit. Coat a baking dish lightly with cooking spray.

- Combine the onion, broccoli and water in a nonstick skillet.

- Sauté over medium heat for approximately 5 to 8 minutes, or until the vegetables are tender.

- Continue to add water as needed to keep the vegetables from drying out, but use as little as possible. When the broccoli is done, drain and set aside.

- Combine the egg substitute, 3/4 cup cheese and milk in a bowl.

- Combine the broccoli mixture and pepper in a medium bowl.

- Stir well to combine.

- Spoon the mixture into the baking dish that has been prepared.

- Place the baking dish in a large pan filled halfway with water.

- Bake, uncovered, for about 45 minutes, or until a knife inserted in the center comes out clean.

- Take the pan out of the oven and sprinkle the top with the remaining 1/4 cup shredded cheese.

- Allow approximately 10 minutes before serving.

Broiled garlic lamb chops

Preparation time-10 minutes | Cook time-15 minutes | Servings-2 to 4 | Difficulty-Easy

Nutritional value: Calories-574 | Proteins-68g | Fat-24g | Carbohydrates-6g

Ingredients

- Eight (4–5-ounce) lamb chops

- Four cloves fresh garlic, finely chopped

- Half tablespoon dried rosemary

- Garlic salt to taste, if desired

- Three tablespoons of Dijon mustard

- Juice from one lemon

- One tablespoon of honey

- Two tablespoons of extra-virgin olive oil

- A quarter teaspoon of red wine vinegar

- Freshly ground pepper to taste

- Fresh mint leaves for garnish

Instructions

- Preheat the oven to broil. Chops should be rinsed in cold water and dried with paper towels. Place them on a broiling pan in a single layer and set them aside.

- In a small mixing dish, combine the garlic and rosemary. Rub the garlic/rosemary mixture onto both sides of the chops, season with garlic salt if preferred, then broil chops for about 4 inches.

- Broil until the desired doneness is reached. While the chops are broiling, combine mustard, honey, lemon juice, vinegar, olive oil, and pepper to taste in a blender and blend until well combined. Remove the chops from the oven and divide them into two serving plates.

- Serve immediately, spooning mustard mixture over chops and garnishing each plate with a mint leaf.

Broiled Garlic Shrimp

Preparation time-10 minutes | Cook time-20 minutes | Servings-4 | Difficulty-Easy

Nutritional value- Calories-140 | Fat-4g | Carbohydrates-14g | Protein-10.4g

Ingredients

- 1/8 teaspoon of pepper

- Half cup of melted unsalted margarine

- Two teaspoons of lemon juice

- One lb. of Shrimp in shells

- One tablespoon of chopped fresh parsley

- Two tablespoons of chopped onion

- One minced clove of garlic

Instructions

- Preheat the broiler in the oven. Washing, drying, and peeling shrimp are all options. Combine the Margarine, lemon juice, onion, garlic, and pepper on a baking dish.

- Add the shrimp and cover with a lid.

- Cook for 5 minutes under the broiler. Broil for another 5 minutes, on the other hand.

- Serve on a tray with the pan juices diluted. Serve with a parsley garnish.

Broiled mango chicken breast fillets

Preparation time-10 minutes | Cook time-15 minutes | Servings-2 to 4 | Difficulty-Easy

Nutritional value: Calories-297 | Proteins-36g | Fat-8g | Carbohydrates-18g

Ingredients

- Four (4–5-ounce) skinless, boneless chicken breast fillets

- Salt and freshly ground pepper to taste

- Four large bay leaves, crumbled

- Two teaspoons of finely chopped fresh garlic

- Six large pitted black olives halved

- Three tablespoons of dry cream sherry

- One tablespoon of extra-virgin olive oil

- Two ripe but firm mangos, peeled and cut into wedges

Instructions

- Rinse fillets under cold water and pat dry with paper towels. Place fillets in a single layer in a shallow baking dish.

- Sprinkle tops of fillets with salt and pepper, as desired. Scatter crumbled bay leaves, garlic, and olives over fillets.

- In a small bowl, combine sherry and olive oil. Whisk to blend and drizzle over fillets.

- Scatter mango wedges over and around fillets. Place the baking dish in the oven and bake at 350 degrees for about 8–10 minutes or until juices run clear when fillets are pierced with a fork. Set oven to broil.

- Transfer baking dish to top rack about 4 inches under heat and broil tops of fillets until lightly browned.

- Serve hot, drizzled with juices from the baking dish and topped with pieces of mangos.

Broiled spicy turkey burgers

Preparation time-10 minutes | Cook time-15 minutes | Servings-2 to 4 | Difficulty-Easy

Nutritional value: Calories-219 | Proteins-22g | Fat-9g | Carbohydrates-12g

Ingredients

- One pound of freshly ground turkey breast
- Two cloves fresh garlic, finely chopped
- Three scallions, finely chopped
- Half cup of fresh spinach, chopped
- Half cup of Italian-seasoned bread crumbs
- Half teaspoon of red hot pepper sauce
- Half teaspoon of Worcestershire sauce
- Two whole wheat pita loaves cut in half with pockets opened
- Alfa sprouts, sliced tomato, lettuce, mustard, etc., as desired, for garnish

Instructions

- Turn on the oven broiler. In a large bowl, combine ground turkey, garlic, scallions, spinach, bread crumbs, hot pepper sauce, and Worcestershire sauce.
- Stir to mix thoroughly and form into four equal-size patties. Place patties on a broiler pan and place in oven about 4 inches under the broiler.
- Broil burgers on each side for roughly 6 minutes, turning only once. Cook until centers are no longer pink. Remove from oven. Place each burger inside a pita pocket and garnish as desired.

Broiled tuna and tomato

Preparation time-10 minutes | Cook time-10 minutes | Servings-2 to 4 | Difficulty-Easy

Nutritional value: Calories-224 | Proteins-20g | Fat-18g | Carbohydrates-2g

Ingredients

- Four (3-ounce) tuna fillets
- Four tablespoons of extra-virgin olive oil
- Two large cloves of fresh garlic, minced
- One tablespoon of chopped fresh parsley
- Salt and freshly ground pepper to taste
- One and a half teaspoons of white wine vinegar
- Eight (Half-inch) slices of fresh tomato
- Fresh Italian parsley, chopped, for garnish

Instructions

- Rinse fillets, pat dry, and set aside. Combine in a covered container Two tablespoons of olive oil, garlic, parsley, and salt and pepper. Add fillets, turning to coat well.
- Marinate fillets at room temperature for 2 hours. In another bowl, combine remaining olive oil, vinegar, salt and pepper, if desired.
- Arrange sliced tomatoes in a flat container in one layer and pour oil mixture over tomatoes; marinate at room temperature for 2 hours.
- Heat broiler, place tuna on grilling pan about 4 inches below heat and broil each side of fillets for about 2–3 minutes.
- Arrange two slices of tomato on each plate; add tuna fillets to the top of tomatoes and garnish with parsley. Serve while hot.

Brown Sugar, Beef, and Broccoli Stir-Fry

Preparation time-5 minutes | Cook time-15 minutes | Servings-4 | Difficulty-Easy

Nutritional value: Calories-152 | Fat-6g | Carbohydrates-10g | Protein-15g

Ingredients

- Half tablespoon of soy sauce
- Two tablespoons of brown sugar
- One cup of sliced yellow onion
- Two cups of chopped broccoli florets
- Nonstick cooking spray
- Eight ounces of stir-fry beef pieces
- Two tablespoons of coconut aminos
- One tablespoon of extra-virgin olive oil

Instructions

- Heat the oil over medium heat. Cook the beef until browned. Set aside
- With cooking spray, coat the skillet. Add onion and broccoli and stir every 30 seconds. Let it cook until the onion becomes translucent.
- Add some soy sauce, brown sugar, cooked beef, and coconut aminos. Then mix well.
- Take off the broccoli and beef from heat and serve.

Buffalo Chicken Wrap

Preparation time-15 minutes | Cook time-0 minutes | Servings-5 | Difficulty-Easy

Nutritional value- Calories-200 | Fat-7g | Carbohydrates-14g | Protein-28g

Ingredients

- 1 tomato, diced
- 5 small 100% whole-grain low-carb wraps
- Chopped raw celery (optional)

- A quarter cup of Buffalo wing sauce

- ½ red onion, finely sliced

- Two cups of chopped romaine lettuce

- A quarter cup of Creamy Peppercorn Ranch Dressing

- 3 cups cooked grilled, canned, or rotisserie chicken breast

Instructions

- Mix lettuce, chicken, onion, tomato, wing sauce, celery (if preferred), and dressing.

- Put one cup of the mixture on each wrap. Fold the sides and close the wrap tightly. Place toothpicks to keep them in place if necessary. Serve warm.

Cajun Chicken Stuffed with Pepper Jack Cheese and Spinach

Preparation time-25 minutes| Cook time-50 minutes| Servings-4 |Difficulty-Hard

Nutritional value- Calories-241| Fat-9g |Carbohydrates-2g| Protein-32g

Ingredients

- One pound of chicken breasts, boneless, skinless

- One cup of frozen spinach thawed and drained (or fresh cooked)

- Two tablespoons of Cajun seasoning (see recipe below if you want to make homemade)

- One tablespoon of bread crumbs

- Three ounces of reduced-fat pepper jack cheese (shredded)

- Toothpicks

Cajun Seasoning

- 3/4 teaspoon of onion powder

- 3/4 tablespoon of paprika

- A quarter teaspoon of ground black pepper

- A quarter teaspoon of cumin

- A quarter teaspoon of ground white pepper

- A quarter teaspoon of fresh ground thyme

- Half teaspoon of freshly ground cayenne pepper

- A quarter teaspoon of freshly ground oregano

Instructions

- Preheat the oven to 350 degrees Fahrenheit.

- Flatten the chicken to a thickness of 1/4 inch.

- Combine the salt, spinach, pepper jack cheese, and pepper in a medium bowl.

- In a small bowl, combine the Cajun seasoning and breadcrumbs.

- Distribute approximately 1/4 cup of the spinach mixture evenly among the chicken breasts. Each chicken breast should be tightly rolled and the seams secured with several toothpicks.

- Drizzle olive oil over each chicken breast. Evenly distribute the Cajun seasoning mixture overall.

- Garnish chicken with any remaining spinach and cheese as an option.

- Arrange the chicken seam-side up on a baking sheet lined with tin foil (for easy cleanup).

- Bake for 35–40 minutes, or until the chicken is fully cooked.

- Before serving, remove the toothpicks. Count to ensure that every toothpick has been removed.

- Slice into medallions or serve whole.

Calamari in spicy red sauce

Preparation time-10 minutes |Cook time-One hour |Servings-2 to 4|Difficulty-Hard

Nutritional value: ~Calories-224|Proteins-26g| Fat-5g|Carbohydrates-16g

Ingredients

- Three cups of low-sodium canned tomato sauce

- One (28-ounce) can peeled Italian tomatoes, broken into pieces

- One cup of Chianti wine

- Two tablespoons of freshly squeezed lemon juice

- One tablespoon of extra-virgin olive oil

- Three cloves fresh garlic, chopped

- One small onion, chopped

- One teaspoon of black pepper

- Salt to taste (optional)

- Half teaspoon of cayenne pepper

- Six fresh basil leaves, chopped

- 1/3 cup of grated Romano cheese

- Two pounds of cleaned calamari, cut in Half-inch rings

Instructions

- In a large deep skillet, add tomato sauce, tomato pieces, wine, lemon juice, olive oil, garlic, onion, pepper, salt to taste, cayenne, basil, and Romano cheese.

- Simmer on medium-low heat for about 30 minutes to allow alcohol to burn off and infuse other ingredients with its flavor.

- Add calamari rings and continue to simmer for an additional 20–30 minutes, occasionally stirring. Calamari is cooked when it plumps and becomes opaque in color.

- Do not overcook calamari; it becomes tough. This goes well with cooked fettuccine.

Cheeseburger Scramble

Preparation time-5 minutes| Cook time-10 minutes| Servings-4 |Difficulty-Easy

Nutritional value: Calories-218| Fat-13g |Carbohydrates-2g| Protein-21g

Ingredients

- A quarter teaspoon of salt

- Half cup of canned diced tomatoes, drained

- Half cup of shredded Cheddar cheese

- Four large eggs

- Eight ounces of lean ground beef

- Nonstick cooking spray

Instructions

- With some cooking spray, oil a large skillet. Now over medium heat, cook the ground beef until it's fully browned.

- Then discard the fat and put the beef aside.

- Over medium heat, put the skillet back and oil it again. Put the eggs into a bowl and whisk well. Put the eggs into the hot skillet and cook the eggs till they are set.

- Lower the heat. Throw in some beef, Cheddar cheese, salt, and tomato, and mix well until the cheese is melted.

- Turn off the heat, serve and enjoy.

Cheesy Crustless Quiche

Preparation time-20 minutes| Cook time-45 minutes| Servings-9 |Difficulty-Hard

Nutritional value: Calories-176| Fat-9g |Carbohydrates-3g| Protein-19g

Ingredients

- 9-inch pie pan

- One cup of skim milk

- Four ounces of cubed baby Swiss (low-fat)

- Oregano to season (if desired)

- Ten ounces of reduced-fat mozzarella cheese, shredded

- Nonstick cooking spray

- Three large eggs

- Six ounces of grilled chicken breast, cut into 1-inch cubes

Instructions

- Preheat the oven to 400 degrees Fahrenheit.

- Using a nonstick cooking spray, coat the pie pan.

- Layer the cubed chicken breast and cubed baby Swiss in the pie-pan.

- Evenly distribute the shredded mozzarella cheese over the whole mixture.

- Season with oregano to taste.

- In a new bowl, whisk the skim milk and eggs together.

- Distribute the cheese and chicken evenly.

- Bake for 41 minutes at 400 degrees (Top will be lightly browned in color when finished).

Allow to cool before serving or cover with tin-foil, refrigerate it.

Cherry Sauce Meatballs

Preparation time-30 minutes |Cook time-15 minutes |Servings-2 to 4 |Difficulty-Easy

Nutritional value: ~Calories-76|Proteins-6g| Fat-4g|Carbohydrates-8g

Ingredients

- One cup of bread crumbs, seasoned

- One small chopped onion

- One large, lightly beaten egg

- Three minced garlic cloves

- One teaspoon of salt

- Half teaspoon of pepper

- Sixteen ounces 90% lean ground beef

- Sixteen-ounce ground pork

Sauce

- One 20-ounces can consist of cherry pie filling

- 1/3 cup of sherry (or substitute chicken broth)

- 1/3 cup of cider vinegar

- A quarter cup of steak sauce

- Two tablespoons of brown sugar

- Two tablespoons of soy sauce, reduced-sodium

- One teaspoon of honey

Instructions

- Preheat your oven to 400 degrees F.

- Mix the first six ingredients and mix well. Add the ground meat and mix thoroughly. Shape the mixture into 1-inch balls. Arrange in a shallow baking pan over a greased rack.

- Bake for 11 to 13 minutes or until cooked through. Drain juice on a paper towel.

- In a large-size saucepan, combine all sauce ingredients. Boil the sauce over medium heat. Simmer uncovered within 2 to 3 minutes or until it thickens.

- Add the meatballs stir gently until heated through.

Chicken piccata

Preparation time-10 minutes | Cook time-25 minutes | Servings-2 to 4 | Difficulty-Easy

Nutritional value: Calories-223 | Proteins-21g | Fat-11g | Carbohydrates-4g

Ingredients

- Four (3-ounce) skinless, boneless chicken breast fillets, lightly pounded

- Salt and freshly ground pepper to taste (optional)

- Two teaspoons of extra-virgin olive oil, divided

- Three cloves of fresh garlic, minced

- One cup of canned low-sodium, fat-free chicken broth

- Two tablespoons of dry white wine

- Four teaspoons of lemon juice

- One tablespoon of all-purpose flour

- Two tablespoons of chopped fresh parsley

- One tablespoon of capers

- Lemon wedges for garnish

Instructions

- Rinse chicken breast fillets under cold water and pat dry, then place breasts between layers of wax paper and lightly pound fillets with a meat mallet.

- Lightly sprinkle each fillet with salt and pepper, if desired. Heat one teaspoon of olive oil in a large, heavy skillet over medium heat, add chicken fillets and cook until fillets are lightly browned and centers cooked (juice will run clear).

- Transfer fillets to a serving platter and put them in a low-temperature oven to keep warm. Add the remaining teaspoon of olive oil and garlic to the same skillet and cook for 30 seconds to soften. Combine chicken broth, wine, lemon juice, and flour in skillet. Stir to blend and continue stirring until the mixture thickens.

- Add parsley and capers to the sauce. Remove chicken from the oven, place each fillet on a plate, and spoon mixture over fillets. Garnish with lemon wedges.

- Serve with cooked spinach linguine or pasta of choice.

Chicken and eggplant

Preparation time-10 minutes | Cook time-55 minutes | Servings-2 to 4 | Difficulty-Hard

Nutritional value: Calories-376 | Proteins-37g | Fat-24g | Carbohydrates-12g

Ingredients

- One medium eggplant, peeled and cut into one and a half-inch cubes

- Half cup of plus two tablespoons of extra-virgin olive oil, divided

- Two pounds skinless, boneless chicken

- One large onion, chopped

- Two cloves of fresh garlic, chopped

- One teaspoon of mixed spices

- Two large tomatoes, peeled, seeded, and chopped

- Two teaspoons of Thick Pomegranate Molasses

- Three tablespoons of freshly squeezed lemon juice

- Salt and freshly ground pepper to taste

- Two tablespoons of finely chopped fresh parsley

To make mixed spices combine

- Two teaspoons of allspice

- One teaspoon of ground cinnamon

- One teaspoon of ground cloves

- One teaspoon of fresh cilantro

- One teaspoon of ground cumin

- A quarter teaspoon of freshly ground pepper

Instructions

- Salt eggplant pieces generously and let drain in a colander for about 30 minutes (this rids eggplant of its bitter juices).

- After 30 minutes, rinse pieces under running cold water, gently squeeze pieces with hands to remove excess moisture, and pat dry with paper towels.

- In a large, heavy skillet, heat half a cup of olive oil over medium heat. Add half of the eggplant pieces and sauté, frequently turning until golden brown.

- With a slotted spoon, transfer pieces to paper towels to drain and soak up excess oil. Repeat procedure with remaining eggplant, adding more olive oil if necessary.

- Pour olive oil from the skillet, allow the skillet to cool, and wipe clean.

- Rinse chicken pieces under cold water and pat dry with paper towels.

- Place chicken in the skillet with two tablespoons of olive oil and sauté, turning to brown evenly on all sides.

- Transfer pieces to plate. Pour off all but three tablespoons of drippings from the skillet.

- Add onions and sauté over medium heat until golden brown. Add garlic and mixed spices and sauté for about 30 seconds while stirring.

- Add tomatoes, thick Pomegranate Molasses, lemon juice, and salt and pepper to taste. Return chicken and any juices from plate to skillet, spooning tomato mixture around pieces. Bring to a boil and reduce to low. Cover and simmer for about 45 minutes or until the chicken is tender.

- Stir in sautéed eggplant and parsley, cover, and simmer for an additional 10 minutes. Adjust seasonings to taste.

- Serve with a side dish of pasta (optional).

Chicken and feta

Preparation time-10 minutes | Cook time-40 minutes | Servings-2 to 4 | Difficulty-Easy

Nutritional value: Calories-259 | Proteins-41g | Fat-7g | Carbohydrates-2g

Ingredients

- One cup of plain low-fat Greek yogurt

- One tablespoon of freshly squeezed lemon juice

- Half tablespoon chopped fresh oregano

- Half tablespoon chopped fresh rosemary

- A quarter teaspoon of freshly ground pepper

- Two large cloves of fresh garlic, minced

- Four (4-ounce) skinless, boneless chicken breasts

- Olive oil cooking spray

- 1/3 cup of crumbled feta cheese

- One tablespoon of chopped fresh parsley for garnish

Instructions

- Combine the first six ingredients in a resealable plastic baggie. Add chicken and toss to coat. Refrigerate marinated chicken for at least 30 minutes.

- Preheat oven to broil. Remove chicken from bag and reserve the marinade. Place chicken on a oven/broiler pan coated with cooking spray. Place pan 6 inches below heat and broil for about 7-8 minutes.

- Turn chicken, then add reserved marinade to the chicken, and top with feta cheese. Continue to broil chicken for an additional 7 minutes or until chicken is cooked through.

- Remove from oven, sprinkle top with parsley, and serve.

Chicken and spicy hummus

Preparation time-10 minutes | Cook time-15 minutes | Servings-2 to 4 | Difficulty-Easy

Nutritional value: Calories-435 | Proteins-43g | Fat-22g | Carbohydrates-17g

Ingredients

- A quarter cup of olive oil

- One tablespoon of finely chopped fresh garlic

- Half teaspoon of ground cumin

- Half teaspoon of freshly ground pepper

- One and a half pounds skinless, boneless chicken breast, cut into 2-inch cubes

- One red bell pepper, sliced lengthwise into 1-inch-wide strips

- One yellow banana pepper, sliced lengthwise into 1-inch-wide strips

- One red onion, cut into strips

- Salt to taste

- Half cup of prepared spicy hummus

- Four lemon wedges for garnish

- Pita wedges (optional)

Instructions

- Combine olive oil, garlic, cumin, black pepper, chicken, red and yellow peppers, onion, and salt in a resealable plastic baggie. Toss all ingredients until chicken is well coated with olive oil and seasonings.

- Line a broiler pan with tin foil and spread the chicken mixture out in a single layer. Place pan 4–6 inches under heat and broil ingredients for roughly 8–10 minutes, stirring once, until chicken is cooked through and veggies are lightly blackened.

- Divide the hummus and chicken mixture each into equal portions. Place hummus on plate and top with chicken mixture. Garnish plate with a lemon wedge and serve with toasted pita wedges, if desired.

Chicken and wild rice with garden vegetables

Preparation time-10 minutes | Cook time-15 minutes | Servings-2 to 4 | Difficulty-Easy

Nutritional value: Calories-518 | Proteins-35g | Fat-14g | Carbohydrates-59g

Ingredients

- One and a half cups of balsamic vinegar

- Half cup of canola or olive oil

- Half cup of honey

- 1/3 cup of chopped fresh oregano

- 1/3 cup of chopped fresh sage

- Half teaspoon of ground cumin

- Four skinless, boneless chicken breasts (about one and a half pounds)

- Four tablespoons of trans fat–free canola/olive oil spread

- Two cups of canned low-sodium, fat-free chicken broth

- One cup of long grain wild rice

- Half cup of fresh or frozen peas

- Half cup of fresh or frozen corn

- Half cup of diced celery

- Three scallions, thinly sliced

- Salt and freshly ground pepper to taste

Instructions

- In a large, resealable plastic baggie, combine vinegar, oil, honey, oregano, sage, cumin, and chicken breasts. Turn to coat chicken with ingredients and refrigerate for at least 3 hours. When the chicken has marinated, remove with tongs, allowing excess marinade to drip off. Transfer to a plate and discard the remaining marinade.

- In a large skillet, melt canola/olive oil spread over medium-high heat. Add chicken and cook until browned on both sides and well done (juices will run clear when cooked through).

- Transfer to a warmed plate and cover with foil. In the same skillet, pour in the broth, scraping up loose chicken pieces and drippings to blend with broth. Add in rice, peas, corn, celery, and scallions.

- Bring to a boil, then reduce heat to a simmer. Stir to mix ingredients, then cover and cook until liquid is absorbed and rice is tender. Slice chicken and serve over rice and vegetable mixture. Add salt and pepper to taste if needed.

Chicken Breasts Ranch with Cheese

Preparation time- 5 minutes| Cook time- 20 minutes| Servings-2 |Difficulty-Easy

Nutritional value: Calories-295| Fat-3g |Carbohydrates-2g| Protein-19g

Ingredients

- Two lb of Chicken breasts

- Two spoons of sugar

- One tablespoon of salt

- Half teaspoon of garlic melted

- Half teaspoon of cayenne pepper paste

- Half teaspoon of ground black peppercorns

- Half teaspoon of ranch seasoning blend

- Half cup of Ricotta cheese

- Half cup of Monterey-Jack cheese

- Four slices of bacon

- A quarter cup of minced scallions

Instructions

- Preheat your oven to 370 ° Fahrenheit.

- Sprinkle melted butter over the chicken. Season the chicken with salt and garlic powder, a seasoning blend of cayenne Pepper, Black Pepper, and ranch.

- Set a cast-iron skillet over moderate heat. Boil, the chicken for 3 to 5 minutes. Place the chicken in a lightly oiled baking dish. Add bacon and cheese. Bake for 12 minutes. Put scallions on end right before serving.

Chicken cacciatore

Preparation time-10 minutes |Cook time-45 minutes |Servings-2 to 4 |Difficulty-Moderate

Nutritional value: Calories-455|Proteins-29g| Fat-13g|Carbohydrates-31g

Ingredients

- Four chicken thighs

- Two chicken breasts, with skin and bones and halved

- Salt and freshly ground pepper to taste

- One cup of all-purpose flour

- Three tablespoons of olive oil

- One green bell pepper, seeded and sliced

- One red bell pepper, seeded and sliced

- One onion, chopped

- One carrot, finely chopped

- One celery stalk, finely chopped

- Three cloves fresh garlic, finely chopped

- 2/3 cup of white wine

- One (28-ounce) can of chopped tomatoes, undrained

- Three tablespoons of capers

- One and a half teaspoons of dried oregano

Instructions

- Rinse chicken and pat dry with paper towels. Combine salt and pepper with flour in a bowl and lightly dredge chicken in flour mixture.

- Heat olive oil in a large skillet over medium-high heat. Add chicken and sauté for about 5 minutes per side. Remove from skillet and set aside.

- In the same skillet, combine green and red bell peppers, onion, carrot, celery, and garlic and sauté until tender. Add wine and let simmer until reduced by half, about 5 minutes. Add tomatoes and juices, capers, oregano, and salt and pepper to taste.

- Return chicken to skillet, cover, and let simmer for roughly 30 minutes, often stirring, until chicken is completely cooked through. Divide into equal portions and serve.

Chicken Cauliflower Fried Rice

Preparation time-10 minutes | Cook time-45 minutes | Servings-8 | Difficulty-Moderate

Nutritional value- Calories-126 | Fat-5g | Carbohydrates-8g | Protein-12g

Ingredients

- Eight teaspoons of coconut aminos
- A quarter teaspoon of salt or Two teaspoons of soy sauce
- Two large eggs
- One teaspoon of ginger powder
- Eight ounces of boneless, skinless chicken breast
- One teaspoon of garlic powder
- One cup of chopped yellow onion
- One cup of peeled, diced carrot
- Two cups of cauliflower rice
- One tablespoon of extra-virgin olive oil

Instructions

- Put the chicken breast in a medium pot and submerge it in water to cover the chicken. Now boil it over medium-high heat for half an hour.
- Take it off heat; discard the hot water, and run cold water on it. Then shred the chicken and leave it there.
- Heat the olive oil in a large skillet over medium heat. Now sauté the onion and carrot cauliflower rice until softened.
- Incorporate the eggs and mix with the veggies for 1 to 2 minutes.
- Now throw in the shredded chicken with ginger powder, garlic powder, coconut aminos, and salt. Now cook for another 1 to 2 minutes and serve.

Chicken Cheese-Steak Wrap

Preparation time-5 minutes | Cook time-7 minutes | Servings-1 | Difficulty-Easy

Nutritional value: Calories-264 | Fat-6g | Carbohydrates-17g | Protein-33g

Ingredients

- A quarter-pound of skinless and boneless chicken breast
- A quarter cup of sliced green pepper
- A quarter cup of mushrooms, sliced
- A quarter cup of chopped onion

- One wedge (3/4-ounce) Laughing Cow Original light swiss cheese or equivalent
- Two teaspoons of sliced pickled hot chili peppers
- One whole-wheat flour, low-carb tortilla

Instructions

- Place the chicken breasts to ¼ inch thickness on a cutting board and slice them into thin strips.
- Mist a skillet with cooking spray and heat over medium-high heat.
- Cook until the onions are translucent and the chicken is no longer pink throughout.
- Add the mushrooms and green peppers to the pan and cook, occasionally stirring until the peppers and mushrooms are soft.
- Fold the tortilla in half and sandwich it between two damp paper towels. Microwave for a total of 20 seconds.
- Lay the warm tortilla flat and spread an even strip of cheese down the center.
- Add chicken, peppers, onions, and mushrooms to the top.
- If using, add chili peppers.
- Fold the tortilla's sides over the center. Serve right away.

Chicken Cordon Bleu

Preparation time-15 minutes | Cook time-30 minutes | Servings-6 | Difficulty-Easy

Nutritional value- Calories-174 | Fat-7g | Carbohydrates-3g | Protein-24g

Ingredients

- Six slices of reduced-fat Swiss cheese (3 ounces total), halved
- Two tablespoons of grated Parmigiano-Reggiano cheese
- A quarter cup of whole-wheat bread crumbs
- One tablespoon of water
- Six boneless, skinless chicken breasts
- Two large eggs
- Six slices of lean deli ham
- Nonstick cooking spray

Instructions

- Preheat the oven to 450°F. Coat a baking sheet with some cooking spray.
- Pound the chicken breasts until it becomes ¼ inch thick.

- On each chicken breast, place 1 slice of ham and 1 slice of cheese. Then roll the chicken. Now put them on the baking sheet with the seam-side down.

- Now, gently beat the eggs. Then combine Parmigiano-Reggiano cheese and bread crumbs in another bowl.

- Now brush each roll with egg wash and sprinkle the bread crumb and cheese mix on top.

- Bake until the chicken is cooked well and turns golden on top.

Chicken Lettuce Wraps

Preparation time- 5 minutes| Cook time- 30 minutes| Servings-2 |Difficulty-Easy

Nutritional value: Calories- 246| Carbohydrates- 5.8g| Protein- 33.5g| Fat- 9.2g

Ingredients

For Chicken

- One tablespoon of avocado oil

- Half small finely chopped onion

- Half teaspoon of minced fresh ginger

- One minced clove of garlic

- Half pound of ground chicken

- Salt and freshly ground black pepper, to taste

For Wraps

- Five romaine lettuce leaves

- Half cup of peeled and julienned carrot

- Half tablespoon of finely chopped fresh parsley

- Half tablespoon of fresh lime juice

Instructions

- In a skillet, heat the oil over medium heat and sauté the onion, ginger, and garlic for about 4-5 minutes. Add the ground chicken, salt, and black pepper, and cook over medium-high heat for about 7-9 minutes, breaking up the meat into smaller pieces with a wooden spoon.

- Remove from the heat and set aside to cool.

- Arrange the lettuce leaves onto serving plates.

- Place the cooked chicken over each lettuce leaf and top with carrot and cilantro.

- Drizzle with lime juice and serve it.

Chicken pesto wrap

Preparation time-10 minutes |Cook time-5 minutes |Servings-2 |Difficulty-Easy

Nutritional value: Calories-249|Proteins-27g| Fat-9g|Carbohydrates-17g

Ingredients

- Olive oil cooking spray

- Four (4-ounce) skinless, boneless chicken tenderloins

- Salt and freshly ground pepper to taste

- Four tablespoons of market-fresh pesto sauce

- Two (8-inch) whole-grain wraps

- Eight slices of sundried tomato, packed in olive oil

- Fresh arugula

Instructions

- Lightly spray a heavy-bottomed skillet with cooking oil. Heat skillet over medium heat, add chicken, season with salt and pepper to taste and cook tenders until cooked through.

- Spread two tablespoons of pesto onto each wrap and add 2–3 slices of sundried tomatoes and a handful of arugula to each wrap.

- Top each wrap with two chicken tender pieces and roll up wrap, folding in ends of the wrap. Slice each wrap in half on a diagonal and serve.

Chicken Rollantini with Spinach ala Parmigiana

Preparation time-25 minutes| Cook time-30 minutes| Servings-9 |Difficulty-Moderate

Nutritional value: Calories-212| Fat-6g |Carbohydrates-16g| Protein-32g

Ingredients

- Six tablespoons of egg whites/egg beaters, divided

- Five ounces of frozen spinach, thawed and squeezed dry of any liquid

- Half cup of whole-wheat breadcrumbs (Italian seasoned)

- Eight chicken breast cutlets, three ounces each (pounded thin)

- Six ounces of part-skim mozzarella, shredded, divided

- Six tablespoons of part-skim ricotta cheese

- One cup of marinara sauce

- A quarter cup of grated and divided parmesan cheese

- Nonstick cooking spray

Instructions

- Preheat the oven to 450 degrees Fahrenheit.

- Using a nonstick cooking spray, coat a 9x13 glass baking dish.

- Season with salt and pepper chicken cutlets.

- Combine breadcrumbs and Two tablespoons of grated parmesan cheese in a small bowl.

- In a separate bowl, place 1/4 cup egg whites.

- Combine a medium mixing bowl of 1.5 ounces of mozzarella cheese, spinach, remaining parmesan cheese, Two tablespoons of egg whites, and ricotta cheese.

- Arrange seasoned, pounded chicken cutlets on a work surface and spread each with 2 tbsp spinach-cheese mixture.

- Using a toothpick or two, loosely roll each cutlet, keeping the seam side down.

- Coat the chicken rolls in egg whites and then in the bread crumb mixture, then place seam-side down in a greased baking dish.

- Repeat with the remainder of the chicken.

- Coat chicken rollatini lightly with nonstick spray.

- Bake for 25 minutes, or until an instant-read thermometer registers 165°F.

- Remove from oven and top with remaining marinara sauce and shredded mozzarella cheese.

- Bake an additional 3 minutes, or until the cheese is melted and bubbly.

- Serve with additional sauce and grated parmesan cheese on the side.

Chicken Sausage and Peppers

Preparation time-10 minutes | Cook time-20 minutes | Servings-2 to 4 | Difficulty-Easy

Nutritional value: Calories-173 | Proteins-22g | Fat-5g | Carbohydrates-7g

Ingredients

- Two tablespoons of extra-virgin olive oil
- Four Italian chicken sausage links
- One onion, thinly sliced
- One red bell pepper, seeded and thinly sliced
- One green bell pepper, seeded and thinly sliced
- Three garlic cloves, minced
- Half cup of dry white wine
- Half teaspoon of sea salt
- A quarter teaspoon of freshly ground black pepper
- Pinch red pepper flakes

Instructions

- In a huge skillet over medium-high heat, heat the olive oil until it shimmers.
- Add the sausages and cook for 5 to 7 minutes, occasionally turning until browned, and they reach an internal temperature of 165°F. With tongs, remove the sausage from the pan and set it aside on a platter, tented with aluminum foil to keep warm.
- Return the skillet to heat and add the onion, red bell pepper, and green bell pepper. Cook for 5 to 7 minutes, occasionally stirring, until the vegetables begin to brown.
- Add the garlic and cook for 30 seconds, stirring constantly.
- Stir in the wine, sea salt, pepper, and red pepper flakes.
- Use the top of a spoon to ground and fold in any browned bits from the pan's bottom.
- Simmer for about 4 minutes more, stirring, until the liquid reduces by half. Spoon the peppers over the sausages and serve.

Chicken shawarma pitas

Preparation time-10 minutes | Cook time-30 minutes | Servings-2 to 4 | Difficulty-Moderate

Nutritional value: Calories-320 | Proteins-39.8g | Fat-15.7g | Carbohydrates-6g

Ingredients

- ¾ tablespoon of cumin
- ¾ tablespoon of coriander
- ¾ tablespoon of turmeric powder
- One sliced onion
- ¾ tablespoon of garlic powder
- Half teaspoon of cloves
- ¾ tablespoon of paprika
- One tablespoon of lemon juice
- Half teaspoon of cayenne pepper
- Eight boneless chicken pieces
- Salt to taste
- 1/3 cup of olive oil
- Pita bread
- Tahini sauce

Instructions

- In a bowl, add sliced chicken pieces, onions, cumin, garlic, cloves, olive oil, turmeric, paprika, lemon juice, salt, and coriander. Toss well to coat chicken evenly. Set aside for three hours in the refrigerator.
- Transfer the chicken pieces along with the marinade in a baking tray sprayed with oil.
- Bake in a preheated oven at 425 degrees F for 30 minutes.
- Spread tahini sauce in pita bread and add baked chicken pieces. You can also add your favorite salad.
- Serve and enjoy it.

Chicken Stir Fry with Eggplant and Basil

Preparation time- 5 minutes | Cook time-20 minutes | Servings-4 | Difficulty-Easy

Nutritional value: Calories-257 | Fat-9g | Carbohydrates-14g | Protein-9g

Ingredients

- A quarter cup of fresh basil, coarsely chopped
- Two tablespoons of fresh mint, chopped
- 3/4 cup chicken stock or broth (low-sodium)
- Three green (spring) onions, including tender green tops, two coarsely chopped and one thinly sliced
- Two tablespoons of low-sodium soy sauce
- One tablespoon of peeled and chopped fresh ginger
- Two tablespoons of extra-virgin olive oil
- Two cloves of garlic
- Half cup of yellow onion, coarsely chopped
- Four cups of eggplant, peel and diced
- One yellow bell pepper, seeded and cut into julienne
- One pound of skinless, boneless chicken breasts, cut into strips 2 inches long and 1/2 inch wide

- One red bell pepper, seeded and cut into julienne

Instructions

- Combine the mint, basil, 1/4 cup of the stock, garlic, onions, green and ginger in a blender or food processor. Pulse the mixture until it is finely minced but not pureed. Place aside.

- In a large nonstick frying pan over medium-high heat, heat one tablespoon of the olive oil. Sauté the yellow onion, eggplant and bell peppers for about 8 minutes, or until the vegetables are just tender. Transfer to a bowl and keep warm by covering with a kitchen towel.

- Heat the pan over medium-high heat with the remaining one tablespoon of olive oil. Add the basil mixture and cook, constantly stirring for approximately 1 minute. Add the chicken strips and soy sauce and sauté for about 2 minutes, or until the chicken is almost opaque throughout. Bring to a boil the remaining half cup of stock. Return the eggplant mixture to the pan and cook, constantly stirring for about 3 minutes, or until heated through. Transfer to a warmed serving dish and top with the green onion slices.

- Serve right away.

Chicken Stuffed Potatoes

Preparation time- 5 minutes| Cook time-20 minutes| Servings-4 |Difficulty-Easy

Nutritional value: Calories-312| Fat-8g |Carbohydrates-35g| Protein-22g

Ingredients

- A quarter cup of water

- Four red potatoes, 6-ounce

- Two cans no-salt-added chicken breast, 5-ounce (drained)

- 1/8 teaspoon of salt

- ⅓ cup of store-bought salsa

- Half teaspoon of chili powder

- One tablespoon of cilantro

- Half cup of cheese, shredded

- Two ounces of Monterey Jack (less-fat)

Instructions

- Using a thin knife, cut a thin slice off one side of each potato. Punctuate with a fork and transfer to a microwave-safe container. 1/4 cup water Microwave on high for 10-12 minutes, uncovered.

- In a separate bowl, whisk together chicken salt. And chili powder. Microwave for 1 minute or until thoroughly heated.

- Scoop a few spoonfuls from the potato's interior. Fill potato shell halfway with chicken mixture.

- Garnish with salsa and shredded cheese.

- Alternatively, heat for 30 seconds to soften the cheese. Garnish with cilantro.

Chicken Tikka Masala

Preparation time-25 minutes| Cook time-5 hours| Servings-10 |Difficulty-Hard

Nutritional value: Calories-270| Fat-8g |Carbohydrates-12g| Protein-45g

Ingredients

- Three pounds of boneless chicken, skinless breast

- Two tablespoons of fresh ginger, minced

- One large onion, diced

- Four cloves of garlic, minced

- Two bay leaves

- One and a half cups of plain Greek yogurt

- Two tablespoons of olive oil

- One 29-ounce can of tomato puree

- One tablespoon of cumin

- Two tablespoons of Gram masala

- Half tablespoon of paprika

- 3/4 teaspoon of ground black pepper

- 3/4 teaspoon of cinnamon

- Chopped cilantro for topping

- One to three teaspoons of cayenne pepper

Instructions

- In a large bowl, combine everything except the bay leaves.

- Using a spatula, combine all ingredients and coat the chicken thoroughly.

- Gently place in a slow cooker and top with bay leaves.

- Cover and cook on low for 8 hours or on high for 4 hours.

- Discard bay leaves and garnish with cilantro.

Chicken with pomegranate sauce

Preparation time-10 minutes |Cook time-37 minutes |Servings-2 to 4 |Difficulty-Moderate

Nutritional value: Calories-364|Proteins-50g| Fat-14g|Carbohydrates-8g

Ingredients

- Four pounds of skinless, boneless chicken breast, cut into small pieces

- Two teaspoons of paprika

- Salt and freshly ground pepper to taste

- A quarter cup of extra-virgin olive oil

- Four cloves of fresh garlic, minced

- Two medium yellow onions, chopped

- A quarter cup of chopped fresh parsley

- One small hot banana pepper, finely chopped

- Three tablespoons of Thick Pomegranate Molasses

- Four cups of canned chunky tomatoes, undrained

Instructions

- Wash chicken, remove fat and cut into small pieces. Sprinkle with paprika and salt and pepper. Heat olive oil in a saucepan, add chicken pieces and stir-fry for about 2–3 minutes.

- Add garlic and stir-fry for another 2–3 minutes. Add onions, parsley, hot banana pepper, Thick Pomegranate Molasses, and tomatoes with liquid; cover and bring to boil. Cook over medium-low heat for about 30 minutes until chicken is tender.

- Serve with rice.

Chickpea pita pockets

Preparation time-10 minutes | Cook time-0 minutes | Servings-2 to 4 | Difficulty-Easy

Nutritional value: ~Calories-152 | Proteins-7g | Fat-3g | Carbohydrates-29g

Ingredients

- One (15-ounce) can of chickpeas, rinsed and drained

- One cup of shredded fresh spinach

- 2/3 cup of halved seedless red grapes

- Half cup of finely chopped red bell pepper

- 1/3 cup of thinly sliced celery

- Half medium cucumber, diced

- A quarter cup of finely chopped onion

- A quarter cup of light mayonnaise

- One tablespoon of balsamic syrup

- Half tablespoon poppy seeds

- Four (6-inch) whole-wheat pita loaves, cut in half

Instructions

- In a large bowl, combine chickpeas, spinach, grapes, red bell pepper, celery, cucumber, and onion. Whisk together mayonnaise, balsamic syrup, and

- poppy seeds. Add poppy seed mixture to chickpea mixture and stir until well blended. Lightly toast pita halves and fill with chickpea filling. Serve.

Chipotle Shredded Pork

Preparation time-10 minutes | Cook time-6 hours | Servings-8 | Difficulty-Hard

Nutritional value: Calories-260 | Fat-11g | Carbohydrates-5g | Protein-20g

Ingredients

- Two pounds of pork shoulder, without extra fat

- One tablespoon of ground cumin

- Juice of one lime

- One can of chipotle peppers

- One tablespoon of dried oregano

- One and a half tablespoons of apple cider vinegar

Instructions

- Puree the adobo sauce, oregano, apple cider vinegar, chipotle peppers, lime juice, and cumin.

- Add pork to the slow cooker, and cover with sauce.

- Close it and cook for 6 hours on low.

- Shred the pork with two forks while still in the pot. If it's still not dried up, let it cook on low for 20 minutes to absorb the leftover liquid.

Classic Tangy Chicken Drumettes

Preparation time- 10 minutes | Cook time- 40 minutes | Servings-2 | Difficulty-Moderate

Nutritional value: Calories-209 | Fat-12.2g | Carbohydrates-3g | Protein-18.1g

Ingredients

- One pound of chicken drumettes

- One spoon of olive oil

- Two spoonsful of butter, melted

- One Garlic Clove, chopped

- Juice of half lemon

- Two teaspoons of white wine

- Salt & Ground Black Pepper

- One spoonful of freshly scallions to try, sliced

Instructions

- Preheat your oven to 440 ° Fahrenheit.

- Place the Chicken in a Baking pan covered with parchment. Sprinkle with melted butter and olive oil. Add the garlic, ginger, oil, vinegar & black pepper.

- Cook for about 35 minutes in the preheated oven. Serve freshly garnished scallions.

Cod with Lemon and Capers

Preparation time-5 minutes| Cook time-30 minutes| Servings-4 |Difficulty-Easy

Nutritional value: Calories-168| Fat-4g |Carbohydrates-2g| Protein-31g

Ingredients

- Four cod fillets, each 6 ounces
- One cup of hot tap water
- One tablespoon of soft butter
- Four teaspoons of capers, rinsed and drained
- Two lemons
- One tablespoon of all-purpose (plain) flour
- One teaspoon of chicken-flavored bouillon granules (low-sodium)

Instructions

- Preheat the oven to 351 degrees Fahrenheit. Cooking spray four corners of foil.
- Arrange one cod-fillet per foil-square. Cut 2 lemons in half. Then squeeze half of the lemon over the fish. Cut the remaining half of the lemon into slices and arrange it above the fish before sealing the foil.
- Bake for about 20 minutes, or until the fish is opaque throughout when tested with the tip of a knife.
- Remove the peel from the second lemon while the fish is cooking. Take care not to cut the pith but only the peel. Peel the peel and cut it into 1/4-inch-wide strips. Place aside.
- Combine the chicken bouillon granules and hot tap water in a small bowl. Stir until the granules are completely dissolved. Set aside.
- In a separate small bowl, combine the butter and flour. Transfer to a large heavy-bottomed saucepan. Over low heat, constantly stir until the butter-flour mixture melts.
- Continue to stir the bouillon into the butter mixture until it thickens. Remove from the heat and stir in the capers. Serve alongside the fish, garnished with lemon peel.

Crab patty burgers

Preparation time-10 minutes |Cook time-10 minutes |Servings-2 to 4|Difficulty-Easy

Nutritional value: Calories-375|Proteins-27g| Fat-26g|Carbohydrates-5g

Ingredients

- One pound of crabmeat, well-drained
- A quarter cup of diced celery
- One tablespoon of chopped green bell pepper
- One tablespoon of chopped white onion

- One teaspoon of Worcestershire sauce
- One teaspoon of hot red pepper sauce (optional)
- Half teaspoon of salt (optional)
- Dash of Old Bay seasoning
- One cup of light mayonnaise
- Half cup of grated cheddar cheese
- The scant amount of canola oil cooking spray
- Lemon wedges for garnish

Instructions

- Mix all ingredients in a large bowl, except lemon wedges. Form into four patties and place on broiling sheet lightly sprayed with cooking oil.
- Place under broiler and broil for about 2 minutes or until patties are lightly browned. Garnish with lemon wedges and serve.

Creamy Beef Stroganoff with Mushrooms

Preparation time-10 minutes| Cook time-30 minutes| Servings-6 |Difficulty-Easy

Nutritional value: Calories-351| Fat-9g |Carbohydrates-30g| Protein-31g

Ingredients

- Half pound of mushrooms, sliced
- Half cup of Greek yogurt
- Half teaspoon of dried thyme
- One teaspoon of Worcestershire sauce
- Two tablespoons of finely chopped fresh parsley for garnish
- Two tablespoons of whole-wheat flour
- One cup of water
- Half teaspoon of dried dill
- One cup of low-sodium beef broth
- One medium onion, chopped
- One teaspoon of extra-virgin olive oil
- One and a half pounds of extra-lean beef sirloin, cut into ½-inch strips
- Nonstick cooking spray

Instructions

- Spray a pan with cooking and put over medium-high heat. Add beef and cook for 5 minutes.
- Heat the oil over medium-high heat. Now cook onions until tender.
- Add mushrooms and cook for 3 minutes.
- Add the flour and mix with onion and mushrooms.

- Mix in the Worcestershire sauce, water, thyme, dill, and broth, and boil it. Now cook for about 10 minutes.

- Add yogurt and beef and mix well. Garnish with the parsley and enjoy.

Creamy Chicken Soup with Cauliflower

Preparation time-15 minutes| Cook time-40 minutes| Servings-4 |Difficulty-Moderate

Nutritional value- Calories-164| Fat-3g |Carbohydrates-5g| Protein-25g

Ingredients

- Two cups of non-fat or 1% milk

- One cup of fresh spinach, chopped

- Two and a half cups of fresh cauliflower florets

- Two cups of low-sodium chicken broth

- One teaspoon of dried thyme

- Two cups of water

- One teaspoon of freshly ground black pepper

- One and a half pounds (3 or 4 medium) cooked chicken breast, diced

- One celery stalk, diced

- One carrot, diced

- Half yellow onion, diced

- One teaspoon of extra-virgin olive oil

- One teaspoon of minced garlic

Instructions

- Place a pot over medium-high heat. Sauté the garlic and olive oil for 1 minute.

- Then add celery, onion, carrots and sauté for 3 to 5 minutes.

- Add the black pepper, broth, water, chicken breast, cauliflower, and thyme. Simmer it, lower the heat to medium-low, and cook for 30 minutes.

- Throw in some spinach and cook for 5 minutes.

- Add in milk and serve hot.

Crispy Pesto Chicken

Preparation time-15 minutes |Cook time-50 minutes | Servings-2| Difficulty-Moderate

Nutritional value: Calories-378| Proteins-29.7g| Fat-16g| Carbohydrates-30g

Ingredients

- Twelve ounces of small red potatoes, scrubbed and diced into 1-inch pieces

- One tablespoon of olive oil

- Half teaspoon of garlic powder

- A quarter teaspoon of salt

- One (8-ounce) boneless, skinless chicken breast

- Three tablespoons of prepared pesto

Instructions

- Heat your oven to 425°F (220°C). Line a baking sheet with parchment paper.

- Combine the potatoes, olive oil, garlic powder, and salt in a medium bowl. Toss well to coat.

- Arrange the potatoes on the parchment paper and roast for 10 minutes. Flip the potatoes and roast for an additional 10 minutes.

- Meanwhile, put the chicken in the same bowl and toss with the pesto, coating the chicken evenly.

- Check the potatoes to make sure they are golden brown on the top and bottom. Toss them again and add the chicken breast to the pan.

- Turn the heat down to 350°F (180°C) and roast the chicken and potatoes for 30 minutes. Check to make sure the chicken reaches an internal temperature of 165°F (74°C), and the potatoes are fork-tender.

- Let cool for 5 minutes before serving.

Crunchy Tuna Patty

Preparation time-10 minutes| Cook time-5 minutes| Servings-8 |Difficulty-Easy

Nutritional value- Calories-80| Fat-1g |Carbohydrates-4g| Protein-12g

Ingredients

- Four cans tuna in water, 3-ounce

- Sixteen Wheat Thins crushed crackers

- Four egg whites

- A quarter cup of carrot, grated

- One tablespoon of minced onion (if tolerated)

- A quarter cup of chopped water chestnuts, capers or diced red pepper

- Pepper, dill and dried mustard (to taste)

Instructions

- Combine all ingredients in a mixing bowl.

- Using your hands, shape the mixture into eight patties.

- Coat a medium skillet with nonstick cooking spray and set aside.

- Cook patties on both sides until golden brown, about 2 to 3 minutes per side.

Crusted chicken breasts

Preparation time-10 minutes |Cook time-15 minutes |Servings-2 to 4 |Difficulty-Easy

Nutritional value: Calories-246|Proteins-40g| Fat-5g|Carbohydrates-2g

Ingredients

- Four (4-ounce) skinless, boneless chicken breasts, pounded to Half-inch thickness

- Two tablespoons of light mayonnaise

- Salt and freshly ground pepper to taste

- Half cup of grated Pecorino cheese

Instructions

- Preheat oven to 500 degrees F. Line a baking sheet with foil and stand a roasting rack inside the sheet.

- With a spatula, lightly coat chicken with mayonnaise, season with salt and pepper to taste, and sprinkle with Pecorino cheese.

- Place chicken on rack and bake for roughly 5 minutes.

- Switch oven to broil. Broil chicken until cooked through and cheese is golden brown.

Curried Pork Tenderloin with Apple Cider

Preparation time-20 minutes| Cook time-25 minutes| Servings-4 |Difficulty-Easy

Nutritional value- Calories-70| Fat-6g |Carbohydrates-19g| Protein-24g

Ingredients

- Sixteen ounces of pork tenderloin, cut into 6 pieces

- One and a half tablespoons of curry powder

- One tablespoon of extra-virgin olive oil

- Two medium yellow onions, chopped (Two cups)

- Two cups of apple cider, divided

- One tart apple, peeled, seeded and chopped into chunks

- One tablespoon of cornstarch

Instructions

- Sprinkle the pork tenderloin with the curry powder & set aside for 16 minutes to marinate.

- In a large skillet over high heat, heat up the olive oil. Cook, turning once until tenderloin is browned on both sides, about 5 to 10 minutes. Remove and set aside the meat from the skillet.

- Add the onions to the skillet and cook, occasionally stirring until soft and golden. Reduce to low heat and add one and a half cups of apple cider; reduce to low heat and simmer until the liquid has reduced to half its volume.

- Combine the chopped apple, cornstarch, and remaining half cup of apple cider in a medium bowl. Stir and cook for approximately 2 minutes, or until the sauce thickens. Reintroduce the tenderloin to the skillet and continue to cook for an additional 5 minutes.

- Arrange tenderloin on a serving platter or divide it among individual plates to serve. Serve immediately with the thickened sauce.

Curry Salmon with Mustard

Preparation time-10 minutes |Cook time-10 minutes |Servings-2 to 4 |Difficulty-Easy

Nutritional value: -Calories-325|Proteins-34g| Fat-18g|Carbohydrates-2.7g

Ingredients

- A quarter teaspoon of ground red pepper or chili powder

- A quarter teaspoon of ground turmeric

- A quarter teaspoon of salt

- One teaspoon of honey

- 1/8 teaspoon of garlic powder or one clove of garlic minced

- Two teaspoons of whole grain mustard

- Four 6-ounces salmon fillets

Instructions

- In a small bowl, mix well salt, garlic powder, red pepper, turmeric, honey, and mustard.

- Preheat the oven to broil and grease a baking dish with cooking spray.

- Place salmon on a baking dish with skin side down and spread the mustard mixture evenly on top of the salmon.

- Pop in the oven and broil until flaky, around 8 minutes.

DZ's Grilled Chicken Wings

Preparation time-15 minutes| Cook time-20 minutes| Servings-18 |Difficulty-Easy

Nutritional value- Calories-82| Fat-6g |Carbohydrates-1g| Protein-7g

Ingredients

- One teaspoon of extra-virgin olive oil

- One cup of buffalo wing sauce

- One teaspoon of garlic powder

- Freshly ground black pepper

- One and a half pounds of frozen chicken wings

Instructions

- Preheat the grill to 350°F.

- Season the wings with some black pepper and garlic powder.

- Grill the wings on each side for 15 minutes. They should be crispy and browned when done.

- Coat the wings in olive oil and buffalo wing sauce. Serve hot.

Egg Bacon and Cheese Sandwich

Preparation time-5 minutes| Cook time-5 minutes| Servings-6 |Difficulty-Easy

Nutritional value- Calories-280| Fat-21g |Carbohydrates-2g| Protein-19g

Ingredients

- Twelve slices of turkey bacon (low sodium)

- Two teaspoons of olive oil

- Six eggs

- Six whole-grain flatbread sandwich thins

- Six slices of low-fat cheese slices (or thinly sliced cheese)

- Two cups of raw spinach

- Siracha or other condiments to taste

Instructions

- Cook turkey bacon according to the package directions.

- In a frying pan over low to medium heat, heat approximately 12 teaspoon oil.

- In a frying pan, crack three eggs and cook for 4-5 minutes, or until the eggs are firm on all sides.

- Turn eggs over and continue cooking until the yolk is firm.

- Repeat the same with the remaining olive oil and three additional eggs.

- If desired, thinly split and toast the sandwich.

- On one half of the thin sandwich, arrange 1 cooked egg, 1 slice of cheese, 2 slices of turkey bacon, and 3 baby spinach leaves.

- Drizzle with sriracha or other desired condiments.

- Complete the sandwich assembly by placing the other half of the sandwich thin on top and serving.

Egg Roll

Preparation time-10 minutes| Cook time-20 minutes| Servings-6 |Difficulty-Easy

Nutritional value- Calories-133| Fat-3g |Carbohydrates-8g| Protein-19g

Ingredients

- Two scallions, finely chopped, for garnish

- One cup of fresh bean sprouts or 1 (14-ounce) can drain and rinse

- One and a half cups of shredded carrots

- Four cups of green cabbage, chopped or shredded into 1-inch ribbons

- Two teaspoons of ground ginger

- Half teaspoons of freshly ground black pepper

- Half cup of low-sodium beef broth

- One and a half tablespoons of low-sodium soy sauce or Bragg Liquid Aminos

- One pound of extra-lean ground chicken or turkey

- One onion, finely diced

- One teaspoon of minced garlic

- Two teaspoons of sesame oil, divided

Instructions

- Over medium-high heat, put a large skillet. Add garlic and one teaspoon of sesame oil. Mix for a minute. Now cook the onion until tender. Then add and cook chicken until browned, breaking up into smaller chunks.

- While the meat is browning, combine soy sauce, black pepper, remaining one teaspoon of sesame oil, ginger, and broth.

- Once the chicken is done, add the sauce. Add carrots, bean sprouts, and cabbage and combine well. Simmer for up to 7 minutes.

- Serve in a bowl. Top with soy sauce and scallions.

Flank Steak, Broccoli and Green Bean Stir-Fry

Preparation time-15 minutes | Cook time-15 minutes | Servings-2 to 4 | Difficulty-Moderate

Nutritional value: Calories-388 | Proteins-29g | Fat-15g | Carbohydrates-35g

Ingredients

- Three cups of cooked brown rice

- Two tablespoons of vegetable oil

- Two tablespoons of rice vinegar

- One and a quarter pound of lean beef flank steak

- One cup of beef broth

- One tablespoon of cornstarch

- One head broccoli, cut into florets (about Six cups)

- One cup of shredded carrot

- Half teaspoon of red pepper flakes

- Half teaspoon of Chinese five-spice powder

- Half pound of thin green beans, trimmed

- Half large onion, sliced

- Half cup of sliced almonds

- A quarter teaspoon of salt

- A quarter cup of reduced-sodium soy sauce

Instructions

- Combine the soy sauce, broth, 5-spice powder, vinegar, cornstarch, & the red chili flakes in a cup and place it aside.

- Take a non-stick frypan, add one tablespoon of oil to it, and heat it. Pepper the salted stir-fry flank steak & for 4 minutes. Remove to a tray.

- Add the remaining one tablespoon. Of oil in it, and then add broccoli, cabbage, green beans, & carrot. Stir-cook for 9 minutes or till it becomes soft & crisp.

- Add a quarter cup of water at the last two minutes of cooking time.

- Now add a mixture of soya sauce& broth in it and then boil & simmer it for 2 minutes, until well dense. Stir in some stored juices & beef & heat up.

- Decorate with the almonds & serve with the cooked brown rice instantly.

Florentine roasted pork

Preparation time-10 minutes | Cook time-Two hours 20 minutes | Servings-2 to 4 | Difficulty-Hard

Nutritional value: Calories-352 | Proteins-47g | Fat-17g | Carbohydrates-2g

Ingredients

- Four pounds of lean loin pork

- Four cloves of fresh garlic, sliced thin

- Half teaspoon of dried rosemary

- Four cloves of fresh garlic, whole

- Six tablespoons of water

- Eight tablespoons of hearty red wine (do not use a glass of cooking wine)

- Salt and freshly ground pepper to taste

Instructions

- If the skin of the loin has not already been scored, cut lines into the skin about 1/8 inch apart. Cut through the flesh to the bone on one side and insert the

- garlic slices and rosemary. Press the whole garlic cloves into the scored skin of the loin and place the loin into a roasting pan in a 350-degree F oven with water and wine.

- Sprinkle loin generously with salt and pepper and roast for two and a half hours or until meat is very tender but still moist, basting occasionally. Serve with a variety of your favorite vegetables.

Ginger Beef Stir Fry

Preparation time-25 minutes | Cook time-35 minutes | Servings-5 | Difficulty-Moderate

Nutritional value- Calories-275 | Fat-8g | Carbohydrates-25g | Protein-17g

Ingredients

- Six ounces of fat-free beef broth

- Two medium garlic cloves

- One pound of flank steak (cut into 1/4 strips)

- A quarter cup of hoisin sauce

- One tablespoon of cornstarch

- One 8-ounce can of sliced water chestnuts

- Half cup of instant brown rice

- One teaspoon of canola oil

- Three tablespoons of soy sauce

- Three ounces of broccoli florets

- A quarter teaspoon of red pepper flakes, crushed

- Two medium-stalks bok choy (cut into 1/2" slices)

- Half medium yellow, green bell or red bell pepper cut into strips

Instructions

- Combine garlic, steak, and ginger in a mixing bowl. Place aside.

- Prepare the rice according to the package directions.

- In a bowl, whisk together soy sauce, hoisin sauce, broth, and cornstarch. Stir until completely dissolved.

- Heat up oil & red pepper flakes in a wok or skillet over medium heat.

- Cook steak for 3–5 minutes on each side or until brownish. Constantly stir. Place aside.

- In a large skillet, combine bell pepper, broccoli, and carrot. Cook for 3-4 minutes over medium-high heat or until tender-crisp. Then Stir. (Add one to two tablespoons of water if the mixture turns dry.

- Add the water, bok choy, chestnuts and toss to combine. Continue cooking for an additional 2–3 minutes, or until the bok choy is tender-crisp. Stir constantly.

- In the center of the pan, make a well & pour in the broth.

- Cook for 1 to 2 minutes, or until broth thickens, stirring occasionally.

- Stir in the beef. Cook for 1 to 2 minutes, or up to heat through. Serve with rice.

Goat cheese and pesto sandwich

Preparation time-10 minutes |Cook time-0 minutes |Servings-2 |Difficulty-Easy

Nutritional value: Calories-294|Proteins-19g| Fat-16g|Carbohydrates-25g

Ingredients

- Four slices of light whole grain bread

- Olive oil cooking spray

- Two tablespoons of goat cheese

- Two tablespoons of market-fresh pesto sauce

- Four thin slices of tomato

- Four thin slices of red bell pepper

- Salt and freshly ground pepper to taste

Instructions

- Lightly spray bread slices with cooking oil. Toast slices until slightly crusty. Set aside to cool. When cooled, divide goat cheese and pesto into two portions.

- Lightly spread top of each slice with a layer of soft goat cheese, followed by pesto sauce. Add tomato and red bell pepper slices.

- Add salt and pepper to taste. Serve as an open sandwich.

Greek Meatballs with Yogurt Sauce

Preparation time-10 minutes| Cook time-40 minutes| Servings-6 |Difficulty-Moderate

Nutritional value- Calories-310| Fat-13g |Carbohydrates-23g| Protein-23g

Ingredients

- Two 14.5-ounce cans of low-sodium diced tomatoes

- One tablespoon of minced garlic

- One tablespoon of olive oil

- A quarter cup of fresh minced mint

- One egg lightly beaten

- Two teaspoons of dried oregano leaves

- Two tablespoons of chopped green onion

- A quarter cup of crumbled reduced-fat feta cheese

- One pound of lean ground beef

- A quarter cup of non-fat milk

- One cup of bread crumbs

Yogurt Sauce

- A quarter teaspoon of black pepper

- Two tablespoons of lemon juice

- A quarter cup of non-fat Greek yogurt

- A quarter cup of crumbled reduced-fat feta cheese

Instructions

- Mix feta, green onion, egg bread crumbs, mint, oregano, and milk. Add ground beef and mix lightly. Make 12 meatballs out of it of about 1 inch in diameter each.

- Warm-up oil over medium-high heat. Add meatballs

and cook on all sides till browned. Remove from heat and close with foil to keep the heat inside.

- Now, sauté garlic for a minute. Mix in tomatoes and cook for 10 minutes. Put meatballs back in the pan and cook for 5 minutes.

- For the yogurt sauce, mix all ingredients well. Cover and chill until ready to be eaten. Serve alongside meatballs.

Greek Yogurt Chicken

Preparation time-15 minutes| Cook time-45 minutes| Servings-4 |Difficulty-Easy

Nutritional value- Calories-266| Fat-4g |Carbohydrates-3g| Protein-46g

Ingredients

- Half cup of grated Parmesan cheese

- Four boneless skinless chicken breasts, 4 ounces each

- One and a half teaspoons of seasoning salt
- One teaspoon of garlic powder
- One cup of plain Greek yogurt
- Half teaspoon of pepper

Instructions

- Preheat the oven to 375 degrees Fahrenheit.
- In a bowl, combine cheese, Greek yogurt, and seasonings.
- Prepare a baking sheet by lining it with foil and spraying it with cooking spray.
- Coat each chicken breast with the Greek yogurt mixture and arrange it on a foil-lined baking sheet.
- Bake at 350 degrees F for 45 minutes.

Green Beans, Spring Onions & Garlic Tofu with Soya-Chili Dressing

Preparation time- 5 minutes| Cook time- 25 minutes| Servings-1 |Difficulty-Easy

Nutritional value- Calories-252|Fat- 8g| Carbohydrates-18g| Protein- 6g

Ingredients

- One and a quarter cups of green beans
- 2/3 cup of plain cubed tofu
- One teaspoon of Garlic paste or crushed garlic
- Three squirts of oil spray
- Four thinly sliced spring onions

For Dressing

- One tablespoon of gluten-free soy sauce
- One teaspoon of olive oil
- A quarter teaspoon of apple cider vinegar or wine
- Chili sauce a few drops (optional)

Instructions

- Steam the green beans until they are only tender, then rinse them under cold water.
- Cook the tofu in the oil spray till golden brown in a nonstick frying pan or wok. Cook for around one minute after adding the spring onions.
- Combine the dressing ingredients in a mixing bowl.
- Toss in the beans, tofu cubes, and spring onion with the seasoning before serving.

Grilled Tangy Balsamic Chicken Thighs

Preparation time-5 minutes| Cook time-20 minutes| Servings-4 |Difficulty-Easy

Nutritional value- Calories-194| Fat-11g |Carbohydrates-10g| Protein-16g

Ingredients

- Freshly ground black pepper
- Salt
- Two garlic cloves, minced
- Half tablespoon of chili powder
- Two tablespoons of brown sugar
- A quarter cup of lime juice
- A quarter cup of balsamic vinegar
- One tablespoon of extra-virgin olive oil
- Four boneless, skinless chicken thighs, trimmed

Instructions

- Mix the chicken, sugar, lime juice, vinegar, olive oil, garlic, and chili powder in a sealable bag. Then season with pepper and salt and mix well. Now marinate in the fridge overnight for a minimum of 1 hour.
- Preheat a grill to medium-high heat. Cook for 5 to 8 minutes and serve.

Ground Lamb with Peas

Preparation time-10 minutes| Cook time- One hour and 5 minutes| Servings-2 |Difficulty-Moderate

Nutritional value-Calories- 297| Carbohydrates- 10.7g| Protein- 35g| Fat- 12.2g

Ingredients

- One chopped onion
- Half tablespoons of olive oil
- Two minced garlic cloves
- Half-inch minced piece of fresh ginger
- Half teaspoon of ground cumin
- One teaspoon of ground coriander
- Half teaspoon of ground turmeric
- One cup of water
- One pound of lean ground lamb
- Half cup of chopped tomato,
- One tablespoon of whipped Greek yogurt (Fat-free)
- Half cup of fresh shelled green peas
- Salt and black pepper to taste
- A quarter cup of fresh chopped cilantro

Instructions

- Heat the oil in a Dutch oven over moderate flame and sauté the onion for 3-4 minutes.

- Then sauté for 1 minute with the garlic, ginger, bay leaf, and ground spices.

- Add lamb and cook for 5 minutes. Then add the tomato and simmer, stirring regularly, for around 10 minutes.

- Add the green peas and water and boil it. Reduce the heat and simmer for 25-30 minutes after covering it with a lid.

- Cook for 4-5 minutes after adding the salt, cilantro, yogurt, and black pepper.

- Extract the bay leaf and serve warm.

Halibut with Creamy Parmesan-Dill Sauce

Preparation time- 5 minutes | Cook time- 20 minutes | Servings-4 | Difficulty-Easy

Nutritional value- Calories-345 | Fat-12g | Carbohydrates-6g | Protein-31g

Ingredients

- ⅓ cup of low-fat sour cream

- Three scallions, finely chopped

- Half teaspoon of dried dill

- Half teaspoon of garlic powder

- Freshly ground black pepper

- Salt

- ⅓ cup of low-fat, plain Greek yogurt

- ⅓ cup of Parmesan cheese

- Juice of half lemon

- Four (6-ounce) fresh halibut fillets (1-inch thick)

Instructions

- Preheat the oven to 400°F.

- Place fillets on a large baking dish; now drizzle lemon juice. Season with some pepper and salt.

- Now mix the yogurt, garlic powder, cheese, scallions, dill, and sour cream. Cover the fish with this mixture.

- Bake until the internal temperature is 145°F, the fish flakes easily with a fork, it becomes opaque, and the cheese turns golden and served.

Herb Crusted Loin with Parsley Sauce

Preparation time- 10 minutes | Cook time- One hour and 40 minutes | Servings-8 | Difficulty-Moderate

Nutritional value- Calories-255 | Fat- 8.3g | Carbohydrates- 9g | Protein- 11.1g

Ingredients

- Two pounds of boneless pork loin

- Two minced cloves of garlic

- Two teaspoons of olive oil

- One tablespoon of Dried sage

- One tablespoon of dried thyme

- Pepper & salt as per taste

Instructions

- Preheat the oven to 350 degrees F.

- Combine oil, salt, sage, thyme, garlic, and pepper in a small bowl. Cook for 1 hour and 15 minutes after coating the pork (exceeding an internal temperature of 155 degrees F). Allow 15 minutes to rest before slicing.

Meanwhile, in a mixer, mix both sauce ingredients and serve.

Herb-Crusted Salmon

Preparation time-10 minutes | Cook time-20 minutes | Servings-2 | Difficulty-Easy

Nutritional value- Calories-197 | Fat-10g | Carbohydrates-9g | Protein-27g

Ingredients

- Half teaspoon of dried thyme

- Four tablespoons of grated Parmigiano-Reggiano cheese

- Two teaspoons of freshly squeezed lemon

- One tablespoon of dried parsley

- Two teaspoons of minced garlic

- Two (4-ounce) salmon fillets

Instructions

- Preheat the oven to 425°F. Line a baking sheet.

- On the baking sheet, arrange the salmon with skin-side down and place the second piece of parchment paper on top. Now bake for 10 minutes.

- In a small dish, combine the Parmigiano-Reggiano cheese, lemon juice, thyme, parsley, and garlic.

- Remove the top parchment paper. Brush the fillets with the herb-cheese mixture.

- Now bake the uncovered salmon for about 5 more minutes. When it is done, serve right away.

Herb-Roasted Turkey Breast

Preparation time-15 minutes | Cook time-One hour 30 minutes | Servings-2 to 4 | Difficulty-Hard

Nutritional value: ~Calories-392 | Proteins-54g | Fat-6g | Carbohydrates-2g

Ingredients

- Two tablespoons of extra-virgin olive oil

- Four garlic cloves, minced

- Zest of one lemon

- One tablespoon of chopped fresh thyme leaves

- One tablespoon of chopped fresh rosemary leaves

- Two tablespoons of chopped fresh Italian parsley leaves

- One teaspoon of ground mustard

- One teaspoon of sea salt

- A quarter teaspoon of freshly ground black pepper

- One (6-pound) bone-in, skin-on turkey breast

- One cup of dry white wine

Instructions

- Preheat the oven to 325°F.

- In a small bowl, whisk the olive oil, garlic, lemon zest, thyme, rosemary, parsley, mustard, sea salt, and pepper.

- Spread the herb mixture evenly over the turkey breast's surface, loosen the skin, and rub underneath as well. Place the turkey breast in a roasting pan on a rack, skin-side up.

- Pour the wine into the pan. Roast for 1 to 1½ hours until the turkey reaches an internal temperature of 165°F.

- Remove from the oven and let rest for 20 minutes, tented with aluminum foil to keep it warm, before carving.

Home-Style Meatloaf with Tomato Gravy

Preparation time-15 minutes| Cook time-One hour 30 minutes| Servings-8 |Difficulty-Hard

Nutritional value- Calories-290| Fat-15g |Carbohydrates-16g| Protein-26g

Ingredients

- Two pounds lean ground beef

- One medium onion, diced small

- Two large egg whites, beaten

- Half cup of finely chopped flat-leaf parsley

- Four tablespoons of ketchup

- One teaspoon of olive oil

- One cup of wheat bran

- Half teaspoon of black pepper

- Two teaspoons of dried thyme

- One tablespoon of Worcestershire sauce

- Three cloves garlic

Tomato Gravy

- A quarter teaspoon of chopped fresh thyme

- One teaspoon of chopped fresh parsley

- One 16-ounce canned no-salt-added tomato purée

Instructions

- Preheat the oven to 350 degrees.

- Spray a 9x5x3" loaf pan.

- Heat the olive oil and sauté garlic and onion until translucent. Add the pepper and thyme and sauté again for 2 minutes. Allow pan to cool.

- Mix the Worcestershire sauce, parsley, bean, ground beef, egg whites, and ketchup. Mix in the sautéed onions.

- Bake the loaf for around 1 hour 20 minutes or until the core temperature, reaches 160 degrees. Serve with Tomato Gravy.

- For Tomato Gravy, in a pan over medium-high heat, heat the oil. Throw in the onion and sauté for a minute.

- Add tomato purée, parsley, black pepper, and fresh thyme. Simmer it for 5 minutes. Serve with meatloaf.

Honey mustard shrimp

Preparation time-10 minutes |Cook time-10 minutes |Servings-2 to 4|Difficulty-Easy

Nutritional value: ~Calories-202|Proteins-23g| Fat-8g|Carbohydrates-8g

Ingredients

- One tablespoon of olive oil

- Two cloves fresh garlic, minced

- 3/4 canned cup of low-sodium, fat-free chicken broth

- One pound of raw medium shrimp (about 30–32 shrimp), peeled and deveined

- A quarter cup of fresh honey mustard salad dressing, store-bought

- Half teaspoon of garlic powder

- Salt and freshly ground pepper to taste

Instructions

- In a large skillet, heat olive oil and add garlic. Sauté until garlic is soft. Add broth and shrimp and cook until shrimp becomes pink and cooked through.

- Reduce heat to very low to keep shrimp warm. In a saucepan, warm the honey mustard dressing with garlic powder and salt and pepper.

- Drain liquid from shrimp and add the warmed mustard mixture to shrimp, then return to very low heat while stirring to coat shrimp and incorporate flavors, about 5 minutes. Serve immediately.

Horseradish-encrusted salmon

Preparation time-10 minutes |Cook time-25 minutes |Servings-2 |Difficulty-Easy

Nutritional value: ~Calories-292 | Proteins-35g | Fat-11g | Carbohydrates-7g

Ingredients

- Olive oil cooking spray
- Two (6-ounce) salmon fillets, skin intact
- 1/3 cup of plain dried bread crumbs
- One tablespoon of low-fat sour cream
- Two tablespoons of prepared fresh horseradish
- Two tablespoons of chopped fresh dill
- Aged balsamic vinegar to drizzle (optional)

Instructions

- Lightly spray a shallow baking pan with cooking oil. Rinse fillets under cold water, pat dry with paper towels, and place skin side down in a baking pan.
- In a food processor, combine bread crumbs, sour cream, horseradish, and dill. Pulse ingredients at low speed into a thick paste.
- Divide into two portions and top each fillet with mixture.
- Place fillets in the oven and bake at 350 degrees until fillets flake easily and topping crusts to a golden brown (about 12–15 minutes).
- Serve hot and drizzle with a small amount of balsamic vinegar, if desired.

Italian Chicken Pasta

Preparation time-10 minutes | Cook time-9 minutes | Servings-2 to 4 | Difficulty-Moderate

Nutritional value: ~Calories-328 | Proteins-23.7g | Fat-8.5g | Carbohydrates-42.7g

Ingredients

- One lb of chicken breast, skinless, boneless, and cut into chunks
- Half cup of cream cheese
- One cup of mozzarella cheese, shredded
- One and a half teaspoons of Italian seasoning
- One teaspoon of garlic, minced
- One cup of mushrooms, diced
- Half onion, diced
- Two tomatoes, diced
- Two cups of water
- Sixteen ounces of whole wheat penne pasta
- Pepper
- Salt

Instructions

- Add all the ingredients except cheeses into the inner pot of the instant pot and stir well.
- Cook on high for 9 minutes. Add cheeses stir well, and serve.

Italian chicken wrap

Preparation time-10 minutes | Cook time-20 minutes | Servings-2 to 4 | Difficulty-Moderate

Nutritional value: ~Calories-610 | Proteins-27g | Fat-36g | Carbohydrates-42g

Ingredients

- Two tablespoons of butter
- Half cup of mayonnaise
- A half lb of boneless chicken breasts
- A quarter cup of shredded Parmesan cheese
- Two cups of shredded romaine lettuce
- Four flour tortillas
- Two sliced Roma tomatoes
- Half cup of crushed croutons
- Sixteen basil leaves

Instructions

- Cook chicken over medium flame in melted butter for 20 minutes.
- Slice the chicken into strips.
- Whisk cheese and mayonnaise and pour over the tortilla.
- Place lettuce followed by chicken, basil, tomato, and croutons on tortilla and wrap.
- Serve and enjoy it.

Italian Halibut

Preparation time-5 minutes | Cook time- 20 minutes | Servings-6 | Difficulty-Easy

Nutritional value- Calories-180 | Fat-5g | Carbohydrates-6g | Protein-26g

Ingredients

- Half cup of shredded part-skim mozzarella cheese
- One cup of prepared spaghetti sauce
- A quarter cup of sliced black olives
- Half cup of sliced mushrooms
- One and a half pounds of halibut fillets, cut into 6 equal pieces

Instructions

- Preheat the oven to 400 degrees. Now coat a baking pan with nonstick cooking spray and arrange halibut fillets on it.

- Top with black olives and mushrooms and drizzle the spaghetti sauce over it. Then bake the fillets for 10 minutes.

- Take out of the oven and cover with cheese on top. Then bake again until the cheese melts and fish flakes easily with a fork.

Lamb and black olives

Preparation time-10 minutes |Cook time-15 minutes |Servings-2 to 4 |Difficulty-Hard

Nutritional value: Calories-461|Proteins-62g| Fat-21g|Carbohydrates-4g

Ingredients

- Two tablespoons of extra-virgin olive oil

- Three cloves fresh garlic, crushed

- Two sprigs of fresh parsley

- Two pounds of lean ground lamb

- Two tomatoes, peeled and chopped

- Half teaspoon of dried rosemary

- Ten to twelve pitted black olives halved

- One cup of dry white wine

Instructions

- Heat olive oil in a large skillet; add garlic and parsley, and sauté until golden brown.

- Add lamb, continue to cook, and often stir until lamb is browned. Add tomatoes, rosemary, olives, and wine. Stir, cover, and cook 3–5 minutes or until lamb is cooked through and most of the liquid has evaporated.

- Serve with rice.

Lamb Chops Curry

Preparation time-15 minutes |Cook time-30 minutes |Servings-2 |Difficulty-Easy

Nutritional value: ~Calories-337|Proteins-30g| Fat-17g|Carbohydrates-15g

Ingredients

- Four (4 ounces) bone-in loin chops of lamb

- One tablespoon of canola oil

- 3/4 cup of orange juice

- Two tablespoons of teriyaki sauce reduced-sodium

- Two teaspoons of grated orange zest

- One teaspoon of curry powder

- One garlic clove, minced

- One teaspoon of cornstarch

- Two tablespoons of cold water

Instructions

- Brown lamb chops on both sides over canola oil.

- Combine the other five ingredients and pour them over the skillet. Cover and let it simmer for 15 to 20 minutes or until lamb turns tender. Remove from heat and keep warm.

- Combine the last two ingredients until smooth. Mix into the pan drippings and boil for 2 minutes or until it thickens.

- Serve with steamed rice if desired.

Lamb wrap

Preparation time-40 minutes |Cook time-0 minutes |Servings-2 to 4 |Difficulty-Easy

Nutritional value: ~Calories-462|Proteins-21g| Fat-6g|Carbohydrates-43g

Ingredients

- 1/3 cup of medium-grain bulgur

- Half cup of diced tomatoes

- Half cup of finely chopped fresh parsley

- A quarter cup of finely chopped fresh mint leaves, no stems

- Two scallions, thinly sliced

- Two and a half tablespoons of extra-virgin olive oil, divided

- Juice from a half lemon

- Two cloves of fresh garlic, minced

- Half pound lean ground lamb

- Salt and freshly ground pepper to taste

- Four ounces of plain non-fat yogurt

- 3/4 cup of diced cucumber

- One tablespoon of chopped fresh mint

- Four (6-inch) whole-wheat pita loaves (do not split open)

- One cup of chopped fresh spinach leaves

- Four ounces of crumbled fat-free feta cheese

Instructions

- Cover bulgur in a bowl with fresh cold water to a depth of roughly a half-inch. Let stand until water is absorbed (about 30 minutes). Fluff with a fork to separate grains. Grains should be plump and slightly moist; if too moist, spread grains on the towel, fold the towel and squeeze to remove excess water.

- Combine tomatoes, parsley, mint, scallions, and two tablespoons of olive oil. Add bulgur and toss gently. Squeeze lemon juice over tabbouleh mixture and refrigerate.

- Heat remaining olive oil and sauté garlic, lamb, and salt and pepper over medium-high heat until browned, constantly stirring to crumble. Drain well and set aside.

- Combine yogurt, cucumber, and mint in a small bowl, stir well and set aside. Stack pita rounds and wrap in waxed paper; microwave on high for 45 seconds. In a bowl, combine lamb mixture, spinach, and feta cheese.

- Spoon a half cup of tabbouleh mixture and 1/4 lamb mixture in the center of each pita round.

- Top with yogurt mixture and roll up pita. To secure, wrap the bottom portion of the pita roll-up with waxed paper.

Lemon Garlic Dover Sole

Preparation time- 5 minutes| Cook time-10 minutes|Servings-4 |Difficulty-Easy

Nutritional value- Calories-140| Fat-5g |Carbohydrates-1g| Protein-21g

Ingredients

- One lemon wedge

- One pound of Dover sole fillets

- One teaspoon of lemon pepper

- Two teaspoons of minced garlic

- One tablespoon of butter

Instructions

- In a large skillet, melt some butter over medium-high heat and add in some garlic.

- With lemon pepper, season the fish on both sides. Now cook on one side. Now turn the fillets and cook for another minute or two, just until it flakes easily with a fork.

- Sprinkle the fillets with some lemon juice.

Lemon-Parsley Crab Cakes

Preparation time-15 minutes| Cook time-10 minutes|Servings-4 |Difficulty-Easy

Nutritional value- Calories-148| Fat-4g |Carbohydrates-5g| Protein-21g

Ingredients

- Nonstick cooking spray

- One egg lightly beaten

- Juice of half lemon

- Two teaspoons of chopped fresh parsley

- A quarter teaspoon of ground cayenne pepper

- One and a half tablespoons of olive oil-based mayonnaise

- Two cans (6-ounce) lump crabmeat, drained, and cartilage removed

- Half teaspoon of Dijon mustard

- Three tablespoons of whole-wheat bread crumbs

Instructions

- Mix egg mayonnaise, mustard, bread crumbs, parsley, lemon juice, and cayenne pepper.

- Slowly add the crabmeat and mix gently.

- Turn the meat into 4 patties with a ¼-cup measuring cup. Refrigerate the patties for 30 minutes.

- Preheat the oven to 500°F.

- Arrange the crab cakes on the baking sheet, put the sheet at the center rack of the oven, and bake for 10 minutes. Serve immediately.

Lemon-Pepper Chicken Bake

Preparation time-10 minutes| Cook time-One hour| Servings-4 |Difficulty-Hard

Nutritional value- Calories-131| Fat-5g |Carbohydrates-6g| Protein-17g

Ingredients

- Freshly ground black pepper

- One teaspoon of seasoned salt

- One tablespoon of extra-virgin olive oil

- One medium red onion, quartered

- One medium tomato, quartered

- One lemon, sliced

- One cup of sliced zucchini

- Eight ounces of skinless chicken breast tenders

Instructions

- Preheat the oven to 400°F.

- Arrange the chicken breasts in a casserole dish, and place the onion, tomato, lemon, and zucchini slices around the chicken. Drizzle thoroughly with olive oil and mix everything to coat the chicken and veggies well with oil.

- Then, season the dish with salt and pepper.

- Bake for about 1 hour until the chicken is cooked through and the veggies are slightly scorched. Cool and serve.

Lemony Chicken and vegetables

Preparation time~10 minutes | Cook time~15 minutes | Servings~2 to 4 | Difficulty-Easy

Nutritional value: ~Calories-255 | Proteins-29g | Fat-15g | Carbohydrates-8g

Ingredients

- Three tablespoons of juice from fresh lemon halves plus extra halves for garnish

- One tablespoon of freshly grated lemon peel

- Two tablespoons of extra-virgin olive oil

- A quarter teaspoon of salt (optional)

- A quarter teaspoon of freshly ground pepper

- Four cloves of fresh garlic, freshly crushed

- One teaspoon of paprika

- One and a half pounds skinless, boneless dark meat chicken

- 3/4 pound of yellow squash, quartered lengthwise

- 3/4 pound of zucchini, quartered lengthwise

- A quarter cup of chopped fresh chives

Instructions

- Whisk together lemon juice, lemon peel, olive oil, salt, and pepper. Reserve Two tablespoons of mixture in a separate cup.

- Add garlic and paprika to the original mixture and pour over chicken; marinate in a covered container in the refrigerator for 3–4 hours. When chicken is marinated, heat grill to medium-high heat.

- Remove chicken from marinade and place on the grill along with squash, zucchini,

- and juiced lemon halves. Close grill top and cook for 10–12 minutes or until juices from the chicken run clear when pierced. Turn chicken one time while grilling.

- Cook squash, zucchini, and lemon halves until tender and brown. Remove chicken from grill and cut into 1-inch-wide pieces. Cut squash and zucchini pieces in half.

- Place chicken and vegetables on a platter and pour reserved marinade over vegetables; sprinkle with chives. Garnish platter with grilled lemon halves and serve.

Lettuce Wrap Beef Tacos

Preparation time~5 minutes | Cook time~15 minutes | Servings~4 | Difficulty-Easy

Nutritional value- Calories-185 | Fat-10g | Carbohydrates-8g | Protein-15g

Ingredients

- Four tablespoons of non-fat plain Greek yogurt

- One teaspoon of ground cumin

- Half cup of avocado

- Four iceberg lettuce leaves

- A quarter teaspoon of salt

- One teaspoon of garlic powder

- A quarter cup of water

- One cup of cauliflower rice

- One cup of chopped yellow onion

- Eight ounces of lean ground beef

- One tablespoon of extra-virgin olive oil

Instructions

- Warm up the oil over medium heat. Cook the beef and onion until the onion becomes translucent.

- Add the garlic powder, cumin, water, salt, and cauliflower rice. Close the lid and let the cauliflower steam for 5 to 7 minutes until softened.

- Turn off the heat and stuff the mixture into every lettuce leaf. Drizzle with Two tablespoons of avocado and one tablespoon of non-fat Greek yogurt for each taco. Pour hot sauce (optional) and enjoy.

Lightly breaded grilled grouper

Preparation time~10 minutes | Cook time~15 minutes | Servings~2 to 4 | Difficulty-Easy

Nutritional value: ~Calories-159 | Proteins-24g | Fat-4g | Carbohydrates-4g

Ingredients

- Half cup of ripe pitted Kalamata olives

- A quarter cup of plain bread crumbs

- One tablespoon of capers, rinsed and drained

- One teaspoon of extra-virgin olive oil

- One teaspoon of lemon juice

- One clove of fresh garlic

- Four (4-ounce) grouper fillets

- Eight lime wedges for garnish

Instructions

- Heat grill to high heat; place oil-rubbed fish-grilling pan on grill rack to heat.

- In a food processor, process olives, bread crumbs, capers, olive oil, lemon juice, and garlic until smooth.

- Brush each side of fillets with olive oil mixture and place fillets on a hot grill pan. Grill fillets uncovered for 5 minutes.

- Before turning fillets over, brush with olive oil mixture, then turn and grill for five additional minutes or until fillets flake easily.

- Remove fillets from grill, place on platter, and serve immediately, garnished with lime wedges.

- This dish goes well with seasoned rice or couscous.

Lunch Stuffed Peppers

Preparation time-10 minute| Cook time-40 minutes|Servings-4 | Difficulty- Moderate

Nutritional value-Calories-285|Fat-4.3g |Carbohydrates-1.5g| Protein-9.4g

Ingredients

- Four big banana peppers cut into halves lengthwise

- One tablespoon of ghee

- Salt and black pepper to the taste

- Half teaspoon of herbs de Provence

- One pound of chopped sweet sausage

- Three tablespoons of chopped yellow onions

- Some marinara sauce

- A drizzle of olive oil

Instructions

- Season the banana peppers with pepper and salt, drizzle with the oil, rub well and bake for 20 minutes in the oven at 325 ° F.

- Meanwhile, over medium, prepare, heat a skillet, add the pieces of sausage, mix and cook for 5 minutes.

- Combine the onion, herbs, salt, pepper and ghee, mix well and simmer for 5 minutes.

- Take the peppers out of the oven, load them with the sausage mix, place them in a dish that is oven-proof, drizzle them with the marinara sauce, place them back in the oven and bake for another 10 minutes.

- Serve and enjoy.

Magically Moist Chicken

Preparation time-15 minutes| Cook time-45 minutes| Servings-12 |Difficulty-Moderate

Nutritional value- Calories-233| Fat-5g |Carbohydrates-8g| Protein-37g

Ingredients

- One whole-wheat Italian bread crumbs (1/4 cups)

- Three pounds of chicken breasts (skinless, boneless)

- Half cup of Smart Balance Omega Plus Light Mayonnaise Dressing (or any light mayo of choice)

Instructions

- Preheat the oven to 425 degrees Fahrenheit.

- Brush chicken with mayonnaise.

- On a large plate, spread bread crumbs and roll chicken until completely coated.

- Bake chicken breasts in a foil-lined baking dish for 40–45 minutes, or until a meat thermometer reads 165 degrees F.

Maryland-style Vegetable Crab Soup

Preparation time-10 minutes| Cook time-One hour 20 minutes|Servings-6 |Difficulty-Hard

Nutritional value- Calories-105| Fat-2g |Carbohydrates-8g| Protein-13g

Ingredients

- A quarter teaspoon of salt

- Three teaspoons of Old Bay seasoning

- One (15-ounce) can of diced tomatoes, drained

- Six cups of reduced-sodium beef or vegetable broth

- One cup of chopped yellow onion

- One pound of claw blue crab meat

- Two cups of peeled, sliced carrot

- One tablespoon of extra-virgin olive oil

Instructions

- Warm-up oil in a medium saucepan over medium heat. Then add and cook onion and carrot for about 7 minutes. Then put the veggies in a large pot.

- Add crab meat, Old Bay seasoning broth, tomato, and salt. Simmer for about an hour on low-medium heat before serving. Simmer longer to enhance the flavor if preferred.

Mediterranean Turkey Meatloaf

Preparation time-10 minutes| Cook time-55 minutes| Servings-4 |Difficulty-Hard

Nutritional value- Calories-298| Fat-8g |Carbohydrates-10g| Protein-31g

Ingredients
For the Topping

- One teaspoon of extra-virgin olive oil

- Juice of half lemons

- Two to three tablespoons of minced fresh basil

- One large tomato, chopped

- Half small cucumber, peeled, seeded, and chopped

For the Meatloaf

- A quarter teaspoon of dried oregano

- Half teaspoon of dried basil
- A quarter cup of chopped fresh parsley
- Two teaspoons of minced garlic
- A quarter cup of minced red onion
- A quarter cup of Kalamata olives pitted and halved
- A quarter cup of fat-free feta cheese
- A quarter cup of whole-wheat bread crumbs
- A quarter cup plus two tablespoons of hummus, such as Lantana Cucumber Hummus, divided
- One large egg lightly beaten
- One pound of extra-lean ground turkey
- Nonstick cooking spray

Instructions

For Meatloaf

- Preheat the oven to 350°F. Take an 8x4" loaf pan and coat with some cooking spray.
- In a large bowl, mix the egg parsley, bread crumbs, ground turkey, olives, feta cheese, onion, basil, Two tablespoons of hummus, oregano, and garlic. Then mix with hands.
- Spread the meatloaf mix in the loaf pan. Put A quarter cup of hummus on top and bake for 1 hour

For Topping

- Combine the tomato, lemon juice, basil, and olive oil cucumber. Refrigerate before serving.
- Once it reaches a temperature of 165°F inside, the meatloaf is done. Cool it down for 5 minutes. Then slice it and garnish with the topping. Enjoy.

Mexican Taco Skillet with Red Peppers and Zucchini

Preparation time-10 minutes| Cook time-20 minutes| Servings-6 |Difficulty-Easy

Nutritional value- Calories-162| Fat-7g |Carbohydrates-8g| Protein-18g

Ingredients

- Half cup of chopped scallions
- One cup of chopped fresh cilantro
- One teaspoon of low-sodium taco seasoning
- Half cup of shredded mild Cheddar cheese
- One pound of boneless, skinless chicken breast
- One large zucchini halved lengthwise and diced
- One (14.5-ounce) can of diced tomatoes
- One tablespoon of ground cumin
- Two medium red bell peppers, diced
- One jalapeño pepper, seeded and finely chopped
- One tablespoon of minced garlic
- One large onion, finely chopped
- Two teaspoons of extra-virgin olive oil

Instructions

- Heat the olive oil. Add the garlic, red bell peppers, onion, and jalapeño. Sauté the veggies until they're tender.
- Then throw in the cumin, chicken, and taco seasoning and mix until the veggies and chicken are well coated.
- Add in some tomatoes and boil them. Now cook for 10 minutes.
- Add the zucchini and cook until it is tender.
- Remove the skillet from the heat. Add in the scallions, cheese, and cilantro. Enjoy.

Mom's Turkey Meatloaf

Preparation time-10 minutes| Cook time-One hour| Servings-4 |Difficulty-Hard

Nutritional value- Calories-258| Fat-10g |Carbohydrates-17g| Protein-25g

Ingredients

- Nonstick cooking spray
- A quarter teaspoon of freshly ground black pepper
- Half teaspoon of salt
- One tablespoon of Italian seasoning
- One garlic clove
- One large egg
- Half cup of old-fashioned rolled oats
- Half medium onion, minced
- One pound of lean ground turkey
- Two teaspoons of Worcestershire sauce
- A quarter cup plus two tablespoons of ketchup, divided

Instructions

- Preheat the oven to 350°F.
- Then Mix and Worcestershire sauce with Two tablespoons of ketchup.
- Mix egg onion, turkey, oats, garlic, salt, pepper, Italian seasoning and the leftover A quarter cup of ketchup. Don't over mix the meat.
- Put it in an oiled loaf pan and place it on a baking pan. Pour the sauce over it.

- Bake for 1 hour. The temperature will reach 165°F when it's done.
- Take out of the oven and allow to cool before serving.

Mustard and smoked paprika baked chicken

Preparation time-10 minutes |Cook time-35 minutes |Servings-2 to 4 |Difficulty-Easy

Nutritional value: Calories-299|Proteins-40g| Fat-5g|Carbohydrates-2g

Ingredients

- One and a half pounds of skinless, bone-in chicken
- Four tablespoons of trans fat–free canola/olive oil spread, melted
- Four tablespoons of Dijon mustard
- Two tablespoons of freshly squeezed lemon juice
- Two teaspoons of light brown sugar
- One teaspoon of smoked paprika
- One teaspoon of dried basil
- Half teaspoon of dried parsley
- Salt and freshly ground pepper to taste

Instructions

- Preheat oven to 400 degrees. Arrange chicken pieces in an oven-safe casserole dish.
- In a bowl, combine canola/olive oil spread, mustard, lemon juice, sugar, paprika, basil, parsley, and salt and pepper to taste. Brush half of the mixture over the tops of the chicken and bake at 400 degrees for 15 minutes.
- Remove casserole from the oven, carefully turn chicken over, and coat surface with remaining mustard mixture. Return chicken to oven to bake for additional 15 minutes. Test for doneness by piercing the thick part of chicken with the tines of a fork; juices should run clear.

One Pan Shrimp and Broccoli

Preparation time-20 minutes| Cook time-25 minutes|Servings-6 |Difficulty-Moderate

Nutritional value- Calories-110| Fat-6g |Carbohydrates-9g| Protein-19g

Ingredients

- One head of broccoli, cut into florets
- One pound of raw shrimp (peeled & deveined)
- One teaspoon of Italian seasoning
- Two tablespoons of cooking oil
- A quarter teaspoon of onion powder
- Two tablespoons of garlic, minced
- A quarter teaspoon of salt

- A quarter teaspoon of paprika
- Two tablespoons of chicken stock (low sodium)
- Juice of half lemon

Instructions

- Preheat the oven to 425 degrees Fahrenheit.
- Cut two large sheets of aluminum foil and lay one flat on the counter.
- Chop broccoli into small pieces and set aside.
- Combine Italian seasoning onion powder and paprika in a small bowl.
- Arrange shrimp on a plate and drizzle with spice mixture, coating completely.
- Arrange shrimp on foil near the center, followed by broccoli on one side of the shrimp.
- Sprinkle garlic on top of broccoli and shrimp.
- Drizzle with lemon juice and season with salt and pepper to taste.
- Add one tablespoon of stock.
- Wrap foil tightly into packets and crimp the edges.
- Arrange sealed side up on a baking sheet and bake for 15-20 minutes.
- Unwrap carefully, and serve!

One-pan baked halibut and vegetables

Preparation time-10 minutes |Cook time-15 minutes |Servings-2 to 4 |Difficulty-Easy

Nutritional value: -Calories-390|Proteins-17g| Fat-31g|Carbohydrates-8.8g

Ingredients

For the Sauce

- Zest of two lemons
- Two teaspoons of dried oregano
- Half teaspoon of black pepper
- One cup of Olive oil
- Four tablespoons of lemon juice
- One teaspoon of seasoned salt
- One tablespoon of minced garlic
- Two teaspoons of dill
- ¾ teaspoons of coriander

For the Fish

- One sliced yellow onion
- One lb of green beans

- One lb of sliced halibut fillet

One lb of cherry tomatoes

Instructions

- Whisk olive oil, onions, oregano, salt, dill, pepper, tomatoes, lemon zest, green beans,

- juice, coriander, and garlic in a bowl.

- Spread vegetable mixture over one side of the baking tray.

- Coat halibut fillets with the sauce and place them on a baking tray.

- Pour the leftover sauce over the vegetable mixture and fillets.

- Bake in a preheated oven at 425 degrees F for 15 minutes.

One-Pan Tuscan Chicken

Preparation time-10 minutes | Cook time-25 minutes | Servings-2 to 4 | Difficulty-Easy

Nutritional value: -Calories-271 | Proteins-14g | Fat-2g | Carbohydrates-29g

Ingredients

- A quarter cup of extra-virgin olive oil, divided

- One pound of boneless, skinless chicken breasts, cut into ¾-inch pieces

- One onion, chopped

- One red bell pepper, chopped

- Three garlic cloves, minced

- Half cup of dry white wine

- One (14-ounce) can of crushed tomatoes, undrained

- One (14-ounce) can diced tomatoes, drained

- One (14-ounce) can of white beans, drained

- One tablespoon of dried Italian seasoning

- Half teaspoon of sea salt

- 1/8 teaspoon of freshly ground black pepper

- 1/8 teaspoon of red pepper flakes

- A quarter cup of chopped fresh basil leaves

Instructions

- In a large skillet over medium-high heat, heat Two tablespoons of olive oil until it shimmers.

- Add the chicken and cook for about 6 minutes, stirring, until browned. Remove the chicken from the skillet and set it aside on a platter, tented with aluminum foil to keep warm.

- Return the skillet to heat and heat the remaining two tablespoons of olive oil until it shimmers.

- Add the onion and red bell pepper. Cook for about 5 minutes, occasionally stirring, until the vegetables are soft.

- Add the garlic and cook for 30 seconds, stirring constantly.

- Stir in the wine, and use the spoon's side to scrape and fold in any browned bits from the bottom of the pan. Cook for 1 minute, stirring.

- Add the crushed and chopped tomatoes, white beans, Italian seasoning, sea salt, pepper, and red pepper flakes. Bring to a simmer and reduce the heat to medium. Cook for 5 minutes, occasionally stirring.

- Return the chicken and any juices that have collected to the skillet. Cook for 1 to 2 minutes until the chicken heats through. Remove from the heat and stir in the basil before serving.

Orangalicious Drink

Preparation time-5 minutes | Cook time-0 minutes | Servings-1 | Difficulty-Easy

Nutritional value- Calories-150 | Fat-0g | Carbohydrates-29g | Protein-9g

Ingredients

- 1/3 cup of ice

- 1/8 teaspoon of lemon extract

- A quarter cup of mandarin oranges

- 1/3 cup nonfat dry powdered milk

- Half cup of orange juice

Instructions

- Mix the powdered milk and orange juice and put it aside for 2 to 3 minutes. Then place all ingredients in a blender and blend well.

Oven-Baked Chicken Tenders

Preparation time-10 minutes | Cook time-20 minutes | Servings-4 | Difficulty-Easy

Nutritional value- Calories-212 | Fat-6g | Carbohydrates-8g | Protein-32g

Ingredients

- One large egg beaten

- A quarter teaspoon of ground cayenne pepper

- One pound of skinless chicken breast tenders

- Freshly ground black pepper

- Salt

- One teaspoon of garlic powder

- Half cup of whole-wheat panko bread crumbs

- Half cup of grated Parmesan cheese

- Nonstick cooking spray

Instructions

- Preheat the oven to 400°F.

- On a baking sheet, put an oven-safe wire rack and coat with cooking spray.

- Combine cayenne, garlic powder, pepper, bread crumbs, salt and cheese, and pepper to taste.

- Submerge each chicken tender in the beaten egg mixture and coat with bread crumb mixture. Move them to the prepared wire rack.

- Bake until the tenders reach an internal temperature of 165°F.

Pan-fried Fish Fillet

Preparation time-10 minutes| Cook time-10 minutes|Servings-2 |Difficulty-Easy

Nutritional value- Calories-240| Fat-10g |Carbohydrates-10g| Protein-25g

Ingredients

- Three tablespoons of yellow cornmeal

- Eight ounces of fish fillets

- Two teaspoons of olive oil

- A quarter teaspoon of ground celery seeds

- One and 1/3 tablespoon of parsley, chopped

- One pinch of salt

- A quarter teaspoon of ground black pepper

Instructions

- Rinse and clean fish fillets. Ascertain that all bones have been removed. Allow airing to dry.

- Combine salt, cornmeal, pepper, chopped parsley and celery seed in a mixing bowl.

- Press cornmeal mixture onto fish and cover with cornmeal mixture.

- In a nonstick skillet, heat the olive oil.

- Cook fish for 2–3 minutes on each side.

- Brown and crisp, the fish should flake when pierced with a fork.

Pan-seared halibut with lemon-caper sauce

Preparation time-10 minutes |Cook time-20 minutes |Servings-2 to 4|Difficulty-Easy

Nutritional value: ~Calories-272|Proteins-35g| Fat-14g|Carbohydrates-0g

Ingredients

- Four (6-ounce) halibut steaks

- Pinch of salt and freshly ground pepper (optional)

- Two tablespoons of olive oil, divided

- One tablespoon of trans fat–free canola/olive oil spread

- One clove of fresh garlic, finely minced

- Two lemons, 1 to juice and zested to make a half teaspoon of lemon zest and one quartered for garnish

- Two tablespoons of freshly squeezed lemon juice

- Four teaspoons of capers, drained, rinsed, and chopped

- Four tablespoons of chopped fresh parsley

Instructions

- Rinse steaks under cold water and pat dry. Season one side of each steak with a pinch of salt and pepper, if desired.

- In a large, heavy-bottomed skillet, heat one tablespoon of olive oil and canola/olive oil spread over medium-high heat. Cook halibut steaks in skillet until golden brown on both sides, about 7 minutes. Set aside but keep warm.

- Heat remaining olive oil in a small skillet, then add garlic, lemon zest and juice, and capers. Let simmer for 30–40 seconds.

- Add parsley and drizzle mixture over seared halibut steaks. Garnish with lemon wedges and serve immediately.

Pan-seared lemon-pepper tilapia

Preparation time-10 minutes |Cook time-15 minutes |Servings-2 |Difficulty-Easy

Nutritional value: ~Calories-278|Proteins-46g| Fat-11g|Carbohydrates-0g

Ingredients

- Four (3–4 ounces) tilapia fillets

- Ground lemon pepper seasoning to taste

- One tablespoon of extra-virgin olive oil

- One tablespoon of trans fat–free canola/olive oil spread

- One lemon, quartered

Instructions

- Rinse fillets under cold water, pat dry with paper towels, and generously coat one side

- of each fillet with lemon pepper seasoning.

- In a large skillet, add olive oil and canola/olive oil spread over medium-high heat. Use a cooking brush to mix them together and spread evenly on the bottom of the skillet.

- When the oil mixture is hot, reduce heat to medium and place fillets lemon-pepper side down in skillet to cook (about 3 minutes, depending on the thickness of fillets).

- Generously sprinkle the other side of each fillet with lemon pepper seasoning and turn fillets. Continue cooking until fish flakes.

- Remove fillets from heat and serve immediately. Garnish with lemon wedges.

Parmesan Baked Haddock

Preparation time-10 minutes| Cook time-20 minutes|Servings-4 |Difficulty-Easy

Nutritional value- Calories-120| Fat-2g |Carbohydrates-2g| Protein-23g

Ingredients

- Half teaspoon of paprika

- A quarter teaspoon of pepper

- A quarter teaspoon of salt

- Four teaspoons of grated Parmesan cheese

- One egg white

- One pound of haddock fillets cut into four equal pieces

- Half cup of all-purpose flour

Instructions

- Preheat the oven to 375 degrees. On a small plate, put all-purpose flour and coat the fillets fish on each side.

- Whisk the egg white with a fork until firm. Dip the fillets in egg white.

- Coat a baking sheet with some nonstick cooking spray and arrange the fillets on the baking sheet. Then season them with salt, pepper, Parmesan cheese, and paprika.

- Bake for 15 to 20 minutes. The fillets will be golden brown and would flake easily with a fork.

Parmesan-crusted fish

Preparation time-20 minutes |Cook time-15 minutes |Servings-2 to 4|Difficulty-Easy

Nutritional value: -Calories-283|Proteins-32g| Fat-14g|Carbohydrates-4g

Ingredients

- Olive oil cooking spray

- 1/3 cup of panko bread crumbs

- A quarter cup of finely shredded Parmesan cheese

- Salt and freshly ground pepper to taste

- Four codfish fillets (about one and a half pounds)

- A quarter cup of melted trans fat–free canola/olive oil spread

- Half tablespoon fresh garlic paste blend

Instructions

- Preheat oven to 350 degrees F. Lightly sprays a baking sheet with cooking oil.

- In a large, shallow baking dish, mix together panko bread crumbs, Parmesan cheese, and salt and pepper to taste. Roll fillets in the mixture to coat all sides. Blend together melted canola/olive oil spread and garlic paste in a small bowl.

- Place fillets on the baking sheet and drizzle garlic-butter mixture over top of fillets. Bake uncovered for 4–6 minutes for each Half-inch thickness until crumbs are golden brown and fish flakes easily.

Pear, cream cheese, and red onion sandwich

Preparation time-10 minutes |Cook time-0 minutes |Servings-2 |Difficulty-Easy

Nutritional value: Calories-207|Proteins-12g| Fat-9g|Carbohydrates-22g

Ingredients

- Four slices of light whole grain bread

- Olive oil cooking spray

- Four tablespoons of light cream cheese

- Two thin slices of red onion

- Eight slices of Bosc or Anjou pear

- Two tablespoons of crumbled blue cheese

- Four fresh basil leaves, cut into thin strips

Instructions

- Lightly spray bread slices with cooking oil and toast in oven or toaster oven until lightly crispy. Spread one tablespoon of cream cheese on each slice

- of bread. Top one slice with onion, pear slices, blue cheese, and basil. Top with the remaining slice of bread. Repeat for other bread.

Pimento Cheese and Tomato Wrap

Preparation time-5 minutes| Cook time-0 minutes| Servings-2 |Difficulty-Easy

Nutritional value- Calories-231| Fat-10g |Carbohydrates-17g| Protein-17g

Ingredients

- Two 6-inch whole-wheat tortillas

- Four slices of ripe tomato

- A quarter teaspoon of onion powder

- One teaspoon of chopped pimento

- Two tablespoons of light mayonnaise

- One cup of shredded low-fat cheddar cheese

Instructions

- Put mayonnaise, cheese, onion powder and pimento in a food blender for 15 seconds.

- Put a half cup of this mixture on a tortilla and top with 2 tomato slices. Tightly roll the tortilla. Continue with the rest of the ingredients.

Rigatoni with ground lamb

Preparation time-10 minutes |Cook time-15 minutes |Servings-2 to 4 |Difficulty-Hard

Nutritional value: Calories-340|Proteins-20g| Fat-8g|Carbohydrates-45g

Ingredients

- One pound of lean ground lamb

- One whole onion, minced

- Half teaspoon of crushed red hot pepper flakes

- One and a half cups of frozen peas

- Two tablespoons of Spicy Garlicky Pesto Sauce

- Salt and freshly ground pepper to taste

- One pound of whole-grain rigatoni pasta

- Three tablespoons of fresh chopped mint for garnish

Instructions

- In a heavy-bottomed saucepan, cook lamb, onion, and hot pepper flakes for about 8 minutes, until lamb is cooked, occasionally stirring to break up meat. Add peas and cook for another 2–4 minutes. Add Spicy Garlicky Pesto Sauce and salt and pepper to taste, mix well, and set aside; keep warm.

- Cook rigatoni in boiling water until al dente, drain pasta and toss with lamb pesto sauce. Garnish with mint.

Roasted Leg Lamb

Preparation time-15 minutes |Cook time-Two hours 30 minutes |Servings-2 to 4|Difficulty-Hard

Nutritional value: Calories-246|Proteins-33g| Fat-11g|Carbohydrates-2g

Ingredients

- One and a half ounces of bone-in lamb leg, trimmed

- One cup of chicken broth

Marinade

- 1/3 cup of fresh minced rosemary

- Two tablespoons of Dijon mustard

- Two tablespoons of olive oil

- Eight minced garlic cloves

- One teaspoon of soy sauce reduced-sodium

- Half teaspoon of salt

- Half teaspoon of pepper

Instructions

- Preheat your oven to 325° F.

- Combine marinade ingredients and coat the lamb. Refrigerate with cover overnight.

- Place the lamb on a rack using a shallow roasting pan with the fat side up.

- Bake without cover for 1 ½ hour. Pour the broth, then cover loosely using foil. Bake for another 1 ½ hours or until the meat turns to your desired doneness.

- Let the lamb cool for 10 to 15 minutes before slicing.

Roasted Rack of Lamb

Preparation time-15 minutes| Cook time-30 minutes| Servings-8 |Difficulty-Moderate

Nutritional value- Calories-210| Fat-12g |Carbohydrates-0g| Protein-23g

Ingredients

- One tablespoon of olive oil

- Two pounds of a rack of lamb chops

- One teaspoon of black pepper

- One teaspoon of salt

- Two teaspoons of fresh thyme

Instructions

- Preheat the oven to 350 degrees F.

- Mix salt, pepper, and thyme in a bowl and season the meat.

- Heat olive oil in a skillet over high heat. Brown the lamb for 3 minutes per side.

- Roast the lamb in the middle of the oven with the fat side up until the inside temperature is 130 degrees.

- Transfer the lamb to a serving dish and cool it a bit for 10 minutes. Now cut into lamb chops and serve.

Roasted Turkey Breast and Root Vegetables

Preparation time-10 minutes| Cook time-One hour 30 minutes| Servings-4 |Difficulty-Easy

Nutritional value- Calories-164| Fat-5g |Carbohydrates-11g| Protein-18g

Ingredients

- One cup of chopped yellow onion

- Eight ounces of boneless, skinless turkey breast

- A quarter teaspoon of salt

- One cup of peeled, cubed sweet potato

- One tablespoon of extra-virgin olive oil

- Two cups of baby carrots

- Nonstick cooking spray

Instructions

- Preheat the oven to 350°F. Then line a medium to large roasting pan with aluminum foil and spray it with some nonstick cooking spray.

- Mix sweet potatoes, onion, carrots, salt, and oil to coat the veggies.

- Then, place veggies with turkey breast and cook for an hour and a half until the temperature reaches 165°F.

- Cut the turkey and serve alongside veggies. Enjoy.

Rosemary Baked Chicken Drumsticks

Preparation time-5 minutes |Cook time-One hour |Servings-2 to 4 |Difficulty-Hard

Nutritional value: Calories-163 |Proteins-26g| Fat-7g |Carbohydrates-3g

Ingredients

- Two tablespoons of chopped fresh rosemary leaves

- One teaspoon of garlic powder

- Half teaspoon of sea salt

- 1/8 teaspoon of freshly ground black pepper

- Zest of one lemon

- Twelve chicken drumsticks

Instructions

- Preheat the oven to 350°F.

- In a small bowl, combine the rosemary, garlic powder, sea salt, pepper, and lemon zest.

- Place the drumsticks in a 9-by-13-inch baking dish and sprinkle with the rosemary mixture—Bake for about 1 hour, or until the chicken reaches an internal temperature of 165°F.

Sage-Spiced Turkey and Cauliflower Rice

Preparation time-10 minutes| Cook time-15 minutes| Servings-4 |Difficulty-Easy

Nutritional value- Calories-144 | Fat-8g |Carbohydrates-6g| Protein-12g

Ingredients

- Half cup of water

- A quarter teaspoon of salt

- Half teaspoon of ground sage

- One teaspoon of garlic powder

- One cup of cauliflower rice

- Eight ounces of lean ground turkey

- Half cup of chopped sweet yellow onion

- One cup of peeled, chopped carrot

- One tablespoon of extra-virgin olive oil

Instructions

- Warm up some oil over medium heat. Then sauté the onion and carrot for about 5 to 7 minutes.

- Add the cauliflower rice, sage, salt, garlic powder, and ground turkey to the skillet. Then put in some water and move turkey and veggies until the cauliflower rice is cooked and the water evaporates. Add more water before it is finished cooking if it starts to stick to the pan.

- Serve warm.

Salmon cakes with sour cream dill sauce

Preparation time-10 minutes |Cook time-20 minutes |Servings-2 to 4 |Difficulty-Easy

Nutritional value: -Calories-251 |Proteins-24g| Fat-15g |Carbohydrates-3g

Ingredients

- Two (12 ounces) cans of salmon

- Two tablespoons of extra-virgin olive oil, divided

- 3/4 cup of chopped scallions

- Three cloves fresh garlic, minced

- Half teaspoon of crushed red hot pepper flakes

- Two eggs

- Half tablespoon lime juice

- Three tablespoons of cornstarch

- Salt and freshly ground pepper to taste

- One cup of fat-free or low-fat sour cream (optional)

- Four tablespoons of finely chopped fresh dill (optional)

Instructions

- Drain and separate salmon; set aside.

- In a heavy-bottomed skillet over medium-low heat, add two teaspoons of olive oil, scallions, garlic, and hot pepper flakes. Sauté until scallions are soft, then set aside.

- In a bowl, whisk together eggs, lime juice, cornstarch, and salt and pepper. Add egg mixture to scallion mixture and gently fold in salmon.

- Form the salmon mixture into equal-sized cakes and refrigerate for about 30 minutes. Pour remaining olive oil into a large skillet over medium-low heat and add chilled salmon cakes.

- Slowly sauté cakes for about 2–3 minutes on each side until heated through.

- Mix sour cream and dill together and serve each salmon cake garnished with a tablespoon of our cream and dill sauce, if desired.

Salmon kabobs

Preparation time-10 minutes | Cook time-10 minutes | Servings-2 to 4 | Difficulty-Easy

Nutritional value: ~Calories-267 | Proteins-35g | Fat-11g | Carbohydrates-7g

Ingredients

- One and a half lb of sliced Salmon fillet
- One sliced red onion
- One sliced zucchini
- Kosher salt to taste
- Black pepper to taste

Marinade

- 1/3 cup of Olive Oil
- Zest of one lemon
- Two tablespoons of lemon juice
- Two minced garlic cloves
- One teaspoon of chili pepper
- Two teaspoons of dry oregano
- Two teaspoons of chopped thyme leaves
- One teaspoon of cumin
- Half teaspoon of coriander

Instructions

- Mix all the ingredients of margination in a bowl.
- In another bowl, add pepper, onions, salt, salmon, and zucchini and mix well.
- Add marinade and mix well. Set aside for 20 minutes.
- Thread onions, salmon, and zucchini in skewers.
- Place skewers overheated grill, cover them, and grill for eight minutes.
- When salmons are ready, serve and enjoy them.

Salmon Patties

Preparation time-10 minutes | Cook time-10 minutes | Servings-4 | Difficulty-Easy

Nutritional value- Calories-246 | Fat-16g | Carbohydrates-9g | Protein-18g

Ingredients

- Two teaspoons of canola oil
- A quarter cup of bread crumbs
- A quarter cup of finely chopped celery
- Two 6-ounce cans of salmon, without bones and skin, drained and flaked
- A quarter teaspoon of Old Bay seasoning
- A quarter cup of chopped green onion
- A quarter cup of nonfat milk
- Two eggs, beaten

Honey Mustard Sauce

- One teaspoon of honey
- One teaspoon of Dijon mustard
- A quarter cup of light mayonnaise

Instructions

- Simply mix milk, Old Bay seasoning, green onions, eggs, and celery in a medium bowl. Add bread crumbs to the salmon and combine well. Make 4 thin patties evenly.
- In a large sauté pan, heat oil over medium heat. Cook the patties for about 3 minutes until
- they brown.
- For Honey Mustard Sauce, mix all the ingredients in a small bowl and serve with patties.

Salmon with Honey- Garlic-Caramelized Onions

Preparation time-10 minutes | Cook time-35 minutes | Servings-4 | Difficulty-Moderate

Nutritional value- Calories-290 | Fat-18g | Carbohydrates-7g | Protein-24g

Ingredients

- Pepper (to taste)
- One lb of Salmon fillets
- One clove of garlic
- Two teaspoons of honey
- One tablespoon of Balsamic vinegar
- One chopped Onion
- One tablespoon of Butter

Instructions

- Preheat your oven to 400 degrees F.
- Over medium-high heat, melt some butter in a skillet and add onion rings.
- Now, lower the heat and sauté onions for 10 minutes. Lower the heat further and cook again for 10 minutes. Now add honey, garlic, and vinegar.
- Arrange salmon on the sprayed baking sheet while onions are cooking. Season with some salt and pepper. Bake for 10 to 15 minutes. Serve with cooked onions.

Salmon with smoked paprika

Preparation time-20 minutes |Cook time-10 minutes |Servings-2 to 4|Difficulty-Easy

Nutritional value: ~Calories-202|Proteins-22g| Fat-11g|Carbohydrates-2g

Ingredients

- A quarter cup of orange juice

- One tablespoon of olive oil

- One teaspoon of thyme

- Four (4–5-ounce) salmon fillets, skinless

- Half tablespoon smoked paprika

- Half tablespoon brown sugar

- Half teaspoon of cinnamon

- One teaspoon of orange zest

Instructions

- In a shallow dish, stir to mix orange juice, olive oil, and thyme.

- Add salmon, turning to coat fillets with juice mixture. Cover dish with plastic wrap and refrigerate.

- When fillets have marinated for at least 30 minutes, place a shallow cast-iron skillet on the top oven rack and preheat the oven to 450 degrees. In a small pinch bowl, mix together paprika, brown sugar, cinnamon, and zest.

- When the oven reaches desired heat, remove fillets from the marinade and rub the tops of fillets with paprika mixture. Place fillets in a heated skillet and cook for 3–4 minutes.

- Turn fillets over once and continue cooking until fish flakes easily.

Saucy Boston Butt

Preparation time-10 minutes |Cook time-One hour 20 minutes |Servings-2 to 4|Difficulty-Hard

Nutritional value: ~Calories-369|Proteins-41.3g| Fat-20.2g|Carbohydrates-3.6g

Ingredients

- One tablespoon of lard, room temperature

- Two pounds of Boston butt, cubed

- Salt and freshly ground pepper

- Half teaspoon of mustard powder

- A bunch of spring onions, chopped

- Two garlic cloves, minced

- Half tablespoon of ground cardamom

- Two tomatoes, pureed

- One bell pepper, deveined and chopped

- One jalapeno pepper, deveined and finely chopped

- Half cup of unsweetened coconut milk

- Two cups of chicken bone broth

Instructions

- In a wok, melt the lard over moderate heat. Massage the pork belly with salt, pepper, and mustard powder.

- Sear the pork for 8 to 10 minutes, stirring periodically to ensure cooking; set aside, and keep it warm.

- In the same wok, sauté the spring onions, garlic, and cardamom. Spoon the sautéed vegetables along with the reserved pork into the slow cooker.

- Add in the remaining ingredients, cover with the lid and cook for 1 hour 10 minutes over low heat.

Sautéed shrimp and zucchini

Preparation time-8 minutes |Cook time-7 minutes |Servings-2 to 3|Difficulty-Easy

Nutritional value: ~Calories-216|Proteins-33g| Fat-6g|Carbohydrates-7g

Ingredients

- One lb of shrimp

- One teaspoon of salt

- Two zucchinis

- Two tablespoons of chopped garlic

- One tablespoon of butter

- Black pepper to taste

- One and a half tablespoons of lemon juice

- Two tablespoons of chopped parsley

- Olive oil as required

Instructions

- Add salt, shrimp, and pepper to a bowl. Mix them well.

- Cook shrimps in heated oil over medium flame for two minutes from each side. Shift cooked shrimp on a plate.

- Cook zucchini in heated oil in the same pan for two minutes, then sprinkle pepper and salt.

- Transfer shrimps to the pan and mix. Add garlic and sauté for two minutes.

- Add butter and cook to melt it. When shrimps, garlic, and zucchini are cooked, add lemon juice and mix well.

- Drizzle parsley and serve.

Sautéed Shrimp with Asparagus Tips

Preparation time-5 minutes| Cook time-10 minutes|Servings-4 |Difficulty-Easy

Nutritional value- Calories-200| Fat-7g |Carbohydrates-5g| Protein-24g

Ingredients

- One tablespoon of chopped fresh parsley
- One tablespoon of olive oil
- Two tablespoons of garlic, minced
- One teaspoon of butter
- One pound of raw medium shrimp
- Two tablespoons of white wine
- One teaspoon of red pepper flakes
- A quarter teaspoon of salt
- One cup of raw asparagus tips (the top two inches of each spear)
- One tablespoon of lemon juice

Instructions

- Heat up the oil. Then add asparagus tips and cook for around 4 minutes.
- Now add garlic, lemon juice, pepper flakes, shrimp, wine, and salt. Then close the skillet lid and cook for 3 minutes.
- Then, remove the lid and add some butter. Take off from the stove and mix in the parsley.

Sea Bass with Herb-Spiced Pecans

Preparation time-10 minutes| Cook time-15 minutes|Servings-4 |Difficulty-Easy

Nutritional value- Calories-230| Fat-12g |Carbohydrates-4g| Protein-22g

Ingredients

- One large tomato, chopped
- A quarter teaspoon of Spice Mixture
- One pound of sea bass, skinned and filleted
- One tablespoon of melted butter
- Two tablespoons of fat-free half-and-half
- Two tablespoons of finely chopped onion
- Two tablespoons of white wine vinegar
- A quarter cup of dry white wine

Spicy Pecans

- A quarter teaspoon of Spice Mixture
- Two teaspoons of butter
- 1/8 teaspoon of allspice
- A quarter teaspoon of dried oregano
- A quarter teaspoon of dried thyme
- A quarter cup of coarsely chopped pecans

Spice Mixture

- 1/8 teaspoon of crushed rosemary
- 1/8 teaspoon of dried oregano
- 1/8 teaspoon of dry mustard
- A quarter teaspoon of dried thyme
- Half teaspoon of garlic powder
- A quarter teaspoon of white pepper
- A quarter teaspoon of dried basil
- A quarter teaspoon of onion powder
- One teaspoon of paprika

Instructions

- Take a small saucepan and boil vinegar, onion, and wine over high heat until most liquid evaporates.
- Add ¾ tomato and fat-free half-and-half. Now simmer for about 6 minutes.
- Heat the grill to medium-high heat.
- Coat the fillets with some butter and season with the Spice Mixture. Now grill for 2 to 3 minutes on each side.
- For Spicy Pecans, in a small bowl, combine the ingredients except for the butter. Then in a small skillet over medium heat, melt the butter and add pecans with spices. Toast until pecans are golden brown. Move to a small dish.
- Transfer the cooked sauce to a serving plate and place the fillets over the sauce. Top with Spicy Pecans and the leftover chopped tomatoes.

Seared Salmon with Lemon Cream Sauce

Preparation time-10 minutes |Cook time-20 minutes | Servings-2 to 4 |Difficulty-Easy

Nutritional value: Calories-310|Proteins-29g| Fat-18g|Carbohydrates-7g

Ingredients

- Four (5-ounce) salmon fillets
- Sea salt and freshly ground black pepper
- One tablespoon of extra-virgin olive oil
- Half cup of low-sodium vegetable broth
- Juice and zest of one lemon
- One teaspoon of chopped fresh thyme
- Half cup of fat-free sour cream
- One teaspoon of honey
- One tablespoon of chopped fresh chives

Instructions

- Preheat the oven to 400°F.
- Season the salmon casually on both sides with salt and pepper.
- Place a large ovenproof frypan on medium-high heat and add the olive oil.
- Sear the salmon fillets on each side until golden, about 3 minutes per side.
- Handover the salmon to a baking dish and bake in the preheated oven until just cooked through for about 10 minutes.
- Meanwhile, whisk together the vegetable broth, lemon juice and zest, and thyme in a small saucepan over medium-high heat wait until the liquid reduces by about one-quarter, about 5 minutes.
- Whisk in the sour cream and honey.
- Stir in the chives and serve the sauce over the salmon.

Sheet Pan Fajitas

Preparation time-5 minutes| Cook time-25 minutes| Servings-4 |Difficulty-Easy

Nutritional value- Calories-176| Fat-6g |Carbohydrates-8g| Protein-24g

Ingredients

- Two tablespoons of Taco Seasoning
- One tablespoon of extra-virgin olive oil
- One red bell pepper, sliced
- One yellow onion, sliced
- One yellow bell pepper, sliced
- One pound of chicken breast, cut into strips

Instructions

- Preheat the oven to 350°F.
- Mix onion, taco seasoning chicken, peppers, and oil.

- Spread the veggies and chicken evenly on one or two baking sheets.
- Bake until the veggies are soft and the chicken is fully cooked. Serve hot.

Shrimp Ceviche

Preparation time-10 minutes| Cook time-30 minutes|Servings-4|Difficulty-Easy

Nutritional value- Calories-206| Fat-8g |Carbohydrates-11g| Protein-25g

Ingredients

- One jalapeño pepper, seeds and veins removed, minced
- Half cup of chopped fresh cilantro
- One avocado pitted and diced into half-inch chunks
- Salt
- A quarter cup of freshly squeezed lime juice
- A quarter cup of freshly squeezed lemon juice
- Half cup of finely chopped red onion
- One cup of diced tomatoes
- One pound of cooked jumbo shrimp, peeled, deveined, and diced

Instructions

- Combine tomatoes, jalapeño, shrimp, and red onion in a large bowl.
- Add some lime juice and lemon, salt, and cilantro to taste. Mix everything to coat.
- Cover the bowl and refrigerate it for at least 30 minutes to enhance the flavor.
- Top with avocado and serve

Shrimp in spicy black bean sauce

Preparation time-10 minutes |Cook time-20 minutes |Servings-2 to 4|Difficulty-Easy

Nutritional value: Calories-211|Proteins-19g| Fat-9g|Carbohydrates-16g

Ingredients

- Two jumbo cloves fresh garlic, minced
- Two tablespoons plus two teaspoons of extra-virgin olive oil, divided
- Three teaspoons of chili powder
- Three teaspoons of ground cumin
- Two cups of canned black beans, rinsed and drained
- One and a half cups of canned low-sodium, fat-free chicken broth
- Twenty-four jumbo shrimp, peeled and deveined

- Salt and freshly ground pepper to taste
- Fresh parsley, chopped for garnish

Instructions

- Sauté all but two teaspoons of garlic in one tablespoon of olive oil until almost browned. Add chili powder and cumin and sauté for another minute.
- Add beans to garlic mixture, frequently stirring, and cook for another 3–4 minutes. Stir in chicken broth and transfer the mixture to a food processor or blender.
- Puree mixture and return to skillet. Simmer sauce for 5 minutes, often stirring. Set aside, but keep warm.
- Rinse shrimp and pat dry; season with salt and pepper. Heat remaining olive oil and sauté shrimp with remaining garlic.
- Cook until shrimp are lightly browned outside and cooked through inside, turning often. Remove shrimp from olive oil with a slotted spoon and set aside. Warm sauce and pour onto serving platter.
- Arrange shrimp on top of the sauce and garnish with parsley. Serve immediately, with rice, if desired.

Shrimp Scampi with Zucchini Noodles

Preparation time-10 minutes | Cook time-10 minutes | Servings-4 | Difficulty-Easy

Nutritional value- Calories-244 | Fat-12g | Carbohydrates-9g | Protein-25g

Ingredients

- Freshly ground black pepper
- Salt
- A quarter teaspoon of red pepper flakes
- Freshly grated Parmesan for garnishing
- Four medium zucchinis
- Juice of half lemons
- One tablespoon of minced garlic
- A quarter cup of fresh parsley
- One pound of peeled and deveined jumbo shrimp
- One tablespoon of butter
- Two tablespoons of extra-virgin olive oil
- A quarter cup of white wine

Instructions

- Warm up the butter. Add red pepper flakes and garlic, and then cook for 1 minute.
- Add and cook shrimp for around 3 minutes. Move the shrimp to a bowl; keep the juices in the skillet.

- Put the skillet back on the stove; add the lemon juice and wine. Then deglaze the pan. Now throw in zoodles and sauté for about 2 minutes.
- Put back the shrimp and mix. Sprinkle with pepper and salt, and serve hot. Top with Parmesan and parsley if you like.

Sloppy Joes

Preparation time-10 minutes | Cook time-30 minutes | Servings-8 | Difficulty-Easy

Nutritional value- Calories-269 | Fat-5g | Carbohydrates-32g | Protein-24g

Ingredients

- One tablespoon of brown sugar
- Two tablespoons of Dijon mustard
- Two tablespoons of Worcestershire sauce
- ⅓ cup of catsup (free of high-fructose corn syrup)
- One (8-ounce) can of tomato sauce
- One cup of chopped celery
- One cup of chopped onion
- Two tablespoons of white vinegar
- One and a half pounds of supreme lean ground beef
- Nonstick cooking spray

Instructions

- With some cooking spray, oil a large skillet and put it over medium heat. Now brown the beef until it is no longer raw. Discard any liquid.
- Now cook celery and onion for 2 to 3 minutes.
- Mix the catsup, Worcestershire sauce, vinegar, brown sugar, tomato sauce, and mustard. Simmer it and lower the heat. Cook until the sauce is thick.
- Put ¾ cup of sloppy joe on your plate and enjoy.

Sloppy Joe–Style Ground Pork

Preparation time-5 minutes | Cook time-10 minutes | Servings-4 | Difficulty-Easy

Nutritional value- Calories-172 | Fat-9g | Carbohydrates-10g | Protein-13g

Ingredients

- One teaspoon of salt
- One tablespoon of brown sugar
- One tablespoon of apple cider vinegar
- One cup of canned diced tomatoes, drained
- One cup of chopped yellow onion
- Eight ounces of lean ground pork
- One tablespoon of extra-virgin olive oil

Instructions

- Warm up the oil over medium heat in a large skillet. Cook onion and pork until cooked through. Put the skillet off the heat and discard the pork fat.
- In the skillet, add apple cider vinegar, salt, tomatoes, and brown sugar. Simmer for 2 minutes on low heat and serve.

Slow Cooker Barbecue Shredded Chicken

Preparation time-5 minutes| Cook time-8 hours 30 minutes| Servings-4 |Difficulty-Easy

Nutritional value- Calories-188| Fat-3g |Carbohydrates-16g| Protein-22g

Ingredients

- One tablespoon of white vinegar
- Three tablespoons of Worcestershire sauce
- A quarter teaspoon of red pepper flakes
- Half teaspoon of dried mustard
- One tablespoon of dried onions
- One tablespoon of freshly squeezed lemon juice
- Half cup of water
- One cup of catsup (free of high-fructose corn syrup)
- Four (4-ounce) boneless, skinless chicken breasts

Instructions

- Put the chicken breasts in a slow cooker.
- Now, Beat together the lemon juice, Worcestershire sauce, catsup dried onions, dried mustard, white vinegar, water, and red pepper flakes. Now add this in the slow cooker to the chicken.
- Put on low and cook for 6 to 8 hours.
- Take out the chicken and shred it with a fork. Put it back in the slow cooker, and cook for 30 minutes on low. Then serve.

Slow Cooker Salsa Chicken

Preparation time-5 minutes| Cook time-4 hour| Servings-8 |Difficulty-Hard

Nutritional value- Calories-176| Fat-6g |Carbohydrates-8g| Protein-24g

Ingredients

- Two cups of any good salsa
- Four chicken breasts (about 2 pounds total)

Instructions

- Put the chicken breasts in a slow cooker and add salsa on top. Now mix it well to ensure complete coating of the chicken.
- Then cook for 4 hours on high or for 6 to 8 hours on low.
- Once the chicken is done, shred it with a fork while still in the slow cooker. Move everything around to mix it well with the juices and salsa in the pot. Serve hot.

Slow Cooker Turkey Chili

Preparation time-10 minutes| Cook time-8 hours| Servings-16 |Difficulty-Hard

Nutritional value- Calories-140| Fat-4g |Carbohydrates-12g| Protein-14g

Ingredients

- One (8-ounce) can of tomato juice
- Three tablespoons of chili powder
- Two tablespoons of ground cumin
- Two celery stalks, finely chopped
- One teaspoon of dried oregano
- One can diced tomatoes
- Nonstick cooking spray
- Four teaspoons of minced garlic
- One green bell pepper, finely chopped
- One large onion, finely chopped
- One (8-ounce) can of tomato puree
- Two (14.5-ounce) cans of kidney beans, drained and rinsed
- Two pounds of extra-lean ground turkey

Instructions

- Coat a large skillet with some cooking spray. Throw in the ground turkey and break it into smaller chunks. Then cook for 7 to 9 minutes.
- Then, put the tomatoes, celery, oregano, beans, onion, bell pepper, garlic, tomato puree, chili powder, cumin and tomato juice in the slow cooker. Mix in the cooked ground turkey.
- Close the lid and cook for 8 hours on low.
- Top with shredded Cheddar cheese, Greek yogurt, and scallions (optional).

Slow-Cooked Turkey and Brown Rice

Preparation time-15 minutes |Cook time-Three hours10 minutes |Servings-2 to 4 |Difficulty-Hard

Nutritional value: Calories-499|Proteins-36.4g| Fat-17g|Carbohydrates-56.7g

Ingredients

- One tablespoon of extra-virgin olive oil
- One and a half pounds of ground turkey
- Two tablespoons of chopped fresh sage, divided
- Two tablespoons of chopped fresh thyme, divided
- One teaspoon of sea salt
- Half teaspoon of ground black pepper
- Two cups of brown rice
- One (14-ounce) can stewed tomatoes, with the juice
- A quarter cup of pitted and sliced Kalamata olives
- Three medium zucchinis, sliced thinly
- A quarter cup of chopped fresh flat-leaf parsley
- One medium yellow onion, chopped
- One tablespoon plus one teaspoon of balsamic vinegar
- Two cups of low-sodium chicken stock
- Two garlic cloves, minced
- Half cup of grated Parmesan cheese for serving

Instructions

- Warm up the olive oil in a non-stick skillet over medium-high heat until shimmering.
- Add the ground turkey and sprinkle with one tablespoon of sage, one tablespoon of thyme, salt, and ground black pepper.
- Sauté for 10 minutes or until the ground turkey is lightly browned.
- Pour them into the slow cooker, then pour in the remaining ingredients, except for the Parmesan. Stir to mix well.
- Cook on high within 3 hours or until the rice and vegetables are tender.
- Put it into a large bowl, then spread with Parmesan cheese before serving.

Slow-cooker Provencal Chicken

Preparation time-25 minutes| Cook time-5 hours| Servings-4 |Difficulty-Easy

Nutritional value- Calories-315| Fat-2g |Carbohydrates-36g| Protein-38g

Ingredients

- Two (1 1/2 pounds) boneless cut in half lengthwise, skinless chicken breast halves
- Two teaspoons of dried basil
- One can diced tomatoes, 14 ½-ounce (untrained)
- A quarter teaspoon of black pepper
- A quarter teaspoon of salt
- One cup of diced yellow bell pepper
- One can navy beans, 16-ounce (rinsed and drained)
- Optional: Fresh or dried basil leaves

Instructions

- In an electric slow cooker or crockpot, place the chicken.
- In a large mixing bowl, combine black pepper, salt, bell pepper, tomatoes, beans and dried basil; stir well.
- Distribute mixture evenly over chicken.
- Cook on low for 5-6 hours, or until the chicken reaches a temperature of 165 degrees.
- Spoon the tomato and bean mixture over each chicken breast half.
- If desired, garnish with fresh or dried basil leaves.

Slow-Roasted Pesto Salmon

Preparation time-5 minutes| Cook time-20 minutes|Servings-4 |Difficulty-Easy

Nutritional value- Calories-182| Fat-10g |Carbohydrates-1g| Protein-20g

Ingredients

- Four tablespoons of Perfect Basil Pesto
- One teaspoon of extra-virgin olive oil
- Four (6-ounce) salmon fillets

Instructions

- Preheat the oven to 275°F. With aluminum foil, line a rimmed baking sheet and brush the foil with olive oil.
- Arrange the salmon fillets on the baking sheet with their skin sides down.
- Put one tablespoon of pesto on every single fillet.
- Now, roast the fillets until they become opaque in the middle. Serve hot.

Southwest Deviled Eggs

Preparation time-5 minutes| Cook time-30 minutes| Servings-6 |Difficulty-Easy

Nutritional value- Calories-83| Fat-5g |Carbohydrates-1g| Protein-7g

Ingredients

- Half teaspoon of Taco Seasoning
- ⅛ teaspoon of salt
- A quarter teaspoon of spicy mustard
- Two tablespoons of low-fat, plain Greek yogurt
- Six large hard-boiled eggs

Instructions

- Peel and halve the eggs vertically.
- Take out the yolks, and move them to a small bowl. Now put the egg whites aside.
- Add the spicy mustard, taco seasoning yogurt, and salt to the egg yolks and squash everything.
- Fill the egg white halves with the mixture and serve.

Spicy Chicken Breasts

Preparation time-15 minutes | Cook time-30 minutes | Servings-2 to 4 | Difficulty-Moderate

Nutritional value: ~Calories-239 | Proteins-34.6g | Fat-6g | Carbohydrates-6g

Ingredients

- One pound of chicken breasts
- One bell pepper, deveined and chopped
- One leek, chopped
- One tomato, pureed
- Two tablespoons of coriander
- Two garlic cloves, minced
- One teaspoon of cayenne pepper
- One teaspoon of dry thyme
- A quarter cup of coconut amino
- Sea salt
- Ground black pepper

Instructions

- Rub each chicken breast with garlic, cayenne pepper, thyme, salt, and black pepper. Cook the chicken in a saucepan over medium-high heat.
- Sear for about 5 minutes until golden brown on all sides. Fold in the tomato puree and coconut amino, and bring it to a boil. Add in the pepper, leek, and coriander.
- Reduce the heat to simmer. Continue to cook, partially covered, for about 20 minutes.

Spicy chicken with couscous

Preparation time-10 minutes | Cook time-20 minutes | Servings-2 to 4 | Difficulty-Easy

Nutritional value: ~Calories-340 | Proteins-34g | Fat-4g | Carbohydrates-38g

Ingredients

- A quarter teaspoon of ground cumin
- A quarter teaspoon of ground turmeric
- One teaspoon of ground cayenne
- One pound of skinless, boneless chicken breasts, cut into 1-inch strips
- One teaspoon of extra-virgin olive oil
- Five cloves of fresh garlic, finely minced
- One (16-ounce) can of low-sodium, fat-free chicken broth
- One cup of fresh peas
- One large white onion, diced
- One medium red bell pepper, diced
- Salt and freshly ground pepper to taste
- One cup of couscous
- A quarter cup of chopped fresh cilantro for garnish

Instructions

- Combine cumin, turmeric, and cayenne, and sprinkle evenly over chicken strips, then set aside. In a non-stick skillet, heat olive oil over medium-high heat until hot.
- Add chicken and garlic and cook about 3 minutes until chicken is lightly browned. Add broth, peas, onion, red bell pepper, and salt and pepper to taste to skillet; bring to boil, reduce heat, and simmer about 2–3 minutes, until chicken is cooked through.
- Stir in couscous, cover, and remove from heat. Let stand until liquid is absorbed. Garnish with cilantro.

Spicy hummus in toasted pita loaves

Preparation time-10 minutes | Cook time-2 minutes | Servings-2 to 4 | Difficulty-Easy

Nutritional value: ~Calories-152 | Proteins-3g | Fat-3g | Carbohydrates-27g

Ingredients

- One (15-ounce) can chickpeas, well rinsed and drained
- Juice from one lemon
- A quarter cup of water
- One large clove of fresh garlic
- Two tablespoons of tahini paste
- Dash of salt
- Pinch of crushed red hot pepper flakes
- Three (6-inch) whole-wheat pita loaves

- Eight slices of tomato, 1/4-inch thick

- Half cucumber, peeled and thinly sliced

- Alfalfa sprouts

Instructions

- In a food processor, add chickpeas, lemon juice, and water, and blend to desired consistency.

- Add garlic, tahini paste, salt, and hot pepper flakes;

- blend again.

- Cut pita loaves in half and toast lightly.

- Divide mixture into equal portions and stuff loaves with mixture. Top each half loaf with tomato, cucumber, and alfalfa sprouts.

Stuffed sesame chicken breasts

Preparation time-10 minutes | Cook time-40 minutes | Servings-2 to 4 | Difficulty-Moderate

Nutritional value: ~Calories-237 | Proteins-37g | Fat-8g | Carbohydrates-4g

Ingredients

- Salt and freshly ground pepper to taste

- Half red bell pepper, deseeded and thinly sliced

- Four tablespoons of lime juice

- A quarter cup of sesame seeds

- Four fresh tarragon sprigs for garnish

- Four (4–5-ounce) skinless, boneless chicken breasts

- One tablespoon of dried tarragon or four sprigs of fresh tarragon

- Half green bell pepper, deseeded and thinly sliced

- A quarter small red chili pepper, finely minced (optional)

- Extra-virgin olive oil to drizzle

Instructions

- Breasts should be rinsed under cold water and patted dry with paper towels before cooking. Split open one side of the breasts with a sharp knife to create a pocket. Repeat on the other side. Salt and pepper the inside of the breasts to taste and season with tarragon (about a quarter tablespoon of dried tarragon per breast or one full sprig stuffed inside the pocket of each breast) before roasting them.

- Insert slices of green and red bell peppers into each breast pocket and close the pockets with a toothpick to keep the peppers from falling out. Combine the lime juice and chilli pepper in a small bowl and set aside. Place the breasts in a single layer on a nonstick baking sheet and sprinkle with a generous amount of sesame seeds. Bake for 30 minutes or until done.

- Bake at 400 degrees for about 30 minutes, or until chicken is tender and cooked through, basting the tops of the breasts with the lime/chili mixture. Preheat the

oven to broil and drizzle a small amount of olive oil over the top of each breast.

- Bake chicken breasts until the sesame seeds are golden brown on a baking sheet under the grill or under the broiler. Garnish with fresh sprigs of tarragon before serving.

Stuffing with Cranberries

Preparation time-20 minutes | Cook time-35 minutes | Servings-6 | Difficulty-Moderate

Nutritional value- Calories-147 | Fat-2g | Carbohydrates-29g | Protein-5g

Ingredients

- One cup of celery, chopped

- One cup of chicken broth (low-sodium)

- Eleven slices of whole-wheat bread (toasted and cut into cubes)

- Half cup of onion, chopped

- A quarter cup of parsley, chopped

- Half teaspoon of paprika

- One teaspoon of dried tarragon

- One cup of apple, chopped

- 1/8 teaspoon of ground nutmeg

- One cup of whole water chestnuts

- Half cup of fresh cranberries, chopped

Instructions

- Preheat the oven to 350 degrees Fahrenheit.

- Spray a 2-quart baking dish lightly with cooking spray.

- In a large skillet over medium heat, heat the chicken broth.

- Add the celery and onion and sauté for about 5 minutes, or until the vegetables are tender. Take the pan off the heat.

- Combine the parsley, tarragon, paprika, bread cubes, nutmeg water chestnuts, cranberries and chopped apples in a large mixing bowl. Combine the celery and onion. Stir well to ensure even distribution.

- Spoon stuffing into the baking dish that has been prepared. Bake for 20 minutes, covered with aluminum foil. Uncover and bake for an additional 10 minutes. Serve right away.

Sweet and Sour Pork

Preparation time-20 minutes | Cook time-40 minutes | Servings-2 | Difficulty-Moderate

Nutritional value- Calories-248 | Fat-3g | Carbohydrates-36g | Protein-18g

Ingredients

- One pound of lean pork tenderloin (cut into thin strips)

- Cooking spray

- Half cup of water

- Two tablespoons of corn starch

- Half teaspoon of table salt

- A quarter cup of Splenda brown sugar blend

- One tablespoon of soy sauce (low-sodium)

- One small sliced onion (as tolerated)

- Three cups of cooked brown rice

- Two medium sliced green peppers (as tolerated)

- 1/3 cup of wine vinegar

- One canned, 15-ounce (unsweetened pineapple chunks)

Instructions

- Over medium-high heat, coat a nonstick skillet with cooking spray.

- Add the pork and cook, occasionally stirring until it is golden brown. Take the skillet out of the heat and set it aside. Empty the skillet of any remaining fat.

- Reserve pineapple juice after draining pineapple chunks; set aside.

- In a small bowl, whisk together the vinegar, cornstarch, sugar, soy sauce, salt, pineapple and water juice that has been reserved. Add to skillet and cook for approximately 2 minutes, or until sauce has thickened.

- Add pork to skillet and cook, occasionally stirring for approximately 30 minutes, or until tender meat. Cook for an additional 5 minutes before adding the onion, peppers and pineapple chunks.

- Arrange on top of rice.

Tuna and Zucchini Patties

Preparation time-10 minutes | Cook time-15 minutes | Servings-2 to 4 | Difficulty-Easy

Nutritional value: -Calories-757 | Proteins-17g | Fat-51g | Carbohydrates-27g

Ingredients

- Three slices whole-wheat sandwich bread, toasted

- Two (5-ounce) cans of tuna in olive oil, drained

- One cup of shredded zucchini

- One large egg, lightly beaten

- A quarter cup of diced red bell pepper

- One tablespoon of dried oregano

- One teaspoon of lemon zest

- A quarter teaspoon of freshly ground black pepper

- A quarter teaspoon of kosher or sea salt

- One tablespoon of extra-virgin olive oil

- Salad greens or four whole-wheat rolls, for serving (optional)

Instructions

- Crumble the toast into bread crumbs with your fingers (or use a knife to cut into ¼-inch cubes) until you have one cup of loosely packed crumbs. Pour the crumbs into a large bowl. Add the tuna, zucchini, beaten egg, bell pepper, oregano, lemon zest, black pepper, and salt. Mix well with a fork.

- Using your hands, form the combination into four (½-cup-size) patties. Place them on a plate, and press each patty flat to about ¾-inch thick.

- In a frypan over medium-high heat, heat the oil until it's very hot, about 2 minutes.

- Add the patties to the hot oil, then reduce the heat down to medium. Cook the patties for 5 minutes, flip with a spatula, and cook for an additional 5 minutes. Serve the patties on salad greens or whole-wheat rolls, if desired.

Turkey Lettuce Wrap

Preparation time-10 minutes | Cook time-15 minutes | Servings-4 | Difficulty-Easy

Nutritional value- Calories-260 | Fat-15g | Carbohydrates-5g | Protein-25g

Ingredients

- Eight thin tomato slices

- One cup of Greek Yogurt Caesar Dressing

- Two ounces of Swiss cheese

- Four romaine lettuce leaves

- Eight ounces of boneless, skinless turkey breast tenderloin, cut into 2-ounce strips

- One tablespoon of extra-virgin olive oil

Instructions

- Warm up the oil and sauté the turkey on each side for about 5 minutes. Take off the heat.

- In the center of each lettuce leaf, put a turkey strip. Add ½ a slice of Swiss cheese and 2 thin tomato slices. Then add two tablespoons of the dressing on top.

- Wrap the lettuce well and serve.

Turkey meatball

Preparation time-10 minutes | Cook time-15 minutes | Servings-12 | Difficulty-Easy

Nutritional value- Calories-280 | Fat-5g | Carbohydrates-18g | Protein-20g

Ingredients

- One pound of ground turkey lean

- 3/4 cup of Panko bread crumbs

- A quarter cup of chopped sweet onion purple

- One large, lightly beaten egg

- Two cloves of chopped or pressed garlic

- Three tablespoons of Worcestershire sauce

- One tablespoon of soy sauce

- One tablespoon of yellow mustard

- One teaspoon of red pepper flakes

- One and a half teaspoons of cajun seasoning

- Half teaspoon of ground cumin

- Half teaspoon of ground sea salt

- Half teaspoon of ground pepper

- Two tablespoons of butter

- One tablespoon of olive oil

Instructions

- Use a mixing bowl to add the ground turkey and all the ingredients.

- With a wooden spoon, stir in the turkey meatballs.

- With clean hands or a wooden spoon, combine well.

- Create little balls of golf size with your own hands

- Make meatballs for turkey by hand

- Place them on a dish or tray.

- Heat the butter and olive oil on a wide scale over medium heat.

- Attach the turkey meatballs and cook them on each side for a couple of minutes.

- Cook the turkey meat in butter and olive oil in a cast-iron skillet pan.

- Using a wooden spoon, turn them over. Rotate them so that they are uniformly cooked.

- You want to get them deep, dipped golden brown (sometimes they look almost free, but they don't look!). Turkey meatballs can get very dark.

- Cover the pan until each side is browned and cook for a further 5 minutes.

- In a cast-iron scallop, turkey meat is cooked.

- Use the meat thermometer, and you can remove the meatballs from the pan when it hits 120-135 degrees F.

- Cut a ball of meat in half and check if it has been finished, to be extra sure. Cooking the meat perfectly with the turkey is important.

Turkey Turnovers

Preparation time-12 minutes| Cook time-17 minutes| Servings-24 |Difficulty-Easy

Nutritional value- Calories-155| Fat-7g |Carbohydrates-13g| Protein-9g

Ingredients

- One pound of ground turkey (breast meat only)

- One cup of 2% low-fat cheese, shredded

- One envelope of dry onion soup

- Three tubes refrigerated crescent rolls (reduced-fat)

Instructions

- Preheat the oven to 350 degrees Fahrenheit.

- In a skillet, combine meat & soup and brown thoroughly.

- Stir in the cheese.

- Unroll the dough, separate the rolls, and halve each triangle.

- Fill the center of each triangle with a spoonful of meat mixture.

- Fold over and seal the edges before placing them on a cookie sheet.

- Bake in the oven for 15 minutes. Then serve!

Turkey-Vegetable Burger

Preparation time-10 minutes| Cook time-15 minutes| Servings-4 |Difficulty-Easy

Nutritional value- Calories-142| Fat-9g |Carbohydrates-2g| Protein-12g

Ingredients

- Nonstick cooking spray

- Eight ounces of lean ground turkey

- A quarter teaspoon of salt

- One large egg

- One teaspoon of ground cumin

- One teaspoon of garlic powder

- A quarter cup of shredded carrot

- A quarter cup of diced yellow onion

- A quarter cup of diced bell pepper

- One tablespoon of extra-virgin olive oil

Instructions

- Heat the oil in a medium skillet over medium heat. Then sauté the onion, bell pepper, and carrot until the onion becomes mildly translucent.

- Then mix the ground turkey, egg garlic powder, salt, cooked vegetables, and cumin. Make 4 patties of the turkey mix.

- Oil a skillet and put it over medium heat.

- Let the patties cook on each side for 4 to 6 minutes. Serve hot.

White Bean Chicken Chili

Preparation time-10 minutes | Cook time-6 hours | Servings-12 | Difficulty-Hard

Nutritional value- Calories-172 | Fat-4g | Carbohydrates-2g | Protein-19g

Ingredients

- One yellow onion, ½ cups (¼-inch dice)

- One boneless chicken breast skinless, ¼ pound

- One green bell pepper, diced

- Two tablespoons of olive oil

- One teaspoon of kosher salt

- Four cloves of garlic, minced

- One tablespoon of cumin

- Two and a half cups of canned white beans (low sodium, divided, drained)

- One cup of roasted mild green chilies (divided, canned & rinsed)

- One cup of unsalted divided chicken stock

- A teaspoon of black pepper

- Fat-free sour cream (Optional)

Instructions

- In a frying pan, warm olive oil on low-medium heat.

- Cook until the diced onions, diced pepper, and cumin are translucent, about 4-5 minutes.

- Stir in garlic and continue cooking for an additional 2-3 minutes, or until fragrant.

- To the slow cooker, add the cooked onions, pepper, cumin, garlic mixture, chicken breasts, 12 cup roasted chilies, 12 cup white beans, and 12 cup chicken stock.

- Puree the remaining twelve cups of roasted green chilies, one cup of beans, and twelve cups of chicken stock in a blender until smooth, about 46 seconds.

- Combine in the slow cooker.

- Season the slow cooker with salt and pepper.

- Cover and cook for 3 hours on high or 6 hours on low.

- Remove chicken from pan and shred or cube.

- Return all ingredients to the slow cooker and stir to combine.

- Season chili with salt and pepper as desired.

- Serve chili with desired toppings.

White beans and smoked paprika shrimp

Preparation time-10 minutes | Cook time-20 minutes | Servings-2 to 4 | Difficulty-Easy

Nutritional value: ~Calories-289 | Proteins-33g | Fat-4g | Carbohydrates-25g

Ingredients

- Four tablespoons of olive oil, divided, plus more to drizzle

- Six cloves fresh garlic, minced and divided

- Three dried red chilies

- Two bay leaves, best to use fresh leaves if possible

- One (28-ounce) can of diced tomatoes, fully drained

- Two tablespoons of tomato paste

- Two (15-ounce) cans of cannellini beans, rinsed and drained

- One cup of canned low-sodium, fat-free chicken broth

- One pound of large raw shrimp, peeled and deveined

- One teaspoon of smoked paprika

- Garlic salt and freshly ground pepper to taste

- Two tablespoons of chopped flat-leaf parsley for garnish

- Four slices of toasted crusty bread (optional)

Instructions

- Preheat broiler. Heat two teaspoons of olive oil in a heavy-bottomed skillet over medium heat. Add three cloves of garlic, chilies, and bay leaves.

- Cook, stirring continuously, until fragrant, about 2–3 minutes. Add diced tomatoes. With the back of a spoon, smash tomatoes until they are completely broken into a mash and cook for about 5 minutes.

- Add tomato paste, constantly stirring until sauce is a deep red, about 3–5 minutes. Stir in beans and broth, bring to a simmer, and cook until juices are slightly reduced and thickened, about 4–5 minutes.

- Transfer bean mixture to an oven-safe casserole dish. In a bowl, add remaining olive oil and garlic, shrimp, and paprika. Season with garlic, salt and pepper to taste. Toss shrimp until evenly coated.

- Scatter shrimp over bean mixture in an even layer. Place casserole under the broiler and broil until shrimp are golden and cooked through about 3–5 minutes. Remove from heat and drizzle a scant amount of olive oil over shrimp and beans and garnish with chopped parsley.

- Serve with crusty bread, if desired.

Whole Herbed Roasted Chicken

Preparation time-10 minutes| Cook time-7 hours| Servings-4 |Difficulty-Hard

Nutritional value- Calories-191| Fat-8g |Carbohydrates-1g| Protein-29g

Ingredients

- Two lemon wedges
- Two sprigs of fresh rosemary
- One (4-pound) whole chicken
- One teaspoon of dried thyme
- Half teaspoon of dried sage
- One teaspoon of paprika
- Half teaspoon of ground black pepper
- One teaspoon of onion powder
- One teaspoon of garlic powder

Instructions

- Combine thyme, black pepper, onion powder, sage, paprika, and garlic powder.
- From the chicken cavity, take out any giblets and wash the chicken cavity with cold water. Now put the chicken in the slow cooker.
- Coat the chicken with the herb blend. Try to get under the skin as much as possible.
- Stuff the chicken with lemon wedges and rosemary.
- Cook for 7 hours, or until the innermost temperature of the thickest part of the breast reaches 165°F.

Zucchini Boat

Preparation time-20 minutes| Cook time-25 minutes| Servings-4 |Difficulty-Moderate

Nutritional value- Calories-101| Fat-2g |Carbohydrates-13g| Protein-17g

Ingredients

- One pound of ground turkey breast
- A quarter teaspoon of pepper
- Half cup of chopped onion
- Four medium zucchinis
- One egg beaten
- One large tomato, diced
- Half pound of sliced mushrooms
- 3/4 cup of spaghetti sauce
- A quarter teaspoon of salt
- A quarter cup of seasoned whole-wheat bread crumbs

- One cup of shredded low-fat mozzarella cheese (4 ounces)

Instructions

- Cut zucchini in half lengthwise; with a sharp knife, make a thin slice from the bottom to allow the zucchini to sit flat.
- Scoop pulp from shells, leaving 1/4-inch shells behind. Set aside pulp.
- Arrange shells in a 3-quart microwave-safe dish that has not been greased. Microwave covered for 3 minutes on high or until drain and set aside until crisp-tender.
- Cook ground turkey and onion in a large skillet over medium heat until meat is no longer pinkish; drain. Take the pan off the heat.
- In a large mixing bowl, combine the beaten egg zucchini pulp, the spaghetti sauce, the mushrooms, the bread crumbs, salt tomato, half cup of cheese, pepper, and cooked ground turkey are all good additions.
- Fill each shell halfway with about a quarter cup of mixture.
- Sprinkle remaining cheese on top.
- Uncovered, bake at 350 degrees F for 20 minutes or until brown.

Zucchini Noodles with Turkey Sauce

Preparation time-10 minutes| Cook time-15 minutes| Servings-12 |Difficulty-Easy

Nutritional value- Calories-120| Fat-5g |Carbohydrates-4g| Protein-11g

Ingredients

- Half cup of Parmesan cheese
- Three medium zucchinis
- Four cloves of garlic, minced
- One pound of lean ground turkey
- Half cup of parsley or basil, chopped
- One tablespoon of Italian seasoning (low sodium)
- One chopped red onion
- One tablespoon of cooking oil
- 28-ounce can of tomatoes, crushed

Instructions

- Prepare zucchini by spiralizing or grating it. Place aside.
- Preheat a large skillet over low heat. Cook for 5 minutes with the oil and onion. Garlic and Italian seasonings should be added at this point. 1 minute cook time.

- Add turkey and cook, occasionally stirring until browned.

- Cook, constantly stirring until tomatoes are thickened, about 5 minutes. Add basil or parsley if desired.

- Place zucchini in a microwave-safe dish to steam. Wrap the container in a lid or plastic wrap. Two cups at a time, microwave on High for about 2 minutes or until soft.

- To serve, arrange a zucchini serving on a plate and drizzle with sauce and cheese.

Chapter 8~Appetizer, Snacks and Sides Recipes

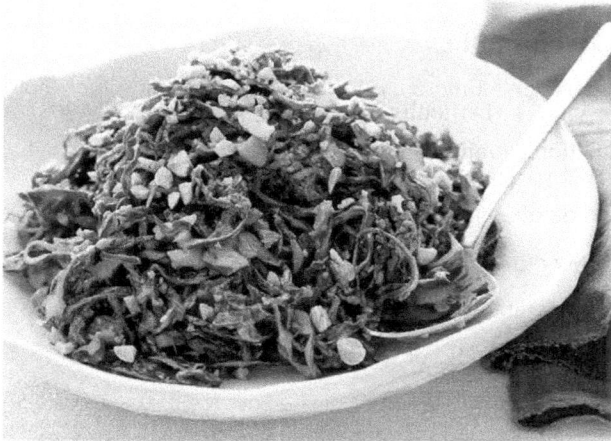

Asian red cabbage slaw with peanuts

Preparation time~15 minutes |Cook time~0 minutes |Serving~6 |Difficulty- Easy

Nutritional value: - Calories-124| Fat-9g| Protein-4g| Carbohydrates-8g

Ingredients

- One tablespoon of spicy mustard
- One tablespoon of soy sauce
- Two teaspoons honey
- Six cups of packed thinly sliced red cabbage
- Two tablespoons of chopped fresh cilantro
- Two tablespoons of roasted no-salt-added creamy peanut butter
- One tablespoon of toasted sesame oil
- Two tablespoons of new ginger, peel and rub
- Juice of one lime
- A quarter cup of thinly sliced fresh basil
- Three thinly sliced scallions, green and white parts
- Two to three tablespoons of chopped roasted unsalted peanuts

Instructions

- Combine the mustard, peanut butter, sesame oil, honey ginger, soy sauce, and lime juice in a large bowl. To coat, add the cilantro, basil, cabbage, and scallions and toss.
- Transfer to a dish, sprinkle with peanuts and serve right away

Asian Cabbage Slaw

Preparation time~10 minutes |Cook time~10 minutes |Serving~4 |Difficulty- Easy

Nutritional value: Calories-123| Fat-6g| Protein-6g| Carbohydrates-16g

Ingredients

- One (14-ounce) package coleslaw
- One red bell pepper, thinly sliced
- One large carrot, grated
- A quarter cup of diced scallions
- A quarter cup of chopped fresh cilantro
- A quarter cup of chopped peanuts
- ⅓ cup of Spicy Peanut Dressing, plus more if desired

Instructions

- In a large bowl, combine coleslaw, bell pepper, carrot, scallions, cilantro, and peanuts.
- Toss with the dressing, add more as desired, and serve.

Baked cauliflower

Preparation time~5 minutes |Cook time~20 minutes |Servings~2 to 4 |Difficulty-Easy

Nutritional value: Calories-108|Proteins-3g| Fat-8g|Carbohydrates-7g

Ingredients

- Five cloves garlic
- Two teaspoons of thyme leaves
- A quarter teaspoon of red pepper
- One head cauliflower
- A quarter cup of olive oil
- Two teaspoons of kosher salt

Instructions

- Preheat microwave to 450 degrees F.
- Toss the cauliflower along with olive oil, red pepper & garlic on a baking sheet, sprinkle with salt & thyme. Toss again.
- Roast till it is golden & tender (20 minutes). Transfer in serving bowl & now serve.

Baked potato fingers with shallots and fresh herbs

Preparation time-10 minutes |Cook time-45 minutes |Servings-2 to 4 |Difficulty-Moderate

Nutritional value: Calories-179|Proteins-3g| Fat-7g|Carbohydrates-27g

Ingredients

- Four large Yukon Gold potatoes
- Two tablespoons of olive oil
- Two large shallots, finely minced
- One tablespoon of finely chopped rosemary (Fresh)
- Salt and freshly ground pepper to taste
- One tablespoon of finely chopped sage leaves (Fresh)
- Olive oil cooking spray

Instructions

- Preheat oven to 375 degrees F. Scrub skins of potatoes with a vegetable brush and pat dry. Cut potatoes in half lengthwise.
- Cut each half into four lengthwise slices. In a small bowl, combine olive oil, shallots, sage, rosemary, and salt and pepper. Stir to blend.
- Spray a shallow baking sheet with cooking oil. Arrange potato fingers in a single layer on a baking sheet and generously brush them with the shallot-herb mixture.
- Place in oven and roast for 40 minutes, turning once after about 20 minutes.

Roast until fingers are browned and tender. Remove from oven and serve.

Baked sweet potato fries with basil pesto

Preparation time-10 minutes |Cook time-10 minutes |Servings-2 |Difficulty-Easy

Nutritional value: ~Calories-221|Proteins-4g| Fat-7g|Carbohydrates-34g

Ingredients

- Two (6-ounce) sweet potatoes
- One tablespoon of fresh Basil Pesto Sauce or market-fresh basil pesto
- Salt and freshly ground pepper to taste
- Low-fat or fat-free sour cream, for garnish (optional)

Instructions

- Clean the skins of sweet potatoes under cold running water and pat potatoes dry with paper towels. Cut potatoes in half and then each half into fry strips.
- Place fries in a single layer on a non-stick baking sheet and brush with pesto sauce. Add salt and pepper to taste.
- Place baking sheet in oven and bake fries at 400 degrees F until tender and lightly browned around edges. Divide fries into two servings and garnish with a dollop of sour cream, if desired.

Baked tofu bites

Preparation time-5 minutes |Cook time-One hour |Serving-4 |Difficulty-Hard

Nutritional value: ~ Calories-124| Fat-9g| Protein-4g| Carbohydrates-8g

Ingredients

- Six ounces of extra-firm tofu
- One tablespoon of sesame seeds
- A quarter cup of soy sauce
- A quarter teaspoon of garlic powder
- Three tablespoons of sugar-free maple syrup
- A quarter teaspoon of ground black pepper
- Two tablespoons of ketchup
- A quarter teaspoon of salt
- One teaspoon of toasted sesame oil
- One tablespoon of rice wine vinegar
- Two teaspoons of Worcestershire sauce
- One dash of sweet chili sauce or hot sauce

Instructions

- Drain tofu of excess liquid. Cover with a paper towel, place in Ziploc bag (or on a plate) and refrigerate overnight.
- Preheat oven to 375 F.
- Cut tofu into ½-1 inch cubes.
- In a bowl, whisk the rest of the ingredients. Gently stir tofu cubes into the sauce. Cover and marinate for at least 5 minutes (or up to 2 hours).
- Place tofu on a baking sheet. Bake 10-20 minutes, turn tofu and bake 10-20 minutes more (until toasty). Turn off the oven and leave Bites in the oven for 20 minutes more. (The exact baking time will depend on the size of the Bites. They are done when they look toasted and dried out.) Don't forget to refrigerate leftovers!

Baked Zucchini Fries

Preparation time-15 minutes | Cook time-30 minutes | Servings-6 | Difficulty-Easy

Nutritional value- Calories-89 | Fat-3g | Carbohydrates-10g | Protein-5g

Ingredients

- One teaspoon of onion powder
- One teaspoon of garlic powder
- A quarter cup of shredded Parmigiano-Reggiano cheese
- One cup of whole-wheat bread crumbs
- Two large eggs
- Three large zucchinis

Instructions

Cover a large baking sheet with tin foil.

- Cut each zucchini in half and keep cutting them into fries of ½ inch in diameter. Now, whisk the eggs gently.
- Then mix the Parmigiano-Reggiano cheese, bread crumbs, onion powder, and garlic powder.
- Now dip each zucchini strip in the egg and cover with the bread crumbs. Arrange on the baking sheet.
- Let them roast for 30 minutes, flipping them midway. They'll be done when they're crispy and brown. Serve and enjoy.

Balsamic Roasted Green Beans

Preparation time-5 minutes | Cook time-20 minutes | Servings-2 | Difficulty-Easy

Nutritional value: ~Calories-93 | Proteins-4g | Fat-5g | Carbohydrates-12g

Ingredients

- One lb of Green beans
- Two Chopped Garlic Cloves
- One tablespoon of Balsamic vinegar
- One tablespoon of Olive oil
- ⅛ teaspoons of Salt
- ⅛ teaspoons of Pepper

Instructions

- Preheat oven to 425°F.
- Mix green beans along with olive oils, pepper & salt in a large bowl.
- Evenly spread green beans on a foil or parchment paper-lined on a baking sheet.
- Bake them for 10-12 minutes in the oven until it turns light brown

- Spread garlic with green beans & mix well to combine. Then again, bake it for another 5 minutes till beans are warm & browned.

Remove from oven & toss with balsamic vinegar.

Barbeque Chicken Pizza

Preparation time-20 minutes | Cook time-15 minutes | Servings-4 | Difficulty-Easy

Nutritional value- Calories-384 | Fat-6g | Carbohydrates-48g | Protein-21g

Ingredients

- One thin pizza crust (12-inch)
- One cup of tomato sauce (no salt added)
- One sliced tomato
- Four tablespoons of barbecue sauce
- Eight green pepper rings
- One cup of sliced mushrooms
- Four ounces of cooked chicken breast (sliced about 1-inch thick)
- One cup of shredded mozzarella cheese(reduced-fat)

Instructions

- Preheat the oven to 400 degrees Fahrenheit.
- Evenly distribute the sauce over the pizza crust. Combine the tomato, pepper, mushrooms, and chicken in a medium bowl.
- Drizzle barbecue sauce on top and sprinkle with cheese.
- Bake for approximately 12 to 14 minutes. Serve immediately after slicing the pizza into eight slices.

Basil tomato rice

Preparation time-10 minutes | Cook time-30 minutes | Servings-2 to 4 | Difficulty-Easy

Nutritional value: Calories-113 | Proteins-3g | Fat-5g | Carbohydrates-14g

Ingredients

- One tablespoon of olive oil
- Two cloves garlic salt to taste
- Black pepper to taste
- Half cup of onion
- One cup of white rice
- One ripe tomato
- Two cups of chicken broth
- Three tablespoons of grated parmesan cheese
- Two tablespoons of basil

Instructions

- Take a frying pan, add onions & olive oil to it and cook it for four minutes. Then add rice in it & cook it for 2-3 minutes more.

- Add tomatoes, chicken broth, sale, black pepper & garlic to it.

- Cover it and boil & reduce heat to a simmer. Cook for 20 minutes. Without raising the lid.

- Please remove it from the stove & rest it for five minutes before removing the lid. Add parmesan cheese & basil & mix well.

- Place this in a bowl and garnish it with remaining parmesan cheese along with basil & tomatoes if required.

Bell Pepper Nachos

Preparation time-10 minutes | Cook time-20 minutes | Serving-4 | Difficulty- Easy

Nutritional value: Calories-348 | Fat-17g | Protein-31g | Carbohydrates-15g

Ingredients

- One pound of lean ground beef (93%)

- ⅓ cup of salsa

- Two tablespoons of Taco Seasoning (store-bought or homemade)

- Nonstick cooking spray

- 20 to 25 mini bell peppers, halved lengthwise, trimmed, and seeded

- One cup of Mexican shredded cheese

Instructions

- Preheat the oven to 400°F.

- In a large skillet over medium heat, brown the meat until no longer pink, breaking it up as it cooks, 7 to 10 minutes. Drain the meat, and stir in the salsa and taco seasoning. Simmer for 3 to 5 minutes until the liquid has cooked down.

- Spray a large baking sheet with cooking spray and arrange the peppers on the sheet cut-side up.

- Fill the peppers with the beef, and sprinkle with the cheese.

- Bake until the cheese is melted, about 5 minutes, and serve immediately.

Black Bean Chipotle Hummus

Preparation time-5 minutes | Cook time-5 minutes | Servings-2 | Difficulty-Easy

Nutritional value- Calories-52 | Fat-2g | Carbohydrates-6g | Protein-2g

Ingredients

- A quarter cup of chopped fresh cilantro

- Two tablespoons of extra-virgin olive oil

- Two teaspoons of ground cumin

- One teaspoon of minced garlic

- One teaspoon of adobo sauce

- One chipotle pepper in adobo sauce

- Juice of one lime

- One (15-ounce) canned black beans, drained and rinsed

Instructions

- Puree the chipotle pepper, cumin, adobo sauce, cilantro, olive oil, lime juice, garlic, and black beans in a blender on high. Pulse until everything's very smooth.

- Add one to two tablespoons of water in case the hummus is thicker than normal.

- Serve right away, or store in an airtight container for up to 7 days.

Boiled fresh red beets

Preparation time-10 minutes | Cook time-10 minutes | Servings-2 | Difficulty-Easy

Nutritional value: ~Calories-45 | Proteins-2g | Fat-0g | Carbohydrates-10g

Ingredients

- Eight medium red beets, unpeeled

- Water to cover beets

- Salt and freshly ground pepper, to taste

- Butter-flavored cooking spray (optional)

Instructions

- Wear disposable gloves or kitchen gloves to prevent hands from staining since fresh red beets' skins and juices will stain skin and clothing as well as porous items. Cut stems and root end from beets.

- Wash beets, gently rubbing skins to extract as much dirt from beets as possible.

- Place unpeeled beets in a large pot and cover with water. Boil on medium-high heat until beets are tender. Remove from heat and strain off juice through a strainer; if you like beetroot juice, reserve.

- Hold beets in a pot under running cool water and gently peel off skins from beets, again using gloves to avoid beet stains.

- Season with salt and pepper and a spray of butter, if desired, and serve.

Broccoli and Cheddar Biscuits

Preparation time-10 minutes | Cook time-35 minutes | Servings-12 | Difficulty-Easy

Nutritional value: Calories-123 | Proteins-4g | Fat-14g | Carbohydrates-8g

Ingredients

- Four cups of broccoli florets
- One and a half cups of almond flour
- One teaspoon of paprika
- Salt and black pepper to the taste
- Two eggs
- A quarter cup of coconut oil
- Two cups of grated cheddar cheese
- One teaspoon of garlic powder
- Half teaspoons of apple cider vinegar
- Half teaspoons of baking soda

Instructions

- In your food processor, place the broccoli florets, add some pepper and salt and combine well.
- Mix pepper, salt, paprika, baking soda and garlic powder with almond flour in a bowl and stir.
- Apply the coconut oil, cheddar cheese, vinegar and eggs and stir.
- Attach the broccoli and stir some more.
- Shape twelve patties, arrange them on a baking sheet, put them at 375 degrees F in the oven and bake for 20 minutes.
- Switch the broiler in the oven and broil the biscuits for another 5 minutes.
- Arrange and serve on a platter.

Broccoli with almonds and olives

Preparation time-10 minutes | Cook time-0 minutes | Servings-2 to 4 | Difficulty-Easy

Nutritional value: Calories-113 | Proteins-3g | Fat-9g | Carbohydrates-9g

Ingredients

- Two tablespoons of extra-virgin olive oil
- One clove of fresh garlic, minced
- Two teaspoons of grated lemon zest
- Half tablespoon freshly squeezed lemon juice
- Twelve pitted Kalamata olives, chopped
- 1/8 teaspoon of crushed red hot pepper flakes
- A quarter cup of chopped toasted almonds
- One fresh head broccoli, florets only, blanched

- One and a half tablespoons of chopped fresh parsley
- Salt and freshly ground pepper to taste

Instructions

- Combine olive oil, garlic, lemon zest, lemon juice, olives, hot pepper flakes, and almonds in a large bowl.
- Add blanched broccoli florets, parsley, and salt and pepper to taste. Toss to coat and serve warm.

Broiled avocado halves and cheddar cheese

Preparation time-10 minutes | Cook time-10 minutes | Servings-2 | Difficulty-Easy

Nutritional value: -Calories-185 | Proteins-5g | Fat-15g | Carbohydrates-8g

Ingredients

- Two ripe-but-firm avocados halved and pitted, with skin on
- A quarter cup of reduced-fat shredded extra-sharp cheddar cheese
- One small jalapeno pepper, finely minced
- Salt and freshly ground pepper to taste
- One tablespoon of fresh lime juice
- One lime, quartered, for garnish

Instructions

- Preheat broiler. Place avocado halves on a lined baking sheet cut side up. In a small mixing bowl, combine cheddar cheese, jalapeno, salt and pepper, and lime juice.
- Divide the cheese mixture among the tops of avocado halves. Place baking sheet 3–4 inches under heat and broil for about 3–5 minutes or until cheese bubbles and begins to brown. Serve halves warm with lime wedges.

Brown rice

Preparation time-10 minutes | Cook time-10 minutes | Servings-2 | Difficulty-Easy

Nutritional value: -Calories-249 | Proteins-7g | Fat-9g | Carbohydrates-38g

Ingredients

- Four cups of canned low-sodium, low-fat chicken broth
- Two cups of brown rice
- Six cloves fresh garlic
- Half cup of pine nuts
- Six scallions, white and green parts, trimmed and sliced
- Eight pitted large black olives, drained and coarsely chopped

- Half tablespoon extra-virgin olive oil

- Salt and freshly ground pepper to taste

- Chopped chives for garnish

Instructions

- In a saucepan, bring broth and rice to a boil; reduce heat to medium, cover, and continue boiling until all liquid is absorbed, occasionally stirring if needed.

- While rice is boiling, sauté garlic, pine nuts, scallions, and olives in olive oil until garlic is soft and pine nuts are lightly toasted. When rice is ready, fluff with a fork and stir in garlic and pine nut mixture; add salt and pepper to taste.

- Transfer to a serving platter and garnish with chives.

Brussels Sprouts with Pistachios

Preparation time-15 minutes | Cook time-15 minutes | Servings-2 | Difficulty-Easy

Nutritional value: ~Calories-126 | Proteins-6g | Fat-7g | Carbohydrates-14g

Ingredients

- One pound of Brussels sprouts, tough bottoms trimmed, halved lengthwise

- Four shallots, peeled and quartered

- One tablespoon of extra-virgin olive oil

- Sea salt

- Freshly ground black pepper

- Half cup of chopped roasted pistachios

- Zest of half lemon

- Juice of half lemon

Instructions

- Preheat the oven to 400°F.

- In a bowl, toss the Brussels sprouts and shallots with the olive oil until well coated.

- Season with pepper and sea salt, and then spread the vegetables evenly on the sheet.

- Bake for 15 minutes or until tender and lightly caramelized.

- Take away from the oven and transfer to a serving bowl.

- Toss with the pistachios, lemon zest, and lemon juice. Serve warm.

Butternut Squash Fries

Preparation time-10 minutes | Cook time-10 minutes | Servings-2 | Difficulty-Easy

Nutritional value: ~Calories-46 | Proteins-2g | Fat-3g | Carbohydrates-10g

Ingredients

- One butternut squash

- One tablespoon of extra virgin olive oil

- Half tablespoon of grapeseed oil

- 1/8 teaspoon of Sea salt

Instructions

- Remove seeds from the squash and cut them into thin slices. Coat with extra virgin olive oil and grapeseed oil. Add a sprinkle of salt and toss to coat well.

Arrange the slices of squash onto three baking sheets and then bake for 10 minutes until crispy.

Cajun onion rings

Preparation time-15 minutes | Cook time-10 minutes | Serving-3 | Difficulty- Easy

Nutritional value: ~ Calories-124 | Fat-9g | Protein-4g | Carbohydrates-8g

Ingredients

- One and a half cups of sour cream

- One and a half cups of milk

- Two tablespoons of hot pepper sauce

- Two large (sliced into rings) red onions

- One teaspoon of celery salt

- One teaspoon of onion powder

- One teaspoon of garlic powder

- One teaspoon of mustard powder

- One teaspoon of paprika

- One tablespoon of chili powder

- One teaspoon of white pepper

- Salt

- Two cups of self-rising flour

- Vegetable oil

Instructions

- Sprinkle the whipped cream, milk and hot sauce together in a large bowl. In the flour season, add the onion rings and separate. In a broad baking dish or pie dish, mix celery salt, onion powder, garlic powder, mustard powder, paprika, chili powder, white pepper, salt and flour.

- In a big Dutch oven, heat about 3 inches of oil at 350 degrees Fahrenheit.

- From the liquid mixture, remove the onion rings and dredge them into the flour mixture. Repeat the double-coat process on the rings. Place the onion rings in batches and fry them in oil for around 5 minutes.

- Remove the paper towel rings from the paper towel plate and season with salt when heating, then switch to a serving dish. Serve with Crab Burgers and Rimled Celery Root.

Cajun Roll-Ups

Preparation time-5 minutes | Cook time-5 minutes | Serving-4 | Difficulty- Easy

Nutritional value: Calories-152 | Fat-9g | Protein-10g | Carbohydrates-6g

Ingredients

- Four slices nitrate-free Cajun deli turkey
- Four teaspoons of spicy mustard, divided
- Four slices of pepper Jack cheese
- Half steak tomato, seeded and diced
- A quarter red onion, thinly sliced
- Two cups of shredded lettuce
- Half avocado, diced
- A quarter cup of chopped banana peppers

Instructions

- On a cutting board, lay out 1 slice of deli turkey and spread with one teaspoon of mustard.
- Top with one slice of cheese, one quarter each of the diced tomato and red onion slices, a quarter cup of shredded lettuce, and one quarter each of the diced avocado and banana peppers.
- Wrap the deli turkey tightly, but delicately, around the filling, and pin it with a toothpick.
- Repeat the process 3 times with the remaining ingredients, and serve.

Caprese Salad Bites

Preparation time-10 minutes | Cook time-15 minutes | Serving-12 | Difficulty- Easy

Nutritional value: Calories-39 | Fat-3g | Protein-1g | Carbohydrates-3g

Ingredients

For the bites

- Twenty-four cherry tomatoes
- Twelve mozzarella balls
- Twelve fresh basil leaves

For the balsamic glaze

- Half cup of balsamic vinegar
- Two tablespoons of extra-virgin olive oil
- One garlic clove, minced
- One teaspoon of Italian seasoning

Instructions

To make the bites

- Using 12 toothpicks or short skewers, assemble each with 1 cherry tomato, 1 mozzarella ball, 1 basil leaf, and another tomato.
- Place on a serving platter or in a large glass storage container that can be sealed.

To make the glaze

- In a small saucepan, bring the balsamic to a simmer. Simmer for 15 minutes or until syrupy. Set aside to cool and thicken.
- In a small bowl, whisk olive oil, garlic, Italian seasoning, and cooled vinegar.
- Drizzle the olive oil and balsamic glaze over the skewers. Serve immediately or keep in the refrigerator for a tasty snack.

Caramelized brussels sprouts with garlic and red chili peppers

Preparation time-10 minutes | Cook time-25 minutes | Servings-2 | Difficulty-Easy

Nutritional value: ~Calories-138 | Proteins-5g | Fat-9g | Carbohydrates-13g

Ingredients

- Two tablespoons of trans fat-free canola/olive oil spread
- Two tablespoons of olive oil
- Four cloves fresh garlic, thinly sliced
- Half red chili pepper or to taste, deseeded and cut into 1/8-inch thick slices
- Two pounds of fresh brussels sprouts halved from the top through stem
- Salt and freshly ground pepper to taste

Instructions

- In a 12-inch heavy-bottomed skillet, melt canola/olive oil spread with olive oil over medium-low heat. Add slices of garlic and red chili pepper and sauté until brown and crisp. With a slotted spoon, remove garlic and chili pepper slices, reserving them.
- Turn heat to low and place brussels sprouts cut side down in skillet, keeping the cut side in direct contact with the pan. Cook sprouts (do not turn) for 10–15 minutes or until they are well caramelized.
- If the skillet becomes dry, drizzle with small amounts of olive oil as needed. Remove sprouts and skillet juices, place them into a warm bowl and toss with the reserved garlic and red chili pepper slices. Sprinkle with salt and pepper to taste.

Caramelized onions and roasted kale

Preparation time-10 minutes | Cook time-35 minutes | Servings-2 | Difficulty-Easy

Nutritional value: ~Calories-70 | Proteins-0g | Fat-8g | Carbohydrates-6g

Ingredients

- Three large red onions
- Four tablespoons of olive oil, divided
- Salt and freshly ground pepper to taste
- Half cup of canned low-sodium, fat-free chicken broth
- Three tablespoons of balsamic vinegar
- One tablespoon of trans fat–free canola/olive oil spread
- Two bunches of kale stems were removed, and leaves were coarsely chopped
- Four cloves fresh garlic, minced
- 1/8 teaspoon of crushed red hot pepper flakes

Instructions

- Preheat oven to 375 degrees F. Cut onions into wedges. In a large skillet, heat one tablespoon of olive oil, then add onions, salt and pepper to taste.
- Cook over medium-high heat for about 5 minutes, often stirring, until onions begin to brown. Reduce heat to medium and add broth and vinegar.
- Cover and cook until onions are soft. Add canola/olive oil spread, increase heat to high, and cook 2–4 minutes longer, stirring onions with a wooden spoon as they caramelize. Scrape the bottom of the pan with a spoon to loosen any bits of onion. Set aside.
- Using heavy tinfoil, place kale leaves in the center of foil and curl up sides of foil to form a basket. Drizzle remaining olive oil over leaves, add garlic and hot pepper flakes, and season with salt and pepper to taste.
- Toss mixture and roast uncovered in the oven for 15–20 minutes, tossing kale several times during roasting. Remove from oven and toss with onion mixture. Serve while hot.

Cauliflower Breadsticks

Preparation time-10 minutes | Cook time-30 minutes | Servings-2 | Difficulty-Moderate

Nutritional value: ~Calories-56 | Proteins-5g | Fat-1g | Carbohydrates-5g

Ingredients

- Four lb of cauliflower
- Two egg whites
- One and a half cups of Mozzarella cheese, shredded
- Italian seasoning
- One teaspoon of Pinch of salt
- A quarter teaspoon of black pepper
- Marinara sauce for dipping
- Cooking spray

Instructions

- Toast blended cauliflower in oven at 375 degrees F for 20 minutes.
- Mix roasted cauliflower with egg whites, cheese, herbs, salt, pepper in a bowl.
- Bake the mixture in the oven at 450 degrees F for 18 minutes.
- Bring in sticks, shape, and serve.

Cauliflower Fried Rice

Preparation time-15 minutes | Cook time-15 minutes | Serving-4 | Difficulty- Easy

Nutritional value: Calories-121 | Fat-7g | Protein-6g | Carbohydrates-9g

Ingredients

- One teaspoon of sesame oil, plus one tablespoon
- Two large eggs, beaten
- Four cups of cauliflower rice (or florets of one head of cauliflower rice in a food processor)
- One cup of frozen mixed vegetables
- Two garlic cloves, minced
- Two tablespoons of low-sodium soy sauce
- Two scallions, diced

Instructions

- In a large skillet over medium heat, heat one teaspoon of sesame oil. Add the eggs, and stir until they are cooked. Set aside.
- In the same skillet over medium heat, heat the remaining tablespoon of oil. Add the cauliflower rice, mixed vegetables, garlic, soy sauce, scallions, and eggs. Cook, stirring, until well combined and the cauliflower is soft, about 4 minutes, and serve. Make sure to not overcook the cauliflower, or it will become soggy.

Cheeseburger Muffins

Preparation time-10 minutes | Cook time-40 minutes | Servings-2 | Difficulty-Moderate

Nutritional value: ~Calories-249 | Proteins-7g | Fat-9g | Carbohydrates-38g

Ingredients

- Half cups of flaxseed meal
- Half cups of almond flour
- Salt and black pepper to the taste
- Two eggs
- One teaspoon of baking powder
- A quarter cup of sour cream

For the filling

- Half teaspoons of onion powder
- Sixteen ounces of ground beef
- Salt and black pepper to the taste
- Two tablespoons of tomato paste
- Half teaspoons of garlic powder
- Half cups of grated cheddar cheese

- Two tablespoons of mustard

Instructions

- Mix the almond flour with the flaxseed meal, pepper, salt and baking powder in a bowl and whisk together.
- Add the sour cream and eggs and stir very well.
- Divide it into a greased muffin pan and use your fingers to press well.
- Over medium-high heat, heat a pan, add beef, stir and brown for a couple of minutes.
- Stir well and add pepper, salt, garlic powder, onion powder and tomato paste.
- Cook for an additional 5 minutes and take the heat off.
- Fill the crusts with this mixture, place them in the oven at 350 degrees F and bake for fifteen minutes
- Spread the cheese on top, put it in the oven again and cook the muffins for another 5 minutes.
- Serve with mustard and your preferred toppings.

Cheesy crab bites

Preparation time-10 minutes | Cook time-15 minutes | Servings-2 | Difficulty-Easy

Nutritional value: Calories-62 | Proteins-5g | Fat-1g | Carbohydrates-2g

Ingredients

- Two ounces of low-fat cream cheese softened
- A quarter cup of low-fat shredded cheddar cheese
- Two tablespoons of light mayonnaise
- One teaspoon of freshly squeezed lemon juice
- Half teaspoon of seafood seasoning mix (such as Old Bay)
- Half teaspoon of garlic powder
- One scallion, thinly sliced
- One (13-ounce) can of crabmeat, picked through and flaked apart
- One (2-ounce) box mini phyllo shells
- Dash of paprika

Instructions

- Preheat oven to 350 degrees F.
- In a bowl, gently blend together cream cheese, cheddar cheese, mayonnaise, and lemon juice. Fold seafood seasoning, garlic powder, scallions, and crabmeat into the mixture.
- Fill phyllo shells with mixture, add a dash of paprika on top of each shell, and place shells on a flat baking sheet.
- Bake for roughly 15 minutes, or until shells are golden brown and the mixture is heated through. Serve warm.

Cheesy thyme waffles

Preparation time-10 minutes | Cook time-8 minutes | Servings-2 | Difficulty-Easy

Nutritional value: ~Calories-412 | Proteins-5g | Fat-56g | Carbohydrates-33g

Ingredients

- Two eggs
- 1/3 cup of parmesan cheese
- One teaspoon of garlic powder
- Two teaspoons of thyme
- One cup of collard greens
- One tablespoon of olive oil
- Two stalks onion
- Half cauliflower
- Half teaspoon of salt
- One cup of shredded mozzarella cheese
- One tablespoon of sesame seeds
- Half teaspoon of black pepper

Instructions

- Cut cauliflower & slice onions.
- Add cauliflower to the blender.
- Add onions, thyme & collard greens to the blender & pulse again.
- Now add the processed mixture to a bowl.
- Mix it well to form a smooth batter.
- Heat the waffle iron.
- Pour the mixture into the waffle iron, ensuring that it is spread properly.
- Cook well & serve hot.

Cherry Tomato Bruschetta

Preparation time-15 minutes | Cook time-0 minutes | Servings-2 | Difficulty-Easy

Nutritional value: ~Calories-100 | Proteins-4g | Fat-6g | Carbohydrates-11g

Ingredients

- Eight ounces of assorted cherry tomatoes halved
- 1/3 cup of fresh herbs, chopped (such as basil, parsley, tarragon, dill)
- One tablespoon of extra-virgin olive oil
- A quarter teaspoon of kosher salt
- 1/8 teaspoon of freshly ground black pepper
- A quarter cup of ricotta cheese
- Four slices whole-wheat bread, toasted

Instructions

- Combine the tomatoes, herbs, olive oil, salt, and black pepper in a medium bowl and mix gently.
- Spread one tablespoon of ricotta cheese onto each slice of toast—spoon one-quarter of the tomato mixture onto each bruschetta. If desired, garnish with more herbs.

Cilantro crackers

Preparation time-15 minutes | Cook time-18 minutes | Servings-2 | Difficulty-Moderate

Nutritional value: ~Calories-76 | Proteins-5g | Fat-3g | Carbohydrates-11g

Ingredients

- Two cups of blanched almond flour
- One tablespoon of tapioca flour
- fine sea salt and ground black pepper
- Two tablespoons of chopped fresh cilantro
- Two large eggs, beaten
- Two tablespoons of tahini (sesame seed paste)
- One tablespoon of extra-virgin olive oil

Instructions

- Preheat the oven to 350°F.
- Mix together the almond flour, tapioca flour, and a pinch of salt and pepper in a large mixing bowl.
- Mix the cilantro, eggs, tahini, and olive oil in another bowl. Pour the wet ingredients into the flour mixture and mix thoroughly.
- Form the dough into a ball with your hands, put the ball on a large piece of parchment paper, and cover it with another large sheet of parchment paper.
- Roll out the dough until it is about 1/8 inch thick.
- Remove the top parchment paper and cut the dough into 1-inch squares with a sharp knife.
- Leaving the dough on the parchment paper, transfer it to a baking sheet and bake for 15 to 18 minutes, until golden brown.
- Let the crackers cool for 5 minutes, then carefully separate the squares. Store in an airtight container for 3 to 5 days.

Citrus-Marinated Olives

Preparation time-5 minutes | Cook time-0 minutes | Servings-2 | Difficulty-Easy

Nutritional value: ~Calories-133 | Proteins-2g | Fat-14g | Carbohydrates-3g

Ingredients

- Two cups of mixed green olives with pits
- A quarter cup of red wine vinegar
- A quarter cup of extra-virgin olive oil
- Four garlic cloves, finely minced
- Zest and juice of one large orange
- One teaspoon of red pepper flake
- Two bay leaves
- Half teaspoon of ground cumin
- Half teaspoon of ground allspice

Instructions

- Incorporate the olives, vinegar, oil, garlic, orange zest and juice, red pepper flakes, bay leaves, cumin, and allspice and mix well.
- Seal and chill for 4 hours or up to a week to allow the olives to marinate. Toss it again before serving.

Classic spinach and pine nuts

Preparation time-10 minutes | Cook time-10 minutes | Servings-2 | Difficulty-Easy

Nutritional value: ~Calories-149 | Proteins-4g | Fat-12g | Carbohydrates-10g

Ingredients

- A quarter cup of golden raisins
- Four tablespoons of pine nuts
- Two tablespoons of extra-virgin olive oil
- Four cloves fresh garlic, chopped
- One and a half (10-ounce) bags of fresh spinach, cleaned
- Fresh lemon juice
- Extra-virgin olive oil to taste
- Salt and freshly ground pepper to taste

Instructions

- Place raisins in a bowl and cover with boiling water.
- Let stand for approximately 10 minutes until raisins are plump; drain well. In a skillet over medium heat, toast pine nuts, constantly stirring for about 1–2 minutes. Remove from heat and set aside in a large skillet, heat olive oil.
- Add garlic and sauté for 1–2 minutes, until golden. Add spinach a little at a time until it all becomes wilted (about 3–5 minutes), stirring constantly.
- Pour raisins over spinach and mix well. With a slotted spoon, transfer spinach to a serving dish, and sprinkle

pine nuts over the top. Serve immediately or, if serving at room temperature, add fresh lemon juice and olive oil and salt and pepper to taste.

Coffee with butter

Preparation time-5 minutes | Cook time-5 minutes | Servings-2 | Difficulty-Easy

Nutritional value: ~Calories-230 | Proteins-0g | Fat-25g | Carbohydrates-0g

Ingredients

- Two cups of hot coffee
- Four tablespoons of butter
- Two tablespoons of coconut oil

Instructions

- Combine all the items in a blender and serve in two cups.

Couscous with turnips and greens

Preparation time-10 minutes | Cook time-15 minutes | Servings-2 | Difficulty-Easy

Nutritional value: ~Calories-205 | Proteins-14g | Fat-19g | Carbohydrates-18g

Ingredients

- Two and a half cups of canned low-sodium, fat-free chicken broth
- Three tablespoons of olive oil, divided
- One and a half cups of pearl couscous
- One bunch baby turnips with greens, peeled and quartered
- Half teaspoon of cumin seeds
- Two cloves fresh garlic, minced
- Half medium white onion, finely chopped
- Salt and freshly ground pepper to taste

Instructions

- In a medium saucepan, add broth and one tablespoon of olive oil and bring to boil. Remove from heat, stir in couscous, cover, and let stand.

- Cut turnips from greens and wash both heads and greens well, removing any brown or wilted leaves. Tear greens into roughly 1-inch pieces, trim turnips, and cut into halves. Set greens and turnips aside.

- Add remaining olive oil to a large skillet over medium-high heat. Add cumin and cook for 1 minute until fragrant. Add garlic and continue to cook until soft and fragrant, about one more minute. Add onion, then stir and cook until soft.

- Add turnips, cover pan, and cook until crispy tender, occasionally stirring. Uncover the pan, add greens and salt and pepper, and cook until greens wilt.

- Fluff couscous with a fork and transfer to a large bowl, add cooked vegetable mixture, fluff all again, and serve immediately.

Couscous, tomatoes, and black beans

Preparation time-10 minutes | Cook time-10 minutes | Servings-2 | Difficulty-Easy

Nutritional value: ~Calories-210 | Proteins-8g | Fat-3g | Carbohydrates-37g

Ingredients

- One and a half cups of canned low-sodium vegetable broth

- One cup of couscous

- One tablespoon of extra-virgin olive oil

- Two cloves fresh garlic, minced

- A quarter cup of fresh lemon juice

- A quarter teaspoon of freshly ground pepper

- One and a half cups of canned black beans, rinsed and drained

- Four large plum tomatoes, chopped

- Half cup of red onion, finely chopped

- Fresh parsley, finely chopped for garnish

Instructions

- In a saucepan, bring broth to a boil. Stir in couscous, remove from heat, cover, and let stand until liquid is absorbed.

- In a small skillet over medium heat, add olive oil and garlic and sauté until golden brown. Remove skillet from heat, add lemon juice and pepper, and mix ingredients through.

- Transfer couscous to a large serving bowl. Fluff grains with fingers to separate. Add in garlic mixture, black beans, tomatoes, and onion; stir gently to mix.

- Garnish with parsley and serve.

Creamy Greek Yogurt and Cucumber

Preparation time-5 minutes | Cook time-10 minutes | Servings-2 | Difficulty-Easy

Nutritional value: ~Calories-31 | Proteins-5g | Fat-0g | Carbohydrates-4g

Ingredients

- Two English cucumbers, thinly sliced

- Small bunch of dill

- One and a half cups of low-fat Greek yogurt

- Two tablespoons of fresh lemon juice

- One and a half teaspoons of mustard seeds

- Coarse salt and ground pepper

Instructions

- Combine all your ingredients in a bowl until combined well, and dig in!

Crispy tender broccolini

Preparation time-10 minutes | Cook time-10 minutes | Servings-2 to 4 | Difficulty-Easy

Nutritional value: ~Calories-95 | Proteins-3g | Fat-7g | Carbohydrates-6g

Ingredients

- One pound of (roughly two bunches) broccolini

- Two tablespoons of olive oil

- Two teaspoons of finely chopped fresh garlic

- Half teaspoon of crushed red hot pepper flakes

- Two tablespoons of freshly squeezed lemon juice

- Zest from half of a lemon

- Salt and freshly ground pepper to taste

Instructions

- Rinse broccolini under cold water. If stems are thick, peel back skins to remove the tough skin in a large skillet; heat olive oil over medium-high heat.

- Add garlic and sauté until fragrant. Add broccolini and sauté for about 3 minutes. Cover with water, add hot pepper flakes, and steam for about 3 minutes or until broccolini is crispy tender.

- Squeeze lemon juice over broccolini, sprinkle with lemon zest, add salt and pepper to taste, and serve.

Cucumber Bites

Preparation time-10 minutes | Cook time-0 minutes | Servings-2 | Difficulty-Easy

Nutritional value: ~Calories-132 | Proteins-3g | Fat-4g | Carbohydrates-7g

Ingredients

- One English cucumber, sliced into 32 rounds
- Ten ounces of hummus
- Sixteen cherry tomatoes halved
- One tablespoon of parsley, chopped
- One ounce of feta cheese, crumbled

Instructions

- Spread the hummus on each cucumber round.
- Divide the tomato halves on each, sprinkle the cheese and parsley on top, and serve as an appetizer.

Cucumber Hummus Sandwiches

Preparation time-10 minutes |Cook time-0 minutes |Servings-2 |Difficulty-Easy

Nutritional value: ~Calories-54|Proteins-2g| Fat-21g|Carbohydrates-8g

Ingredients

- Ten round slices of cucumber
- Five teaspoons of hummus

Instructions

- Add one teaspoon of hummus to one slice of cucumber.
- Top with another slice and serve.

Cucumber olive rice

Preparation time~30 minutes |Cook time-55 minutes |Servings-2 to 4|Difficulty-Hard

Nutritional value: ~Calories-223|Proteins-4.5g| Fat-12.7g|Carbohydrates-24.7g

Ingredients

- Three garlic clove
- One lb of heirloom
- Eight ounces of feta
- One cup of parsley leaves
- Seven tablespoons of olive oil
- Kosher salt to taste
- Black pepper to taste
- One and a half cups of brown rice
- One chopped onion
- Three chopped cucumbers
- Three tablespoons of sherry vinegar
- One cup of mint leaves

Instructions

- Add two tablespoons of oil to a heated frying pan.

- Then add garlic along with salt and cook it for five minutes. At the same time, stir till it gives aroma & transparent. Transfer this into a bowl.
- Take frying pan again, heat it and add one tablespoon of oil & rice. Cook this for three minutes while stirring till it turns golden & nutty.
- Add water to the bowl and boil it. Mix it only one time & then decrease the heat to low temperature and then cover it. Cook till rice is delicate & water has been soaked up. Please remove it from the stove and let it cool for five minutes.
- Move rice into a bowl along with the mixture of onion and let it cool for 20 minutes.
- Mix cucumbers, tomatoes, vinegar, & remaining oil. Season with sea salt & black pepper.
- Finally, Coat with cheese, parsley, & mint and serve it.

Cucumber Sandwich Bites

Preparation time-5 minutes |Cook time-0 minutes |Servings-2 |Difficulty-Easy

Nutritional value: ~Calories-187|Proteins-9g| Fat-12.4g|Carbohydrates-5g

Ingredients

- One cucumber, sliced
- Eight slices of whole wheat bread
- Two tablespoons of cream cheese, soft
- One tablespoon of chive, chopped
- A quarter cup of avocado, peeled, pitted, and mashed
- One teaspoon of mustard
- Salt and black pepper to the taste

Instructions

- Spread the mashed avocado on each bread slice.
- Also, spread the rest of the ingredients except the cucumber slices.
- Divide the cucumber slices into the bread slices.
- Cut each slice in thirds, arrange on a platter and serve.

Edamame Hummus

Preparation time-10 minutes |Cook time-10 minutes |Serving-Two cups |Difficulty- Easy

Nutritional value: ~Calories-115| Fat-9g| Protein-4g| Carbohydrates-6g

Ingredients

- One and a half cups of frozen edamame, thawed, rinsed, and drained
- A quarter cup of tahini
- Two tablespoons of extra-virgin olive oil

- Two garlic cloves, peeled

- Half teaspoon of ground cumin

- Three to four teaspoons freshly squeezed lemon juice (juice of one lemon)

- Salt

- Freshly ground black pepper

- Two to four tablespoons of water

- Raw veggies, for serving

Instructions

- In a food processor, combine the edamame, tahini, olive oil, garlic, cumin, and lemon juice. Process until smooth, stopping to scrape down the sides as needed.

- Add salt and pepper to taste. Process again until combined.

- To thin, if desired, add one tablespoon of water and process. Repeat this step until you reach your desired consistency.

- Transfer to a serving bowl, and serve with raw veggies.

Everything Parmesan Crisps

Preparation time-10 minutes |Cook time-10 minutes |Serving-12 |Difficulty- Easy

Nutritional value: ~ Calories-23| Fat-2g| Protein-2g| Carbohydrates-0g

Ingredients

- One teaspoon of poppy seeds

- One teaspoon of sesame seeds

- One teaspoon of garlic flakes

- One teaspoon of onion flakes

- Twelve tablespoons of grated Parmesan cheese

Instructions

- Preheat the oven to 400°F.

- In a small bowl, mix the poppy seeds, sesame seeds, garlic flakes, and onion flakes together.

- Line a sheet pan with a silicone baking mat or parchment paper. Pour one tablespoon of Parmesan onto the mat, and gently pat down with your fingers to make a 2- to 2½-inch round.

- Repeat 11 more times, making sure to keep at least 1 inch between each round.

- Bake for 3 minutes. Remove from the oven, and sprinkle A quarter teaspoon of the seasoning over each Parmesan round.

- Bake for another 3 to 5 minutes, or until golden and crisp, and serve.

Feta and mixed beans

Preparation time-10 minutes |Cook time-10 minutes |Servings-2 |Difficulty-Easy

Nutritional value: ~Calories-151|Proteins-11g| Fat-3g|Carbohydrates-26g

Ingredients

- One (16-ounce) can of light red kidney beans

- One (16-ounce) can of cannellini beans, rinsed and drained

- One (16-ounce) can chickpeas, rinsed and drained

- Three ounces of fresh feta cheese, crumbled

- One cup of finely chopped red onion

- Three tablespoons of chopped fresh mint

- One and a half tablespoons of non-caloric sweetener

- Two cloves fresh garlic, finely chopped

- A quarter teaspoon of salt or to taste

- A quarter teaspoon of freshly ground pepper

- Two tablespoons plus one teaspoon of fresh-squeezed lemon juice

- One tablespoon of balsamic vinegar

- One teaspoon of extra-virgin olive oil

- Four cups of mixed greens

Instructions

- Combine all beans, feta cheese, onion, mint, and sweetener and mix well. Add garlic, salt and pepper, lemon juice, vinegar, and olive oil to the bean mixture.

- Toss again. Place one cup of greens on each plate; divide bean mixture into equal servings, top each plate of greens with bean mixture, and serve.

Frozen yogurt pops

Preparation time-15 minutes |Cook time-0 minutes |Serving-3 |Difficulty- Easy

Nutritional value: ~ Calories-124| Fat-9g| Protein-4g| Carbohydrates-8g

Ingredients

- One small package of sugar-free gelatin, strawberry flavored

- One cup of boiling water

- One medium ripe banana

- One cup of light vanilla yogurt

- One scoop of protein powder (optional but recommended)

- Eight to ten small paper cups

- Eight to ten plastic spoons

Instructions

- Carefully pour hot water into the blender. Add gelatin and blend until combined. (Remember to remove the cork on the top of your blender, so it doesn't explode!)

- Add banana and yogurt, blending until smooth and creamy. If using protein powder, add to blender last and process until smooth.

- Fill each paper cup almost full with the yogurt mixture. Place cups on a flat surface in the freezer. When pops are partially frozen (somewhere around 30 minutes to 1 hour), insert a plastic spoon into each, positioned, so it is sticking straight up. Freeze for four hours or overnight. When ready to eat, peel away the paper cup!

Fresh stewed tomatoes

Preparation time-10 minutes |Cook time-15 minutes |Servings-2 |Difficulty-Easy

Nutritional value: ~Calories-54|Proteins-1g| Fat-4g|Carbohydrates-6g

Ingredients

- One tablespoon of olive oil

- Half cup of diced white onion

- Half cup of chopped celery

- 1/8 cup of finely diced green bell pepper

- One tablespoon of freshly minced garlic

- A quarter teaspoon of crushed red hot pepper flakes

- One teaspoon of dried basil

- Two large tomatoes, peeled and quartered

- One and a half teaspoons of low-calorie baking sweetener

- A quarter cup of chopped fresh parsley

- Salt and freshly ground pepper to taste

Instructions

- In a large pot, add olive oil, onion, celery, green bell pepper, garlic, hot pepper flakes, and basil. Cook on medium-low heat, often stirring, until vegetables are soft.

- Add tomatoes, sweetener, parsley, and salt and pepper to taste. Continue cooking on medium-low heat, often stirring, until tomatoes become very soft and fall apart. Serve as a side with meat, chicken, or fish.

Fried Queso

Preparation time-10 minutes |Cook time-20 minutes |Servings-6 |Difficulty-Easy

Nutritional value: ~Calories-249|Proteins-7g| Fat-9g|Carbohydrates-38g

Ingredients

- Two ounces of pitted and chopped olives,

- Five ounces of cubed and freeze queso Blanco

- A pinch of red pepper flakes

- One and a half tablespoons of olive oil

Instructions

- Over medium-high heat, heat a pan with the oil, add cheese cubes and fry until the lower part melts a bit.

- Flip the spatula cubes and sprinkle on top with black olives.

Let the cubes cook a little more, flip and sprinkle with the red flakes of pepper and cook until crispy.

Flip, cook until crispy on the other side, then move to a chopping board, cut into tiny blocks, and then serve.

Garlic rice

Preparation time-10 minutes |Cook time-15 minutes |Servings-2 |Difficulty-Easy

Nutritional value: ~Calories-194|Proteins-5g| Fat-3g|Carbohydrates-38g

Ingredients

- Half tablespoon extra-virgin olive oil

- Four cloves fresh garlic, minced

- One cup of basmati long-grain rice

- Two cups of canned low-sodium, fat-free chicken broth

- A quarter cup of grated Parmesan cheese

- Two tablespoons of chopped fresh parsley

- Three jumbo cloves roasted fresh garlic, cut into small pieces

- Salt and freshly ground pepper to taste

- Fresh chopped parsley or cilantro for garnish

Instructions

- In a skillet, heat olive oil and sauté fresh garlic until golden brown.

- Bring rice in chicken broth to a boil, cover tightly, reduce heat to simmer, and cook until liquid is absorbed.

- Remove rice from heat and add olive oil and sautéed garlic, Parmesan cheese, parsley, roasted garlic, and salt and pepper to taste; toss well.

- Garnish with parsley or cilantro and serve.

Garlic roasted cauliflower

Preparation time-10 minutes |Cook time-35 minutes |Servings-2 |Difficulty-Easy

Nutritional value: ~Calories-91|Proteins-4g| Fat-7g|Carbohydrates-7g

Ingredients

- One jumbo fresh garlic clove, finely chopped

- One medium head of cauliflower (about 3 pounds), cut into one and a half-inch florets

- Two tablespoons of extra-virgin olive oil

- Garlic salt or seasoning of choice to taste (optional)

Instructions

- Place garlic, florets, and olive oil in a large resealable plastic baggie and toss to coat florets. Arrange florets in a single layer in a shallow baking pan and sprinkle with seasoning, if desired.

- Place pan on the middle rack of a 425-degree oven and roast cauliflower until tender and golden brown (about 20–30 minutes). Stir and turn florets over occasionally while roasting.

Garlicky cannellini beans

Preparation time-10 minutes |Cook time-10 minutes |Servings-2 to 4 |Difficulty-Easy

Nutritional value: ~Calories-123|Proteins-6g| Fat-5g|Carbohydrates-18g

Ingredients

- Two (15-ounce) cans of cannellini beans

- Five large cloves of fresh garlic, minced

- Two tablespoons of extra-virgin olive oil

- Half cup of canned low-sodium, fat-free chicken broth

- Salt and freshly ground pepper to taste

- Pita wedges (optional)

Instructions

- Rinse and drain beans.

- Cook garlic and olive oil in a skillet over medium heat until garlic softens, then add chicken broth and beans and simmer until most of the liquid is evaporated.

- Season with salt and pepper and serve with toasted pita.

Garlic-Parmesan Cauliflower Mash

Preparation time-15 minutes |Cook time-10 minutes |Serving-2 |Difficulty- Easy

Nutritional value: ~ Calories-169| Fat-9g| Protein-12g| Carbohydrates-13g

Ingredients

- Four cups of cauliflower florets

- One teaspoon of extra-virgin olive oil

- Three garlic cloves, minced

- ⅓ cup of grated Parmesan cheese

- One tablespoon of low-fat cream cheese

- Half teaspoon of salt

Instructions

- In a large pot, bring A quarter cup of water to a boil. Add the cauliflower florets. Cook, covered, for 3 to 8 minutes, or until fork-tender. Drain and discard the steaming liquid.

- In a small skillet over medium heat, heat the oil. Add the garlic, and sauté until aromatic, 1 to 2 minutes.

- In a food processor or high-speed blender, blend the cauliflower, garlic, cheeses, and salt until smooth. Serve warm.

German braised cabbage

Preparation time-20 minutes |Cook time-15 minutes |Servings-2|Difficulty-Easy

Nutritional value: ~Calories-94|Proteins-2g| Fat-3g|Carbohydrates-15g

Ingredients

- Two tablespoons of olive oil

- One-fourth chopped sweet onion

- Five cups of shredded red cabbage

- One pear, peeled & chopped

- Three tablespoons of vinegar

- Half teaspoons of dry mustard

- One tablespoon of sugar

- Half teaspoons of caraway seeds

Instructions

- Heat olive oil on moderate heat in a frying pan.

- Add cabbage, onion & pear. sauté till tendered for 10 minutes.

- Stir together vinegar, caraway seed sugar & mustard in a bowl.

- Combine cabbage and vinegar mixture and stir. Cover for 5 minutes.

- Now Serve hot.

Green beans and baby portobellos

Preparation time-10 minutes |Cook time-20 minutes |Servings-2 |Difficulty-Easy

Nutritional value: ~Calories-74|Proteins-2g| Fat-5g|Carbohydrates-7g

Ingredients

- Twelve ounces of fresh green beans ends snipped

- One and a quarter cup of s sliced baby portobello mushrooms

- One and a half tablespoons of finely chopped fresh garlic

- Half teaspoon of onion powder

- Two tablespoons of trans fat–free canola/olive oil spread

- Salt and freshly ground pepper to taste

Instructions

- In a medium saucepan, add beans and mushrooms plus enough water to fill 1/3 of the pan. Bring to a boil, then reduce heat and cook until beans are tender.

- Drain well and transfer beans and mushrooms to a large heavy-bottomed skillet. Add chopped garlic, onion powder, and canola/olive oil spread, and heat over low heat to melt spread, often stirring to coat beans and mushrooms. Continue to cook on low heat for at least 15 minutes to marry flavors.

- Add salt and pepper to taste.

Green Beans with Pine Nuts and Garlic

Preparation time~10 minutes | Cook time~20 minutes | Servings~2 to 4 | Difficulty~Easy

Nutritional value: ~Calories~165 | Proteins~4g | Fat~13g | Carbohydrates~12g

Ingredients

- One pound of green beans, trimmed

- One head of garlic (10 to 12 cloves), smashed

- Two tablespoons of extra-virgin olive oil

- Half teaspoon of kosher salt

- A quarter teaspoon of red pepper flakes

- One tablespoon of white wine vinegar

- A quarter cup of pine nuts, toasted

Instructions

- Preheat the oven to 425°F.

- In a large bowl, blend the green beans, garlic, olive oil, salt, and red pepper flakes and mix—put it in a single layer on the baking sheet. Roast for 10 minutes, stir, and roast for another 10 minutes, or until golden brown.

- Mix the cooked green beans with the vinegar and top with the pine nuts.

Green Chili and Cheese Cornbread Muffins

Preparation time~5 minutes | Cook time~25 minutes | Serving~8 | Difficulty~ Easy

Nutritional value: ~ Calories~93 | Fat~2.5g | Protein~4g | Carbohydrates~13g

Ingredients

- Half cup of all-purpose flour

- Half cup of coarse yellow cornmeal

- One teaspoon of baking powder

- Half teaspoon of baking soda

- A quarter teaspoon of salt

- One and a half teaspoons of onion powder

- Half cup of low-fat buttermilk

- One egg

- Two tablespoons of diced mild green chilies, drained

- Half cup of reduced-fat shredded Cheddar cheese

Instructions

- Preheat the oven to 400°F.

- Spray a muffin tin with cooking spray.

- In a large mixing bowl, combine the flour, baking powder, salt, cornmeal, baking soda, and onion powder. Stir to combine.

- In a medium mixing bowl, whisk together the buttermilk, egg, chiles, and cheese, just enough to combine.

- Fill the muffin cups two-thirds full with batter.

- Bake for 5 minutes until a toothpick inserted into the middle of a muffin comes out clean.

- Let the muffins cool for 15 minutes before turning the tin over to release the muffins.

Grilled eggplant

Preparation time~10 minutes | Cook time~10 minutes | Servings~2 | Difficulty~Easy

Nutritional value: ~Calories~74 | Proteins~5g | Fat~6g | Carbohydrates~10g

Ingredients

- One tablespoon of extra-virgin olive oil

- Two tablespoons of fresh oregano leaves

- Two plum tomatoes, diced

- One and a half pounds eggplant cut lengthwise into Half-inch thick slices

- Olive oil cooking spray

- Two large cloves of fresh garlic, finely minced

- One teaspoon of chopped dried rosemary

- Salt and freshly ground pepper to taste

- A quarter cup of crumbled feta cheese

- Lemon wedges

- Fresh oregano sprigs for garnish

Instructions

- Heat olive oil in a saucepan, add oregano leaves, then remove the pan from heat. Add tomatoes to oregano and allow to bathe in hot olive oil until ready to serve.

- Meanwhile, spray both sides of eggplant slices with cooking oil, sprinkle with garlic, rosemary, salt and pepper, and place on a medium-hot grill. Cover grill and cook eggplant until tender and browned on both sides, turning once.

- Remove eggplant to a platter, drizzle with oregano tomato oil, and top with feta cheese. Garnish with lemon wedges and oregano sprigs.

Grilled jumbo portobello mushrooms

Preparation time-10 minutes | Cook time-16 minutes | Servings-2 | Difficulty-Easy

Nutritional value: ~Calories-101 | Proteins-1g | Fat-9.8g | Carbohydrates-2g

Ingredients

- Four large (4–6-inch) portobello mushrooms

- One tablespoon of balsamic vinegar

- One tablespoon of Worcestershire sauce

- 1/3 cup of extra-virgin olive oil

- Salt and freshly ground pepper to taste

Instructions

- Wash and clean mushrooms. Mix liquid ingredients together, place mushrooms in a resealable plastic baggie, and pour marinade over mushrooms.

- Seal bag and gently toss mushrooms and marinade to cover mushrooms. Refrigerate and marinate for 1–2 hours. Heat grill, place mushrooms on the grill, and brush tops with remaining marinade.

- Grill, each side for 5–6 minutes or until mushrooms are soft. Turn mushrooms over once, brushing marinade mixture onto the other side.

Grilled polenta with cheddar cheese and sundried tomatoes

Preparation time-10 minutes | Cook time-25 minutes | Servings-2 | Difficulty-Easy

Nutritional value: ~Calories-208 | Proteins-5g | Fat-7g | Carbohydrates-28g

Ingredients

- Six cups of water

- Salt to taste

- One and 3/4 cups of yellow cornmeal

- One and a half tablespoons of chopped fresh oregano

- One and a half tablespoons of chopped fresh basil

- Three tablespoons of trans fat–free canola/olive oil spread

- Six ounces of reduced-fat shredded cheddar cheese

- Six sundried tomato slices

Instructions

- In a heavy saucepan, bring water to a boil and add salt. Gradually whisk in cornmeal. Reduce heat to low and cook cornmeal mixture until it thickens, often stirring for about 15 minutes.

- Remove from heat, add oregano, basil, and canola/olive oil spread, and stir until melted into the mixture.

- Transfer to a lightly oiled 7-inch baking dish, spreading out evenly to about 3/4-inch thickness. Refrigerate until cold and firm, at least 2–3 hours.

- When firm, invert polenta onto a clean surface and cut into 2x2-inch pieces. Heat grill to medium heat. Oil both sides of polenta with olive oil and sear each side until golden brown

- (about 3 minutes).

- Remove from heat, and while hot, sprinkle with cheddar cheese and top with a sundried tomato slice. Serve immediately.

Homestyle Refried Beans

Preparation time-5 minutes | Cook time-15 minutes | Serving-2 | Difficulty- Easy

Nutritional value: ~ Calories-292 | Fat-8g | Protein-14g | Carbohydrates-42g

Ingredients

- One tablespoon of extra-virgin olive oil

- A quarter onion, diced

- One garlic clove, minced

- Half teaspoon of ground cumin

- A quarter teaspoon of chili powder

- One (15-ounce) can of pinto beans, drained and rinsed

- Half cup of chicken broth

Instructions

- In a small skillet over medium heat, heat the oil. Add the onion, garlic, cumin, chili powder, and sauté until the onion is soft, about 3 minutes.

- Add the beans and broth, and bring to a simmer.

- Mash the beans with a potato masher.

Continue to simmer until well mashed, leaving some chunks if desired, and serve.

Hummus and Olive Pita Bread

Preparation time-10 minutes |Cook time-0 minutes |Servings-2 |Difficulty-Easy

Nutritional value: ~Calories-225 |Proteins-9g| Fat-6g |Carbohydrates-39g

Ingredients

- Seven pita bread cut into six wedges each
- One (7 ounces) container of plain hummus
- One tablespoon of Greek vinaigrette
- Half cup of Chopped pitted Kalamata olives

Instructions

- Spread the hummus on a serving plate—Mix vinaigrette and olives in a bowl and spoon over the hummus.
- Enjoy with wedges of pita bread.

Jalapeno Balls

Preparation time-10 minutes |Cook time-30 minutes |Servings-3 |Difficulty-Easy

Nutritional value: ~Calories-249 |Proteins-7g| Fat-9g |Carbohydrates-38g

Ingredients

- Three slices of bacon
- Three ounces of cream cheese
- A quarter teaspoon of onion powder
- Salt and black pepper as per taste
- One chopped jalapeno pepper
- Half teaspoons of dried parsley
- A quarter teaspoon of garlic powder

Instructions

- Over medium-high heat, heat a skillet, add bacon, cook until crispy, switch to paper towels, remove the fat and crumble.
- Reserve the pan's bacon fat.
- Combine the jalapeno pepper, cream cheese, garlic powder and onion, parsley, pepper and salt in a bowl and stir thoroughly.
- Use this blend to mix bacon crumbles and bacon fat, stir softly, form balls, and serve.

Kale with orange-mustard dressing

Preparation time-10 minutes |Cook time-10 minutes |Servings-2 to 4 |Difficulty-Easy

Nutritional value: ~Calories-157 |Proteins-4g| Fat-12g |Carbohydrates-13g

Ingredients

- One tablespoon of olive oil
- Two bunches of fresh kale stems removed, leaves cut to bite-sized pieces
- Two radishes, sliced thin
- One avocado, deseeded, peeled, and chopped

For Dressing

- Two large oranges, peeled, pith removed, and segments separated
- Two tablespoons of grainy mustard
- A quarter cup of extra-virgin olive oil
- One teaspoon of chopped fresh thyme leaves
- Salt and freshly ground pepper to taste

Instructions

- In a large skillet, heat olive oil over medium heat. Add kale, a handful at a time, and sauté, frequently stirring until wilted.
- Transfer to serving bowl, add radishes, avocado, remaining orange segments from dressing, and dressing. Toss to coat kale mixture, divide into equal portions, and serve warm.

Dressing

- In a small bowl, squeeze enough orange segment membranes to make Three tablespoons of juice. Set remaining segments aside.
- Whisk mustard and olive oil into the juice until combined. Add thyme salt and pepper to taste. Set dressing aside.

Lemon garlic asparagus

Preparation time-10 minutes | Cook time-10 minutes | Servings-2 | Difficulty-Easy

Nutritional value: ~Calories-134 | Proteins-8g | Fat-11g | Carbohydrates-3g

Ingredients

- Three tablespoons of extra-virgin olive oil
- Two pounds fresh asparagus, cleaned, with ends trimmed
- One clove of fresh garlic, crushed
- Salt and freshly ground pepper to taste
- Two tablespoons of sweet orange juice
- 3/4 teaspoon of grated lemon peel
- One cup of shredded fresh Parmesan cheese

Instructions

- In a large non-stick skillet, heat olive oil over medium heat. Add asparagus, garlic, salt and pepper; turn several times to coat asparagus with olive oil.
- Cover skillet and cook for 6–7 minutes or until asparagus is tender and lightly browned. Remove from heat.
- Sprinkle with orange juice and lemon peel. Transfer to serving platter and top with Parmesan cheese.

Low sodium herbed grilled corn

Preparation time-5 minutes | Cook time-20 minutes | Servings-2 to 3 | Difficulty-Easy

Nutritional value: ~Calories-182 | Proteins-3g | Fat-12.6g | Carbohydrates-18g

Ingredients

- Half cup of Unsalted butter
- Two tablespoons of chopped parsley
- Two tablespoons of chopped chives
- One teaspoon of dried thyme
- Half teaspoon of Cayenne pepper
- Eight Sweet corn
- Two limes

Instructions

- Take a small bowl. Beat 1 st five ingredients till they are fully blended. Spread one tablespoon mixture on each ear of corn.
- Wrap the corn individually into the heavy foil.
- Grill the corn and cover it properly. Heat it for 15 minutes on moderate heat till it is tendered. Open the foil carefully to allow the steam to escape.

Maple and Pecan Bars

Preparation time-10 minutes | Cook time-30 minutes | Servings-12 | Difficulty-Moderate

Nutritional value: ~Calories-157 | Proteins-4g | Fat-12g | Carbohydrates-13g

Ingredients

- Half cups of flaxseed meal
- Two cups of pecans, toasted and crushed
- One cup of almond flour
- Half cups of coconut oil
- A quarter teaspoon of stevia
- Half cups of coconut, shredded
- A quarter cup of maple syrup

For the maple syrup

- A quarter cup of erythritol
- Two and a quarter teaspoons of coconut oil
- One tablespoon of ghee
- A quarter teaspoon of xanthan gum
- 3/4 cups of water

Two teaspoons of maple extract

- Half teaspoons of vanilla extract

Instructions

- Combine ghee with two and a quarter teaspoons of xanthan gum and coconut oil in a heat-proof bowl, stir, put in your oven and heat up for 1 minute.

- Add the extract of erythritol, water, maple and vanilla, mix well and fire for 1 minute more in the microwave.

- Mix the flaxseed meal and the coconut and almond flour in a bowl and stir.

- Add the pecans, and stir them again.

- Apply a quarter of a cup of maple syrup, stevia, and half a cup of coconut oil, and mix well.

- Spread this in a baking dish, push well, position it at 350 degrees F in the oven and cook for 25 minutes.

- To cool off, leave it aside, break into 12 bars and act as a keto snack.

Marinated Feta and Artichokes

Preparation time-10 minutes | Cook time-10 minutes | Servings-2 | Difficulty-Easy

Nutritional value: ~Calories-235 | Proteins-4g | Fat-23g | Carbohydrates-4g

Ingredients

- Four ounces of drained artichoke hearts quartered lengthwise

- Zest and juice of one lemon

- Four ounces of traditional Greek feta, cut into half-inch cubes

- 1/3 cup of extra-virgin olive oil

- Two tablespoons of fresh rosemary (roughly chopped)

- Half teaspoon of black peppercorns

- Two tablespoons of fresh parsley(roughly chopped)

Instructions

- Combine the feta and artichoke hearts in a glass bowl. Toss gently to coat with the lemon zest, olive oil, juice, parsley, rosemary, and peppercorns, being careful not to break the feta.

- Allow for 4 hours of cooling time or up to 4 days. Remove 30 minutes before serving from the refrigerator.

Mashed Cauliflower

Preparation time-10 minutes | Cook time-5 minutes | Servings-3 cups | Difficulty-Easy

Nutritional value- Calories-64 | Fat-2g | Carbohydrates-8g | Protein-3g

Ingredients

- ⅓ cup of low-fat buttermilk

- One tablespoon of extra-virgin olive oil

- One tablespoon of minced garlic

- A quarter cup of water

- One large head cauliflower

Instructions

- Breakaway the cauliflower into small florets. Put it in a bowl with the water and microwave it until the cauliflower softens. Discard the liquid.

- Over medium speed, blend the garlic, cauliflower, buttermilk, and olive oil in a blender until everything's creamy.

- Serve right away.

Mashed parsnips and carrots

Preparation time-10 minutes | Cook time-15 minutes | Servings-2 to 4 | Difficulty-Easy

Nutritional value: ~Calories-191 | Proteins-4g | Fat-0g | Carbohydrates-13g

Ingredients

- Two pounds parsnips, cleaned, peeled, and chopped

- One pound of carrots, cleaned, peeled, and chopped

- Three cloves fresh garlic, chopped

- One medium onion, chopped

- Salt and freshly ground pepper to taste

Instructions

- In a pot, add all vegetables and cover them with water. Bring to a boil, reduce heat to medium-high, and cook until carrots are soft.

- Drain off liquid and transfer vegetable mixture to a food processor and process until smooth.

- Remove from the processor with a rubber spatula and serve hot or warm, seasoned with salt and pepper to taste.

Mexican Cheese Cubes

Preparation time- 5 minutes| Cook time- 0 minutes|Servings-2 |Difficulty-Easy

Nutritional value- Calories-170| Fat-12g |Carbohydrates-4g| Protein-15g

Ingredients

- A quarter teaspoon of cumin powder
- A quarter teaspoon of onion powder
- A quarter teaspoon of garlic powder
- A quarter teaspoon of chili powder
- Half cup of small cubes reduced-fat Monterey Jack cheese

Instructions

- In a small bowl, add and mix all the ingredients. Refrigerate until you serve.

Mini Caprese Bites

Preparation time-20 minutes| Cook time-0 minutes|Servings-10-12 |Difficulty-Easy

Nutritional value- Calories-264| Fat-20g |Carbohydrates-2.1g| Protein-18.9g

Ingredients

- One pint of halved grape tomatoes
- Ten to twelve small mozzarella cheese balls
- Thirty-two (4 inches) wooden skewers
- A quarter cup of extra virgin olive oil
- Two tablespoons of balsamic vinegar
- A quarter teaspoon of kosher salt
- A quarter teaspoon of pepper
- Six (thinly sliced) fresh basil leaves
- Kosher salt and pepper

Instructions

- Mix half a tomato halve, 1 slice of cheese and one more tomato halve in each slice and put the skewers in a shallow serving dish.
- Shake the oil and the 3 ingredients that follow. Sprinkle with salt and pepper and basil. Rain oil mixture on skewers.
- It is possible to replace a package of fresh mozzarella sliced into 1 (8- oz.) 1/2-inch cubes.

Mini pitas

Preparation time-10 minutes |Cook time-20 minutes |Servings-2 |Difficulty-Easy

Nutritional value: ~Calories-123|Proteins-5g| Fat-3g|Carbohydrates-12g

Ingredients

For plain pita

- One large egg
- One tablespoon of extra-virgin olive oil
- A quarter teaspoon of apple cider vinegar
- One tablespoon of coconut flour
- A quarter cup plus Two tablespoons of blanched almond flour
- Two tablespoons of ground golden flax seeds
- Half teaspoon of baking soda
- A quarter teaspoon fine sea salt
- One teaspoon of garlic powder
- A quarter teaspoon of ground black pepper

For garlic & herb pita

- (add to plain pita recipe)
- One teaspoon of garlic powder
- One tablespoon of chopped fresh cilantro

For chili & paprika pita

- (add to plain pita recipe)
- One teaspoon of paprika
- A quarter teaspoon of chili powder

For a cashew version

- Use cashew meal instead of almond flour and increase the water to half a cup.

Instructions

- Preheat the oven to 350°F. Line a baking sheet with parchment paper.
- Whisk the egg, olive oil, vinegar, and A quarter cup of water in a small bowl.
- In another bowl, combine the coconut flour, almond flour, flax, baking soda, salt, spices and/or herbs. Pour the egg mixture into the dry mixture and stir to combine.
- Scoop a spoonful of the batter onto the parchment and spread it into a 3-inch circle that's about 1/2 inch thick. Repeat until all the batter is used.
- Bake the pitas for 15 to 18 minutes, until firm to the touch. Cool on the baking sheet for 5 minutes, then serve and enjoy.

Nachos

Preparation time-10 minutes |Cook time-10 minutes |Servings-2 |Difficulty-Easy

Nutritional value: ~Calories-140|Proteins-3g| Fat-7g|Carbohydrates-19g

Ingredients

- Four ounces of restaurant-style corn tortilla chips

- One medium green onion, thinly sliced (about one tablespoon)

- One (4 ounces) package of finely crumbled feta cheese

- One finely chopped and drained plum tomato

- Two tablespoons of Sun-dried tomatoes in oil, finely chopped

- Two tablespoons of Kalamata olives

Instructions

- Mix an onion, plum tomato, oil, sun-dried tomatoes, and olives in a small bowl.

- Arrange the tortillas chips on a microwavable plate in a single layer topped evenly with cheese—microwave on high for one minute.

- Rotate the plate half turn and continue microwaving until the cheese is bubbly. Spread the tomato mixture over the chips and cheese and enjoy.

Naturally Nutty & Buttery Banana Bowl

Preparation time-5 minutes |Cook time-0 minutes |Servings-2 |Difficulty-Easy

Nutritional value: ~Calories-370|Proteins-23g| Fat-11g|Carbohydrates-48g

Ingredients

- Two cups of vanilla Greek yogurt

- Two medium-sized bananas, sliced

- A quarter cup of creamy and natural peanut butter

- One teaspoon of ground nutmeg

- A quarter cup of flaxseed meal

Instructions

- Divide the yogurt equally between two big serving bowls. Top each yogurt bowl with the banana slices.

- Put the peanut butter inside a microwave-safe bowl. Melt the peanut butter in your microwave for 40 seconds. Drizzle one tablespoon of the melted peanut butter over the bananas for each bowl.

- To serve, sprinkle over with the ground nutmeg and flax-seed meal.

Oven-roasted potato wedges

Preparation time-10 minutes |Cook time-30 minutes |Servings-2 |Difficulty-Easy

Nutritional value: ~Calories-170|Proteins-4g| Fat-7g|Carbohydrates-24g

Ingredients

- One and a half pounds russet potatoes, scrubbed and cut lengthwise into wedges

- A quarter cup of olive oil

- Half teaspoon of smoky paprika

- A quarter teaspoon of garlic salt or to taste

- Cayenne pepper to taste

- Freshly ground pepper to taste

Instructions

- Preheat oven to 450 degrees F. Combine potato wedges, olive oil, paprika, garlic salt, cayenne, and pepper in a large, resealable plastic baggie.

- Toss well to coat all sides of potatoes with olive oil and seasonings. Remove from bag, place wedges in a single layer on a foil-lined baking sheet, and bake, turning once after 10–15 minutes, until edges are golden and crispy (about 25–30 minutes).

Parmesan Popcorn Delight

Preparation time-5 minutes| Cook time-5 minutes|Servings-2 |Difficulty-Easy

Nutritional value- Calories-80| Fat-3g |Carbohydrates-12g| Protein-3g

Ingredients

- 1/8 teaspoon of black pepper

- Two teaspoons of grated parmesan cheese

- Two cups of popped light-butter microwave popcorn

Instructions

- Pop the popcorn according to directions. Once ready, fill Two cups, add some parmesan cheese and pepper and mix well.

Peanut Butter Honey over Rice Cakes

Preparation time-5 minutes| Cook time-0 minutes|Servings-2 |Difficulty-Easy

Nutritional value- Calories-180| Fat-9g |Carbohydrates-21g| Protein-5g

Ingredients

- One tablespoon of natural creamy peanut butter
- Half teaspoon of honey
- A quarter teaspoon of vanilla extract
- Two brown rice cakes

Instructions

- Take a small bowl and mix honey, peanut butter, and vanilla extract. Now spread it over the rice cakes and enjoy.

Pears and Gorgonzola

Preparation time-5 minutes | Cook time-0 minutes | Servings-2 | Difficulty-Easy

Nutritional value- Calories-110 | Fat-2g | Carbohydrates-24g | Protein-2g

Ingredients

- One small pear, peeled
- 1/8 teaspoon of black pepper
- One teaspoon of fat-free cream cheese softened
- Two teaspoons of Gorgonzola crumbles

Instructions

- Mix gorgonzola, pepper, and cream cheese in a small bowl. Serve alongside pear slices.

Pepper Nachos

Preparation time-10 minutes | Cook time-30 minutes | Servings-6 | Difficulty-Easy

Nutritional value- Calories-164 | Fat-8g | Carbohydrates-12g | Protein-3g

Ingredients

- One pound of halved mini bell peppers
- Salt and black pepper as per the taste
- One teaspoon of garlic powder
- One teaspoon of sweet paprika
- Half teaspoons of dried oregano
- A quarter teaspoon of red pepper flakes
- One pound of ground beef meat
- One and a half cups of shredded cheddar cheese
- One tablespoon of chili powder
- One teaspoon of ground cumin
- Half cups of chopped tomato
- Sour cream for serving

Instructions

- Mix the chili powder, pepper, salt, paprika, oregano, cumin, flakes of pepper and garlic powder in a bowl and stir.
- Over medium heat, heat a pan, add beef, mix and brown for 10 minutes.
- Add the mixture of chili powder, stir and take the heat off.
- On a lined baking sheet, arrange the pepper halves, stuff them with the beef mix, sprinkle the cheese, place in the oven at 400 degrees F and cook for 10 minutes.
- Remove the peppers from the oven, sprinkle with the tomatoes, divide among the plates and serve with sour cream.

Pepper Tapenade

Preparation time-10 minutes | Cook time-0 minutes | Servings-2 | Difficulty-Easy

Nutritional value: ~Calories-200 | Proteins-5g | Fat-6g | Carbohydrates-14g

Ingredients

- Seven ounces of roasted red peppers, chopped
- Half cup of parmesan, grated
- 1/3 cup of parsley, chopped
- Fourteen ounces of canned artichokes, drained and chopped
- Three tablespoons olive oil
- A quarter cup of capers, drained
- One and a half tablespoons of lemon juice
- Two garlic cloves, minced

Instructions

- In your blender, combine the red peppers with the Parmesan and the rest of the ingredients and pulse well. Divide into cups and serve as a snack.

Pesto and garlic shrimp bruschetta

Preparation time-10 minutes | Cook time-15 minutes | Servings-2 | Difficulty-Easy

Nutritional value: ~Calories-168 | Proteins-5g | Fat-7g | Carbohydrates-19g

Ingredients

- Eight ounces of shrimp
- Black pepper to taste
- Two tablespoons of butter
- Four tablespoons of olive oil
- Twenty basil leaves
- One bread
- Four minced garlic cloves

- Three ounces of pesto
- Two ounces of capers
- Three ounces of sun-dried tomatoes
- One ounce of feta cheese
- Kosher salt to taste
- Balsamic glaze for garnishing

Instructions

- Sprinkle salt and pepper over shrimps in a bowl. Set aside for ten minutes.
- Add olive oil and butter of about two tablespoons of each in the pan and cook for 2 minutes over medium flame.
- Stir in garlic and sauté for one more minute.
- Mix shrimps and cook for four minutes.
- Remove from flame and let it set.
- Slice the bread and place in a baking tray, drizzle oil, and toast in the oven for five minutes.
- Spread pesto sauce over each bread slice followed by sun-dried tomatoes, shrimp, caper, cheese, basil, and balsamic glaze and serve.

Pesto Crackers

Preparation time-10 minutes| Cook time-17 minutes|Servings-6 |Difficulty-Easy

Nutritional value- Calories-124| Fat-7g |Carbohydrates-8g| Protein-6g

Ingredients

- Half teaspoons of baking powder
- Salt and black pepper to the taste
- One and a quarter cups of almond flour
- A quarter teaspoon of basil, dried
- One minced garlic clove
- Two tablespoons of basil pesto
- A pinch of cayenne pepper
- Three tablespoons of ghee

Instructions

- Mix the pepper, salt, almond flour and baking powder together in a bowl.
- Stir in the garlic, basil and cayenne.
- Add whisk the pesto.
- Also, add ghee and with your finger, mix your dough.
- Spread this dough on a baking sheet and bake it at 325 degrees F in the oven for 17 minutes.

- Leave your crackers aside to cool down, cut them and serve.

Pickle Roll-Ups

Preparation time-20 minutes| Cook time- 20 minutes|Servings-20 |Difficulty-Easy

Nutritional value- Calories-86| Fat-7g |Carbohydrates-4g| Protein-4g

Ingredients

- A quarter-pound of deli ham (nitrate-free), thinly sliced (about 8 slices)
- Eight ounces of Neufchâtel cheese, at room temperature
- One teaspoon of dried dill
- One teaspoon of onion powder
- Eight whole kosher dill pickle spears

Instructions

- Put the ham on the cutting board and spread some Neufchâtel cheese on.
- Season with onion powder and dill.
- Put one pickle on each slice and gently roll.

Now make ½ to 1-inch rolls.

Place a toothpick in the middle and serve.

Pistachio-Stuffed Dates

Preparation time-10 minutes |Cook time-0 minutes |Servings-2 |Difficulty-Easy

Nutritional value: ~Calories-220|Proteins-4g| Fat-7g|Carbohydrates-41g

Ingredients

- Half cup of unsalted pistachios shelled
- A quarter teaspoon of kosher salt
- Eight Medjool dates pitted

Instructions

- In a food processor, add the salt and pistachios. Process until combined with chunky nut butter, 3 to 5 minutes.
- Split open the dates and spoon the pistachio nut butter into each half.

Pork Ginger Kebabs

Preparation time-10 minutes| Cook time-20 minutes|Servings-10-12 |Difficulty-Easy

Nutritional value- Calories-60| Fat-2g |Carbohydrates-4g| Protein-8g

Ingredients

- One pound of pork tenderloin, cut into twenty-four ½-inch cubes

- Twelve cherry tomatoes

- Twelve 1-inch cubes of fresh peeled and cored pineapple

- One teaspoon of freshly grated ginger

- One tablespoon of canola oil

- Two tablespoons of fresh lemon juice

- Half teaspoon of salt

- Half teaspoon of garlic powder

- Half teaspoon of paprika

- Twelve 6-inch wooden skewers soaked in water

Instructions

- Mix all the ingredients into a medium bowl (except for skewers) and marinate for 30 minutes.

- Preheat your oven to 350 degrees F. Take each skewer and place a piece of pork, one cherry tomato, another piece of pork, and lastly, a pineapple chunk.

- Then, on a dry cookie sheet, arrange the ready skewers and bake until the pork is cooked thoroughly. Serve right away.

Pumpkin Muffins

Preparation time-20 minutes| Cook time-20 minutes|Servings-18 |Difficulty-Moderate

Nutritional value- Calories-181| Fat-6g |Carbohydrates-13g| Protein-3g

Ingredients

- A quarter cup of sunflower seed butter

- 3/4 cups of pumpkin puree

- Two tablespoons of flaxseed meal

- A quarter cup of coconut flour

- Half cup of erythritol

- Half teaspoons of ground nutmeg

- One teaspoon of ground cinnamon

- Half teaspoons of baking soda

- One egg

- Half teaspoons of baking powder

A pinch of salt

Instructions

- Mix the butter with the pumpkin puree and egg in a bowl and mix well.

- Stir well and add coconut flour, flaxseed meal, erythritol, baking powder, baking soda, nutmeg, cinnamon and a pinch of salt.

- Spoon this into an oiled muffin pan, add in the oven at 350 degrees F and cook for 15 minutes.

- Let the muffins cool and serve them as a snack.

Red Pepper Hummus

Preparation time-10 minutes |Cook time-0 minutes |Servings-2 |Difficulty-Easy

Nutritional value: ~Calories-255|Proteins-7g| Fat-8g|Carbohydrates-18g

Ingredients

- Four ounces of roasted red peppers, peeled and chopped

- Sixteen ounces of canned chickpeas, drained and rinsed

- A quarter cup of Greek yogurt

- Three tablespoons tahini paste

- Juice of one lemon

- Three garlic cloves, minced

- One tablespoon of olive oil A pinch of salt and black pepper

- One tablespoon of parsley, chopped

Instructions

- In your food processor, combine the red peppers with the rest of the ingredients. Do not include the oil and the parsley and pulse well.

- Add the oil, pulse again, divide into cups, sprinkle the parsley on top, and serve as a party spread.

Roast Asparagus

Preparation time-15 minutes |Cook time-5 minutes |Servings-2 |Difficulty-Easy

Nutritional value: ~Calories-123|Proteins-3g| Fat-11g|Carbohydrates-5g

Ingredients

- One tablespoon of Extra virgin olive oil

- One medium lemon

- Half teaspoon of freshly grated nutmeg

- Half teaspoon of black pepper

- Half teaspoon of Kosher salt

Instructions

- Warm the oven to 500°F. Put the asparagus on an aluminum foil drizzle with extra virgin olive oil, and toss until well coated.

- Roast the asparagus in the oven for about five minutes; toss and continue roasting until browned. Sprinkle the roasted asparagus with nutmeg, salt, zest, and pepper.

Roasted broccoli

Preparation time-10 minutes |Cook time-25 minutes |Servings-2 |Difficulty-Easy

Nutritional value: ~Calories-154 | Proteins-1g | Fat-12g | Carbohydrates-9g

Ingredients

- One and a quarter pounds of fresh broccoli florets
- Three and a half tablespoons of olive oil, divided
- Four cloves of fresh garlic, minced
- A quarter teaspoon of crushed red hot pepper flakes
- Salt and freshly ground pepper to taste
- Grated Parmesan cheese to sprinkle (optional)

Instructions

- Preheat oven to 450 degrees F. Combine broccoli and Three tablespoons of olive oil in a resealable plastic baggie and toss to coat the broccoli. Transfer broccoli to a baking sheet and roast for 15 minutes. Remove from oven and set aside.
- Combine remaining olive oil, garlic, and hot pepper flakes in a small bowl and drizzle mixture over broccoli, tossing to coat. Return broccoli to oven and roast until florets begin to brown, about 6–8 minutes.
- Season with salt and pepper and serve immediately with a sprinkling of Parmesan cheese, if desired.

Roasted Garden Vegetables

Preparation time-5 minutes | Cook time-30 minutes | Serving-6 | Difficulty- Easy

Nutritional value: Calories-75 | Fat-5g | Protein-0g | Carbohydrates-8g

Ingredients

- One medium bell pepper, cut into strips
- One small onion halved then sliced
- One small zucchini, sliced into rounds
- One pint of grape tomatoes
- Two tablespoons of extra-virgin olive oil
- Salt
- Freshly ground black pepper

Instructions

- Preheat the oven to 400°F.
- Using 1 or 2 large baking sheets, arrange the vegetables, so they are lying flat, lightly touching each other.
- Evenly pour the olive oil over the vegetables, and gently toss to coat, using either a spoon or your hands. Add salt and pepper to taste.
- Roast for 20 to 30 minutes, or until soft and lightly charred, stirring halfway through, and serve.

Roasted Parmesan Broccoli

Preparation time-10 minutes | Cook time-10 minutes | Servings-2 | Difficulty-Easy

Nutritional value: ~Calories-154 | Proteins-9g | Fat-3g | Carbohydrates-11g

Ingredients

- Two heads broccoli, cut into small florets
- Two tablespoons of extra-virgin olive oil
- Two teaspoons of minced garlic
- Zest of one lemon
- Juice of one lemon
- Pinch sea salt
- Half cup of grated Parmesan cheese

Instructions

- Preheat the oven to 400°F.
- Lightly grease a baking sheet using olive oil and set it aside.
- In a large bowl, toss the broccoli with two tablespoons of olive oil, garlic, lemon zest, lemon juice, and sea salt
- Spread the combination on the baking sheet in a single layer and sprinkle with the Parmesan cheese.
- Bake for about 10 minutes or until tender. Transfer the broccoli to a serving dish and serve.

Roasted peppers

Preparation time-10 minutes | Cook time-20 minutes | Servings-2 to 4 | Difficulty-Easy

Nutritional value: ~Calories-108 | Proteins-1g | Fat-10g | Carbohydrates-7g

Ingredients

- Four large red bell peppers
- Two cloves of fresh garlic, peeled and sliced
- Four tablespoons of extra-virgin olive oil
- Salt and freshly ground pepper to taste

Instructions

- Clean peppers and pat dry. Place peppers on a moderately hot grill or on a rack under a broiler 1–2 inches from heat, often turning until skin is charred and blistered.
- Charring of the entire skin takes about 15–20 minutes. Remove from grill or broiler and place peppers aside to cool. When cool enough to handle, rub off blackened skins. Cut each pepper in half, remove stalk and seeds, and cut into Half-inch strips.
- Place strips in a bowl and add garlic, olive oil, salt and pepper to taste.
- Toss and set aside for about 30 minutes before serving.

Roasted Root Vegetables

Preparation time-15 minutes| Cook time-45 minutes|Servings-6 |Difficulty-Easy

Nutritional value- Calories-68| Fat-3g |Carbohydrates-11g| Protein-1g

Ingredients

- Two teaspoons of dried thyme
- Four teaspoons of minced garlic
- Two tablespoons of extra-virgin olive oil
- One medium red onion
- One medium butternut squash, peeled and seeded
- Two large carrots, peeled
- Two large parsnips, peeled
- Two medium red beets, peeled
- Nonstick cooking spray

Instructions

- Preheat the oven to 425°F. Coat a baking sheet with some nonstick cooking spray.
- Gently cut the carrots, parsnips, butternut squash, and beets into 1-inch chunks. Now slice the onion into 4 pieces.
- On the baking sheet, place the veggies evenly. Now sprinkle them with thyme garlic and drizzle some olive oil. Toss the veggies thoroughly to coat them with seasonings and oil.
- Now, roast them for 45 minutes or until they become tender. Keep moving the veggies every 15 minutes in the middle.
- Serve warm.

Roasted Rosemary Olives

Preparation time-10 minutes |Cook time-25 minutes |Servings-2 |Difficulty-Easy

Nutritional value: ~Calories-101|Proteins-0g| Fat-9g|Carbohydrates-4g

Ingredients

- One cup of mixed variety olives pitted and rinsed
- Two tablespoons of lemon juice
- One tablespoon of extra-virgin olive oil
- Six garlic cloves, peeled
- Four rosemary sprigs

Instructions

- Preheat the oven to 400°F.
- Combine the olive oil, olives, lemon juice, and garlic in a medium bowl and mix.
- Spread in a single layer on the prepared baking sheet. Sprinkle on the rosemary—roast for 25 minutes, tossing halfway through.
- Take away the rosemary leaves from the stem and place them in a serving bowl. Add the olives and mix before serving.

Roasted tomatoes with thyme and feta

Preparation time-5 minutes |Cook time-20 minutes |Servings-2 |Difficulty-Easy

Nutritional value: ~Calories-195|Proteins-2g| Fat-7.3g|Carbohydrates-4g

Ingredients

- Half teaspoon of dried thyme
- Sixteen ounces of cherry tomatoes
- Black pepper to taste
- Three tablespoons of olive oil
- Salt to taste
- Six tablespoons of feta cheese

Instructions

- In a baking tray, put tomatoes.
- Pour olive oil and drizzle pepper, thyme leaves, and salt over tomatoes and mix well.
- Bake in a preheated oven at 450 degrees F for 15 minutes.
- Drizzle cheese and broil for five minutes and serve when the cheese melts.

Saffron rice

Preparation time-10 minutes |Cook time-25 minutes |Servings-2 |Difficulty-Easy

Nutritional value: ~Calories-282 | Proteins-5g | Fat-2g | Carbohydrates-49g

Ingredients

- Four cups of canned low-sodium, fat-free vegetable broth

- One tablespoon of extra-virgin olive oil

- Four tablespoons of chopped shallots

- Two cloves fresh garlic, minced

- One cup of short-grain rice

- One cup of dry white wine

- A quarter teaspoon of crushed saffron threads

- Half teaspoon of dried thyme

- Salt and freshly ground pepper to taste

- Instructions

- Bring broth to a boil, then reduce heat to a low simmer. In a large skillet, heat olive oil, add shallots and garlic and sauté until soft (about 5 minutes). Add rice and continue to sauté, constantly stirring to keep the mixture from burning.

- Add wine, saffron, and thyme, constantly stirring, scraping in any brown bits from the pan. When wine is absorbed, slowly add simmering broth, constantly stirring as the broth is absorbed and rice has become tender (about 15–20 minutes).

- It's possible some of the broth will be leftover. Add salt and pepper to taste.

Salmon fish sticks

Preparation time-10 minutes | Cook time-20 minutes | Servings-2 | Difficulty-Easy

Nutritional value: ~Calories-102 | Proteins-15g | Fat-6g | Carbohydrates-5g

Ingredients

Fish Sticks

- Two lb of salmon fillet

- A quarter teaspoon of salt

- A quarter teaspoon of black pepper

First coating

- Half teaspoon of garlic powder

- Half teaspoon of dried thyme

- One cup of almond meal

- Half teaspoon of sea salt

- A quarter teaspoon of black pepper

Second coating

- Half teaspoon of salt

- 2/3 cup of chickpea flour

Third coating

- Two eggs

Dipping Sauce

- A quarter teaspoon of salt

- A quarter cup of Greek yogurt

- One teaspoon of lemon juice

- One tablespoon of Dijon mustard

- Half teaspoon of dill

- 1/8 teaspoon of garlic powder

Instructions

- Whisk all the ingredients for the dipping sauce list in a bowl and set aside. The dipping sauce is ready.

- Mix garlic, thyme, and almond meal in a bowl. The first coating is ready.

- Add chickpea flour to another bowl. The second coating is ready.

- Beat the eggs in another bowl. Set aside.

- Sprinkle pepper and salt over sliced fish with removed skin. 6. First, coat the fish with chickpea flour, followed by coating with egg and almond meal coating.

- Align coated fish pieces in a baking sheet covered with parchment paper.

- Bake in a preheated oven at 400 degrees F for 18 minutes.

- Serve baked fish with dipping sauce and serve.

Sautéed garlic spinach

Preparation time-10 minutes | Cook time-10 minutes | Servings-2 | Difficulty-Easy

Nutritional value: ~Calories-56 | Proteins-5g | Fat-1g | Carbohydrates-7g

Ingredients

- One and a half cups of canned low-sodium, fat-free chicken broth
- Six cloves of fresh garlic, chopped
- Three (10-ounce) bags of fresh spinach leaves
- Freshly ground pepper to taste
- Salt to taste

Instructions

- In a heavy-bottomed skillet over medium heat, add chicken broth and garlic. Add handfuls of spinach while stirring, moving wilted leaves to one side until all of the spinach has been added and wilted.
- Reduce heat to low, add pepper, and occasionally stir to blend garlic and spinach until broth has evaporated.
- Add salt to taste. Serve while hot.

Sautéed kale

Preparation time-10 minutes | Cook time-15 minutes | Servings-2 | Difficulty-Easy

Nutritional value: ~Calories-53 | Proteins-4g | Fat-1g | Carbohydrates-8g

Ingredients

- One teaspoon of olive oil
- One medium shallot, finely chopped
- One clove of fresh garlic, minced
- Half cup of canned low-sodium, fat-free chicken broth
- One teaspoon of finely shredded lemon peel
- One (12-ounce) package of fresh kale
- Salt and freshly ground pepper to taste
- Lemon wedges for garnish

Instructions

- In a heavy skillet, heat olive oil over medium heat, add shallots and garlic and sauté until soft.
- Add chicken broth, lemon peel, and handfuls of kale at a time, constantly stirring until leaves wilt. When kale is wilted, add salt and pepper to taste and serve with lemon wedges.

Sautéed kale and spinach with mushrooms and tomato

Preparation time-10 minutes | Cook time-15 minutes | Servings-2 | Difficulty-Easy

Nutritional value: ~Calories-151 | Proteins-11g | Fat-15g | Carbohydrates-27g

Ingredients

- Four tablespoons of olive oil, divided
- Four tablespoons of chopped fresh garlic
- Three bunches of fresh kale leaves only
- Crushed red hot pepper flakes to taste
- One (9-ounce) bag of fresh baby spinach
- A quarter cup of water, if needed
- Salt and freshly ground pepper to taste
- Half large white onion, chopped
- Two (8-ounce) containers of fresh white button mushrooms, halved
- Fifteen grape tomatoes
- Two tablespoons of fresh garlic paste blend

Instructions

- In a large skillet over medium-high heat, add Two tablespoons of olive oil and garlic and sauté until soft and fragrant. Add kale, a handful at a time, and hot pepper flakes, and cook, often stirring, until kale is wilted.
- Add baby spinach and continue to cook until wilted. Add water, if needed, to keep moist. Season with salt and pepper to taste. Reduce heat to very low and keep warm.
- In a separate skillet over medium heat, add the remaining two tablespoons of olive oil. Add onion, mushrooms, grape tomatoes, and garlic paste. Cook, often stirring, until mushrooms are soft and tomatoes begin to break down.
- Add salt and pepper to taste. Combine tomato mixture with spinach mixture and return heat to a simmer, stirring to incorporate ingredients and flavors, about 2 minutes, and serve.

Sautéed portobellos with garlic and parsley

Preparation time-10 minutes | Cook time-10 minutes | Servings-2 | Difficulty-Easy

Nutritional value: ~Calories-82 | Proteins-3g | Fat-8g | Carbohydrates-5g

Ingredients

- Two tablespoons of extra-virgin olive oil
- Twelve ounces of portobello mushrooms, cut into chunks
- Salt and freshly ground pepper to taste
- Four cloves fresh garlic, finely minced
- One tablespoon of finely chopped fresh parsley

Instructions

- In a skillet, heat olive oil and sauté mushrooms over high heat for about 4 minutes. Add salt and pepper to taste.

- Sprinkle with garlic and parsley and serve hot.

Sour candy Grapes

Preparation time~5 minutes |Cook time~10 minutes |Servings~2 |Difficulty~Easy

Nutritional value: ~Calories~67 |Proteins~1g| Fat~0g| Carbohydrates~18g

Ingredients

- One box of Gelatin per three lb of grapes

- One cup of Water

- Lemon juice

Instructions

- Pour the gelatin into the small bowl.

- Poke the toothpick in through a spot where the stem was connected.

- With the help of a toothpick, dip it in the water & roll.

- Put this into the refrigerator until chilled properly.

- Once they are chilled, toothpicks can easily be removed.

- Serve and enjoy the food.

Southwest Deviled Eggs

Preparation time~10 minutes |Cook time~10 minutes |Serving~6 |Difficulty~ Easy

Nutritional value: ~Calories~83| Fat~5g| Protein~7g| Carbohydrates~1g

Ingredients

- Six large hard-boiled eggs

- Two tablespoons of low-fat, plain Greek yogurt

- A quarter teaspoon of spicy mustard

- ⅛ teaspoon of salt

- Half teaspoon of Taco Seasoning (store-bought or homemade)

Instructions

- Peel the eggs, and halve them lengthwise.

- Remove the yolks, and transfer them to a small bowl, setting the whites aside.

- Add the yogurt, spicy mustard, salt, and taco seasoning to the bowl with the yolks, and mash everything together.

- Spoon the mixture into the egg white halves, and serve.

Speedy Sweet Potato Chips

Preparation time~15 minutes |Cook time~One hour |Servings~2 |Difficulty~Hard

Nutritional value: ~Calories~150 |Proteins~2g| Fat~9g| Carbohydrates~17g

Ingredients

- One large sweet potato

- One tablespoon of extra virgin olive oil

- Salt

Instructions

- Preheat the oven at 300°F.

- Slice your potato into nice, thin slices that resemble fries.

- Toss the potato slices with salt and extra virgin olive oil in a bowl.

- Bake for about one hour, flipping every 15 minutes until crispy and browned.

Spiced Maple Nuts

Preparation time~5 minutes |Cook time~10 minutes |Servings~2 |Difficulty~Easy

Nutritional value: ~Calories~175 |Proteins~3g| Fat~18g| Carbohydrates~4g

Ingredients

- Two cups of raw walnuts or pecans

- One teaspoon of extra-virgin olive oil

- One teaspoon of ground sumac

- Half teaspoon of pure maple syrup

- A quarter teaspoon of kosher salt

- A quarter teaspoon of ground ginger

- Two to four rosemary sprigs

Instructions

- Preheat the oven to 350°F.

- In a bowl, combine the nuts, olive oil, sumac, maple syrup, salt, ginger mix. Spread in a sole layer on the prepared baking sheet. Add the rosemary. Roast for 8 to 10 minutes, or wait until golden and fragrant.

- Remove the rosemary leaves from the stems and place them in a serving bowl. Add the nuts and toss to combine before serving.

Spicy Almonds

Preparation time~5 minutes| Cook time~5 minutes| Servings~2 |Difficulty~Easy

Nutritional value- Calories~220 | Fat~19g | Carbohydrates~8g| Protein~7g

Ingredients

- 1/8 teaspoon of red pepper flakes
- 1/8 teaspoon of onion powder
- A dash of salt
- A quarter teaspoon of olive oil
- A quarter cup of whole raw almonds

Instructions

- Preheat your oven to 350 degrees F. Mix everything in a bowl.
- Put the almond mix on an unoiled baking sheet and roast for 5 minutes. Flip the almonds once. Cool them and serve.

Spicy julienned sweet potato fries

Preparation time-10 minutes |Cook time-30 minutes |Servings-2 |Difficulty-Easy

Nutritional value: ~Calories-55|Proteins-1g| Fat-2g|Carbohydrates-5g

Ingredients

- One pound of sweet potatoes, peeled and julienned
- One tablespoon of olive oil
- One tablespoon of light brown sugar
- One teaspoon of salt or to taste
- Half teaspoon of chili powder
- Pinch of cayenne pepper
- A quarter teaspoon of ground cinnamon

Instructions

- Preheat oven to 450 degrees. Line a large baking sheet with foil. In a large, resealable plastic baggie, combine potatoes, olive oil, brown sugar, salt,
- chili powder, cayenne, and cinnamon. Toss well to coat and remove from bag.
- Arrange potatoes in a single layer on a baking sheet and bake for roughly 15 minutes. Turn potatoes over and bake for additional 15 minutes or until crispy.

Spicy Roasted Chickpeas

Preparation time-5 minutes |Cook time-1 hour |Serving-8 to 10 |Difficulty- Hard

Nutritional value: Calories-144| Fat-4g| Protein-7g| Carbohydrates-22g

Ingredients

- Two (15-ounce) cans of organic garbanzo beans (rinsed and drained)
- One and a half tablespoons of chili powder
- One tablespoon of ground cumin

- Two teaspoons of ground cayenne powder
- Two teaspoons of garlic powder
- Two teaspoons of paprika
- One teaspoon of salt
- One tablespoon of extra-virgin olive oil

Instructions

- Preheat the oven to 300°F. Line a baking sheet with aluminum foil.
- In a large bowl, mix the beans, chili powder, cumin, cayenne, garlic powder, paprika, salt, and olive oil, coating the beans well.
- Spread evenly on a baking sheet.
- Bake for 30 minutes, and stir gently.
- Bake for another 20 to 30 minutes, until hard and crunchy, and serve.

Steamed artichokes

Preparation time-10 minutes |Cook time-30 minutes |Servings-2 |Difficulty-Easy

Nutritional value: ~Calories-76|Proteins-5g| Fat-0.5g|Carbohydrates-17g

Ingredients

- Four medium globe artichokes (about 10–11 ounces each)
- Four cups of canned low-sodium, fat-free chicken broth
- Ten cloves of fresh garlic
- Salt and freshly ground pepper to taste
- Extra-virgin olive oil or melted trans fat–free canola/olive oil spread to drizzle (optional)

Instructions

- Wash artichokes under running water. Remove the sharp tips of each leaf with poultry scissors, keeping the globe intact. Place artichokes, broth, and garlic in a large pot. Cover pot and bring to a boil.
- Reduce heat to medium, keep the pot covered, and continue to steam artichokes, turning over once while steaming. If necessary, add water to the pot to keep artichokes bathed in liquid while steaming.
- Steam until you can pierce the globe stem area of the artichoke with a fork without much resistance. Remove chokes with a slotted spoon to serving dishes, sprinkle with salt and pepper, and drizzle with olive oil or melted canola/olive oil spread, if desired. Serve while warm.
- To eat this delectable vegetable, simply pull off the leaves one by one and run the soft flesh of the leaf over your bottom front teeth, extracting the flesh from the inner part of the leaf.
- In the center of all the leaves is the best part; the heart of the choke connected to the stem is also very good.

The only part not considered edible by most people is the crown of fuzzy little leaves that sits directly on top of the heart.

- Simply remove these fuzzy little leaves with your fingers before eating the heart and stem.

Strawberries in Balsamic Yogurt Sauce

Preparation time-15 minutes | Cook time-0 minutes | Servings-2 | Difficulty-Easy

Nutritional value: ~Calories-51 | Proteins-3g | Fat-1g | Carbohydrates-9g

Ingredients

- One tablespoon of honey
- One tablespoon of balsamic vinegar
- One cup of sliced strawberries
- Half cup of yogurt

Instructions

- Mix all the ingredients in a bowl except strawberries.
- Put strawberries on top of each serving and refrigerate for 2-3 hours, then serve.

Stuffed Avocado

Preparation time-10 minutes | Cook time-0 minutes | Servings-2 | Difficulty-Easy

Nutritional value: ~Calories-233 | Proteins-6g | Fat-9g | Carbohydrates-12g

Ingredients

- One avocado halved and pitted
- Ten ounces of canned tuna, drained
- Two tablespoons of sun-dried tomatoes, chopped
- One and a half tablespoons of basil pesto
- Two tablespoons of black olives, pitted and chopped
- Salt and black pepper to the taste
- Two teaspoons of pine nuts, toasted and chopped
- One tablespoon of basil, chopped

Instructions

- Mix the tuna with the sun-dried tomatoes and the rest of the ingredients except the avocado and stir.
- Stuff the avocado halves with the tuna mix and serve as an appetizer.

Stuffed Cabbage Rolls

Preparation time-25 minutes | Cook time-45 minutes | Servings-6 | Difficulty-Easy

Nutritional value- Calories-174 | Fat-5g | Carbohydrates-16g | Protein-6g

Ingredients

- 1/3 cup of brown Minute Rice or other whole grain of choice
- One teaspoon of olive oil
- Two cups of tomato sauce
- One head of cabbage, individual leaves removed
- One pound of 93% lean ground turkey
- Two teaspoons of garlic powder
- Two medium carrots, diced
- Half medium onion, diced (if tolerated)
- Two teaspoons of Italian seasoning or oregano

Instructions

- Preheat the oven to 350 degrees Fahrenheit.
- Rinse & blanch the cabbage that needs to leave for 31 seconds to create them more manageable.
- Prepare rice according to the package directions.
- Meanwhile, heat olive oil in a large skillet over medium heat.
- Stir in the onions and carrots until they are slightly softened and caramelized.
- Cook the turkey in the skillet with the vegetables until browned.
- Add the seasonings and powders.
- Combine meat and rice in a mixing bowl.
- Fill the center of 1 cabbage leaf with 1Two cups of the mixture. Roll up, securing both ends along the way.
- Place cabbage rolls seam side down, side by side in baking dish to avoid them from unrolling.
- Drizzle the tomato sauce over the cabbage rolls, allowing it to drop to the bottom of the dish.
- Bake at 350°F for 35–45 minutes. Allow cooling 5–10 minutes before serving.

Stuffed Celery

Preparation time-15 minutes | Cook time-20 minutes | Servings-2 | Difficulty-Moderate

Nutritional value: ~Calories-64 | Proteins-1g | Fat-6g | Carbohydrates-9g

Ingredients

- Olive oil
- One clove garlic, minced
- Two tablespoons of Pine nuts
- Two tablespoons of dry-roasted sunflower seeds
- A quarter cup of Italian cheese blend, shredded
- Eight stalks of celery leaves

- One (8-ounce) pack of fat-free cream cheese

- Cooking spray

Instructions

- Sauté garlic and pine nuts over a medium setting for the heat until the nuts are golden brown. Cut off the wide base and tops from celery.

- Remove two thin strips from the round side of the celery to create a flat surface.

- Mix Italian cheese and cream cheese in a bowl and spread into cut celery stalks.

- Sprinkle half of the celery pieces with sunflower seeds and a half with the pine nut mixture. Cover the mixture and let it stand for at least 4 hours before eating.

Stuffed Poblano Peppers

Preparation time-20 minutes |Cook time-30 minutes |Servings-2 to 4|Difficulty-Moderate

Nutritional value: ~Calories-302|Proteins-8g| Fat-16g|Carbohydrates-34g

Ingredients

- Half cup of Poblano peppers

- Two cups of water

- One cup quinoa

- Three tablespoons of olive oil

- One diced onion

- Two diced ribs celery

- Two diced carrots

- Two minced garlic cloves

- Half cup of diced red peppers roasted

- One tablespoon of adobo sauce with chipotle

- One cup of peas

- 1/3 cup of chopped pecans

Instructions

- Heat the oven before 375°F.

- With stem, slit each pepper lengthwise. Scoop the seeds out and put them aside.

- Take a medium saucepan, heat water, and add quinoa. Until cooked, boil it and simmer with water immersed. Put it aside.

- Add olive oil in a medium heated skillet.

- Sauté the carrots, onion, and celery for about 8 minutes until softened. Then add garlic and for a minute sauté it.

- Add quinoa cooked before in it and mix well. Add the chipotle, pecans, peas, and roasted red peppers.

- A shallow baking dish places stuffed peppers and bakes them until the peppers are softened for 30 minutes.

- Serve with meat or a side salad. Enjoy!

Summer Squash Ribbons with Lemon and Ricotta

Preparation time-20 minutes |Cook time-0 minutes |Servings-2 |Difficulty-Easy

Nutritional value: ~Calories-90|Proteins-4g| Fat-6g|Carbohydrates-5g

Ingredients

- Two medium zucchini or yellow squash

- Half cup of ricotta cheese

- Two tablespoons of fresh mint, chopped, plus additional mint leaves for garnish

- Two tablespoons of fresh parsley, chopped

- Zest of half lemon

- Two teaspoons of lemon juice

- Half teaspoon of kosher salt

- A quarter teaspoon of freshly ground black pepper

- One tablespoon of extra-virgin olive oil

Instructions

- Using a vegetable peeler, make ribbons by peeling the summer squash lengthwise. The squash ribbons will resemble the wide pasta, pappardelle.

- In a bowl, mix the ricotta cheese, mint, parsley, lemon zest, lemon juice, salt, and black pepper.

- Place mounds of the squash ribbons evenly on four plates, then dollop the ricotta mixture on top. Sprinkle with the olive oil, then garnish with the mint leaves.

Tomato and fresh parmesan cheese bruschetta

Preparation time-10 minutes |Cook time-10 minutes |Servings-2 |Difficulty-Easy

Nutritional value: ~Calories-70|Proteins-3g| Fat-0.3g|Carbohydrates-13g

Ingredients

- Four slices (Half-inch thick) of a French baguette or crusty whole-grain bread

- Two cloves fresh garlic, finely minced

- One teaspoon of extra-virgin olive oil + more for brushing

- One small onion, diced

- One medium tomato, diced

- Pinch dried oregano, crumbled

- Pinch freshly ground pepper

- Two tablespoons of freshly grated Parmesan cheese

Instructions

- Scantly brush slices of bread on both sides with olive oil, then toast. Remove from oven and evenly distribute garlic on one side of bread. Rub garlic into bread with the handle of a knife and set aside; keep warm.

- Heat teaspoon of olive oil in a skillet, add onion, and lightly sauté until golden brown.

- Remove from heat. Preheat broiler. Combine onion, tomato, oregano, and pepper; spread evenly over garlic bread and sprinkle with Parmesan cheese.

- Place bread with Parmesan cheese under the broiler for 1 minute until lightly browned. Serve immediately.

Tomato and garlic bruschetta

Preparation time-10 minutes |Cook time-10 minutes |Servings-2 |Difficulty-Easy

Nutritional value: ~Calories-57|Proteins-2.5g| Fat-0.4g|Carbohydrates-11g

Ingredients

- Four slices (Half-inch thick) of a French baguette or a crusty whole-grain bread

- One teaspoon of extra-virgin olive oil

- One and a quarter cup of chopped plum tomatoes

- One and a half teaspoons of minced fresh garlic

- One teaspoon of balsamic vinegar

- Half teaspoon of dried basil

- A quarter teaspoon of non-caloric sweetener

- A quarter teaspoon of freshly ground pepper

Instructions

- Place slices of bread on an ungreased baking sheet. Brush each slice with olive oil and bake at 500 degrees F for 3–4 minutes until golden brown.

- Combine tomatoes, garlic, vinegar, basil, sweetener, and pepper in a small bowl. Mix well and spoon mixture over bread slices.

Tomato Eggs

Preparation time-5 minutes |Cook time-10 minutes |Servings-2 |Difficulty-Easy

Nutritional value: ~Calories-169|Proteins-11.7g| Fat-12.2g|Carbohydrates-4.2g

Ingredients

- One tomato, chopped

- One teaspoon of sunflower oil

- One cup of fresh parsley, chopped

- Three eggs, beaten

- One ounce of feta cheese, crumbled

Instructions

- Heat sunflower oil in the pan.

- Then add chopped tomatoes and parsley—Cook the ingredients for 2 minutes.

- After this, add eggs and stir the mixture well.

- Cook the dish for 2 minutes more, add feta cheese and stir well.

- Cook the meal for 1 minute more.

Tomato Tarts

Preparation time-10 minutes| Cook time-20 minutes|Servings-4 |Difficulty-Easy

Nutritional value- Calories-174| Fat-5g |Carbohydrates-16g| Protein-6g

Ingredients

- A quarter cup of olive oil

- Two sliced tomatoes

- Salt and black pepper to the taste

For the base

- Five tablespoons of ghee

- One tablespoon psyllium husk

- Half cups of almond flour

- Two tablespoons of coconut flour

- A pinch of salt

For the filling

- Two teaspoons of minced garlic

- Three teaspoons of chopped thyme

- Two tablespoons of olive oil

- Three ounces of crumbled goat cheese

- One small thinly sliced onion

Instructions

- On a lined baking sheet, spread the tomato slices, season with pepper and salt, drizzle with a quarter of a cup of olive oil, place in the oven at 425 degrees F and bake for 40 minutes.

- Meanwhile, mix psyllium husk with almond flour, coconut flour, pepper, salt and cold butter in your food processor and stir until you've got your dough.

- Divide this dough into cupcake molds of silicone, press well, place it in the oven at 350 degrees F and bake for 20 minutes.

- Remove the cupcakes from the oven and leave them aside.

- Also, take slices of tomatoes from the oven and cool them down a bit.

- On top of the cupcakes, divide the tomato slices.

- Heat a saucepan over medium-high heat with two tablespoons of olive oil, add the onion, stir and cook for 4 minutes.

- Add the thyme and garlic, stir, cook for another 1 minute and remove from the heat.

- Spread the mix over the tomato slices.

- Sprinkle with the goat cheese, put it back in the oven and cook for five more minutes at 350 degrees F.

- Arrange and serve on a platter.

Tortilla Chips

Preparation time-5 minutes |Cook time-25 minutes |Servings-6 |Difficulty-Easy

Nutritional value: ~Calories-119|Proteins-8g| Fat-2g|Carbohydrates-8g

Ingredients

For the tortillas

- Two teaspoons of olive oil

- One cup of flaxseed meal

- Two tablespoons of psyllium husk powder

- A quarter teaspoon of xanthan gum

- One cup of water

- Half teaspoons of curry powder

- Three teaspoons of coconut flour

For the chips

- Six flaxseed tortillas

- Salt and black pepper to the taste

- Three tablespoons of vegetable oil

- Fresh salsa for serving

- Sour cream for serving

Instructions

- Combine psyllium powder, flaxseed meal, xanthan gum, olive oil curry powder and water in a bowl and mix until an elastic dough is obtained.

- On a working surface, spread coconut flour.

- Divide the dough into six pieces, place each portion on the work surface, roll it into a circle and cut it into six pieces each.

- Over medium-high heat, heat a pan with vegetable oil, add tortilla chips, cook on each side for 2 minutes and transfer to paper towels.

- Put in a bowl of tortilla chips, season with pepper and salt and serve on the side with sour cream and fresh salsa.

Tuscan braised fennel

Preparation time-10 minutes |Cook time-45 minutes |Servings-2 |Difficulty-Moderate

Nutritional value: ~Calories-174|Proteins-2g| Fat-14g|Carbohydrates-8g

Ingredients

- Two medium fennel bulbs

- Four tablespoons of extra-virgin olive oil

- Two cloves fresh garlic, peeled and sliced

- Salt and freshly ground pepper to taste

- Two cups of canned low-sodium vegetable broth

- Garnish with grated Parmesan cheese

Instructions

- Wash and trim bulbs, then cut off tops and reserve for garnish. Pat bulbs dry and cut into quarters. Place pieces of fennel, flat-side down, in a heavy skillet, together with olive oil, garlic, and salt and pepper to taste.

- Cook over medium heat, turning until fennel pieces are browned. Add broth, bring to a boil, cover, and reduce heat to simmer. Cook another 30–40 minutes until fennel is tender and liquid is absorbed. Sprinkle with Parmesan cheese and serve.

Twice-baked sweet potatoes with cheese and fresh sage

Preparation time-10 minutes | Cook time-One hour 15 minutes | Servings-2 | Difficulty-Hard

Nutritional value: ~Calories-112 | Proteins-2g | Fat-3g | Carbohydrates-18g

Ingredients

- One large sweet potato

- Olive oil to drizzle

- Two tablespoons of freshly grated Parmesan cheese plus some to sprinkle

- One tablespoon of finely chopped fresh sage

- Salt and freshly ground pepper to taste

Instructions

- Preheat oven to 400 degrees F. Place sweet potato in a shallow oven-safe platter and lightly drizzle the top with olive oil. Bake until soft, roughly 45 minutes.

- Remove from oven and allow to cool. Reduce oven temperature to 375 degrees. When the potato is cool enough to touch, cut in half and gently scoop out the flesh from both halves into a bowl, reserving the skins.

- Add Parmesan cheese and sage to bowl, mix well, and return mixture to reserved skins. Sprinkle tops with salt and pepper to taste.

- Return potato halves to the oven and bake at 375 degrees for an additional 15–20 minutes until thoroughly heated. Serve with a sprinkling of Parmesan cheese.

White Bean Bruschetta

Preparation time-10 minutes | Cook time-10 minutes | Servings-2 | Difficulty-Easy

Nutritional value: ~Calories-137 | Proteins-4.1g | Fat-5.5g | Carbohydrates-17.4g

Ingredients

- One to two cloves of garlic, sliced

- One cup of cannellini beans, cooked

- Half teaspoon of red pepper flakes

- Two tablespoons of balsamic vinegar

- Two tablespoons of olive oil

- Two tablespoons of basil leaves

- Six slices of Italian bread garlic

- Salt to taste

- Pepper to taste

Instructions

- Mix all the items in a jar except bread.

- Toast the bread, spread the mixture, and serve.

Chapter 9~Soup and Stew Recipes

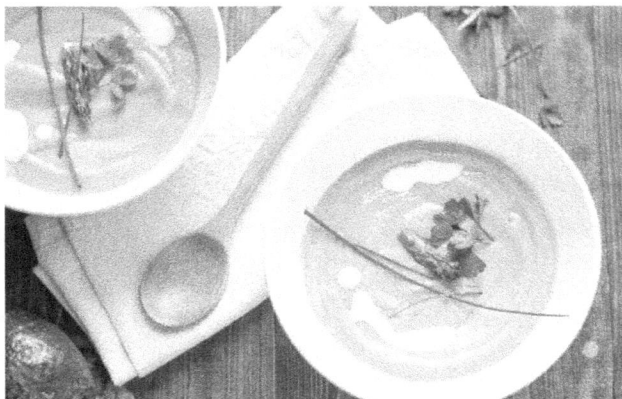

Asparagus Avocado Soup

Preparation time-10 minutes |Cook time-20 minutes |Servings-4 |Difficulty-Easy

Nutritional value: ~Calories-208|Proteins-4g| Fat-11g|Carbohydrates-7g

Ingredients

- One avocado, peeled, pitted, cubed
- Twelve ounces of asparagus
- Half teaspoon of ground black pepper
- One teaspoon of garlic powder
- One teaspoon of sea salt
- Two tablespoons of olive oil, divided
- Half of a lemon, juiced
- Two cups of vegetable stock

Instructions

- Switch on the air fryer, insert fryer basket, grease it with olive oil, then shut with its lid, set the fryer at 425 degrees F and preheat for 5 minutes.
- Meanwhile, place asparagus in a shallow dish, drizzle with one tablespoon oil, sprinkle with garlic powder, salt, and black pepper and toss until well mixed.
- Open the fryer, add asparagus to it, close with its lid and cook for 10 minutes until nicely golden and roasted, shaking halfway through the frying.
- When the air fryer beeps, open its lid and transfer asparagus to a food processor.
- Add remaining ingredients into a food processor and pulse until well combined and smooth.
- Tip the soup in a saucepan, pour in water if the soup is too thick and heat it over medium-low heat for 5 minutes until thoroughly heated.
- Ladle soup into bowls and serve.

Baked Potato-Turkey Bacon Soup

Preparation time-10 minutes| Cook time-30 minutes| Servings-6 |Difficulty-Moderate

Nutritional value- Calories-181| Fat-9g |Carbohydrates-18g| Protein-9g

Ingredients

- Four tablespoons of chopped chives
- Half cup of shredded sharp Cheddar cheese
- Half cup of low-fat plain Greek yogurt
- Three medium unpeeled russet potatoes, cut into 1-inch chunks
- One and a half cups of vegetable or chicken broth
- One and a half cups of 1% milk
- Three tablespoons of whole-wheat flour
- Two tablespoons of extra-virgin olive oil
- Four slices of turkey bacon (nitrate-free)

Instructions

- Put a stockpot on medium heat. Add and cook the turkey bacon on both sides until crispy. Move to a plate lined with a paper towel. Cool it, then chop finely and put it aside.
- In the stockpot, heat the olive oil over medium heat. Add some flour and cook for 2 to 3 minutes. Add some milk and beat until it thickens. Then add the broth and potatoes.
- Boil the mixture and lower the heat. Now simmer the soup until the potatoes soften. Throw in the Greek yogurt and mix well.
- Top with cheese, turkey bacon, Greek yogurt, and chives. Serve.

Barley with Winter Vegetable Soup

Preparation time-5 minutes |Cook time-10 minutes |Servings-6 |Difficulty-Easy

Nutritional value: ~Calories-233|Proteins-4g| Fat-2g|Carbohydrates-29g

Ingredients

- Six cups of veggie broth
- Three cups of water
- Two cups of chopped winter vegetables
- One and a half cups of chopped carrots
- One cup of sliced onions
- One cup of peeled, chopped parsnip
- One cup of pearled barley
- One chopped potato
- Half cup of chopped celery

- Two tablespoons of tamari

- One tablespoon of olive oil

- One tablespoon of miso (dissolved in three tablespoons of water)

- Salt and pepper to taste

Instructions

- Pour oil into a deep-bottomed saucepan with a lid and heat it.

- When hot, cook celery, carrots, and onions until the onions are browning.

- Pour in the broth, and add potato, tamari, parsnip, and barley.

- Close and seal the lid.

- Cook on high heat for 8 minutes.

- Turn off the heat and let it stand for some time.

- Check the barley, and if it isn't cooked through, bring the pot back to pressure for 3-5 minutes.

- When ready, add the miso (dissolved in water).

- Season and serve!

Beef Stew

Preparation time-20 minutes | Cook time-1 hour 40 minutes | Serving-4 | Difficulty- Hard

Nutritional value: ~Calories-376 | Fat-18g | Protein-45g | Carbohydrates-8g

Ingredients

- Two tablespoons of extra-virgin olive oil

- One and ⅓ pounds of chuck roast, cut into 1-inch cubes

- One yellow onion, cut into 1-inch pieces

- Two garlic cloves, minced

- Six cups of beef broth

- One dried bay leaf

- One teaspoon of dried thyme

- Salt

- Freshly ground black pepper

- Three celery stalks, chopped

- One large carrot, peeled and sliced

Instructions

- In a large, heavy-bottomed pan over medium-high heat, heat the olive oil. Add the meat, and sear in batches.

- Add the onion and garlic, lower the heat to medium, and continue to cook until the onion is translucent, 3 to 5 minutes.

- Add the broth, bay leaf, thyme, salt and pepper to taste.

- Bring the stew to a boil. Lower the heat to simmer, cover, and cook for 1 to 1½ hours. Add the celery and carrot halfway through cooking.

- Remove the bay leaf before serving.

Black Bean Soup

Preparation time-5 minutes | Cook time-20 minutes | Servings-6 | Difficulty-Easy

Nutritional value: ~Calories-191 | Proteins-9g | Fat-4g | Carbohydrates-31g

Ingredients

- Four tablespoons of sour cream

- One chopped onion

- One tablespoon of. chili powder

- Fifteen ounces of black beans

- One tablespoon of canola oil

- One teaspoon of cumin

- Half cup of prepared salsa

- A quarter teaspoon of salt

- One tablespoon of lime juice

- Three cups of water

- Two tablespoons of chopped cilantro

Instructions

- In a saucepan, heat oil and add onion.

- Cook the onions for 3 minutes

- Add cumin and chili powder while stirring.

- Then, add salt, water, salsa, and beans and boil at low heat for 10 minutes.

- Turn off the heat and add lime juice.

- Later, blend the mixture in a blender and make a puree.

- Afterward, slightly cook the puree in a pan for 5 minutes.

- Serve it with cilantro or sour cream.

Bone Broth

Preparation time-1 hour | Cook time-12 hours | Serving-1Two cups of | Difficulty- Hard

Nutritional value: ~ Calories-69 | Fat-4g | Protein-6g | Carbohydrates-1g

Ingredients

- Two pounds of beef bones (ideally knuckles and joints)
- One gallon of water
- Two tablespoons of apple cider vinegar
- One onion, roughly chopped
- Two large carrots, roughly chopped
- Two celery stalks, roughly chopped
- One tablespoon of salt
- One teaspoon of peppercorns
- One bunch of fresh parsley (or herbs of your choosing)
- Two garlic cloves

Instructions

- Preheat the oven to 350°F.
- Place the bones on a baking sheet and roast for 30 minutes.
- Transfer the bones to a stockpot, add the water and vinegar, and let sit for 30 minutes.
- Add the onions, carrots, and celery, and bring to a boil.
- Transfer to a slow cooker, and add the salt and peppercorns. Cook on low for 12 to 24 hours, using a spoon to periodically remove any impurities that float to the surface.
- During the last 30 minutes of cooking, add the parsley and garlic.
- Remove from the heat and let cool. Strain with a fine metal strainer.
- Once cooled, skim the fat from the broth (if desired).
- Transfer to air-tight jars. Store in the refrigerator for up to 5 days or in the freezer for up to 3 months. For easy use in recipes, freeze in ice cube trays and then transfer to a large freezer bag.

Cabbage and meatball soup

Preparation time-10 minutes |Cook time-40 minutes |Servings-2 |Difficulty-Easy

Nutritional value: -Calories-263|Proteins-21g| Fat-15g|Carbohydrates-12g

Ingredients

For the soup

- One large head cabbage (about 2 pounds)
- Three tablespoons of unsalted butter, ghee, or coconut oil
- Two medium white onions, diced
- Two teaspoons of minced garlic
- Two teaspoons of chili powder
- One tablespoon of ground cumin

- One teaspoon of paprika
- Fine sea salt and ground black pepper
- Four cups of Beef Broth
- A quarter cup of chopped fresh cilantro for garnish

For the meatballs

- Two pounds of ground beef
- Fine sea salt and ground black pepper
- One tablespoon of garlic powder
- Two tablespoons of chopped fresh cilantro
- Two teaspoons of ground cumin

Instructions

- Cut the cabbage into thin strips and set it aside.
- Make the meatballs: Combine the beef, a pinch of salt and pepper, the garlic powder, cilantro, and cumin in a large bowl and mix well with your hands. Form the meat mixture into 1-inch balls and set aside.
- Make the soup: Melt the fat in a stockpot over medium heat. Add the onions and garlic and cook for 2 minutes. Add the chili powder, cumin, paprika, and a pinch of salt and pepper.
- Sauté the onion mixture for about 2 minutes, then add the sliced cabbage. Continue to cook until the cabbage starts to soften, about 5 minutes.
- Add the broth and meatballs to the pot and cook, uncovered, over medium heat for 30 minutes. Adjust seasoning to taste.
- Ladle the soup into bowls and top with the cilantro.

California soup

Preparation time-10 minutes |Cook time-0 minutes|Servings-6 |Difficulty-Easy

Nutritional value: ~80 Calories| Fat-6g|Protein-4g|Carbohydrates-3g

Ingredients

- One large or two small avocados, very ripe
- One quart of hot chicken broth

Instructions

Pit and peel the avocado, and cut it into big chunks.

Purée in the blender with the broth (use caution when blending hot liquids) until very smooth, and serve.

Caramelized onion soup

Preparation time-15 minutes | Cook time-One hour | Servings-2 | Difficulty-Hard

Nutritional value: ~Calories-213 | Proteins-10g | Fat-8g | Carbohydrates-24g

Ingredients

*   Ten medium white onions (about 2 pounds)
*   Two tablespoons of unsalted butter, ghee, or coconut oil
*   Fine sea salt and ground black pepper
*   Half teaspoon of dried thyme leaves
*   Four cups of Beef Broth (see here)
*   Two bay leaves
*   A quarter cup of apple cider vinegar
*   Four ounces of grated Parmesan cheese for garnish (optional)

Instructions

*   Slice the onions into rings.
*   Melt the fat over medium heat in a stockpot.
*   Add the onions, a pinch of salt and pepper, and the thyme. Cook the onions until golden brown, about 20 to 22 minutes, frequently stirring.
*   Add the beef broth and bay leaves and bring the liquid to a simmer over medium heat. Scrape the bottom of the pot to release any browned bits of onion.
*   Cook the onion broth for an additional 20 minutes, uncovered.
*   Add the vinegar and another pinch of salt and pepper. Let the soup simmer until all the flavors combine, about ten more minutes.
*   If using the Parmesan cheese, turn on the broiler to high and line a baking sheet with parchment paper. Place the cheese on the lined baking sheet in 2-inch mounds. Broil the cheese in the oven for 2 to 3 minutes, until golden brown.
*   Remove the crisped cheese mounds from the parchment paper and let them cool for 5 minutes on a wire rack.
*   Divide the soup equally among serving bowls. Place the crispy cheese wafers on top, if desired.

Cauliflower soup

Preparation time-10 minutes | Cook time-25 minutes | Servings-2 | Difficulty-Easy

Nutritional value: ~Calories-76 | Proteins-2g | Fat-5g | Carbohydrates-5g

Ingredients

*   Two tablespoons of olive oil
*   One large yellow onion, coarsely chopped
*   Two teaspoons of finely chopped fresh garlic
*   Six cups of fresh cauliflower florets (about one large head)
*   Half cup of chopped carrot
*   Half cup of chopped celery
*   One small jalapeño pepper, seeds removed and diced
*   Three and a half cups of low-sodium, fat-free chicken broth
*   One (14.5-ounce) can of diced tomatoes
*   One bay leaf
*   Half teaspoon of ground cumin
*   Salt and freshly ground pepper to taste
*   Large croutons (optional)
*   Crumbled feta cheese for garnish

Instructions

*   Heat olive oil in a large pot over medium heat, add onion and garlic and sauté until soft. Add cauliflower florets, carrot, celery, and jalapeño.
*   Cook until florets begin to brown. Add broth, tomatoes, bay leaf, cumin, salt and pepper, and bring to a boil.
*   Reduce heat to low and cook for 20–25 minutes, occasionally stirring, until cauliflower is tender. Remove from heat, discard bay leaf, and serve with croutons, if desired, and feta cheese.

Chicken, Barley, and Vegetable Soup

Preparation time-15 minutes | Cook time-50 minutes | Servings-8 | Difficulty-Hard

Nutritional value- Calories-198 | Fat-3g | Carbohydrates-9g | Protein-16g

Ingredients

*   Two bay leaves
*   A quarter teaspoon of dried rosemary
*   Half teaspoon of dried thyme
*   Two large carrots, chopped
*   ¾ cup of pearl barley
*   Two cups of water
*   Three celery stalks, chopped
*   Two and a half cups of diced cooked chicken

- Four cups of low-sodium chicken broth
- One large onion, diced
- One (14.5-ounce) can of diced tomatoes
- One teaspoon of minced garlic
- Half teaspoon of dried sage
- One tablespoon of extra-virgin olive oil

Instructions

- Put a large pot on medium-high heat.
- Sauté the garlic and olive oil for 1 minute. Then add celery, onion, carrots and sauté for 3 to 5 minutes.
- Throw in barley, water, sage, broth, rosemary, thyme, bay leaves, chicken, and tomatoes. Simmer and lower the heat to medium-low and cook for 45 minutes. Once the barley becomes soft, the soup is done
- Take out bay leaves and serve hot.

Chicken Stew with Artichokes, Capers, and Olives

Preparation time-20 minutes | Cook time-35 minutes | Servings-2 to 4 | Difficulty-Moderate

Nutritional value: Calories-500 | Proteins-39g | Fat-36g | Carbohydrates-11g

Ingredients

- One and a half pounds of boneless, skinless chicken thighs
- One teaspoon of kosher salt, divided
- A quarter teaspoon of freshly ground black pepper
- Two tablespoons of olive oil
- One onion, julienned
- Four garlic cloves, sliced
- One teaspoon of ground turmeric
- One teaspoon of ground cumin
- Half teaspoon of ground coriander
- Half teaspoon of ground cinnamon
- A quarter teaspoon of red pepper flakes
- One dried bay leaf
- One and a quarter cups of no-salt-added chicken stock
- A quarter cup of white wine vinegar
- Two tablespoons of lemon juice
- One tablespoon of lemon zest
- One (14-ounce) can artichoke hearts, drained
- A quarter cup of olives, pitted and chopped

- One teaspoon of caper, rinsed and chopped
- One tablespoon of fresh mint, chopped
- One tablespoon of fresh parsley, chopped

Instructions

- Season the chicken with a half teaspoon of salt and pepper.
- Heat the olive oil in a large skillet or sauté pan over medium heat. Add the chicken and sauté for 2 to 3 minutes per side. Transfer to a plate and set aside.
- Add the onion to the pan, then sauté until translucent, about 5 minutes. Then add the garlic and sauté for 30 seconds. Add the remaining half teaspoon of salt, turmeric, cumin, coriander, cinnamon, red pepper flakes, and bay leaf and sauté for 30 seconds.
- Add A quarter cup of the chicken stock and increase the heat to medium-high to deglaze the pan, rubbing up any brown bits on the bottom. Add the remaining one cup of stock, the lemon juice, and lemon zest. Cover, lessen the heat to low, then simmer for 10 minutes.

Add the artichokes, olives, and capers and mix well. Add the reserved chicken and nestle it into the mixture. Simmer, uncovered, until the chicken thoroughly cooks through, about 10 to 15 minutes. Garnish with mint and parsley.

Chicken Zoodle Soup

Preparation time-15 minutes | Cook time-30 minutes | Serving-4 | Difficulty- Easy

Nutritional value: ~ Calories-153 | Fat-5g | Protein-17g | Carbohydrates-11g

Ingredients

- Two large zucchinis
- One tablespoon of extra-virgin olive oil
- Half onion, diced
- Two celery stalks, diced
- One large carrot, diced
- One garlic clove, minced
- Half teaspoon of dried basil
- Half teaspoon of dried oregano
- Six to eight cups of chicken broth
- Two chicken breasts, cooked and shredded or finely diced
- Two dried bay leaves
- Salt
- Freshly ground black pepper

Instructions

- Using a spiralizer, spiralize the zucchini. Cut into desired length noodles. Set aside.

- In a large stockpot over medium heat, heat the oil. Add the onions, celery, carrots, garlic, basil, and oregano. Sauté for 3 minutes.

- Add the broth, chicken, and bay leaves. Bring to a boil.

- Simmer for 15 minutes.

- Add the zucchini, and simmer for 5 minutes more. Add salt and pepper to taste. (If preparing the soup for another day, consider adding zucchini when reheating to preserve its freshness.)

- Remove the bay leaves, and serve.

Chicken(less) Soup

Preparation time-10 minutes | Cook time-15 minutes | Servings-4 | Difficulty-Easy

Nutritional value: ~Calories-90 | Proteins-6g | Fat-2g | Carbohydrates-15g

Ingredients

- Six cups of hot water

- One cup of diced potatoes

- Two diced carrots

- One minced onion

- One diced celery rib

- ¾ cup of cubed, extra-firm tofu

- Two bay leaves

- Two tablespoons of seasoning blend

- Two teaspoons of minced garlic

- One teaspoon of salt

- ⅛ teaspoon of dried thyme

- ¾ cup of nutritional yeast flakes

- One and a half tablespoons of onion powder

- One tablespoon of dried basil

- One tablespoon of dried oregano

- One tablespoon of dried parsley

- One teaspoon of salt

- Half teaspoon of celery seed

- A quarter teaspoon of white pepper

Instructions

- To make your seasoning blend, put everything in a blender and process until it has become a fine powder. Don't breathe it in.

- Mix two tablespoons into your water and set aside.

- Heat a deep-bottomed saucepan with a lid and saute the onion until brown.

- Add garlic and cook for another minute.

- Add the rest of the ingredients, including the seasoned water.

- Close and seal the lid.

- Let it boil for around 10 minutes.

- Turn off the heat and let it stand with a closed lid for about 5 minutes.

- Serve!

Chili

Preparation time-10 minutes | Cook time-30 minutes | Serving-8 | Difficulty- Easy

Nutritional value: ~Calories-254 | Fat-8g | Protein-20g | Carbohydrates-27g

Ingredients

- One pound of extra-lean ground beef • Half cup of chopped onion

- Two large tomatoes (or two cups of canned, unsalted tomatoes)

- Four cups of canned kidney beans, rinsed and drained

- One cup of chopped celery

- One teaspoon of sugar

- One and a half tablespoons of chili powder or to taste

- Water, as desired

- Two tablespoons of cornmeal

- Jalapeno peppers, seeded and chopped, as desired

Instructions

- Combine the ground meat and onion in a soup pot. Sauté until the meat is browned and the onion is transparent over medium heat. Drain thoroughly.

- Toss the ground beef mixture with tomatoes, sugar, celery, kidney beans, and chili powder. Cook, covered, for 10 minutes, stirring occasionally.

- Remove the cover and add enough water to achieve the desired consistency. Mix in the cornmeal. Allow for at least another 10 minutes of cooking time to allow the flavors to meld.

- If preferred, garnish with jalapeño peppers and serve in warmed bowls. Serve right away.

Chilled Honeydew Soup with Spearmint

Preparation time-5 minutes | Cook time-0 minutes | Serving-8 | Difficulty- Easy

Nutritional value: ~ Calories-73 | Fat-0.2g | Protein-1g | Carbohydrates-15g

Ingredients

- One honeydew melon

- A quarter cup of lemon juice

- Half cup of cooking sherry or alcohol-free white wine

- Two tablespoons of chopped spearmint leaves

- Eight sprigs of fresh spearmint (optional)

Instructions

- Cut the melon in half and scrape out and discard the seeds.

- Using a tablespoon, scrape all of the flesh into a food processor fitted with a metal S blade. Add the lemon juice, sherry or wine, and chopped spearmint.

- Puree the mixture just until it has a liquid consistency.

- Place it into a 3-quart (3- L) container with an airtight lid and chill it in the refrigerator for at least 1 hour.

- Stir and serve in chilled dessert bowls or martini glasses. Garnish with the spearmint sprigs (if using).

Chinese-style tuna soup

Preparation time-10 minutes |Cook time-15 minutes|Servings-3 |Difficulty-Easy

Nutritional value: ~216 Calories| Fat-9g|Protein-27g|Carbohydrates-3g

Ingredients

- One quart of chicken broth

- Two teaspoons of soy sauce

- One teaspoon of grated fresh ginger root

- Two eggs

- One can (Six ounces) tuna packed in olive oil

- One and a half cups of chopped fresh spinach

- Two scallions, sliced thin

Instructions

- In a big saucepan, combine the chicken broth with the soy sauce and ginger. Put it over medium-high heat, and bring it to a boil, then turn the heat down till the broth is just simmering.

- While the broth is heating, break the eggs into a little glass measuring cup or another container with a pouring lip. Beat them up with a fork.

- When your soup is simmering, pour one-third of the egg into the soup, wait just 1 or 2 seconds, then stir with a fork, drawing out the egg into strands. Repeat with the rest of the egg in 2 or 3 more additions.

- When you're done adding the egg, add the tuna and spinach. Heat through and serve with scallions on top.

Classic Turkey Chili

Preparation time-10 minutes| Cook time-30 minutes| Servings-8 |Difficulty-Easy

Nutritional value: Calories-243| Fat-9g |Carbohydrates-28g| Protein-17g

Ingredients

- One pound of lean ground turkey

- One (14.5-ounce) can of kidney beans

- Two tablespoons of ground cumin

- Three tablespoons of chili powder

- One teaspoon of dried oregano

- Two tablespoons of tomato paste

- One (8-ounce) can tomato purée

- One (28-ounce) can of diced tomatoes

- Four teaspoons of garlic

- Two green bell peppers, finely chopped

- One large onion, finely chopped

- Two tablespoons of extra-virgin olive oil

Instructions

- Heat a large skillet. Put ground turkey in the pan. Now break it into smaller chunks and brown it for7 to 9 minutes.

- Now, heat some olive oil in a medium to a pot over medium heat.

- Throw bell pepper, garlic, spices, and onions in the pot and then sauté them for 5 to 7 minutes.

- Now incorporate turkey in the pot; keep breaking it into smaller chunks.

- Mix the tomato purée, tomato paste, kidney beans, and tomatoes. Now boil them.

- Then cook this mixture for 15 to 20 minutes, and enjoy.

Classic (Vegan) Chili

Preparation time-30 minutes |Cook time-10 minutes |Servings-8 |Difficulty-Moderate

Nutritional value: ~Calories-331|Proteins-25g| Fat-5g|Carbohydrates-51g

Ingredients

- Six cups of tomato juice

- Seven cups of canned kidney beans

- Two cups of textured soy protein

- Two cans of diced tomatoes

- One cup of water

- Five minced garlic cloves

- One diced onion

- Two tablespoons of vegetable oil

- One tablespoon plus one teaspoon of chili powder
- One teaspoon of garlic powder
- One teaspoon of sea salt
- Half teaspoon of cumin
- Salt to taste

Instructions

- In a deep-bottomed saucepan/pot, heat the veggie oil.
- When hot, cook onions until they're soft and about to become clear.
- Add the garlic and cook for a minute or so. Scoop out the onions and garlic.
- Add the tomato juice and seasonings.
- Puree the onion/garlic mixture before returning to the pot.
- Add the rest of the ingredients.
- Close and seal the lid.
- Let it cook for around 7 minutes.
- Turn off the flame and let it stand for 5 minutes.
- Taste and season before serving!

Classic vegetable soup

Preparation time-10 minutes | Cook time-20 minutes | Servings-10 | Difficulty-Easy

Nutritional value: ~Calories-113 | Proteins-2.3g | Fat-1.8g | Carbohydrates-22g

Ingredients

- 3/4 cup of alphabet pasta
- One teaspoon of grapeseed oil
- One medium yellow onion, finely chopped
- Two large stalks of celery, finely chopped
- A quarter large red bell pepper, finely chopped
- One clove of garlic, minced
- One teaspoon of kosher salt
- A quarter teaspoon of ground allspice
- Four cups of vegetable stock
- Two cups of tomato-vegetable juice
- Two cups of frozen mixed vegetables (green beans, peas, carrots, corn)
- Juice of half a lemon

Instructions

- Bring a pot of water to a boil over medium heat, add alphabet pasta, and cook according to the package directions. Drain and set aside.

- In a medium soup pot over medium heat, heat grapeseed oil. Add yellow onion, celery, red bell pepper, garlic, and kosher salt, and cook, frequently stirring, for about 5 minutes or until softened.
- Add allspice, vegetable stock, tomato-vegetable juice, and frozen mixed vegetables, and bring to a boil. Reduce heat to medium, and cook, partially covered, for 10 minutes.
- Stir in cooked pasta and lemon juice, cook for 1 minute or until pasta is heated through, and serve.

Cold Tomato Summer Vegetable Soup

Preparation time-20 minutes | Cook time-0 minutes | Servings-6 | Difficulty-Easy

Nutritional value: ~Calories-89 | Proteins-4g | Fat-0.6g | Carbohydrates-18g

Ingredients

- Half teaspoons of black pepper
- Two minced zucchinis
- Two chopped stalks of celery
- Two teaspoons of sugar
- Two chopped garlic cloves
- Two tablespoons of olive oil
- One chopped cucumber
- Six chopped tomatoes
- Half chopped onion
- One teaspoon of salt
- One chopped red bell pepper
- One teaspoon of chopped dry oregano
- One teaspoon of Vegan Worcestershire sauce
- A quarter cup of sherry vinegar
- Three cups of tomato juice
- One and a half cups of vegetable broth
- One tablespoon of chopped dill
- Hot sauce if needed

Instructions

- Take a big bowl.
- Add all the ingredients and mix them all.
- To adjust the consistency to the desired level, use extra tomato juice.
- Add spices to the taste and serve the next day.

Crab and asparagus soup

Preparation time-10 minutes |Cook time-15 minutes|Servings-4 |Difficulty-Easy

Nutritional value: ~237 Calories| Fat-8g|Protein-31g|Carbohydrates-5g

Ingredients

- Two quarts of chicken broth
- Two teaspoons of grated fresh ginger root
- One pound of asparagus
- Two eggs
- One and a half tablespoons of dry sherry
- One tablespoon of soy sauce
- Two teaspoons of dark sesame oil
- Twelve ounces of lump crabmeat, fresh or canned

Instructions

- In a large, heavy saucepan, start the broth warming over medium heat. Stir in the ginger root.
- Now snap the ends off of your asparagus where it wants to break naturally. Discard the ends, and slice the asparagus on the diagonal into half-inch (1 cm) pieces. When the soup is simmering, add the asparagus to it. Let it simmer for about 3 minutes.
- While that's happening, beat the eggs until blended in a glass measuring cup. When the asparagus is just barely tender-crisp, take a fork in one hand and the cup of beaten egg in the other.
- Pour a stream of egg onto the surface of the soup, then stir with the fork. Repeat. It should take 3 or 4 additions to stir in all the eggs. Now you have lovely egg drops!
- Stir in sherry, soy sauce, and sesame oil. Now add the crab, stir again, and cook for another 5 minutes or so before serving.

Cream of mushroom soup

Preparation time-10 minutes |Cook time-6 hours|Servings-5 |Difficulty-Hard

Nutritional value: ~217 Calories| Fat-19g|Protein-6g|Carbohydrates-5g

Ingredients

- Eight ounces of mushrooms, sliced
- A quarter cup of chopped onion
- Two tablespoons of butter
- One quart of chicken broth
- Half cup of heavy cream
- Half cup of sour cream
- Salt and ground black pepper, to taste

- Guar or xanthan (optional)

Instructions

- In a big, heavy skillet, sauté the mushrooms and onion in the butter until the mushrooms soften and change color.
- Transfer them to your slow cooker. Add the broth. Cover the slow cooker, set it to low, and let it cook for 5 to 6 hours.
- When the time's up, scoop out the vegetables with a slotted spoon and put them in your blender or food processor. Add enough broth to help them process easily and purée them finely.
- Pour the puréed vegetables back into the slow cooker, scraping out every last bit with a rubber scraper.
- Now stir in the heavy cream and sour cream and season with salt and pepper to taste. Thicken a bit with guar or xanthan if you think it needs it. Serve immediately

Cream of salmon soup

Preparation time-10 minutes |Cook time-35 minutes|Servings-4 |Difficulty-Easy

Nutritional value: ~594 Calories| Fat-54g|Protein-23g|Carbohydrates-5g

Ingredients

- One and a half tablespoons of butter

A quarter cup of finely minced onion

A quarter cup of finely minced celery

Two cups of heavy cream

One can (Fourteen ounces) salmon, drained

Half teaspoon of dried thyme

Instructions

- In a heavy saucepan, melt the butter over medium-low heat and add the onion and celery.
- Sauté the vegetables for a few minutes until the onion starts turning translucent.
- Meanwhile, pour the cream into a glass 2-cup (475 ml) measure or any other microwavable container similar in size with a pouring spout. Place it in the microwave and heat it at 50 percent power for 3 to 4 minutes.
- Pour the cream into the saucepan and add the salmon and thyme. Break up the salmon as you stir the soup.
- Heat until simmering, and serve.

Cream of Thyme Tomato Soup

Preparation time-10 minutes |Cook time-20 minutes |Servings-6 |Difficulty-Easy

Nutritional value: ~Calories-310|Proteins-11g| Fat-27g|Carbohydrates-5g

Ingredients

- Two tablespoons of plant-based butter
- Half cup of raw cashew nuts, diced
- Two (twenty-eight ounces) cans of tomatoes
- One teaspoon of fresh thyme leaves plus extra to garnish
- One and a half cups of water
- Salt and black pepper to taste

Instructions

- Cook butter in a pot over medium heat and sauté the onions for 4 minutes until softened.
- Stir in the tomatoes, thyme, water, cashews, and season with salt and black pepper.
- Cover and bring to simmer for 10 minutes until thoroughly cooked.
- Open, turn the heat off, and puree the ingredients with an immersion blender.
- Adjust to taste and stir in the heavy cream.
- Spoon into soup bowls and serve.

Creamy broccoli soup

Preparation time-10 minutes | Cook time-20 minutes | Servings-2 to 3 | Difficulty-Easy

Nutritional value: ~Calories-243 | Proteins-10.5g | Fat-12.7g | Carbohydrates-25.2g

Ingredients

- Two cups of chopped broccoli
- One teaspoon of olive oil
- Half roughly chopped sweet onion
- Four cups of vegetable broth
- A quarter cup of grated parmesan cheese
- Black pepper as per taste
- One cup of rice milk

Instructions

- Heat the olive oil in a medium saucepan over high heat. Add the onion & cook for 3-5 min, until the onion begins to soften. Add broccoli & broth. Season it with pepper.
- Bring a boil & reduce the heat. Then simmer uncovered for 10 min, until broccoli is tendered but bright green.
- Now put the soup mixture into a blender. Add rice milk & process until smooth. Now put in the saucepan, add some parmesan cheese & serve.

Creamy Broccoli Soup with "Chicken" and Rice

Preparation time-30 minutes | Cook time-10 minutes | Servings-8 | Difficulty-Moderate

Nutritional value: ~Calories-193 | Proteins-8g | Fat-5g | Carbohydrates-27g

Ingredients

- Two boxes of mushroom broth
- Two bunches' worth of broccoli florets
- One head's worth of cauliflower florets
- One medium-sized, diced Yukon Gold potato
- Two cups of cooked brown rice
- One package of vegan chicken strips
- One vegan, chicken-flavored bouillon cube
- One cup of water
- One cup of unsweetened almond milk
- Three minced garlic cloves
- One diced white onion
- Two tablespoons of tamari
- One tablespoon of vegetable oil
- Dash of salt
- Dash of black pepper

Instructions

- Heat the oil in a deep-bottomed saucepan with a lid.
- Toss in the onion and cook until soft.
- Add garlic and cook for another minute or so.
- Add the broccoli, cauliflower, and potato.
- Season with the tamari, salt, pepper, and bouillon cube.
- Pour in the liquids (water, milk, and broth) and stir.
- Close and seal the lid.
- Cook on high pressure for 6 minutes.
- Turn off the flame and let it stand for 5 minutes.
- Puree when the soup has cooled a little.
- Before serving, add the vegan chicken strips and cooked rice.

Creamy Cauliflower Soup

Preparation time-15 minutes | Cook time-30 minutes | Servings-6 | Difficulty-Moderate

Nutritional value: ~Calories-214 | Proteins-12g | Fat-17g | Carbohydrates-9g

Ingredients

- Five cups of cauliflower rice
- Eight ounces of vegan cheese, grated

- Two cups of unsweetened almond milk
- Two cups of vegetable stock
- Two tablespoons of water
- Two garlic cloves, minced
- One tablespoon of olive oil

Instructions

- Cook olive oil in a large stockpot over medium heat.
- Add garlic and cook for 1-2 minutes. Add cauliflower rice and water. Cover and cook for 5-7 minutes.
- Now add vegetable stock and almond milk and stir well. Bring to a boil.
- Turn heat to low and simmer for 5 minutes. Turn off the heat.
- Slowly add cheddar cheese and stir until smooth.
- Season soup with pepper and salt.
- Stir well and serve hot.

Creamy corn chowder

Preparation time-10 minutes | Cook time-20 minutes | Servings-4 | Difficulty-Easy

Nutritional value: ~Calories-223 | Proteins-2.3g | Fat-3.8g | Carbohydrates-32g

Ingredients

One cup of blanched almonds

- Two tablespoons of extra-virgin olive oil
- One large yellow onion, finely chopped
- Two small stalks of celery, finely chopped
- Half medium red bell pepper, finely chopped
- One medium carrot, finely chopped
- One teaspoon of kosher salt
- Two tablespoons of all-purpose flour
- Six cups of light vegetable stock
- Three large Yukon gold potatoes, peeled and cut into 1/4 -in. (.5cm) dice
- Six cups of corn kernels (shucked from about 4 ears of corn)
- One tablespoon of plant-based butter
- One teaspoon of freshly squeezed lemon juice
- Half teaspoon of hot sauce, such as Sriracha
- A quarter teaspoon of freshly ground black pepper

Instructions

- Soak almonds in cold water overnight.

- Discard water nuts soaked in, rinse nuts well, and drain. Set aside.
- In a large soup pot over medium heat, heat extra-virgin olive oil. Add yellow onion, and cook, frequently stirring, for 5 minutes.
- Add celery, red bell pepper, carrot, and kosher salt, and cook for 3 more minutes or until vegetables are softened and just beginning to color.
- Add all-purpose flour, and stir for 1 minute.
- Add vegetable stock, stirring vigorously to combine. Bring to a boil, and reserve one cup of stock. Add Yukon gold potatoes and corn.
- In a blender, combine almonds and reserved vegetable stock, and blend until smooth. Stir almond mixture into the soup, and simmer until potatoes are tender. 8 Add plant-based butter, lemon juice, hot sauce, and black pepper. Serve immediately.

Creamy green garden soup

Preparation time-10 minutes | Cook time-30 minutes | Servings-2 | Difficulty-Easy

Nutritional value: ~Calories-163 | Proteins-4g | Fat-8g | Carbohydrates-15g

Ingredients

- Four tablespoons of trans fat–free canola/olive oil spread
- One white onion, chopped
- Four cloves fresh garlic, minced
- One large leek, thinly sliced white parts and sliced green parts, keep separate
- Eight ounces of fresh brussels sprouts, sliced
- Five ounces of fresh green beans, thinly sliced
- Five cups of low-sodium, fat-free vegetable broth
- One and a half cups of frozen peas, defrosted
- One tablespoon of freshly squeezed lemon juice
- One teaspoon of ground coriander
- One cup of low-fat milk
- Four teaspoons of all-purpose flour
- Salt and freshly ground pepper to taste
- Herb-flavored croutons for garnish (optional)

Instructions

- In a large skillet, melt canola/olive oil spread over low heat. Add onion and garlic and cook until soft and fragrant, but do not brown. Add the green parts of the leek, brussels sprouts, and green beans to the skillet. Add broth and bring to a boil. Reduce heat and let simmer for 10 minutes.
- Add peas, lemon juice, and coriander and continue to let simmer for 10–15 minutes more or until vegetables

are tender. Remove vegetable mixture from heat and allow to cool slightly, then transfer to a blender or food processor and process until smooth.

- Return to a saucepan and add white parts of the leek. Bring to a boil over medium-high heat, then reduce to a simmer for about 5 minutes, and reduce again to keep warm.

- In a separate small bowl, whisk together milk and flour until smooth. Add flour mix to soup, stirring to incorporate, and add salt and pepper to taste.

- Serve with a scattering of croutons on top, if desired.

Cumin cauliflower soup

Preparation time-5 minutes |Cook time-20 minutes |Servings-2 |Difficulty-Easy

Nutritional value: ~Calories-153|Proteins-8g| Fat-5g|Carbohydrates-14g

Ingredients

- One large head cauliflower (about 2 pounds), cored and cut into florets

- Four tablespoons of unsalted butter, ghee, or coconut oil, divided

- One medium white onion, minced

- Two teaspoons of minced garlic

- Two teaspoons of ground cumin, plus more for garnish

- One teaspoon of chili powder

- Fine sea salt and ground black pepper

- Four cups of Chicken Broth

- Extra-virgin olive oil, for garnish

Instructions

- Rinse the cauliflower florets, drain, and set aside.

- Melt two tablespoons of the fat in a large saucepan over medium heat. Add the onion and sauté it for 2 to 3 minutes. Add the garlic, cumin, chili powder, and a pinch of salt and pepper, and sauté for about 1 minute until onion is translucent.

- Add the chicken broth and cauliflower to the saucepan and simmer until tender, about 10 minutes. Stir in the remaining two tablespoons of fat.

- Puree the soup with an immersion blender until creamy, or puree in a blender or food processor in batches. Adjust the seasonings to taste.

- Ladle the soup into bowls and top each with a sprinkle of cumin and a drizzle of olive oil.

Curried cauliflower coconut soup

Preparation time-10 minutes |Cook time-30 minutes |Servings-8 |Difficulty-Easy

Nutritional value: ~Calories-113|Proteins-2.3g| Fat-1.8g|Carbohydrates-22g

Ingredients

- One tablespoon of grapeseed oil

- One medium yellow onion, finely chopped

- One large carrot, finely chopped

- Two medium stalks celery, finely chopped

- One clove of garlic, minced

- One teaspoon of kosher salt

- One medium head cauliflower, cut into florets

- Four cups of vegetable stock

- One (15-oz.) can of full-fat coconut milk

- One teaspoon of curry powder

- Half teaspoon of sambal oelek (chili garlic paste)

- Juice of half lime

- Fresh cilantro leaves

Instructions

- In a medium soup pot over medium-high heat, heat grapeseed oil. Add yellow onion, carrot, celery, garlic, and kosher salt, and cook, stirring gently, for about 5 minutes or until the onion is softened.

- Add cauliflower and vegetable stock. Reduce heat to medium-low, cover, and cook for about 10 minutes or until cauliflower is tender.

- Stir in coconut milk, curry powder, and sambal oelek, and cook for 2 more minutes.

- Remove from heat, and stir in lime juice.

- Using an immersion blender, purée soup until smooth, or transfer in batches to a blender to purée. Serve immediately, garnished with a few whole cilantro leaves.

Egg drop soup

Preparation time-10 minutes |Cook time-15 minutes|Servings-4 |Difficulty-Easy

Nutritional value: ~75 Calories| Fat-4g|Protein-8g|Carbohydrates-2g

Ingredients

- One quart of chicken broth, divided

- A quarter teaspoon of guar or xanthan (optional)

- One tablespoon of soy sauce

- One tablespoon of rice vinegar

- Half teaspoon of grated fresh ginger root

- One scallion, sliced

- Two eggs

Instructions

- Put one cup or so of the chicken broth in your blender, turn it on low, and add the guar (if using).

- Let it blend for a second, then put it in a large saucepan with the remaining three cups of broth. (If you're not using guar or xanthan, just put all the broth directly in a saucepan.)

- Add the soy sauce, rice vinegar, ginger, and scallion. Over medium-high heat, bring to a simmer and cook for 5 minutes or so to let the flavors blend.

- Beat your eggs in a glass measuring cup or small pitcher—something with a pouring lip.

- Use a fork to stir the surface of the soup in a slow circle and pour in about one-quarter of the eggs, stirring as they cook and turn into shreds (which will happen almost instantaneously).

- Repeat 3 more times, using up all the eggs. That's it.

Giambotta (Italian summer vegetable stew)

Preparation time-20 minutes |Cook time-One hour |Servings-5 |Difficulty-Hard

Nutritional value: ~Calories-193|Proteins-2.3g| Fat-1.8g|Carbohydrates-22g

Ingredients

- One medium eggplant, quartered and cut in 1 /2 -in. (1.25cm) slices

- Two teaspoons of kosher salt

- Half lb. of flat Italian green beans, trimmed

- Three large white potatoes, unpeeled

- Twelve medium plum tomatoes

- A quarter cup of extra-virgin olive oil

- Two large yellow onions, halved and thinly sliced

- Two cloves of garlic smashed and roughly chopped

- Two red bell peppers, ribs and seeds were removed and thinly sliced

- Two large zucchinis, halved and thinly sliced

- Half teaspoon of freshly ground black pepper

- A quarter cup of fresh basil leaves

Instructions

- In a colander, toss eggplant with one teaspoon of kosher salt, and set aside to drain over a bowl. After 30 minutes, discard liquid, rinse eggplant, and gently squeeze excess water from eggplant. Set aside.

- Bring a medium pot of salted water to a boil over high heat. Add Italian green beans, and cook for 5 minutes. Using a slotted spoon, transfer beans to a bowl of ice water, immediately drain and set aside.

- In the same pot, cook white potatoes with boiling water to cover for about 15 minutes or until tender. Remove to a cutting board to cool slightly.

- Meanwhile, core plum tomatoes and score a small X at the bottom of each.

- When potatoes are done, using the same pot of boiling water and adding a little more if necessary, work in batches to quickly blanch tomatoes, about 1 minute at a time, transferring them to an ice bath immediately after. Peel tomatoes, seed, and cut into slices, reserving tomatoes and juice in a bowl.

- In a 4-quart (4L) stockpot over medium-high heat, heat extra-virgin olive oil. Add yellow onions, and cook for 5 minutes.

- Add garlic, and cook for 1 minute.

- Stir in eggplant, and cook for another 5 minutes, frequently stirring to avoid vegetables sticking while cooking.

- Stir in tomatoes, red bell peppers, zucchini, green beans, and the remaining one teaspoon of kosher salt, reduce heat to medium-low, and simmer for 20 minutes.

- Meanwhile, peel potatoes and cut them into quarters. When vegetables are tender, stir in potatoes and black pepper, and cook for 5 minutes. Remove from heat; stir in basil; and serve hot, warm, or cold.

Ginger kale soup

Preparation time-10 minutes |Cook time-25 minutes |Servings-4 |Difficulty-Easy

Nutritional value: ~Calories-113|Proteins-2.3g| Fat-1.8g|Carbohydrates-22g

Ingredients

- One tablespoon of sesame oil

- One (2-in.) piece fresh ginger, peeled and finely chopped

- Three cloves of garlic, peeled and finely chopped

- Four scallions, thinly sliced, white and green parts separated

- One large carrot, peeled and thinly sliced

- Two large stalks of celery, thinly sliced

- Eight cups of vegetable stock

- One teaspoon of tamari

- Four dried shiitake mushrooms rinsed well

- Six oz. of fresh shiitake mushrooms stems removed, and thinly sliced

- Eight leaves of lacinato kale stemmed and sliced into thin ribbons

- Juice of one lemon

- One teaspoon of Sriracha, or to taste (optional)

- Two cups of cooked basmati or jasmine rice

Instructions

- In a medium saucepan over medium-high heat, heat sesame oil. Add ginger, garlic, and white parts of scallions, and stir for 1 minute.

- Add carrot and celery, and stir for 1 minute.

- Add vegetable stock, tamari, and dried shiitake mushrooms, and simmer the soup for 15 minutes.

- Add fresh shiitake mushrooms and kale, and simmer, covered, for 5 minutes.

- Remove dried shiitake mushrooms and remove the pan from heat. Add lemon juice and Sriracha (if using).

- Divide basmati rice among 4 bowls, and ladle soup over the top. Garnish each bowl with green scallion slices that were reserved, and serve.

Grandma's chicken noodle soup

Preparation time~10 minutes | Cook time~20 minutes | Servings~10 | Difficulty~Easy

Nutritional value: ~Calories~223 | Proteins~6.3g | Fat~4.8g | Carbohydrates~32g

Ingredients

- Two oz. of spaghetti or fettuccine, broken into small pieces

- One tablespoon of extra-virgin olive oil

- One medium yellow onion, finely chopped

- One large carrot, cut in 1/4 -in. (.5cm) dice

- One or two medium stalks celery, cut in 1/4 -in. (.5cm) dice

- One small parsnip, cut in 1/4 -in. (.5cm) dice

- One clove of garlic, minced

- One teaspoon of kosher salt

- Four cups of Golden Chicken-y Stock or vegetable stock

- One teaspoon of nutritional yeast

- Half teaspoon of reduced-sodium tamari

- A quarter teaspoon of freshly ground black pepper

- One tablespoon of finely chopped fresh Italian flat-leaf parsley

- One tablespoon of finely chopped fresh dill

Instructions

- Bring a medium pot of salted water to a boil over high heat, add spaghetti, and cook according to the package directions until pasta is al dente (cooked but firm to the bite). Drain, rinse with cold water and set aside.

- In a large saucepan over medium-high heat, heat extra-virgin olive oil. Add onion, reduce heat to medium, and cook, frequently stirring, for 5 to 10 minutes or until the onion is golden and softened.

- Add carrot, celery, parsnip, garlic, and kosher salt, and cook for 3 minutes.

- Stir in Golden Chicken-y Stock, nutritional yeast, tamari, and black pepper. Increase heat to high, bring to a boil, reduce heat to medium, and simmer for 10 minutes.

- Stir in spaghetti, and cook for 1 more minute. 6 Stir in Italian flat-leaf parsley and dill, and serve immediately.

Green bean soup

Preparation time~10 minutes | Cook time~40 minutes | Servings~2 | Difficulty~Easy

Nutritional value: ~Calories~145 | Proteins~3g | Fat~2g | Carbohydrates~11g

Ingredients

- One tablespoon of unsalted butter, ghee, or coconut oil

- One medium white onion, diced

- One tablespoon of minced garlic

- Fine sea salt and ground black pepper

- One stick cinnamon

- Two bay leaves

- One cup of diced celery

- Four large carrots, diced

- Five cups of Chicken Broth

- Three medium zucchinis

- One pound of green beans, trimmed

- Three tablespoons of tomato paste

- A quarter cup of chopped fresh parsley for garnish

Instructions

- Melt the fat in a stockpot over medium heat.

- Add the onion to the pot and sauté for 1 minute.

- Add the garlic, a pinch of salt and pepper, the cinnamon, and the bay leaves while stirring for 2 minutes. Add the celery and carrots and sauté the mixture for two more minutes.

- Add the chicken broth and bring the soup to a boil. Reduce the heat, cover, and let simmer for 20 minutes.

- Slice the zucchini into quarters lengthwise, then in half crosswise. Add the zucchini, green beans, and tomato paste and stir to incorporate the paste. Simmer the soup, uncovered, until the green beans are soft, about 10 minutes.

- Remove from heat and adjust the seasonings to taste. Remove the cinnamon stick and bay leaves, ladle into bowls, top with parsley, and enjoy.

Green breakfast soup

Preparation time-8 minutes |Cook time-4 minutes |Servings-2 |Difficulty-Easy

Nutritional value: ~Calories-95|Proteins-3g| Fat-3.8g|Carbohydrates-13.2g

Ingredients

- Four cups of spinach
- Four cups of vegetable stock
- Two teaspoons of ground coriander
- One avocado
- Black pepper to taste
- One teaspoon of cumin
- One teaspoon of turmeric

Instructions

- Put all the ingredients in a blender and continue to grind until smooth.
- Transfer the ground mixture to a saucepan and cook until 2-3 minutes. Soup is ready

Green curry vegetable stew

Preparation time-10 minutes |Cook time-20 minutes |Servings-4 |Difficulty-Easy

Nutritional value: ~Calories-113|Proteins-2.3g| Fat-1.8g|Carbohydrates-22g

Ingredients

- Two tablespoons of virgin coconut oil
- Two cloves of garlic, finely chopped
- One (1-or 2-in.) piece ginger, peeled and grated
- Two tablespoons of Thai green curry paste
- One hot chile pepper, such as Serrano, seeded and thinly sliced
- One medium yellow onion halved and thinly sliced
- One (8-oz.) pkg. of shiitake mushrooms, stemmed and thinly sliced
- One teaspoon of kosher salt, plus more to taste
- One (14-oz.) can full-fat, best-quality Thai coconut milk
- One cup of vegetable stock or water
- Two Kaffir lime leaves, or one tablespoon of grated lime zest
- One cup of carrot, thinly sliced
- One large zucchini, halved and thinly sliced
- One (10-oz.) pkg. of baby spinach
- Half cup of thinly sliced scallion, white and light green parts
- A quarter cup of finely chopped fresh cilantro

Instructions

- In a large saucepan over medium-high heat, heat virgin coconut oil. Add garlic, ginger, Thai green curry paste, and hot chile pepper, and stir for 1 minute.
- Add yellow onion, shiitake mushrooms, and kosher salt, and stir for 2 minutes more.
- Stir in coconut milk, vegetable stock, Kaffir lime leaves, and carrot. Bring to a boil, reduce heat to a simmer, and cook for 5 minutes.
- Stir in zucchini, and simmer for 5 minutes.
- Stir in baby spinach, scallion, and cilantro, and cook for 1 more minute. Remove from heat, and serve.

Guacamole Soup

Preparation time-10 minutes |Cook time-10 minutes |Servings-4 |Difficulty-Easy

Nutritional value: ~Calories-239|Proteins-3g| Fat-17g|Carbohydrates-18g

Ingredients

- Four cups of veggie stock
- Three smashed, ripe avocados
- One chopped onion
- Three minced garlic cloves
- One tablespoon of ground cumin
- One bay leaf
- One teaspoon of oregano
- $\frac{1}{8}$ seeded and chopped small habanero
- Two teaspoons of agave syrup
- Salt and pepper to taste

Instructions

- Heat one deep-bottomed saucepan/pot.
- When hot, cook the onions and garlic for about 5 minutes, or until fragrant and the onions are clear.
- Add the rest of the ingredients (minus the agave) to the pot.
- Cook on high heat for 10 minutes.
- Turn off the heat and let it stand for 5 minutes.
- Open the lid and pick out the bay leaf.
- Blend the soup till smooth before adding the agave syrup and a squirt of lime juice.
- Season more to taste, if necessary, before serving.

Gumbo filé

Preparation time-25 minutes | Cook time-One hour 30 minutes | Servings-4 | Difficulty-Hard

Nutritional value: ~Calories-223 | Proteins-6.3g | Fat-4.8g | Carbohydrates-32g

Ingredients

Half cup of grapeseed oil

- Half cup of all-purpose flour
- One large yellow onion, finely chopped
- Four medium stalks celery, finely chopped
- One medium green bell pepper, ribs and seeds removed and finely chopped
- One medium red bell pepper, ribs and seeds removed and finely chopped
- Six cloves of garlic, chopped
- Six cups of vegetable stock
- A quarter cup of extra-virgin olive oil
- Two links veggie Andouille sausage, thinly sliced
- One lb. of oyster mushrooms, roughly chopped
- One teaspoon of sweet paprika
- One teaspoon of kosher salt
- Half teaspoon of Creole seasoning
- Half teaspoon of dried oregano
- Half teaspoon of dried thyme
- Half teaspoon of freshly ground black pepper
- A quarter teaspoon of ground allspice
- Pinch cayenne
- Twelve fl. oz. of amber beer
- One (14-oz.) can dice fire-roasted tomatoes with juice
- One tablespoon of balsamic vinegar
- One tablespoon of vegan Worcestershire sauce
- One teaspoon of Louisiana hot sauce
- Two teaspoons of filé powder
- Half cup of thinly sliced scallions, white and green parts
- A quarter cup of finely chopped fresh Italian flat-leaf parsley
- Two tablespoons of dark rum (optional)

Instructions

- In a large soup pot over medium heat, heat grapeseed oil. Whisk in all-purpose flour until well combined. Using a wooden spoon, stir roux constantly over medium heat until the mixture is a golden, caramel brown color.
- Stir in yellow onion, celery, green bell pepper, and red bell pepper, and cook, frequently stirring, for 10 more minutes. Reduce heat to medium-low if necessary to prevent burning.
- Add 1/2 of garlic, stir for 1 minute, and bring to a simmer.
- Stir in vegetable stock, bring to a boil, and reduce heat to a gentle simmer.
- Meanwhile, in a wide sauté pan over medium heat, heat extra-virgin olive oil. Add sliced veggie Andouille sausage, and stir for 1 minute. Using a slotted spoon, transfer sausage to a bowl.
- Add oyster mushrooms and remaining garlic to the sauté pan, and stir until mushrooms are golden.
- Add sweet paprika, kosher salt, Creole seasoning, oregano, thyme, black pepper, allspice, and cayenne, and stir for 1 minute.
- Add amber beer, increase heat to high, and stir vigorously to deglaze the pan, releasing any browned bits stuck to the pan.
- Stir mushroom mixture into the soup pot along with fire-roasted tomatoes with juice, balsamic vinegar, vegan Worcestershire sauce, and hot sauce. Bring to a boil, reduce heat to low or medium-low, and simmer for 1 hour, stirring occasionally and adjusting heat as necessary.
- Stir in reserved Andouille sausage and filé powder, and simmer for 5 minutes.
- Stir in scallions, Italian flat-leaf parsley, and dark rum (if using).
- Ladle into bowls over hot, cooked rice, or serve with plenty of crusty French bread, passing additional filé powder and hot sauce at the table.

Keto Chicken Enchilada Soup

Preparation time-5 minutes | Cook time-35 minutes | Servings-3 | Difficulty-Moderate

Nutritional value: ~Calories-196 | Proteins-10g | Fat-0g | Carbohydrates-30g

Ingredients

- Six oz. Shredded chicken
- Two teaspoons of Cumin
- One teaspoon of Oregano
- One teaspoon of Chili Powder
- Half teaspoon of Cayenne Pepper
- Half cup of chopped cilantro
- Half medium Lime, juiced
- three tablespoons of Olive Oil
- Three stalks of diced Celery

- One medium diced Red Bell Pepper, diced
- Two teaspoons of garlic, minced
- Four cups of Chicken Broth
- One cup of Diced Tomatoes
- Eight oz. of Cream Cheese

Instructions

- Heat the oil in a pan and add celery and pepper. Add the tomatoes and cook for 2-3 minutes once the celery is soft.
- Add the spices to the pan and mix well.
- Add the chicken broth and the cilantro to the mixture, boil, and then reduce to low for 20 minutes to simmer.
- Then add the cream cheese and bring it back to a boil. Once it has cooked, reduce the heat to low and cover and cook for 25 minutes.
- Scrap the chicken and add it to the pot, then top it with half the lime juice.
- Mix together everything.
- Serve with coriander, sour cream or shredded cheese.

Keto beef stew

Preparation time-10 minutes| Cook time- Two hours and 10 minutes|Servings-6 |Difficulty-Hard

Nutritional value- Calories- 341| Proteins- 31g| Carbohydrates-9g| Fat- 20g

Ingredients

- One and a half lb. of sliced chuck roast
- Six cups of beef broth
- Two tablespoons of tomato paste
- Three teaspoons of salt
- One bay leaf
- Two minced garlic cloves
- One lb. of sliced turnips
- Two sliced carrots
- Two tablespoons of vinegar (red wine)
- One diced onion
- One tablespoon of chopped parsley
- One tablespoon of avocado oil
- One diced celery stalk
- One tablespoon of Worcestershire sauce
- Half teaspoon of xanthan gum

Instructions

- Toss beef with salt and set aside.

- Heat oil in a pan on medium heat.
- Place beef pieces in a single layer in a pan and cook for five minutes or turn brown.
- Dish out beef pieces and keep them aside.
- Pour vinegar and half a cup of broth in the same skillet on medium flame.
- After five minutes, add tomato paste, bay leaf, beef pieces and Worcestershire sauce and boil them all.
- Cover, reduce the flame to low and simmer it for 90 minutes.
- After the beef is tenderized, add carrots, garlic, turnips, salt and celery and mix.
- Mix xanthan gum in half cup of broth taken from the pan and pour in pan and cover.
- Simmer again for 45 minutes with occasional stirring.
- Serve after drizzling parsley over the beef.

Keto Slow Cooker Buffalo Chicken Soup

Preparation time-15 minutes |Cook time-6 hours |Servings-2 |Difficulty-Hard

Nutritional value: ~Calories-223|Proteins-6.3g| Fat-4.8g|Carbohydrates-32g

Ingredients

- Three Chicken Thighs, de-boned and sliced
- One teaspoon of Onion Powder
- One teaspoon of Garlic Powder
- Half teaspoon Celery Seed
- A quarter cup of butter
- Half cup of Frank's Hot Sauce
- Three cups of Beef Broth
- One cup of Heavy Cream
- Two oz. Cream Cheese
- A quarter teaspoon of Xanthan Gum
- Salt and pepper as per taste

Instructions

- Begin by de-boning the chicken thighs, break the chicken into chunks and place the remainder of the ingredients in a slow cooker in the crockpot with the exception of cream, cheese, and xanthan gum.
- Set a low, slow cooker for 6 hours (or a high one for 3 hours) and cook fully.
- Remove the chicken from the slow cooker until it is done, and shred it with a fork.
- Use the slow cooker to combine cream, cheese, and xanthan gum. Combine it all together

- Transfer the chicken to the slow cooker and blend.

- Season it with salt, pepper, and hot sauce. Serve.

Lentil and vegetable dal

Preparation time-10 minutes |Cook time-30 minutes |Servings-4 |Difficulty-Easy

Nutritional value: ~Calories-323|Proteins-6.3g| Fat-4.8g|Carbohydrates-56g

Ingredients

- Two tablespoons of coconut oil

- One large yellow onion, finely chopped

- One tablespoon of finely chopped fresh ginger

- Two cloves of garlic, minced

- Six cups of vegetable stock

- One cup of red lentils picked over and rinsed

- 1 /3 small head cauliflower, separated into florets and finely chopped

- One tablespoon of ground turmeric

- One teaspoon of ground coriander

- Half teaspoon of ground cumin

- A quarter teaspoon of ground cinnamon

- A quarter teaspoon of cayenne

- Two tablespoons of tomato paste

- One bunch of spinach washed well, stemmed, and thinly sliced

- One teaspoon of kosher salt

- Juice of one medium lime

- Two tablespoons of finely chopped fresh cilantro

- Half cup of plant-based plain yogurt

Instructions

- In a large soup pot over medium-high heat, heat coconut oil. Add yellow onion, ginger, and garlic, and cook, frequently stirring, for 5 minutes. Reduce heat if necessary to prevent burning.

- Stir in vegetable stock, red lentils, cauliflower, turmeric, coriander, cumin, cinnamon, and cayenne. Bring to a boil, reduce heat, and simmer for 20 minutes.

- When lentils and cauliflower are tender, place tomato paste in a small bowl. Ladle a little bit of broth into the bowl, stir until smooth, and stir mixture back into the soup pot.

- Add spinach, kosher salt, lime juice, and one tablespoon of cilantro, and simmer for 5 minutes.

- Whisk remaining one tablespoon of cilantro into yogurt, and serve dal warm with a dollop of cilantro yogurt.

- Make Naan serve with dal.

- Before making dal, in a large bowl, whisk together two and a half cups of all-purpose flour with one package of fast-acting instant yeast, two teaspoons of kosher salt, and one teaspoon of baking powder.

- In a medium bowl, whisk together 3 /4 cup warm water, three tablespoons of plain plant-based yogurt, and two tablespoons melted coconut oil. Stir wet ingredients into dry, and knead with your hands for 1 or 2 minutes to form a sticky dough. Let dough rise at room temperature for 45 minutes or until doubled.

- Ten minutes before serving, heat a large cast-iron frying pan over medium heat.

- Divide dough into six balls and stretch into teardrop shapes about 5 inches (12.5cm) long. Dampen dough with a little water, add to the hot pan a few at a time, and cook for about 1 minute per side.

- Brush the pan with 1 /2 teaspoon grapeseed oil to keep naan from sticking if necessary.

Lentil Soup with Cumin and Coriander

Preparation time-10 minutes |Cook time-20 minutes |Servings-8 |Difficulty-Easy

Nutritional value: ~Calories-228|Proteins-14.4g| Fat-0g|Carbohydrates-41g

Ingredients

- Eight cups of veggie broth

- Two cups of uncooked brown lentils

- Two sliced carrots

- Two cubed big Yukon gold potatoes

- Two bay leaves

- Two minced garlic cloves

- One chopped onion

- One chopped celery rib

- One teaspoon of ground coriander

- Half teaspoon of ground cumin

- Black pepper to taste

Instructions

- First, pick through the lentils, throw out any stones, and then rinse.

- Pour the broth into a pressure cooker and heat it up.

- Prepare the vegetables. Add to the pressure cooker, along with everything else.

- Close and seal the pressure cooker.

- Cook on high pressure for 10 minutes. After, wait for 5 minutes before quick-releasing.

- Check the tenderness of the lentils and potatoes.

- If not done, turn the pot back and finish cooking with the lid on, but not sealed or at pressure.

- Pick out the bay leaves and salt to taste.

- Serve with a squirt of lemon juice.

Lentil stew

Preparation time-10 minutes | Cook time-56 minutes | Servings-2 | Difficulty-Moderate

Nutritional value: ~Calories-215 | Proteins-15g | Fat-3.5g | Carbohydrates-36g

Ingredients

- One and a half cups of lentils

- One medium onion, chopped

- Four cloves fresh garlic, chopped

- One tablespoon of extra-virgin olive oil

- Five cups of canned low-sodium fat-free chicken broth

- One tablespoon of Worcestershire sauce

- One (15-ounce) can diced tomatoes, undrained

- One bay leaf

- Half teaspoon of fresh thyme

- Half teaspoon of cayenne

- A quarter teaspoon of freshly ground pepper

- Salt to taste

- Two large potatoes, peeled and chopped

- Four medium carrots, chopped

- One (10-ounce) bag of fresh spinach

- Dollop low-fat sour cream for garnish (optional)

- Multigrain crusty bread (optional)

Instructions

- Rinse lentils and set them aside. In a large deep skillet, sauté onion and garlic in olive oil until tender but not browned. Add lentils, chicken broth, Worcestershire sauce, tomatoes, bay leaf, thyme, cayenne, pepper, and salt to taste. Bring to a boil, cover, and reduce to simmer for 20 minutes.

- Add potatoes, carrots, and spinach, and stir to incorporate all ingredients. Bring to a boil, cover, reduce to medium-high, and cook for 20–30 minutes or until lentils and vegetables are tender and most of the liquid has been absorbed.

- Remove bay leaf and serve stew garnished with a dollop of sour cream and crusty multigrain bread, if desired.

Lime-Mint Soup

Preparation time-10 minutes | Cook time-20 minutes | Servings-4 | Difficulty-Easy

Nutritional value: ~Calories-214 | Proteins-5g | Fat-2g | Carbohydrates-7g

Ingredients

- Four cups of vegetable broth

- A quarter cup of fresh mint leaves

- A quarter cup of scallions

- Three garlic cloves, minced

- Three tablespoons of freshly squeezed lime juice

Instructions

- In a large stockpot, combine the broth, mint, scallions, garlic, and lime juice.

- Bring to a boil over medium-high heat.

- Cover, set heat to low, simmer for 15 minutes, and serve.

Meaty mushroom stew

Preparation time-15 minutes | Cook time-30 minutes | Servings-4 | Difficulty-Moderate

Nutritional value: ~Calories-225 | Proteins-7g | Fat-4.8g | Carbohydrates-31g

Ingredients

- Four tablespoons of extra-virgin olive oil

- Two medium yellow onions, finely chopped

- One small shallot halved and finely chopped

- Two medium stalks celery, finely chopped

- One large carrot, finely chopped

- One (10-oz.) pkg. of tiny white button mushrooms, halved

- Eight oz. of hen of the woods mushrooms, sliced

- Eight oz. of fresh chanterelle mushrooms, sliced

- Three cloves of garlic, finely chopped

- One teaspoon of kosher salt, plus more to taste

- Half teaspoon of freshly ground black pepper, plus more to taste

- One tablespoon of sweet Hungarian paprika

- One teaspoon of dried thyme

- One teaspoon of dried dill

- Two tablespoons of all-purpose flour

- Four cups of Mushroom Stock

- One cup of dry red wine

- One large russet potato, peeled and diced

- A quarter cup of finely chopped fresh Italian flat-leaf parsley

- One tablespoon of balsamic vinegar

Instructions

- In a 4-quart (4L) stockpot over medium-high heat, heat Two tablespoons of extra-virgin olive oil. Add yellow onions and shallot, and cook, frequently stirring, for 5 minutes.

- Add celery, carrot, white button mushrooms, hen of the woods mushrooms, chanterelle mushrooms, and garlic, and cook, frequently stirring, for about 10 minutes or until mushrooms begin to turn golden. Add remaining two tablespoons of olive oil as mushrooms begin to stick to the pan.

- Stir in kosher salt, black pepper, sweet Hungarian paprika, thyme, and dill.

- Add all-purpose flour to mushroom mixture, and stir for 2 minutes.

- Add three cups of Mushroom Stock, red wine, and russet potato, and bring to a boil. Reduce heat to medium, and cook, often stirring, for 10 minutes or until stew is thickened and vegetables are tender. Add additional stock if the stew is too thick for your liking.

- Remove from heat, and stir in Italian flat-leaf parsley and balsamic vinegar. Taste, add more kosher salt and black pepper if needed, and serve.

Meaty Seitan Stew

Preparation time-10 minutes | Cook time-10 minutes | Servings-6 | Difficulty-Easy

Nutritional value: ~Calories-213 | Proteins-2g | Fat-19g | Carbohydrates-29g

Ingredients

- Four cups of veggie broth

- Two cups of cubed seitan

- Six quartered baby potatoes

- Three chopped carrots

- One 15-ounce can of corn

- One 15-ounce can of green beans

- One chopped sweet onion

- Two bay leaves

- Two tablespoons of vegan-friendly Worcestershire sauce

- Two tablespoons of arrowroot powder

- One tablespoon of tomato paste

- One tablespoon of cumin

- One teaspoon of garlic powder

- One teaspoon of onion powder

- One teaspoon of paprika

Instructions

- Dissolve the arrowroot powder in a little bit of water.

- Pour (along with everything else) in the pressure cooker and stir.

- Close and seal the lid.

- Cook on high pressure for 10 minutes.

- Pick out the bay leaves before serving.

- Add some black pepper if desired.

Mexican Baked Potato Soup

Preparation time-5 minutes | Cook time-15 minutes | Servings-4 | Difficulty-Easy

Nutritional value: ~Calories-196 | Proteins-10g | Fat-0g | Carbohydrates-30g

Ingredients

- Four cups of veggie broth

- Four cups of diced potatoes

- Four diced garlic cloves

- One diced onion

- Half cup of salsa

- Half cup of nutritional yeast

- ⅛ cup of seeded jalapeno peppers

- One teaspoon of cumin

- A quarter teaspoon of oregano

- Black pepper to taste

Instructions

- Heat up a deep-bottomed saucepan with a lid.

- When hot, add the onion, jalapeno, and garlic. Stir until browning.

- Add potatoes, salsa, cumin, and oregano, and pour the broth over everything. Stir.

- Close and seal the lid.

- Cook for 10 minutes on high heat.

- Turn off the heat and let it stand for 10 minutes.

- To make the soup creamy, run through a blender.

- Add nutritional yeast and pepper.

- Serve!

Minestrone

Preparation time-15 minutes | Cook time-One hour | Servings-4 | Difficulty-Easy

Nutritional value: ~Calories-411 | Proteins-5.3g | Fat-8.8g | Carbohydrates-55g

Ingredients

- Four tablespoons of extra-virgin olive oil
- One large red onion, cut into small dice
- Three medium carrots, cut into small dice
- Four large stalks of celery, cut in small dice
- Five cloves of garlic, minced
- Three tablespoons of tomato paste
- Six cups of vegetable stock
- One large russet potato, peeled and cut in small dice
- One bay leaf
- One teaspoon of kosher salt, plus more to taste
- Half small head savoy cabbage, thinly sliced
- One (14-oz.) can of cannellini beans, rinsed and drained
- One (14-oz.) can of cranberry beans, rinsed and drained
- One (28-oz.) can of diced tomatoes, with juice
- Four tablespoons of finely chopped fresh Italian flat-leaf parsley
- One tablespoon of red wine vinegar
- Half teaspoon of freshly ground black pepper

Instructions

- In a large soup pot over medium-high heat, heat two tablespoons of extra-virgin olive oil. Add red onion, carrots, and celery, and cook, often stirring, for 5 minutes.
- Add two cloves of garlic, and stir for one minute more.
- Stir in tomato paste, mix well, and add vegetable stock. Bring to a boil.
- Add russet potato, bay leaf, and kosher salt. Reduce heat to a simmer, and cook for 15 minutes.
- Meanwhile, in a wide sauté pan over medium-high heat, heat the remaining two tablespoons of extra-virgin olive oil. Add remaining three cloves of garlic, and stir for 30 seconds.
- Add savoy cabbage, and cook, frequently stirring, for about 10 minutes or until cabbage is softened.
- Add cabbage to the soup pot along with cannellini beans, cranberry beans, tomatoes with juice, and two tablespoons of Italian flat-leaf parsley, and simmer for 30 minutes.

- Stir in red wine vinegar and black pepper. Allow soup to rest for 10 minutes, remove bay leaf, stir in remaining two tablespoons of Italian flat-leaf parsley, and serve.

Miso Soup

Preparation time-5 minutes | Cook time-10 minutes | Servings-4 | Difficulty-Easy

Nutritional value: ~Calories-74 | Proteins-4g | Fat-2g | Carbohydrates-9g

Ingredients

- Four cups of water
- One cup of cubed silken tofu
- Two chopped carrots
- Two chopped celery stalks
- One sliced onion
- Two tablespoons of miso paste
- Dash of vegan-friendly soy sauce

Instructions

- Put the carrots, onion, celery, tofu, wakame, and water in a deep bottomed saucepan with a lid.
- Close and seal.
- Cook on high pressure for 6 minutes.
- Turn off the heat and let it stand for 5 minutes.
- Open the lid and ladle out one cup of broth.
- Add the miso paste to this broth and whisk until completely dissolved.
- Pour back into pot and stir.
- Season with soy sauce and serve!

Miso udon bowl

Preparation time-5 minutes | Cook time-5 minutes | Servings-4 | Difficulty-Easy

Nutritional value: ~Calories-196 | Proteins-10g | Fat-0g | Carbohydrates-30g

Ingredients

- One (8-oz.) pkg. of udon noodles
- Four cups of kombu stock or vegetable stock
- One teaspoon of grapeseed oil
- One (4-oz.) pkg. of shiitake mushrooms, stemmed and thinly sliced
- One (1-in.) piece fresh ginger, finely grated
- One clove of garlic, minced

- One cup of wakame (seaweed)

- Half pkg. of firm silken tofu, cut into 1 /2 -in. (1.25cm) cubes

- Two tablespoons of white (Shiro) miso paste

- One (5-oz.) pkg. of baby spinach

Instructions

- Cook udon noodles in boiling water according to the package directions. Drain in a colander, rinse with cold water, and set aside.

- In a small saucepan over medium-high heat, heat kombu stock until simmering. 3 In a medium saucepan over medium-high heat, heat grapeseed oil. Add shiitake mushrooms, and sauté for 1 minute.

- Add ginger and garlic, and sauté for 30 seconds. Add heated stock, bring to a boil, and reduce heat to a simmer. Stir in wakame and tofu, and cook for 5 minutes.

- Ladle a half cup of soup into a small bowl, and whisk in white (Shiro) miso paste.

- Stir baby spinach and noodles into the soup, and cook for 1 minute or until spinach is wilted. Remove from heat and stir in miso mixture. Serve immediately.

Mushroom & Cardamom, Squash Soup

Preparation time~8 minutes |Cook time~30 minutes |Servings~2 to 3|Difficulty~Easy

Nutritional value: ~Calories-189|Proteins-3.7g| Fat-18.8g|Carbohydrates-4.7g

Ingredients

- One teaspoon of ginger

- One leek

- One teaspoon of Celtic sea salt

- 1/8 cup of coconut cream

- A quarter cup of mushrooms

- A quarter cup of passata

- ¾ cup of water

- A quarter cup of peeled squash

- Four cardamom pods

- One cup of herbs

- Dash of coconut oil

Instructions

- In a bowl, sugar, milk, salt, ginger, and past, cardamom into a squash. Cook and for 15 minutes.

- Blend the mixture.

- Sauté mushrooms in heated oil for five minutes.

- Serve in serving dish by making layers and serve.

Mushroom & Jalapeño Stew

Preparation time~20 minutes |Cook time~50 minutes |Servings~4 |Difficulty~Easy

Nutritional value: ~Calories-65|Proteins-2.8g| Fat-2.8g|Carbohydrates-1g

Ingredients

- Two teaspoons of olive oil

- One cup of leeks, chopped

- One garlic clove, minced

- Half cup of celery stalks, chopped

- Half cup of carrots, chopped

- One green bell pepper, chopped

- One jalapeño pepper, chopped

- Two and a half cups of mushrooms, sliced

- One and a half cups of vegetable stock

- Two tomatoes, chopped

- Two thyme sprigs, chopped

- One rosemary sprig, chopped

- Two bay leaves

- Half teaspoons of salt

- A quarter teaspoon of ground black pepper

- Two tablespoons of vinegar

Instructions

- Set a pot over medium heat and warm oil.

- Add in garlic and leeks and sauté until soft and translucent.

- Add in the black pepper, celery, mushrooms, and carrots.

- Cook as you stir for 12 minutes; stir in a splash of vegetable stock to ensure there is no sticking.

- Stir in the rest of the ingredients.

- Set heat to medium; allow to simmer for 25 to 35 minutes or until cooked through.

- Divide into individual bowls and serve warm.

Mushroom and cabbage borscht

Preparation time~10 minutes |Cook time-One hour 10 minutes |Servings-6 |Difficulty-Hard

Nutritional value: ~Calories-113|Proteins-2.3g| Fat-1.8g|Carbohydrates-22g

Ingredients

- Four small beets

- One tablespoon plus one teaspoon of grapeseed oil

- Two medium yellow onions, halved and thinly sliced

- Two medium carrots, thinly sliced

- Three large stalks of celery, thinly sliced

- One (10-oz.) pkg. of white button mushrooms, thinly sliced

- One tablespoon of sugar

- Two teaspoons of kosher salt

- A quarter teaspoon of freshly ground black pepper

- Two tablespoons of tomato paste

- Eight cups of mushroom stock

- One small head of savoy cabbage, shredded

- Two tablespoons of freshly squeezed lemon juice, or apple cider vinegar

- A quarter cup of finely chopped fresh dill

Instructions

- Preheat the oven to 400°F (200°C).

- Scrub beets, but do not peel. Roast beets on a baking sheet lined with parchment paper for about 30 minutes or until tender. Cool slightly, peel, and cut into 1/4 -inch (.5cm) dice. (Beets can be roasted 1 day in advance.)

- In a large soup pot over medium-high heat, heat the remaining one tablespoon of grapeseed oil. Add yellow onions, carrots, celery, button mushrooms, sugar, and kosher salt. Cook, frequently stirring, for 5 to 10 minutes or until onions are softened and vegetables begin to color.

- Stir in black pepper and tomato paste. Add mushroom stock and reserved beets. Increase heat to high, bring to a boil and stir in savoy cabbage. Reduce heat to medium-low, and cook, partially covered, stirring occasionally, for about 30 minutes or until cabbage is tender.

- Remove from heat, stir in lemon juice and fresh dill, and serve.

Mushroom barley soup

Preparation time-20 minutes |Cook time-One hour |Servings-4 |Difficulty-Hard

Nutritional value: ~Calories-196|Proteins-10g| Fat-0g|Carbohydrates-30g

Ingredients

- Nine cups of vegetable stock

- One oz. of dried Borowik, porcini, or forest mix mushrooms

- Two tablespoons of grapeseed oil

- Two large yellow onions, finely chopped

- Four small stalks of celery, finely chopped

- Two small carrots, finely chopped

- Three cloves of garlic, finely chopped

- Twelve oz. of button mushrooms, thinly sliced

- 3/4 cup of pearl barley

- Four medium yellow potatoes (such as Yukon Gold), peeled and cut in 1/2 -in. (1.25cm) dice

- One bay leaf

- Four tablespoons of finely chopped fresh Italian flat-leaf parsley

- One teaspoon of kosher salt, plus more to taste

- Half teaspoon of freshly ground black pepper

- Juice of half medium lemon

Instructions

- In a small saucepan over medium heat, bring one cup of vegetable stock to a simmer.

- Rinse dried mushrooms, place in a small bowl, and pour the hot stock over the top. Set aside to soften for 10 minutes.

- When mushrooms are softened, lift them out of stock, gently agitating to loosen any remaining soil, and lightly squeeze dry and finely chop. Reserve mushroom soaking liquid.

- In a large, heavy soup pot over medium heat, heat grapeseed oil. Add yellow onions, celery, and carrots, and cook, frequently stirring, for 10 minutes.

- Add chopped dried mushrooms, garlic, and button mushrooms, and cook for 5 minutes.

- Line a fine-mesh strainer with cheesecloth, and pour reserved mushroom soaking liquid through the strainer into the soup pot. Add remaining eight cups of vegetable stock, increase heat to high, and bring to a boil.

- Stir in the pearl barley, yellow potatoes, bay leaf, two tablespoons of Italian flat-leaf parsley, kosher salt, and black pepper. Reduce heat to medium-low, and cook for about 45 more minutes or until barley and vegetables are tender.

- Remove soup from heat, and remove bay leaf. Stir in lemon juice and the remaining two tablespoons of Italian flat-leaf parsley, taste to see if the soup needs more salt, and serve hot.

Mushroom soup

Preparation time-5 minutes |Cook time-45 minutes |Servings-2 to 4 |Difficulty-Moderate

Nutritional value: ~Calories-101|Proteins-11g| Fat-5g|Carbohydrates-7g

Ingredients

- Salt to taste

- Black pepper to taste

- Six sprigs thyme

- Four cups of chicken stock

- Three tablespoons of olive oil

- A quarter cup of whipping cream

- A quarter cup of Cognac

- A quarter cup of chopped chives

- Half cup of minced shallot

- One sprig rosemary

- One lb of mixed mushrooms

- One lb of cremini mushrooms

Instructions

- Chop the mushroom stems roughly, let them simmer, and cover for about an hour in the chicken broth.

- In a large skillet, heat the oil and sauté each shallot until they are transparent. Lightly add the spices, salt, and pepper.

- Chop the mushroom caps beautifully and precisely into the 1/2-inch dice. Add them as they are sliced into the shallots. Keep the heat very low until the mushroom fluid is released and then reabsorbed, and cook gently. Shake the cup so that they do not stick. Remove the rosemary and thyme.

- Turn the heat up, then add the Cognac. Flame it up if you. Cook down the mushroom cap or shallot mixture until well reduced and begin to turn the edges a bit golden.

- Strain the fungus from the broth of the chicken.

- To the filtered broth, apply the wonderful shallot mixture and mushroom cap and heat it gently.

- Swirl in and serve the cream and chives. Or serve, if you like to get fancy, in tiny sipping bowls topped with chives and softly whipped cream.

Not pea soup

Preparation time-10 minutes | Cook time-30 minutes | Servings-5 | Difficulty-Easy

Nutritional value: ~120 Calories | Fat-9g | Protein-5g | Carbohydrates-5g

Ingredients

- Three tablespoons of butter

- Half cup of chopped onion

- Half cup of chopped celery

- One medium carrot, grated

- Four ounces of ham

- Four cans (Fourteen and a half ounces, each) green beans

- Half teaspoon of dried thyme

- Two bay leaves

- Two pinches of cayenne

- Salt and ground black pepper, to taste

Instructions

- In a heavy saucepan, melt the butter and start sautéing the onion, celery, and carrot over medium heat.

- While that's happening, put your ham in your food processor with the S-blade in place, and pulse until it's chopped medium-fine. Scrape this out of the food processor and into the saucepan with the veggies. Give everything a stir while you're there.

- Return the processor bowl to its base, and put the S-blade back in. Dump in the green beans, liquid and all, and run the processor until the beans are pureed quite smooth.

- Go back and look at your sautéing vegetables; when they are soft, add the garlic.

- Sauté it with the vegetables for just a minute.

- Now dump in your green bean puree, and stir everything together. Add the thyme, bay leaves, and cayenne, and stir them in.

- Turn the heat to low, and bring the soup to a simmer. Let it cook for 15 minutes or so.

- Season with salt and pepper to taste, remove the bay leaves, and pour into mugs.

Old Fashioned Salmon Soup

Preparation time-10 minutes | Cook time-30 minutes | Servings-8 | Difficulty-Easy

Nutritional value: ~155 Calories | Fat-7g | Protein-14g | Carbohydrates-8g

Ingredients

- Two tablespoons of unsalted butter

- One medium chopped carrot

- Half cup of chopped celery

- Half cup of chopped onion

- One pound of sockeye salmon, cooked

- Two cups of reduced-sodium chicken broth

- Two cups of 1% low-fat milk

- 1/8 teaspoon of black pepper

- A quarter cup of cornstarch

- A quarter cup of water

Instructions

- Let the butter melt in a 3-quart saucepan on a stovetop burner. Add the vegetables to the saucepan and cook until tender.

- Add the pre-cooked salmon chunks to the pan.

- Stir together in the saucepan the chicken broth, milk, and black pepper. Bring mixture to a near-boil afterward, reduce heat to simmer.

- Combine the cornstarch and water and then slowly pour into broth mixture, stirring, until the soup is thickened.

- Simmer for another five minutes. Serve warm and enjoy!

Olive soup

Preparation time-10 minutes |Cook time-20 minutes|Servings-6 |Difficulty-Easy

Nutritional value: ~189 Calories| Fat-17g|Protein-2g|Carbohydrates-3g

Ingredients

- One quart of chicken broth, divided

- Half teaspoon of guar or xanthan

- One cup of minced black olives (you can buy cans of minced black olives)

- One cup of heavy cream

- A quarter cup of dry sherry

- Salt or Vege-Sal and ground black pepper, to taste

Instructions

- Put half a cup of the chicken broth in the blender with the guar and blend for a few seconds.

- Pour into a saucepan and add the remaining three and a half cups of broth and the olives.

- Heat until simmering, then whisk in the cream. Bring back to a simmer, stir in the sherry, and season with salt and pepper to taste.

Potato-broccoli soup with greens

Preparation time-10 minutes |Cook time-20 minutes |Servings-2 to 4 |Difficulty-Easy

Nutritional value: ~Calories-350|Proteins-17g| Fat-14g|Carbohydrates-42g

Ingredients

- Three medium red-gold potatoes, chopped

- Two cloves fresh garlic, minced

- Two cups of low-sodium, fat-free chicken broth

- Three cups of fresh broccoli florets

- Three scallions, sliced

- Two cups of 2% milk

- Three tablespoons of all-purpose flour

- Two cups of smoked Gouda cheese, shredded plus more for garnish

- Salt and freshly ground pepper to taste

- Two cups of coarsely torn escarole leaves, rinsed and drained

- One cup of peppered seasoned croutons for garnish

Instructions

- In a large pot, combine potatoes, garlic, and broth. Bring to a boil, then reduce heat, and let simmer uncovered until potatoes start to soften.

- With a heavy fork, slightly mash potatoes. Add broccoli, scallions, and milk, and heat to a simmer until florets are crispy tender.

- Reduce heat to very low, then add flour and Gouda cheese, gently stirring until cheese melts and sauce is thickened. Season with salt and pepper to taste. Divide soup into equal portions.

- Top each serving with escarole, additional cheese, and a scattering of croutons, and serve.

Pork, White Bean, and Spinach Soup

Preparation time-10 minutes| Cook time-40 minutes| Servings-4 |Difficulty-Easy

Nutritional value- Calories-156| Fat-4g |Carbohydrates-17g| Protein-17g

Ingredients

- Eight ounces of fresh spinach leaves

- One can of northern beans

- A quarter teaspoon of crushed red pepper flakes

- Half teaspoon of dried thyme

- Three cups of low-sodium chicken broth

- One (14.5 ounces) can of diced tomatoes

- Two (4-ounce) boneless pork chops cut into 1-inch cubes

- 1 medium onion, chopped

- One teaspoon of extra-virgin olive oil

Instructions

- Over medium heat, put a large pot and heat the olive oil.

- Throw in and sauté onion until tender. Add some pork and brown it on both sides.

- Mix in the red pepper flakes, thyme, tomatoes, broth, and beans. Boil it and lower the heat. Then simmer it for 30 minutes.

- Add wilt the spinach for about 5 minutes, and serve.

Red Curry-Coconut Milk Soup

Preparation time-5 minutes | Cook time-8 minutes | Servings-4 | Difficulty-Easy

Nutritional value: ~Calories-553 | Proteins-23g | Fat-24g | Carbohydrates-59g

Ingredients

- Two cups of veggie broth
- One and a half cups of red lentils
- One 15-ounce can of coconut milk
- One 14-ounce can of diced tomatoes (with liquid)
- One diced onion
- Three minced garlic cloves
- Two tablespoons of red curry paste
- ⅛ teaspoon of ground ginger
- Dash of red pepper
- Handful of spinach

Instructions

- Heat a deep-bottomed saucepan/pot.
- When hot, cook onion and garlic until they're beginning to brown.
- Add the curry paste, ground ginger, and red pepper.
- Stir to coat the onion and garlic in spices.
- Pour in the diced tomatoes with their liquid, coconut milk, veggie broth, and lentils.
- Stir before closing and sealing the lid.
- Cook for 6 minutes on high.
- Turn off the heat and let it stand for 10 minutes.
- When the pressure is all gone, throw in the spinach and serve when the leaves have wilted.

Red lentil soup

Preparation time-10 minutes | Cook time-45 minutes | Servings-2 to 4 | Difficulty-Moderate

Nutritional value: ~Calories-366 | Proteins-14.7g | Fat-15.4g | Carbohydrates-47g

Ingredients

- Four minced garlic cloves
- A quarter cup of olive oil
- One teaspoon of curry powder
- Two chopped carrots
- Two teaspoons of ground cumin
- One chopped onion
- Half teaspoon of dried thyme
- One cup of brown lentils
- Twenty-eight ounces of diced tomatoes
- Four cups of vegetable broth
- One teaspoon of salt
- Two cups of water
- One pinch of red pepper flakes
- One cup of chopped kale
- Black pepper to taste
- One and a half tablespoons of lemon juice

Instructions

- Cook carrots and onions in a quarter cup of heated olive oil in a Dutch oven over medium flame for five minutes.
- Stir in thyme, cumin, garlic, and curry powder.
- Cook for half a minute. Add tomatoes and cook for another five minutes.
- Add pepper flakes, broth, salt, lentils, black pepper, and water in a Dutch oven.
- Let it boil. Cover the oven, lower the flame and let it simmer for 30 minutes.
- Blend a portion of soup of about two cups in a food processor and transfer it into the pot again.
- Mix chopped greens and cook for another five minutes.
- Remove from the flame, mix lemon juice, and serve.

Roasted tomato basil soup

Preparation time-10 minutes | Cook time-50 minutes | Servings-2 to 4 | Difficulty-Easy

Nutritional value: ~Calories-114 | Proteins-4.5g | Fat-1g | Carbohydrates-23.7g

Ingredients

- Three lb of halved Roma tomatoes
- Olive oil
- Two chopped carrots
- Salt to taste
- Two chopped yellow onions
- Black pepper to taste
- Five minced garlic cloves
- Two ounces of basil leaves
- One cup of crushed tomatoes
- Three thyme sprigs

- One teaspoon of dry oregano

- Two teaspoons of thyme leaves

- Half teaspoon of paprika

- Two and a half cups of water

- Half teaspoon of cumin

- One tablespoon of lime juice

Instructions

- Mix salt, olive oil, carrot, black pepper, and tomatoes in a bowl.

- Transfer carrot mixture to a baking tray and bake in a preheated oven at 450 degrees for 30 minutes.

- Blend baked tomato mixture in a blender. You can use a little water if needed during blending.

- Sauté onions in heated olive oil over medium flame in a pot for three minutes.

- Mix garlic and cook for one more minute.

- Transfer the blended tomato mixture to the pot, followed by the addition of crushed tomatoes, water, spices, thyme, salt, basil, and pepper.

- Let it boil. Reduce the flame and simmer for 20 minutes.

- Drizzle lemon juice and serve.

Roasted Tomato Soup

Preparation time-20 minutes | Cook time-20 minutes | Servings-6 | Difficulty-Moderate

Nutritional value: ~Calories-126 | Proteins-3g | Fat-6g | Carbohydrates-8g

Ingredients

- Three pounds of tomatoes in a halved manner

- Six garlic(smashed)

- Four teaspoons of cooking oil or virgin oil

- Salt to taste

- A quarter cup of vegan heavy cream(optional)

- Sliced fresh basil leaves for garnish

Instructions

- Oven medium heat of about 427°F, preheat the oven.

- In your mixing bowl, mix the halved tomatoes, garlic, olive oil, salt and pepper

- Spread the tomato mixture on the already prepared baking sheet

- For a process of 20- 28 minutes, roast and stir.

- Then remove it from the oven, and the roasted vegetables should now be transferred to a soup pot.

- Stir in the basil leaves.

- Blend in small portions in a blender.

- Serve immediately.

Roman stew

Preparation time-10 minutes | Cook time-8 hours | Servings-8 | Difficulty-Easy

Nutritional value: ~413 Calories | Fat-31g | Protein-28g | Carbohydrates-5g

Ingredients

- Two pounds of beef round, cut into 1-inch (2.5 cm) cubes

- One large onion, chopped

- Two cans (Six and a half ounces, each) sliced mushrooms

- One and a half cups of beef broth

- Two teaspoons of Worcestershire sauce

- One teaspoon of beef bouillon concentrate

- One teaspoon of paprika

- Eight ounces of cream cheese

- Eight ounces of sour cream

Instructions

- In your big, heavy skillet, over medium-high heat, brown the beef in the oil, working in a few batches. Transfer to a slow cooker.

- Add the celery and garlic, then sprinkle the seasonings over everything. Now pour the canned tomatoes and the wine over everything. Cover the pot, set the slow cooker to low, and cook for 7 to 8 hours.

- You can thicken the pot juices a little if you like, but it's not really necessary.

Root Veggie Soup

Preparation time-10 minutes | Cook time-30 minutes | Servings-8 | Difficulty-Moderate

Nutritional value: ~Calories-256 | Proteins-24g | Fat-14g | Carbohydrates-31g

Ingredients

- Seven cups of veggie broth

- Six cups of peeled and chopped russet potatoes

- Three cups of peeled and chopped carrots

- One cup of Italian-style tomatoes (canned)

- One cup of chopped yellow onion

- Half cup of coconut oil

- Two tablespoons of garlic powder

- One tablespoon of mild chili powder

- One tablespoon of salt

Instructions

- Pour everything in a deep pot with a lid.
- Stir before closing the lid.
- Let it boil and cook for around 30 minutes.
- Turn off the heat and let it stand for around 10 minutes.
- To make the soup creamy, blend until smooth.
- Taste and season more if necessary.

Salmon soup

Preparation time-10 minutes |Cook time-13 minutes |Servings-2 to 4|Difficulty-Easy

Nutritional value: -Calories-388|Proteins-32.4g| Fat-10.7g|Carbohydrates-30.3g

Ingredients

- Olive oil
- Half chopped green bell pepper
- Four chopped green onions
- Four minced garlic cloves
- Five cups of chicken broth
- One ounce of chopped dill
- One lb of sliced gold potatoes
- One teaspoon of dry oregano
- One sliced carrot
- ¾ teaspoons of coriander
- Kosher salt to taste
- Half teaspoon of cumin
- Black pepper to taste
- Zest of one lemon
- One lb of sliced salmon fillet
- One tablespoon of lemon juice

Instructions

- Cook onions, garlic, and bell pepper in heated olive oil in a pot over medium flame for four minutes.
- Stir in the dill and cook for half a minute.
- Pour broth into the pot. Add carrot, potatoes, salt, spices, and pepper.
- Let it boil. Reduce the flame and let it simmer for six minutes.
- Add salmon and cook for five more minutes.
- Add lemon juice and zest and cook for one minute.

- Serve the soup and enjoy it.

Shrimp Gazpacho-Style Soup

Preparation time-10 minutes| Cook time-10 minutes|Servings-4 |Difficulty-Easy

Nutritional value- Calories-109| Fat-4g |Carbohydrates-9g| Protein-11g

Ingredients

- One and a half cups of cooked shrimp
- Half teaspoon of salt
- Four teaspoons of freshly squeezed lemon juice
- Three cups of chopped tomato
- Half cup of diced bell pepper
- One cup of chopped yellow onion
- One tablespoon of extra-virgin olive oil

Instructions

- Oil a medium skillet and put it over medium heat. Add some pepper and onion. Then cook until the onion becomes mildly translucent.
- Then, in a blender, add the pepper, lemon juice, cooked onion, tomato, and salt. Run the blender on high until everything's smooth.
- Pour the soup into a serving bowl, add shrimp on top and serve.

Simple Beef-and-Veggie Soup

Preparation time-5 minutes| Cook time-35 minutes| Servings-4 |Difficulty-Easy

Nutritional value- Calories-175| Fat-8g |Carbohydrates-12g| Protein-13g

Ingredients

- Eight ounces of lean ground beef
- Nonstick cooking spray
- One cup of chopped yellow onion
- Three teaspoons of powdered beef bouillon
- Three cups of water
- Two cups of peeled, chopped carrot
- One teaspoon of garlic powder
- One tablespoon of extra-virgin olive oil

Instructions

- Heat up the oil in a medium pot over medium heat. Cook the onion and carrot until the onion is translucent.
- Add some bouillon, water, and garlic powder. Simmer for about 5 minutes.

- Over medium heat, heat up a small skillet sprayed with cooking spray as the broth simmers. Add and cook the beef until it is no longer raw. Turn off the heat and put beef in the pot with the broth and vegetables.

- Simmer the soup for 20 minutes on medium-low heat until the carrots soften. Serve on a plate and enjoy.

Smoky white bean and tomato soup

Preparation time-10 minutes |Cook time-One hour |Servings-6 |Difficulty-Hard

Nutritional value: ~Calories-383|Proteins-2.3g| Fat-7.8g|Carbohydrates-42g

Ingredients

- Two cups of dry great northern beans or other small white beans soaked 6 hours or overnight

- Eight cups of vegetable stock or filtered water

- Four cloves of garlic, thinly sliced

- One tablespoon of finely chopped fresh rosemary

- One teaspoon of finely chopped fresh thyme or a half teaspoon of dried

- A quarter cup of tomato paste

- One teaspoon of smoked sea salt

- One teaspoon of kosher salt

- One large yellow onion, chopped

- Four small stalks celery, cut in 1 /4 -in. (.5cm) dice

- One (28-oz.) can of diced tomatoes, with juice

- A quarter cup of plus two tablespoons of extra-virgin olive oil

- A quarter teaspoon of crushed red pepper flakes

- A quarter teaspoon of freshly ground black pepper

- One tablespoon of apple cider vinegar

Instructions

- Drain soaked great northern beans, rinse well, and place in a large soup pot. Cover with vegetable stock, add garlic, rosemary, and thyme, and bring to a boil over high heat. Reduce heat to a simmer, and cook, partially covered, for 30 minutes. Taste beans for tenderness; they should be almost completely cooked but slightly al dente at this point. If not, cook for 10 to 15 more minutes.

- Place tomato paste in a small bowl, and ladle in a little of the hot stock. Stir well, and add tomato paste mixture, smoked sea salt, kosher salt, yellow onion, celery, tomatoes with juice, a quarter cup of extra-virgin olive oil, crushed red pepper flakes, and black pepper. Increase heat to high, and return to a boil. Reduce heat to medium-low, and simmer, uncovered, for 30 minutes or until beans are completely tender.

- Remove from heat, and stir in apple cider vinegar and the remaining two tablespoons of olive oil. If desired, remove the half cup of soup to a blender, purée, return

to the pot, and stir (or use an immersion blender to purée slightly). Serve hot.

Sopa tlalpeño

Preparation time-10 minutes |Cook time-30 minutes|Servings-6 |Difficulty-Easy

Nutritional value: ~235 Calories| Fat-13g|Protein-26g|Carbohydrates-4g

Ingredients

- One and a half quarts of chicken broth, divided

- One pound of boneless, skinless chicken breast

- One chipotle chile canned in adobo

- One Hass avocado

- Four scallions, sliced

- Salt and ground black pepper, to taste

- 3/4 cup of shredded Monterey Jack cheese

Instructions

- Pour the chicken broth into a large, heavy-bottomed saucepan, reserving a half cup of it, and place it over medium-high heat.

- While it's heating, cut your chicken breast into thin strips or small cubes, then add to the broth. Let the whole thing simmer for 10 to 15 minutes, or until the chicken is cooked through.

- Put the reserved chicken broth in your blender with the chipotle and blend until the chipotle is puréed. Pour this mixture into the soup and stir.

- Split the avocado in half, remove the seed, peel it, and cut it into Half-inch (1 cm) chunks. Add to the soup, along with the scallions, and salt and pepper to taste.

- Ladle the soup into bowls and top each serving with shredded cheese.

Spicy Chili with Red Lentils

Preparation time-15 minutes |Cook time-20 minutes |Servings-5 |Difficulty-Easy

Nutritional value: ~Calories-420|Proteins-24g| Fat-2g|Carbohydrates-68g

Ingredients

- Seven cups of water

- Two cups of red lentils

- Two diced red peppers

- One diced onion

- 14-ounce can of diced tomatoes

- Five minced garlic cloves

- A quarter cup of brown sugar

- 6-ounce can of tomato paste

- Two tablespoons of apple cider vinegar
- One tablespoon of paprika
- One tablespoon of chili powder
- One teaspoon of cayenne

Instructions

- Prepare your ingredients.
- Throw everything in the dee pot and seal the lid.
- Cook for 17 minutes on high pressure.
- Turn down the flame and wait for 15 minutes before opening up the lid.
- Stir and serve over rice!

Spicy vegetable stew

Preparation time-10 minutes | Cook time-25 minutes | Servings-2 | Difficulty-Easy

Nutritional value: ~Calories-288 | Proteins-12g | Fat-2g | Carbohydrates-43g

Ingredients

- Four cups of fresh cauliflower florets
- Two teaspoons of curry powder
- Half teaspoon of cumin
- One (14.5-ounce) can fiery roasted diced tomatoes, undrained
- Two cloves fresh garlic, finely minced
- One tablespoon of finely chopped Serrano chili pepper
- One (15-ounce) can chickpeas, drained
- 3/4 cup of solid packed canned pumpkin mash
- 3/4 cup of water
- Salt and freshly ground pepper to taste
- One cup of frozen baby peas
- One cup of frozen corn
- Couscous or brown rice, cooked

Instructions

- Place cauliflower florets in a pot and cover them partially with water. Bring to a boil, cover, and steam until florets are almost tender. Remove from heat, drain well, and cut large florets into smaller sizes. Set aside.
- In a large, non-stick skillet over medium heat, add curry powder and cumin and heat until fragrant. Add tomatoes with juices, garlic, chili pepper, chickpeas, pumpkin, and water. Bring to a boil, then reduce heat to a simmer.
- Add florets and salt and pepper to taste and let simmer for about 15 minutes. Add peas and corn and let simmer for 5 minutes longer. Remove from heat and serve over cooked couscous or brown rice.

Spinach feta cheese soup

Preparation time-10 minutes | Cook time-20 minutes | Servings-2 | Difficulty-Easy

Nutritional value: ~Calories-226 | Proteins-10g | Fat-10g | Carbohydrates-24g

Ingredients

- Ten ounces of spinach, washed under running water, divided
- Six cups of low-sodium, fat-free chicken broth, divided
- A quarter cup of fresh cilantro, chopped
- Two tablespoons of extra-virgin olive oil
- One large white onion, coarsely chopped
- Two medium potatoes, peeled and diced
- Four cloves fresh garlic, minced
- One teaspoon of ground cumin
- One (10-ounce) package of frozen baby lima beans, thawed
- 1/3 cup of couscous
- Six ounces of feta cheese, cut into chunks
- Half teaspoon of freshly ground pepper to taste
- Finely chopped fresh parsley for garnish
- Lemon wedges for garnish

Instructions

- Cut half of the spinach leaves into thin ribbons, reserving stems, and set aside.
- Using a food processor or blender, combine the reserved stems and the remaining spinach with one cup of broth and cilantro. Process until smooth and set aside.
- In a large pot, heat olive oil over medium heat, add onion, sauté until golden brown, and then add potatoes, garlic, and cumin; stir to make sure potatoes are well coated. Add remaining five cups of broth.
- Reduce heat to medium and cook until potatoes are tender, roughly 15 minutes. Add ribbon spinach, spinach-cilantro puree, lima beans, couscous, and feta cheese. Cook, until lima beans are crispy tender and cheese has melted through soup. Season soup with freshly ground pepper.
- Divide soup into equal servings. For garnish, sprinkle parsley over soup and add a lemon wedge on the side.

Spinach Soup

Preparation time- 5 minutes | Cook time- 25 minutes | Servings-8 | Difficulty-Easy

Nutritional value- Calories-202 Fat- 4.3g | Carbohydrates-7.3g | Protein- 9.1g

Ingredients

- Two tablespoons of ghee
- Twenty ounces of chopped spinach
- One teaspoon of minced garlic
- Salt and black pepper as per taste
- Forty-five ounces of chicken stock
- Half teaspoons of ground nutmeg
- Two cups of heavy cream
- One chopped yellow onion

Instructions

- Heat a pot over medium heat with the ghee, add the onion, stir and simmer for 4 minutes.
- Stir in the garlic, stir and simmer for a minute.
- Add spinach and stock and simmer for 5 minutes.
- Blend the broth with an immersion mixer and reheat the soup.
- Stir in pepper, nutmeg, salt, and cream, stir and simmer for a further 5 minutes.
- Ladle it into cups and serve.

Split Pea Soup

Preparation time-10 minutes | Cook time-1 hour 10 minutes | Serving-1 gallon | Difficulty- Hard

Nutritional value: ~Calories-92 | Fat-1g | Protein-8g | Carbohydrates-20g

Ingredients

- One tablespoon of extra-virgin olive oil
- Two large carrots, chopped
- One medium onion, diced
- Two garlic cloves, minced
- Four cups of chicken broth
- Two cups of water
- Salt
- Freshly ground black pepper
- Two dried bay leaves
- One (16-ounce) bag of green split peas

Instructions

- In a large stockpot over medium heat, heat the oil.
- Add the carrot, onion, and garlic. Sauté until soft, 5 to 7 minutes.

- Add the broth, water, salt and pepper to taste, bay leaves, and split peas. Stir well, and bring to a boil.
- Reduce to a simmer, cover, and let cook for 1 hour, or until the peas are soft.
- Remove the bay leaves, and serve immediately.

Stracciatella

Preparation time-10 minutes | Cook time-20 minutes | Servings-4 | Difficulty-Easy

Nutritional value: -117 Calories | Fat-7g | Protein-12g | Carbohydrates-2g

Ingredients

- One quart of chicken broth, divided
- Two eggs
- Half cup of grated Parmesan cheese
- Half teaspoon of lemon juice
- Pinch of ground nutmeg
- Half teaspoon of dried marjoram

Instructions

- Put a quarter cup of the broth into a glass measuring cup or small pitcher. Pour the rest into a large saucepan over medium heat.
- Add the eggs to the broth in the measuring cup and beat with a fork. Then add the Parmesan, lemon juice, and nutmeg, and beat with a fork until well blended.
- When the broth in the saucepan is simmering, stir it with a fork as you add small amounts of the egg-and-cheese mixture, until it's all stirred in. (Don't expect this to form long shreds like Chinese egg drop soup; because of the Parmesan, it makes small, fluffy particles instead.)
- Add the marjoram, crushing it a bit between your fingers, and simmer the soup for another minute or so before serving.

Tavern soup

Preparation time-10 minutes | Cook time-8 hours | Servings-8 | Difficulty-Hard

Nutritional value: -274 Calories | Fat-20g | Protein-18g | Carbohydrates-3g

Ingredients

- One and a half quarts of chicken broth
- A quarter cup of finely diced celery
- A quarter cup of finely diced green bell pepper
- A quarter cup of shredded carrot
- A quarter cup of chopped fresh parsley
- Half teaspoon of ground black pepper
- One pound of sharp Cheddar cheese, shredded

- Twelve ounces of light beer
- Half teaspoon of salt or Vege-Sal
- A quarter teaspoon of hot pepper sauce
- Guar or xanthan, as needed

Instructions

- Combine the broth, celery, green pepper, carrot, parsley, and black pepper in your slow cooker. Cover the pot, set the slow cooker to low, and let it cook for 6 to 8 hours.

- When the time's up, either use a handheld blender to purée the vegetables right there in the slow cooker or scoop them out with a slotted spoon, purée them in your blender, and return them to the slow cooker.

- Now whisk in the cheese a little at a time until it's all melted in. Add the beer, salt, and hot pepper sauce, and stir until the foaming stops.

- Use guar as needed to thicken your soup until it's about the texture of heavy cream. Re-cover the pot, turn the slow cooker to high, and let it cook for another 20 minutes before serving.

Tofu Stir Fry with Asparagus Stew

Preparation time-15 minutes |Cook time-30 minutes |Servings-4 |Difficulty-Easy

Nutritional value: ~Calories-138|Proteins-7g| Fat-9g|Carbohydrates-12g

Ingredients

- One pound of asparagus cut off stems
- Two tablespoons of olive oil
- Two blocks of tofu pressed and cubed
- Two garlic cloves, minced
- One teaspoon of Cajun spice mix
- One teaspoon of mustard
- One bell pepper, chopped
- A quarter cup of vegetable broth
- Salt and black pepper, to taste

Instructions

- Using a huge saucepan with lightly salted water, place in asparagus and cook until tender for 10 minutes; drain.
- Set a wok over high heat and warm olive oil; stir in tofu cubes and cook for 6 minutes.
- Place in garlic and cook for 30 seconds until soft.
- Stir in the remaining ingredients, including reserved asparagus, and cook for an additional 4 minutes.
- Divide among plates and serve.

Tom yum soup

Preparation time-15 minutes |Cook time-10 minutes |Servings-4 |Difficulty-Easy

Nutritional value: ~Calories-196|Proteins-10g| Fat-0g|Carbohydrates-30g

Ingredients

- Two large stalks of fresh lemongrass
- One teaspoon of coconut oil or grapeseed oil
- Two tablespoons of finely chopped galangal or ginger
- Three Kaffir lime leaves, fresh or frozen, or the zest of one medium lime
- One small fresh hot red chile pepper, such as Thai bird chile or Serrano, thinly sliced
- Two teaspoons of sambal oelek (chili garlic sauce)
- Five cups of Golden Chicken-y Stock or vegetable stock
- Six oz. of white button mushrooms, sliced
- A quarter lb. of firm silken tofu, cut in 1 /2 -in. (1.25cm) cubes
- Two tablespoons of reduced-sodium tamari
- Juice of one and a half medium limes
- A quarter cup of finely chopped fresh cilantro

Instructions

- Peel tough outer layer from lemongrass stalks and smash stalks with the flat side of your knife to tenderize. Chop finely.
- In a medium saucepan over medium-high heat, heat coconut oil. Add lemongrass, galangal, Kaffir lime leaves, hot red chile pepper, and sambal oelek, and stir for one minute.
- Add Golden Chicken-y Stock, button mushrooms, tofu, and tamari, and bring to a boil.
- Reduce heat to medium, and cook for 10 minutes or until mushrooms are tender.
- Remove from heat, remove and discard lime leaves, stir in lime juice and cilantro, and serve.

Tomato rice soup

Preparation time-10 minutes |Cook time-20 minutes |Servings-8 |Difficulty-Easy

Nutritional value: ~Calories-216|Proteins-10g| Fat-2.7g|Carbohydrates-31g

Ingredients

- Three tablespoons of extra-virgin olive oil
- Two medium leeks, thinly sliced
- One large carrot, finely chopped
- Four medium stalks celery, finely chopped

- Two cloves of garlic, finely chopped

- One teaspoon of kosher salt

- One teaspoon of sweet Hungarian paprika

- Half teaspoon of freshly ground black pepper

- A quarter teaspoon of smoked paprika

- A quarter teaspoon of ground allspice

- A quarter teaspoon of ground cloves

- One bay leaf

- One (28-oz.) can of plum tomatoes, with juice, crushed by hand

- Four cups of vegetable stock or filtered water

- Half cup of white basmati rice

- A quarter cup of dry white wine

- Half teaspoon of hot sauce (optional)

Instructions

- In a medium soup pot over medium-high heat, heat extra-virgin olive oil. Add leeks, carrot, and celery, and cook for about 5 minutes or until leek is reduced and softened.

- Add garlic, kosher salt, sweet Hungarian paprika, black pepper, smoked paprika, allspice, cloves, and bay leaf, and stir for 1 minute.

- Add crushed tomatoes with juice and vegetable stock, bring to a boil, and stir in white basmati rice. Reduce heat to medium, cover, and cook, occasionally stirring, for 15 minutes or until rice is tender.

- Remove bay leaf, and stir in white wine and hot sauce (if using). Serve immediately, or freeze in an airtight container for up to 3 months.

Tomato tortellini soup

Preparation time-10 minutes |Cook time-20 minutes |Servings-2 |Difficulty-Easy

Nutritional value: ~Calories-148|Proteins-5g| Fat-5g|Carbohydrates-20g

Ingredients

- One tablespoon of olive oil

- One white onion, chopped

- Half teaspoon of crushed red hot pepper flakes

- Two teaspoons of chopped fresh garlic

- Two cups of low-sodium, fat-free chicken broth

- One cup of water

- Two teaspoons of beef bouillon base

- One (14.5-ounce) can dice low-sodium tomatoes with basil and garlic

- One (15-ounce) can of low-sodium tomato sauce

- One tablespoon of dry Italian seasoning mix

- Salt and freshly ground pepper to taste

- One (16-ounce) bag cheese tortellini

- Crusty bread

Instructions

- In a large skillet over medium heat, add olive oil, onion, hot pepper flakes, and garlic. Sauté until onion and garlic are soft. Transfer to a large soup pot.

- Add broth, water, and beef base to the pot, and bring to a boil, then reduce heat to a simmer. Add tomatoes, tomato sauce, Italian seasoning, and salt and pepper to taste.

- Let simmer for 15 minutes, then add tortellini, and let simmer for another 5 minutes or until tortellini is soft.

- Serve while hot with crusty bread.

Turkish mussel stew

Preparation time-10 minutes |Cook time-50 minutes |Servings-2 to 4|Difficulty-Moderate

Nutritional value: ~Calories-236|Proteins-14g| Fat-9g|Carbohydrates-20g

Ingredients

- One cup of dry white wine

- One cup of water

- Six dozen mussels, scrubbed and debearded (discard any open mussels)

- Two tablespoons of extra-virgin olive oil

- One medium onion, peeled and sliced

- One leek, white part only, sliced

- Six cloves fresh garlic, coarsely chopped

- Four large tomatoes, peeled and diced

- Two large white potatoes, peeled, sliced about 1/4-inch thick

- Two medium carrots, cleaned and chunked

- Pinch of saffron

- Two bay leaves

- Salt and freshly ground pepper to taste

- A quarter cup of finely chopped fresh flat-leaf parsley

Instructions

- In a large, heavy saucepan, combine wine, water, and mussels. Cover pan and steam mussels until they open (roughly about 7–10 minutes). Remove mussels from liquid and discard any that have not opened. Set mussel liquid aside.

- Remove mussels from shells and add a small amount of liquid to keep them moist. Strain remaining mussel liquid through cheesecloth and set aside.

- In a clean saucepan, add olive oil and gently sauté onion, leek, and garlic until tender, then add tomatoes and cook for another 1–2 minutes.

- Add potato slices, carrots, saffron, bay leaves, and strained mussel liquid; cover the pan and cook over medium-low heat until vegetables are tender (about 30 minutes).

- Add mussels to the mixture and continue cooking until all is heated thoroughly; add salt and pepper to taste. Remove from heat and stir in parsley. Serve while hot.

Turkish Soup

Preparation time-5 minutes |Cook time-10 minutes |Servings-10 |Difficulty-Easy

Nutritional value: ~Calories-531|Proteins-29g| Fat-9g|Carbohydrates-67g

Ingredients

- One cup of red lentils
- One chopped carrot
- One chopped potato
- One chopped onion
- Half cup of celery
- Three minced garlic cloves
- Half tablespoon of rice
- Three teaspoons of olive oil
- Half teaspoon of paprika
- Half teaspoon of coriander
- Salt to taste

Instructions

- Heat a deep-bottomed pot with a lid, add oil.
- While that heats up, prepare your veggies.
- When oil is hot, cook the garlic for a few minutes until fragrant.
- Rinse off the rice and lentils, and put them in the pot.
- Add two and a half cups of water, paprika, salt, and veggies.
- Close and seal the lid.
- Cook on high pressure for 10 minutes.
- Turn down the flame and let it rest for 10 minutes.
- Let the mixture cool for a little while before pureeing in a blender.
- Serve!

Vegetable and tortellini soup

Preparation time-10 minutes |Cook time-20 minutes |Servings-2 |Difficulty-Easy

Nutritional value: ~Calories-213|Proteins-7g| Fat-7g|Carbohydrates-26g

Ingredients

- One large white onion, chopped
- Four cloves fresh garlic, chopped
- Three celery stalks, chopped
- Two tablespoons of olive oil
- Thirty-two ounces low-sodium, fat-free chicken broth
- One cup of frozen corn
- One cup of chopped carrot
- One cup of frozen cut green beans
- One cup of diced raw potato
- One teaspoon of dried sweet basil
- One teaspoon of dried thyme
- One teaspoon of minced chives
- Two (14.5-ounce) cans of diced tomatoes, undrained
- Three cups of fresh chicken-filled tortellini
- Shredded fat-free or low-fat cheddar cheese (optional)
- Crusty croutons for garnish (optional)

Instructions

- In a large pot, sauté onion, garlic, celery, and olive oil until soft and fragrant. Add broth, corn, carrot, beans, potato, basil, thyme, and chives. Bring to a boil.

- Reduce heat, cover, and let simmer for about 15 minutes or until vegetables are tender. Add tomatoes and tortellini and let simmer uncovered for another 5 minutes or until heated through.

- Serve hot with a sprinkling cheddar cheese and a few crusty croutons, if desired.

Veggie-Quinoa Soup

Preparation time-5 minutes |Cook time-5 minutes |Servings-6 |Difficulty-Easy

Nutritional value: ~Calories-201|Proteins-11g| Fat-1.1g|Carbohydrates-37g

Ingredients

- Three cups of boiling water
- Two bags of frozen mixed veggies (12-ounces each)
- One 15-ounce can of white beans
- One 15-ounce can of fire-roasted diced tomatoes
- One 15-ounce can of pinto beans

- A quarter cup of rinsed quinoa

- One tablespoon of dried basil

- One tablespoon of minced garlic

- One tablespoon of hot sauce

- Half tablespoon of dried oregano

- Dash of salt

- Dash of black pepper

Instructions

- Put everything in the pot and stir.

- Close and seal the lid.

- Cook for 2 minutes on high pressure.

- Turn down the heat and let it stand for some time.

- When all the pressure is gone, open the pot and season to taste.

- Serve!

Weeknight Three-Bean Chili

Preparation time-10 minutes |Cook time-8 minutes |Servings-6 |Difficulty-Easy

Nutritional value: ~Calories-167|Proteins-11g| Fat-1g|Carbohydrates-31g

Ingredients

- Three and a half cups of vegetable broth

- One can of black beans

- One can of red beans

- One can of pinto beans

- One 14.5-ounce can of diced tomatoes

- One 14.5-ounce can of tomato sauce

- Two cups of chopped onion

- ¾ cup of chopped carrots

- A quarter cup of chopped celery

- One chopped red bell pepper

- Two tablespoons of mild chili powder

- One tablespoon of minced garlic

- One and a half teaspoons of ground cumin

- One and a half teaspoons of dried oregano

- One teaspoon of smoked paprika

Instructions

- Rinse and drain the canned beans.

- Heat a pressure cooker before throwing in the onion and garlic to sauté for 5 minutes or so.

- Add the rest of the ingredients, except the tomatoes and tomato sauce. Stir.

- Close and seal the lid.

- Cook on high pressure for 6 minutes.

- Let the pressure come down naturally. When the pressure is gone, stir in the tomato sauce and diced tomatoes.

- If you want a thicker chili, spoon out two cups of the chili and blend before returning to the pot.

- Serve with fresh parsley if desired.

Wild Rice Mushroom Soup

Preparation time-20 minutes| Cook time-25 minutes| Servings-4 |Difficulty-Moderate

Nutritional value- Calories-170| Fat-5g |Carbohydrates-20g| Protein-7g

Ingredients

- A quarter cup of carrots, chopped

- A quarter cup of celery, chopped

- One cup of cooked wild rice

- Two and a half cups of fat-free chicken broth (low-sodium)

- Half cup of low-sodium, low-fat chicken broth or a half cup of white wine

- One and a half cups of sliced fresh white mushrooms

- Black pepper

- One tablespoon of olive oil

- Two tablespoons of flour

- Half a white onion, chopped

- A quarter teaspoon of dried thyme

- One cup of fat-free half and half

Instructions

- Bring olive oil to low heat in a stockpot.

- Stir in the celery, onion, and carrots that have been chopped. Cook until the vegetables are tender.

- Combine the white wine, mushrooms, and chicken broth in a medium bowl. Cover and continue heating until thoroughly heated.

- In a large mixing bowl, whisk together half-&-half thyme, flour and pepper.

- Stir and cook wild rice.

- Transfer the rice mixture to a hot stockpot along with the vegetables. Then cook above moderate heat. Continue stirring until the mixture is bubbly and thickened.

Chapter 10-Salad Recipes

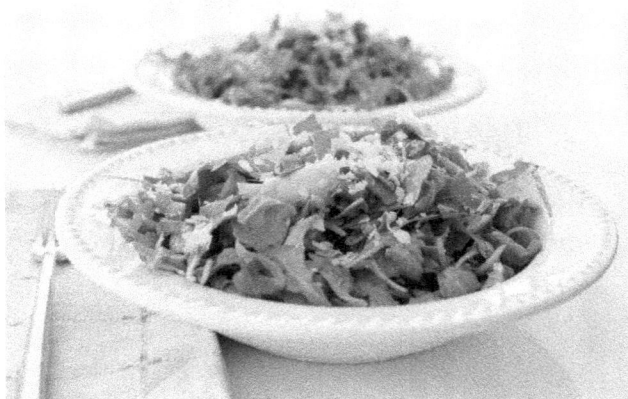

Arugula and artichoke salad with citrus dressing

Preparation time-10 minutes | Cook time-0 minutes | Servings-2 to 4 | Difficulty-Easy

Nutritional value: ~Calories-126 | Proteins-8g | Fat-8g | Carbohydrates-16g

Ingredients

- Ten ounces of arugula
- Half red onion, sliced into 1-inch pieces
- One cup of cherry tomatoes halved
- Half cup of pomegranate seeds
- One and a half cups of canned artichoke hearts that are quartered and drained

For the dressing

- Two tablespoons of orange juice
- Two teaspoons of lemon juice
- Two teaspoons of lime juice
- Six tablespoons of extra-virgin olive oil
- Fine sea salt to taste
- Ground black pepper as per taste

Instructions

- Combine the arugula, onion, tomatoes, pomegranate seeds, and artichoke hearts in a large bowl.
- In a small bowl, whisk together the dressing ingredients.
- Pour the dressing over the salad ingredients and toss to coat thoroughly.

Arugula and Asian pear salad

Preparation time-10 minutes | Cook time-10 minutes | Servings-2 to 4 | Difficulty-Easy

Nutritional value: ~Calories-208 | Proteins-5g | Fat-16g | Carbohydrates-10g

Ingredients

- 1/3 cup of fresh grapefruit juice
- 1/3 cup of fresh orange juice
- Three tablespoons of extra-virgin olive oil plus enough to drizzle
- One small shallot, finely chopped
- Sixteen raw almonds, chopped
- Dash of garlic powder
- One (6-ounce) bag arugula
- One ripe but firm Asian pear halved and cored
- A quarter cup of crumbled blue cheese
- Salt and freshly ground pepper to taste

Instructions

- Whisk together both juices, olive oil, and shallot, and set aside to marry flavors. In a small skillet over medium heat, add chopped almonds, garlic powder, and a drizzle of olive oil.
- Toast almonds but do not burn; set aside. Divide arugula into equal portions on salad plates. Slice pear into slices, and top each plate of arugula with four pear slices.
- Drizzle each salad with dressing, including bits of shallot. Scatter on blue cheese, toasted almonds, and salt and pepper to taste, and serve.

Arugula and Fig Salad

Preparation time-15 minutes | Cook time-0 minutes | Servings-2 | Difficulty-Easy

Nutritional value: ~Calories-517 | Proteins-18.9g | Fat-36.2g | Carbohydrates-30.2g

Ingredients

- Three cups of arugula
- Four fresh, ripe figs (or 4 to 6 dried figs), stemmed and sliced
- Two tablespoons of olive oil
- A quarter cup of lightly toasted pecan halves
- Two tablespoons of crumbled blue cheese
- Two tablespoons of balsamic glaze

Instructions

- Toss the arugula and figs with the olive oil in a large bowl until evenly coated.

- Add the pecans and blue cheese to the bowl. Toss the salad lightly.

- Drizzle with the balsamic glaze and serve immediately.

Arugula Salad

Preparation time-5 minutes | Cook time-0 minutes | Servings-2 to 4 | Difficulty-Easy

Nutritional value: ~Calories-257 | Proteins-7g | Fat-23.3g | Carbohydrates-10g

Ingredients

- Four cups of arugula leaves

- One cup of cherry tomatoes

- A quarter cup of pine nuts

- One tablespoon of rice vinegar

- Two tablespoons of. olive/grapeseed oil

- A quarter cup of grated parmesan cheese

- Black pepper & salt (as desired)

- One large sliced avocado

Instructions

- Peel and slice the avocado. Rinse and dry the arugula leaves, grate the cheese, and slice the cherry tomatoes into halves.

- Combine the arugula, pine nuts, tomatoes, oil, vinegar, salt, pepper, and cheese.

- Toss the salad to mix and portion it onto plates with the avocado slices to serve.

Autumn Wheat Berry Salad

Preparation time-25 minutes | Cook time-Two hours | Servings-4 | Difficulty-Hard

Nutritional value: ~Calories-113 | Proteins-2.3g | Fat-1.8g | Carbohydrates-22g

Ingredients

- Two and a half cups of wheat berries, soaked overnight

- A quarter cup of plus

- Two tablespoons of apple cider vinegar

- A quarter cup of brown rice syrup

- Two celery stalks, thinly sliced

- Half cup of chopped green onion (white and green parts)

- Two tablespoons of minced tarragon

- One Bosc pear, cored and diced

- Half cup of fruit-sweetened dried cranberries

- Salt and freshly ground black pepper to taste

Instructions

- Bring five cups of water to a boil in a medium saucepan and add the wheat berries. Return to a boil over high heat, reduce the heat to medium, cover, and cook until the wheat berries are tender about 1¾ hours. Drain the excess water from the pan and rinse the berries until cool.

- Combine all the other ingredients in a large bowl. Add the cooled wheat berries and mix well. Chill for 1 hour before serving.

Avocado salad

Preparation time-10 minutes | Cook time-0 minutes | Servings-2 to 3 | Difficulty-Easy

Nutritional value: ~Calories-130 | Proteins-2g | Fat-10g | Carbohydrates-10g

Ingredients

- One large ripe avocado pitted and peeled

- One cup of halved cherry tomatoes

- Two tablespoons of chopped fresh parsley

- One small onion, finely chopped

- Half small hot pepper, finely chopped (optional)

- Two teaspoons of fresh lime juice

- Salt and freshly ground pepper to taste

Instructions

- Cut avocado into bite-sized chunks.

- Combine tomatoes, parsley, onion, hot pepper, and lime juice. Toss well; add salt and pepper to taste.

- Add avocado and toss gently.

- Divide into equal portions and serve.

Baby Bok Choy Salad with Sesame Dressing

Preparation time-5 minutes | Cook time-25 minutes | Servings-8 | Difficulty-Easy

Nutritional value: ~Calories-222 | Proteins-3g | Fat-17g | Carbohydrates-16g

Ingredients

Sesame dressing

- A quarter cup of brown sugar

- A quarter cup of olive oil

- Two tablespoons of red wine vinegar

- Two tablespoons of sesame seeds (toasted)

- One tablespoon of soy sauce

Salad

- Two tablespoons of olive oil

- One package of ramen noodles

- A quarter cup of sliced almonds

- One bunch of baby boy choy sliced

- Five chopped scallions

Instructions

To make the dressing

- Combine the olive oil, brown sugar, sesame seeds, vinegar, & soy sauce in a tiny jar/bowl with a tight-fitting cover. Let the flavors mix at room temp as the rest of the salad is being prepared.

To make the salad

- In a wide saucepan, heat the olive oil till it shimmers, on med heat. Lower the heat. Add the ramen noodles & almonds; sauté for around ten min till toasted, stirring regularly to prevent scorching.

- Combine the baby bok choy, the scallions, and the crunchy mix in a wide bowl. Sprinkle salad dressing on the top & toss till evenly mixed. At room temperature, serve.

For toasting sesame seeds

- Warm the sesame seeds in a med pan on med heat till they are golden brown & fragrant, often stirring, for around 3 to 5 mins.

- Take it from heat & move it to a plate instantly to cool fully. Place in an airtight jar in the pantry for six months or up to one year in a freezer.

To make ahead

- Mix the sesame dressing and store it in the fridge.

- Scallions & Baby bok choy can be minced & kept separately in the fridge within the containers.

- The crunchy combination can be toasted in advance, cooled, and kept at room temp.

Baby Lima Bean and Quinoa Salad

Preparation time-5 minutes | Cook time-25 minutes | Servings-4 | Difficulty-Easy

Nutritional value: ~Calories-113 | Proteins-2.3g | Fat-1.8g | Carbohydrates-22g

Ingredients

- Two tablespoons of brown rice syrup

- A quarter cup of brown rice vinegar

- Zest of one lime and juice of two limes

- Four cups of cooked quinoa

- Two cups of cooked baby lima beans or one 15-ounce can drain and rinse

- One cup of shredded red cabbage

- One carrot, peeled and grated

- Half cup of chopped cilantro

- Salt and freshly ground black pepper to taste

Instructions

- Place the brown rice syrup, brown rice vinegar, lime zest and juice in a large bowl and whisk to combine. Add the quinoa, baby lima beans, red cabbage, carrot, cilantro, and salt and pepper and toss until well mixed. Refrigerate before serving.

Bacon and Zucchini Noodles Salad

Preparation time-10 minutes | Cook time-0 minutes | Servings-2 | Difficulty-Easy

Nutritional value: ~217 Calories | Fat-10g | Protein-26g | Carbohydrates-5g

Ingredients

- One cup of baby spinach

- Four cups of zucchini noodles

- 1/3 cup of crumbled bleu cheese

- 1/3 cup of thick cheese dressing

- Half cup of cooked and crumbled bacon

- Black pepper as per taste

Instructions

- Mix the spinach with the bacon, zucchini noodles and the bleu cheese in a salad dish, and toss.

- Apply the black pepper and cheese dressing as per taste, toss well to cover, distribute into two bowls and eat.

Beans and Cucumber Salad

Preparation time-10 minutes | Cook time-0 minutes | Servings-2 to 4 | Difficulty-Easy

Nutritional value: ~Calories-233 | Proteins-8g | Fat-9g | Carbohydrates-13g

Ingredients

- Fifteen ounces of canned great northern beans

- Two tablespoons of olive oil

- Half cup of baby arugula

- One cup of cucumber, sliced

- One tablespoon of parsley, chopped

- Two tomatoes, cubed

- A pinch of sea salt Black pepper

- Two tablespoons of balsamic vinegar

Instructions

- Mix the beans with the cucumber and the rest of the ingredients in a large bowl. Toss and serve cold.

Beet and carrot salad

Preparation time-10 minutes | Cook time-25 minutes | Servings-2 to 4 | Difficulty-Easy

Nutritional value: ~Calories-116 | Proteins-7g | Fat-8g | Carbohydrates-9g

Ingredients

- Five medium red beets
- Five medium carrots
- A quarter cup of apple cider vinegar
- A quarter cup of extra-virgin olive oil
- Half teaspoon of fine sea salt
- A quarter teaspoon of ground black pepper
- A quarter cup of chopped fresh cilantro for garnish

Instructions

- Place the unpeeled beets in a large saucepan filled two-thirds of the way with water. Bring to a boil over medium-high heat and boil the beets for 20 to 25 minutes, until fork-tender.
- Meanwhile, peel and slice the carrots into 1/2-inch circles, then boil them until slightly soft but still firm, about 5 minutes. Drain the cooked carrots and set them aside.
- Rinse the boiled beets under cold running water, allowing the peels to slip off easily in your hands. Cut the beets into bite-sized pieces.
- Arrange the carrots around the edge of a serving platter, then place the beets in the center.
- Mix the vinegar, olive oil, salt, and pepper in a small bowl and pour the dressing over the vegetables. Sprinkle the cilantro on top.
- Serve warm, at room temperature, or chilled.

Beet and tomato salad

Preparation time-10 minutes | Cook time-0 minutes | Servings-2 to 4 | Difficulty-Easy

Nutritional value: ~Calories-225 | Proteins-7g | Fat-11g | Carbohydrates-25g

Ingredients

- Two pounds of tomatoes (preferably heirloom), sliced
- One pint cherry tomatoes halved
- Two (15-ounce) cans of sliced red beets, well-drained
- A quarter cup of crumbled reduced-fat feta cheese
- A quarter cup of torn fresh cilantro leaves, no stems
- A quarter cup of extra-virgin olive oil
- Salt and freshly ground pepper to taste

Instructions

- Arrange tomatoes and beets on a platter. Scatter feta cheese and cilantro over top and drizzle on olive oil.
- Season with salt and pepper to taste.

Bulgur, Cucumber and Tomato Salad

Preparation time-5 minutes | Cook time-25 minutes | Servings-4 | Difficulty-Easy

Nutritional value: ~Calories-211 | Proteins-3.3g | Fat-1.8g | Carbohydrates-32g

Ingredients

- One and a half cups of bulgur
- One cup of cherry tomatoes halved
- One medium cucumber halved, seeded, and diced
- Three cloves garlic, peeled and minced
- Four green onions (white and green parts), sliced
- Zest and juice of two lemons
- Two tablespoons of red wine vinegar
- One teaspoon of crushed red pepper flakes, or to taste
- A quarter cup of minced tarragon
- Salt and freshly ground black pepper to taste

Instructions

- Bring three cups of water to a boil in a medium pot and add the bulgur. Remove the pot from the heat, cover with a tight-fitting lid, and let it sit until the water is absorbed and the bulgur is tender for about 15 minutes. Spread the bulgur on a baking sheet and let cool to room temperature.
- Transfer the cooled bulgur to a bowl, add all the remaining ingredients, and mix well to combine. Chill for 1 hour before serving.

Buttery Garlic Green Beans

Preparation time-10 minutes |Cook time-10 minutes | Servings-4 | Difficulty-Easy

Nutritional value: ~Calories-116 | Proteins-13g | Fat-8.8g | Carbohydrates-9g

Ingredients

- One lb. of green beans
- Three tablespoons of butter
- Three chopped garlic cloves
- Lemon pepper to taste
- Salt

Instructions

- In a big pan, put the green beans & fill them with water; carry to a simmer. Lower the heat to med-low & boil for around five min before the beans begin to soften. Drain the water. Put the butter to the green beans; mix & cook for 2 ~ 3 minutes till the butter is melted.
- Cook & mix garlic only with green beans for 3-4 minutes, till garlic is soft & fragrant.
- Garnish with lemon pepper & salt.

Cashews and Red Cabbage Salad

Preparation time-10 minutes |Cook time-0 minutes | Servings-2 to 4 | Difficulty-Easy

Nutritional value: ~Calories-210 | Proteins-8g | Fat-6.3g | Carbohydrates-5.5g

Ingredients

- One pound of red cabbage, shredded
- Two tablespoons of coriander, chopped
- Half cup of cashews halved
- Two tablespoons of olive oil
- One tomato, cubed
- A pinch of salt and black pepper
- One tablespoon of white vinegar

Instructions

- Mix the cabbage with the coriander and the rest of the ingredients in a salad bowl, toss and serve cold.

Chickpea Salad

Preparation time-15 minutes |Cook time-10 minutes | Servings-2 to 4 | Difficulty-Easy

Nutritional value: ~Calories-163 | Proteins-4g | Fat-7g | Carbohydrates-22g

Ingredients

- Fifteen ounces of cooked chickpeas

- One diced Roma tomato
- Half of one diced green medium bell pepper
- One tablespoon of fresh parsley
- One small white onion
- Half teaspoons of minced garlic
- One lemon, juiced

Instructions

- Chop the tomato, green pepper, and onion. Mince the garlic. Combine each of the ingredients into a salad bowl and toss well.
- Cover the salad to chill for at least 15 minutes in the fridge. Serve when ready.

Chicken Salad with Thai Flavors

Preparation time-25 minutes| Cook time-15 minutes| Servings-4 | Difficulty-Easy

Nutritional value- Calories-368 | Fat-17g | Carbohydrates-14g | Protein-4g

Ingredients

- Three fresh cilantro (or fresh coriander) sprigs plus three tablespoons of chopped cilantro
- Two cups of reduced-sodium vegetable stock, chicken stock or broth
- One green spring onion (halved lengthwise) plus two green onions (thinly sliced)
- One and a quarter pounds of skinless, boneless chicken breasts
- Two stalks of lemongrass, thinly sliced (bottom 6 inches only)
- One tablespoon of fish sauce
- One tablespoon of reduced-sodium soy sauce
- Two tablespoons of rice vinegar
- Two tablespoons of fresh lime juice
- Half-inch piece fresh ginger, thinly sliced
- One tablespoon of peanut butter
- Half small head green cabbage
- One tablespoon of minced shallot
- One garlic clove
- Three tablespoons of extra-virgin olive oil
- Half bunch spinach
- One tablespoon of unsalted dry-roasted peanuts, crushed
- One large carrot, peeled, halved lengthwise, and thinly sliced on the diagonal

Instructions

- Combine the stock, ginger, lemongrass, halved green cilantro and onion sprigs in a large saucepan. Bring to a boil over high heat, then reduce to low heat and continue to cook for 5 minutes. Increase the heat to high and add the chicken breasts. Bring to a boil.

- Reduce the heat to a low setting and continue to simmer the chicken for 3 minutes. Take the pan off the heat and cover. After 5 minutes, remove the cover and allow the chicken to cool in the stock. When the chicken is cool enough to handle, remove it from the stock.

- Stock must be reserved. Shred the chicken against the grain with your fingers into strips about 1/2 inch wide and 2 inches long. Refrigerate covered.

- Strain and discard the solids from the cooled stock. 1 1/Two cups of the stock should be returned to the saucepan; discard the remainder. Bring to a boil over medium heat and cook, uncovered, for 5 to 6 minutes, or until reduced to a half cup of Cool.

- Puree the vinegar, lime juice, fish sauce, shallot, soy sauce, garlic, peanut butter and reduced stock in a blender. Blend until completely smooth. Slowly add the olive oil while the motor is running. The dressing will be quite thin. Place aside.

- Remove the spinach stems and core the cabbage. Separate the cabbage and spinach leaves and cut them into 1/4-inch strips crosswise.

- Toss the cabbage, spinach, shredded chicken, cilantro, carrot and sliced green onions in a large bowl. Half of the dressing should be poured over the salad. Distribute the salad among individual plates evenly. Peanuts can be used as a garnish. Distribute the remaining dressing evenly around the table.

Chickpea and Feta Salad

Preparation time-7 minutes | Cook time-0 minutes | Servings-1 | Difficulty-Easy

Nutritional value- Calories-298 | Fat-16g | Carbohydrates-2.8g | Protein-20.9g

Ingredients

- ¾ cup of chopped raw vegetables
- A quarter cup of Chickpeas
- A quarter cup of Crumbled feta cheese
- A quarter cup of Lemon juice
- A quarter cup of Olive oil
- A quarter cup of Dried oregano
- Dash Each of:
- Dash of Pepper
- Dash of Salt

Instructions

- Use your imagination for the chopped veggies. Include peppers, avocado, tomatoes, onions, and celery, or your favorites.

- Rinse and drain the chickpeas. Combine all of the ingredients and chill in the fridge until ready to serve.

Chickpeas and garden vegetables

Preparation time-10 minutes | Cook time-0 minutes | Servings-2 to 4 | Difficulty-Easy

Nutritional value: ~Calories-195 | Proteins-16g | Fat-7g | Carbohydrates-24g

Ingredients

- Two tablespoons of freshly squeezed lemon juice
- Two cloves fresh garlic, finely minced
- One tablespoon of fresh basil leaf snipped
- 1/8 teaspoon of freshly ground pepper
- One (15-ounce) can chickpeas, rinsed and well-drained
- Two cups of coarsely chopped fresh broccoli
- Half cup of sliced fresh carrots
- One (7-ounce) can diced tomatoes, undrained
- One cup of cubed part-skim mozzarella cheese

Instructions

- In a large serving bowl, combine lemon juice, garlic, basil, and ground pepper.
- Stir in chickpeas, broccoli, carrots, tomatoes with juice, and mozzarella cheese.
- Toss ingredients, mixing well. Cover and refrigerate for at least 4 hours.

Chopped Chef Salad

Preparation time-10 minutes | Cook time-0 minutes | Servings-4 | Difficulty-Easy

Nutritional value- Calories-151 | Fat-10g | Carbohydrates-5g | Protein-10g

Ingredients

- A quarter cup of reduced-fat ranch dressing
- A quarter cup of red onion, chopped
- Two large eggs, hard-boiled and chopped
- A quarter cup of chopped reduced-sodium turkey
- A quarter cup of chopped reduced-sodium ham
- A quarter cup of shredded low-fat cheddar cheese
- A quarter cup of black olives
- A quarter cup of peeled, seeded and chopped cucumber
- A quarter cup of thinly sliced fresh carrots
- Two cups of chopped romaine lettuce

Instructions

Throw in all the ingredients and mix well.

Citrus Green Beans with Pine Nuts

Preparation time- 5 minutes| Cook time-20 minutes| Servings-4 |Difficulty-Easy

Nutritional value- Calories-186| Fat-3.8g |Carbohydrates-12g| Protein-12g

Ingredients

- One lb. of trimmed green beans
- One teaspoon of grated orange rind
- Two teaspoons of olive oil
- 3/4 cup of sliced shallots
- One tablespoon of orange juice fresh
- One tablespoon of toasted pine nuts
- A quarter teaspoon of black pepper
- 1/8 teaspoon of the coarse salt sea

Instructions

- Cook the green beans for 2 minutes in boiling water. Drain under cold running water. Drain well.
- Over medium-high heat, heat a nonstick skillet. In a pan, add oil; swirl to coat. Add shallots; sauté for 2 minutes or until soft. Garnish with green beans; stir well. Add juices, rind, salt, and pepper; sauté for 2 minutes. Spoon it into a dish; sprinkle it with nuts.

Corn and bean salad

Preparation time-10 minutes |Cook time-10 minutes |Servings-2 to 4|Difficulty-Easy

Nutritional value: ~Calories-203|Proteins-8g| Fat-0g|Carbohydrates-30g

Ingredients

- One (10-ounce) bag frozen corn, steamed and well-drained
- One (15-ounce) can of red small kidney beans, drained
- Half cup of chopped green bell pepper
- One (28-ounce) can diced tomatoes with chipotle, drained
- Two tablespoons of chopped fresh cilantro
- One clove of fresh garlic, minced
- Salt and freshly ground pepper to taste
- Eight large iceberg lettuce leaves
- Extra-virgin olive oil to drizzle

Instructions

- In a bowl, combine all ingredients except lettuce leaves and olive oil. Cover and refrigerate for roughly 2 hours.
- To serve, place two lettuce leaves each onto four salad plates.
- Divide the salad mixture into equal portions. Mound salad mixture on top of lettuce.
- Drizzle salad with the scant amount of olive oil and serve.

Crab salad

Preparation time-15 minutes| Cook time- 0 minutes|Servings-2 |Difficulty-Easy

Nutritional value- Calories- 265| Proteins- 9.1g| Carbohydrates-19.6g| Fat- 17.1 g.

Ingredients

- 1/8 cup of chopped scallions
- One cup of chopped mock crab meat
- Three tablespoons of mayonnaise
- Half cup of celery chopped
- One tablespoon of lemon juice
- Salt to taste
- A quarter cup of chopped bell pepper (green)
- Adobo seasoning as required
- Black pepper to taste

Instructions

- Whisk bell pepper, mayonnaise, crab meat, lemon juice, celery, salt, scallions, black pepper and adobo seasoning in a mixing bowl.
- Cover the bowl, place it in the refrigerator for 30 minutes and serve.

Crab Salad Melts

Preparation time-10 minutes | Cook time-5 minutes | Servings-2 | Difficulty-Easy

Nutritional value: Calories-240 | Fat-8g | Carbohydrates-20g | Protein-22g

Ingredients

- One teaspoon of finely chopped fresh cilantro
- One tablespoon of chopped green onion
- A quarter cup of finely chopped red pepper
- A quarter cup of finely chopped celery
- One 6.5-ounce can of crab meat, drained

Instructions

- Preheat the broiler on high. Mix celery, cilantro, Old Bay seasoning, lemon juice, red pepper, green onion, crab, and mayonnaise in a medium bowl.
- Arrange the rice cakes on a baking sheet and put a quarter cup of crab mixture over each one. Then top each one with two tablespoons of shredded cheese. Broil for 3 minutes to melt the cheese. Serve.

Crunchy chicken and fruit salad

Preparation time-10 minutes | Cook time-0 minutes | Servings-2 to 4 | Difficulty-Easy

Nutritional value: ~Calories-286 | Proteins-34g | Fat-11g | Carbohydrates-12g

Ingredients

- A quarter cup of pecans, chopped
- Three cups of chopped roasted chicken, breast meat only
- One large head of Bibb lettuce
- Two ripe tangerines, peeled and sectioned
- Two small Granny Smith apples, cored and coarsely chopped

For Dressing

- 1/3 cup of light mayonnaise
- One orange halved
- Salt and freshly ground pepper to taste

Instructions

- In a small skillet over low heat, toast pecans, frequently stirring until golden brown, and set aside. Divide chicken, lettuce, tangerine slices, and apples into equal portions.
- Arrange on individual plates. Add a sprinkling of toasted pecans and drizzle each serving with dressing.

Dressing

- In a small bowl, add mayonnaise. Squeeze juice from the orange. Stir enough juice into mayonnaise until it has a dressing consistency.

- Add salt and pepper to taste.

Cucumber salad

Preparation time-10 minutes | Cook time-0 minutes | Servings-2 | Difficulty-Easy

Nutritional value: ~Calories-38 | Proteins-1g | Fat-0.5g | Carbohydrates-4g

Ingredients

- One large cucumber, thinly sliced
- One small red onion, thinly sliced
- Aged red wine vinegar
- Salt and freshly ground black pepper to taste

Instructions

- Place cucumber and onion slices in a bowl and cover them with vinegar.
- Cover and chill for at least 1–2 hours. Before serving, sprinkle with salt and pepper to taste.

Curried Chicken Salad

Preparation time-20 minutes | Cook time-0 minutes | Serving-6 | Difficulty- Easy

Nutritional value: ~Calories-190 | Fat-6g | Protein-26g | Carbohydrates-4g

Ingredients

- Half cup of low-fat, plain Greek yogurt
- Half cup of loose cilantro leaves, coarsely chopped
- Two tablespoons of curry powder
- One tablespoon of ground turmeric
- One teaspoon of salt
- One teaspoon of freshly ground black pepper
- The meat of one rotisserie chicken, shredded, skin removed (roughly 3 cups)

Instructions

- In a large bowl, mix the yogurt with the cilantro leaves, curry powder, turmeric, salt, and pepper. Taste and adjust spices if necessary.
- Mix in the chicken, stir well until combined, and serve.

Curried Rice Salad

Preparation time- 5 minutes | Cook time-50 minutes | Servings-4 | Difficulty-Moderate

Nutritional value- Calories-136 | Fat-1.6g | Carbohydrates-23g | Protein-2.3g

Ingredients

- Two cups of brown basmati rice

- Zest and juice of two limes

- A quarter cup of brown rice vinegar

- A quarter cup of brown rice syrup

- Half cup of currants

- Six green onions, finely chopped

- Half small red onion, peeled and minced

- One jalapeño pepper, minced

- One tablespoon of curry powder

- A quarter cup of chopped cilantro

- Salt and freshly ground black pepper to taste

Instructions

- Rinse the rice under cold water and drain. Add it to a pot with four cups of cold water. Bring it to a boil over high heat, reduce the heat to medium, and cook, covered, for 45 to 50 minutes, or until the rice is tender.

- While the rice is cooking, combine the lime zest and juice, brown rice vinegar, brown rice syrup, currants, green onion, red onion, jalapeño pepper, curry powder, cilantro, and salt and pepper in a large bowl and mix well. When the rice is finished cooking, drain off the excess water, add the rice to the bowl, and mix well.

Easy sweet potato salad

Preparation time-10 minutes | Cook time-10 minutes | Servings-2 to 4 | Difficulty-Easy

Nutritional value: ~Calories-116 | Proteins-7g | Fat-8g | Carbohydrates-9g

Ingredients

- Four medium sweet potatoes

- Half teaspoon of fine sea salt

- Half teaspoon of ground black pepper

- Half cup of minced red onion

- One teaspoon of ground ginger

- A quarter cup of extra-virgin olive oil

- Two tablespoons of apple cider vinegar

- A quarter cup of chopped fresh cilantro

Instructions

- Peel the sweet potatoes and cut them into bite-sized pieces.

- Place the sweet potatoes in a steamer pot with Three cups of water over medium heat. Cook until slightly soft or fork-tender but not mushy, about 10 minutes.

- Place the sweet potatoes in a glass bowl and let cool for 5 minutes.

- Make the dressing: In a small bowl, mix together the salt, pepper, onion, ginger, olive oil, vinegar, and cilantro. Pour the dressing over the sweet potatoes and toss.

- Serve warm or chill for 1 hour before serving.

Fennel salad

Preparation time-10 minutes | Cook time-0 minutes | Servings-2 to 4 | Difficulty-Easy

Nutritional value: ~Calories-76 | Proteins-0g | Fat-10g | Carbohydrates-3g

Ingredients

- One large clove of fresh garlic halved

- One large fennel bulb, thinly sliced

- Half English cucumber, thinly sliced

- One tablespoon of minced fresh chives

- Eight large radishes, thinly sliced

- Three tablespoons of extra-virgin olive oil

- Two and a half tablespoons of freshly squeezed lemon juice

- Salt and freshly ground pepper to taste

- Marinated mixed olives (optional)

Instructions

- Rub the inside of a large bowl with garlic.

- Add fennel, cucumber, chives, and radishes. In a separate bowl, whisk together olive oil, fresh lemon juice, and salt and pepper to taste.

- Pour olive oil mixture over salad and toss to mix.

- Garnish with marinated olives, if desired.

Feta Tomato Salad

Preparation time-5 minutes | Cook time-0 minutes | Servings-2 to 4 | Difficulty-Easy

Nutritional value: ~Calories-121 | Proteins-3g | Fat-9g | Carbohydrates-9g

Ingredients

- Two tablespoons of. balsamic vinegar
- One and a half teaspoons of freshly minced basil or dried
- Half teaspoon of salt
- Half cup of coarsely chopped sweet onion
- Two tablespoons of olive oil
- One lb of cherry or grape tomatoes
- A quarter cup of crumbled feta cheese

Instructions

- Whisk the salt, basil, and vinegar. Toss the onion into the vinegar mixture, and wait for about five minutes
- Slice the tomatoes into halves and stir in the tomatoes, feta cheese, and oil to serve.

Fish Taco Salad

Preparation time-10 minutes | Cook time-10 minutes | Serving-4 | Difficulty- Easy

Nutritional value: ~Calories-328 | Fat-11g | Protein-36g | Carbohydrates-23g

Ingredients

For the fish

- 1½ pounds wild-caught cod
- One tablespoon of extra-virgin olive oil
- Two tablespoons of Taco Seasoning (store-bought or homemade)
- Salt
- Freshly ground black pepper

For the salad

- 8 cups shredded lettuce
- Two cups of cauliflower rice, steamed
- Half cup of black beans
- 1 red bell pepper, diced
- 1 avocado, peeled and diced
- Half cup of pico de gallo
- 1 lime, quartered

Instructions

To make the fish

- Cut the fish into 4 equal-size portions. In a large bowl, combine the fish, olive oil, and taco seasoning, and gently toss to coat.
- Heat a grill or skillet over medium heat. When hot, add the fish and cook until it is brown and flakes easily, about 3 minutes per side. Season with salt and pepper as desired.

To make the salad

- Divide the shredded lettuce, cauliflower rice, black beans, bell pepper, avocado, and fish evenly among 4 plates.
- Dress in the pico de gallo and lime wedges for squeezing and serving.

Fresh chopped garden salad

Preparation time-10 minutes | Cook time-0 minutes | Servings-2 to 4 | Difficulty-Easy

Nutritional value: ~Calories-119 | Proteins-2g | Fat-4g | Carbohydrates-16g

Ingredients

- Half head iceberg lettuce, shredded
- One large carrot, cleaned and finely chopped
- Three stalks celery, cleaned and finely chopped
- Half small red onion, finely diced
- Four large red radishes, chopped
- Half (6.5-ounce) can sliced ripe black olives, well-drained
- Half (6.5-ounce) can chickpeas, well-drained
- Four teaspoons of julienne-cut sundried tomatoes in olive oil
- Four tablespoons of oil from the sundried tomato jar
- Half medium ripe-but-firm tomato, diced
- Half large avocado, cut into Half-inch cubes
- Salt and freshly ground pepper to taste
- Seasoned croutons for garnish (optional)

Instructions

- In a large salad bowl, combine lettuce, carrot, celery, onion, radishes, black olives, chickpeas, and sundried tomatoes.
- Drizzle salad with the oil from sundried tomato. Gently toss salad until well mixed.
- Scatter diced tomato and avocado pieces over top of salad, and season with salt and pepper.
- Garnish with croutons, if desired, and serve.

Freshly chopped salad with walnut dressing

Preparation time-10 minutes | Cook time-0 minutes | Servings-2 to 4 | Difficulty-Easy

Nutritional value: -Calories-195 | Proteins-4g | Fat-16g | Carbohydrates-13g

Ingredients

- Three medium ripe tomatoes, seeded and chopped
- One medium cucumber, peeled, seeded, and diced
- One large green bell pepper, seeded and diced
- Five scallions, finely chopped
- One head of iceberg lettuce
- A quarter cup of fresh spearmint leaves, finely chopped
- Twenty pitted Kalamata black olives

For Walnut Dressing

- Two slices of Italian bread, soaked in water, squeezed dry and crumbled
- A quarter cup of finely minced shelled walnuts
- Half teaspoon of finely crushed garlic
- A quarter cup of extra-virgin olive oil
- Lemon juice, freshly squeezed, to taste
- Salt to taste (optional)
- Red hot pepper sauce to taste (optional)

Instructions

- In a large mixing bowl, combine tomatoes, cucumber, green bell pepper, and scallions. Add Walnut Dressing and toss thoroughly. Add salt to taste.
- Line a serving platter with lettuce leaves. Spoon salad mixture over cleaned and separated lettuce leaves, sprinkle with spearmint and garnish with olives. Serve immediately.

Walnut Dressing

- In a blender or food processor, add bread, walnuts, and garlic and blend while slowly adding olive oil. Gradually add lemon juice and beat until the mixture is smooth. Add salt and hot pepper sauce to taste.

Fruited Millet Salad

Preparation time-10 minutes | Cook time-15 minutes | Servings-4 | Difficulty-Easy

Nutritional value- Calories-213 | Fat-1.8g | Carbohydrates-43g | Protein-2.3g

Ingredients

- One cup of millet
- Zest and juice of one orange
- Juice of one lemon
- Three tablespoons of brown rice syrup
- Half cup of dried unsulfured apricots, chopped
- Half cup of currants
- Half cup of golden raisins
- One Gala apple, cored and diced
- Two tablespoons of finely chopped mint

Instructions

- Bring 2 quarts of lightly salted water to a boil over high heat and add the millet. Return to a boil, reduce the heat to medium, cover, and cook for 12 to 14 minutes. Drain the water from the millet, rinse it until cool, and set it aside.
- Place the orange juice and zest, lemon juice, and brown rice syrup in a large bowl. Whisk to combine. Add the apricots, currants, raisins, apple, and mint and mix well. Add the cooked millet and toss to coat. Refrigerate before serving.

Ginger–sesame tofu salad

Preparation time-5 minutes | Cook time-0 minutes | Serving-3 | Difficulty- Easy

Nutritional value: ~ Calories-124 | Fat-9g | Protein-4g | Carbohydrates-8g

Ingredients

- Juice of one small orange
- One tablespoon of soy sauce
- One tablespoon of your favorite sugar alternative
- One teaspoon of toasted sesame oil
- One dash of chili sauce
- Half teaspoon of grated ginger
- Two cloves of garlic, grated
- Six ounces of extra-firm tofu drained and diced into cubes
- One cup of sugar snap peas, chopped
- Two small carrots, peeled into thin strips or grated

One cup of finely shredded red cabbage

- Two tablespoons of chopped peanuts
- One teaspoon of toasted sesame seeds

Instructions

- In a large bowl, mix the orange juice, soy sauce, sweetener, oil, chili sauce, ginger, and garlic. Place tofu cubes into the mixture, and let sit while you fix the rest of the salad.
- Toss the sugar snap peas, carrots, cabbage, and peanuts with the tofu and marinade. Sprinkle the top with toasted sesame seeds and serve!

Goat cheese stuffed tomatoes

Preparation time-10 minutes |Cook time-0 minutes|Servings-2 |Difficulty-Easy

Nutritional value: ~Calories-142|Proteins-7g| Fat-13g|Carbohydrates-7g

Ingredients

- Six to eight leaves arugula
- Two medium ripe tomatoes
- Three ounces of crumbled feta cheese
- Salt and freshly ground pepper to taste
- Balsamic vinegar to drizzle
- Extra-virgin olive oil to drizzle
- One red onion, very thinly sliced for garnish
- Fresh chopped parsley for garnish

Instructions

- Place 3–4 leaves arugula in the center of each salad plate. Cut tops (about 1/4 inch) off the tomatoes.
- With a paring knife, core out the center of the tomatoes, about half-inch deep.
- Fill tomatoes with crumbled feta cheese, add salt and pepper to taste, and drizzle with balsamic vinegar and olive oil.
- Garnish with red onion slices and chopped parsley. Serve at room temperature.

Greek Broccoli Salad

Preparation time-15 minutes| Cook time-0 minutes| Servings-4 |Difficulty-Easy

Nutritional value- Calories-272| Fat-2g |Carbohydrates-17g| Protein-8g

Ingredients

Broccoli salad

- A quarter cup of sliced almonds
- One and a quarter lb. of chopped to bite-sized broccolis
- A quarter cup of chopped shallot/red onion
- ⅓ cup of sun-dried tomatoes chopped
- A quarter cup of crumbled feta cheese/thinly sliced Kalamata olives

Dressing

- Half teaspoon of Dijon mustard
- A quarter cup of olive oil
- One teaspoon of honey or maple syrup or agave nectar
- Pinch red pepper flakes

- One clove garlic, pressed or minced
- Two tablespoons of lemon juice
- Half teaspoon of dried oregano
- A quarter teaspoon of salt, more to taste

Instructions

- Toss the broccoli, red onion, sun-dried tomatoes, olives, and almonds in a serving bowl.
- Whisk together all of the ingredients in a bowl until blended. Drizzle over the salad with the dressing and toss well.
- Let the salad rest 30 minutes before serving the best flavor so that the broccoli marinates in the lemony dressing.

Greek Chop-Chop Salad

Preparation time-15 minutes |Cook time-15 minutes |Serving-6 |Difficulty- Easy

Nutritional value: ~Calories-173| Fat-13g| Protein-4g| Carbohydrates-10g

Ingredients

- 1 medium English cucumber, chopped (Two cups of)
- One cup of halved cherry tomatoes
- 1 red bell pepper, seeded and diced
- ½ red onion, diced
- Half cup of pitted Kalamata olives, roughly chopped
- One cup of crumbled feta cheese
- Half cup of balsamic dressing

Instructions

- In a large bowl, toss the cucumber, tomatoes, bell pepper, onion, olives, and cheese with the dressing, and serve.

Greek Olive and feta cheese pasta Salad

Preparation time-10 minutes |Cook time-10 minutes |Servings-2 to 4|Difficulty-Easy

Nutritional value: ~Calories-235|Proteins-7g| Fat-10g|Carbohydrates-27g

Ingredients

- Four and a half ounces of ziti pasta
- Three ounces of crumbled feta cheese
- Ten small Greek olives pitted and coarsely chopped
- A quarter cup of fresh, coarsely chopped basil leaves
- Two cloves of fresh garlic, finely minced
- One tablespoon of extra-virgin olive oil + more to drizzle
- A quarter teaspoon of finely chopped hot pepper
- Half red bell pepper, diced
- Half yellow bell pepper, diced
- Two plum tomatoes, seeded and diced

Instructions

- Bring water to a boil, add pasta, and cook pasta until al dente.
- Remove from heat, drain pasta, and return to pot, drizzling with the scant amount of olive oil to keep the pasta from sticking together. Set aside.
- In a large serving bowl, combine feta cheese, olives, basil, garlic, olive oil, and hot pepper, then set aside for 30 minutes.
- Add cooked pasta, red and yellow bell peppers, and tomatoes; toss ingredients well.
- Cover and refrigerate for at least 1 hour, until well chilled. Toss again before serving.
- This salad goes well as a side dish to grilled lamb or fish.

Greek-style egg salad

Preparation time-15 minutes | Cook time-0 minutes | Serving-4 | Difficulty- Easy

Nutritional value: Calories-114| Fat-3g| Protein-7g| Carbohydrates-0g

Ingredients

- Four hard-cooked eggs, chopped
- Two tablespoons of finely chopped green onion
- Two tablespoons of sliced Kalamata or black olives
- A quarter cup of diced, seeded tomatoes
- Two tablespoons of reduced-fat mayonnaise
- Two teaspoons of milk
- Salt and black pepper
- Two tablespoons of crumbled Feta cheese

Instructions

- In a medium bowl, combine eggs, onion, olives and tomatoes. Stir in mayonnaise, milk, and seasonings until well mixed.
- Gently stir in cheese. Cover and chill.

Greens with cheese medallions

Preparation time-10 minutes | Cook time-10 minutes | Servings-2 | Difficulty-Easy

Nutritional value: ~Calories-205 | Proteins-6g | Fat-25g | Carbohydrates-6g

Ingredients

- Two ounces soft goat cheese, log style
- A quarter cup of extra-virgin olive oil, divided in half
- 1/8 cup of plain bread crumbs
- Two tablespoons of freshly crushed garlic
- Olive oil cooking spray
- Two cups of mixed greens such as escarole, red and green leaf lettuce, radicchio, and endive, washed and well dried
- Half cup of halved cherry tomatoes
- Two tablespoons of red wine vinegar
- Two teaspoons of Dijon mustard
- Salt and freshly ground pepper to taste
- Finely chopped pecans (optional)

Instructions

- Preheat broiler. Cut goat cheese log into two equal pieces and place cheese medallions in a bowl containing half of the olive oil; lightly swish mixture.
- Transfer the oil-laden cheese medallions to a bowl containing a mixture of bread crumbs and crushed garlic.
- Coat medallions on both sides with bread crumbs and garlic mixture. Lightly spray a baking sheet with cooking oil and place medallions on the sheet; broil until golden brown and crisp, 1–2 minutes per side. Toss greens with tomatoes, divide into two portions and top each portion with a cheese medallion.
- Combine the remaining olive oil, red wine vinegar, and Dijon mustard in a bottle and shake to mix well. Drizzle mixture over salads. Add salt and pepper to taste.
- Garnish with pecans, if desired, before serving.

Grilled Chicken and Pecan Salad

Preparation time- 5 minutes| Cook time-10 minutes| Servings-4 |Difficulty-Easy

Nutritional value- Calories-240| Fat-13g |Carbohydrates-4g| Protein-27g

Ingredients

- A quarter cup of light mayonnaise
- A quarter cup of pecans, chopped
- One teaspoon of olive oil
- A quarter cup of chopped green onions
- One teaspoon of lemon juice
- A quarter cup of minced celery
- One pound of boneless skinless chicken breast
- A quarter teaspoon of salt
- A quarter teaspoon of black pepper
- Half teaspoon of onion powder
- Half teaspoon of garlic powder
- Half teaspoon of paprika
- **Instructions**
- Prep a medium-hot fire in a gas grill.
- Then mix onion powder, garlic, paprika, salt, and black pepper. Coat the chicken with oil and then the spice mixture.
- Grill the chicken for 4 minutes. Turn over and cook again for a couple of minutes. Check doneness by a thermometer till it reads 165 degrees.
- Cool the chicken and cut it into half-inch cubes. Then mix chicken, pecans, lemon juice, green onions, celery, and mayonnaise.
- Refrigerate for 4 to 6 and serve.

Herbed potato salad

Preparation time-10 minutes |Cook time-25 minutes |Servings-2 to 4|Difficulty-Easy

Nutritional value: ~Calories-274|Proteins-8g| Fat-10g|Carbohydrates-41g

Ingredients

- Two pounds of red skin potatoes, cubed
- Fourteen ounces of low-sodium, fat-free chicken broth
- Two cloves fresh garlic, minced
- Half cup of plain low-fat yogurt
- One tablespoon of chopped fresh dill
- One tablespoon of chopped fresh oregano

- Two tablespoons of light mayonnaise
- Two tablespoons of extra-virgin olive oil
- Two tablespoons of white wine vinegar
- Salt and freshly ground pepper to taste

Instructions

- In a large saucepan, add two cups of water, potatoes, chicken broth, and garlic.
- Cook over medium-high heat for about 20 minutes or until potatoes are tender. Drain and allow to cool.
- Whisk together yogurt, dill, oregano, mayonnaise, olive oil, vinegar, and salt and pepper.
- Gently fold potatoes into yogurt mixture and chill for at least 2 hours before serving.

Israeli Quinoa Salad

Preparation time-5 minutes| Cook time-25 minutes| Servings-4 |Difficulty-Easy

Nutritional value- Calories-223| Fat-3.8g |Carbohydrates-32g| Protein-2.3g

Ingredients

- Four and a half cups of quinoa
- A quarter teaspoon of ground cumin
- A quarter teaspoon of turmeric
- One cup of finely chopped tomatoes
- One cup of finely chopped cucumber
- Half cup of finely chopped roasted red bell pepper
- One tablespoon of basil, finely chopped
- Juice of one lemon
- Salt and freshly ground black pepper to taste

Instructions

- Rinse the quinoa under cold water and drain. Bring one and a quarter cups of water to a boil in a medium saucepan over high heat. Add the quinoa, cumin, and turmeric and bring to a boil over medium-high heat.
- Reduce the heat to low, cover, and cook for 10 to 15 minutes, or until all the water is absorbed, stirring occasionally. Remove the pan from the heat, fluff the quinoa with a fork, and allow it to cool for 5 minutes.
- While the quinoa cools, combine the tomato, cucumber, red pepper, basil, and lemon juice in a medium bowl. Stir in the cooled quinoa and season with salt and pepper.

Leftover Salmon Salad

Preparation time-5 minutes |Cook time-0 minutes |Serving-2 |Difficulty- Easy

Nutritional value: ~ Calories-162| Fat-7g| Protein-18g| Carbohydrates-6g

Ingredients

- Six ounces of cold leftover salmon

- Six small black olives, sliced

- One tablespoon of finely chopped celery

- One tablespoon of finely chopped red bell pepper

- One and a half teaspoons of finely chopped red onion

- One teaspoon of chopped fresh parsley

- Two cups of salad greens, washed, drained, and dried with paper towels

- One and a half tablespoons of low-fat, low-carb salad dressing

- One Italian plum tomato, cored and cut into four wedges

Instructions

- Flake the salmon apart with a fork, removing any skin or bones, and place it in a small mixing bowl.

- Add the olives, celery, pepper, onion, and parsley and mix gently, just enough to combine. In a small mixing bowl, place the salad greens.

- Pour the salad dressing over the greens and gently toss to expose all of the surface areas to the dressing. Equally, distribute the greens onto plates and top with the salmon mixture. Garnish each salad with tomato wedges and serve.

Lemon-Dijon Tuna Salad

Preparation time-5 minutes | Cook time-0 minutes | Serving-4 | Difficulty- Easy

Nutritional value: ~Calories-227| Fat-20g| Protein-10g| Carbohydrates-0g

Ingredients

- Two (5-ounce) cans of water-packed tuna, drained

- Half cup of mayonnaise

- Two teaspoons of freshly squeezed lemon juice

- One teaspoon of Dijon mustard

- Two teaspoons of dill pickle juice

- Salt

- Freshly ground black pepper

Instructions

- In a medium bowl, mash the tuna with a fork.

- Add the mayonnaise, lemon juice, mustard, and pickle juice, and season with salt and pepper to taste. Mix until well combined, and serve.

Lime Spinach and Chickpeas Salad

Preparation time-10 minutes | Cook time-0 minutes | Servings-2 to 4 | Difficulty-Easy

Nutritional value: ~Calories-240 | Proteins-12g | Fat-8.2g | Carbohydrates-11.7g

Ingredients

- Sixteen ounces of canned chickpeas, drained and rinsed

- Two cups of baby spinach leaves

- Half tablespoon of lime juice

- Two tablespoons of olive oil

- One teaspoon of cumin, ground

- A pinch of sea salt black pepper

- Half teaspoon of chili flakes

Instructions

- Mix the chickpeas with the spinach and the rest of the ingredients in a large bowl. Toss and serve cold.

Loaded chickpea salad

Preparation time-20 minutes | Cook time-10 minutes | Servings-2 to 4 | Difficulty-Easy

Nutritional value: ~Calories-308 | Proteins-11.1g | Fat-15.3g | Carbohydrates-17.3g

Ingredients

- Olive oil

- One sliced eggplant

- One cup of cooked chickpeas

- Three diced Roma tomatoes

- Three tablespoons of Za'atar spice

- Salt to taste

- Half chopped English cucumber

- One cup of chopped parsley

- One chopped small red onion

- One cup of chopped dill

Garlic Vinaigrette

- Two chopped garlic cloves

- 1/3 cup of extra virgin olive oil

- Two tablespoons of lime juice

- Salt to taste

- Black pepper to taste

Instructions

- Season eggplant with salt and set aside for 30 minutes.

- Dry eggplant and cook in olive oil for five minutes from each side.

- When the eggplant has turned brown from both sides, remove the pan from the flame and keep it aside.

- In a bowl, combine cucumber, onions, tomatoes, dill, zaatar, chickpeas, parsley, and mix well.

- Place all the dressing ingredients in a bowl and toss well.

- Transfer cooked eggplant and chickpeas mixture in one large bowl and pour the dressing over them.

- Serve and enjoy it.

Lunch Caesar Salad

Preparation time-10 minute| Cook time-0 minutes| Servings-2 | Difficulty- Easy

Nutritional value-Calories-261 | Fat-8.5g | Carbohydrates-1.4g | Protein-15.8g

Ingredients

- One pitted, peeled and sliced avocado

- Salt and black pepper to the taste

- Three tablespoons of creamy Caesar dressing

- One cup of cooked and crumbled bacon

- One grilled and shredded chicken breast

Instructions

- Mix the avocado with the chicken breast and bacon in a salad bowl and stir.

- Add salt and pepper, caesar dressing, toss to coat, split into two bowls and serve.

Minty cucumber and tomato salad

Preparation time-10 minutes |Cook time-0 minutes |Servings-2 |Difficulty-Easy

Nutritional value: ~Calories-118 | Proteins-6g | Fat-4g | Carbohydrates-8g

Ingredients

- Two medium cucumbers

- Two Roma tomatoes

- Half cup of plain yogurt (optional)

- Two tablespoons of extra-virgin olive oil

- One teaspoon of minced garlic

- Two tablespoons of chopped fresh mint

- fine sea salt and black pepper to taste

- Two tablespoons of lemon juice

Instructions

- Peel the cucumbers cut them in half lengthwise, and then scoop out the seeds with a spoon. Discard the seeds. Cut the tomatoes in half, scoop out the seeds and discard.

- Dice the cucumbers and tomatoes.

- Combine all of the ingredients in a salad bowl and toss.

- If desired, chill the salad for 1 hour before serving.

Mixed Salad with Balsamic Honey Dressing

Preparation time-15 minutes |Cook time-0 minutes |Servings-2 | Difficulty-Easy

Nutritional value: ~Calories-337 | Proteins-4.2g | Fat-26.1g | Carbohydrates-22.2g

Ingredients

Dressing

- A quarter cup of balsamic vinegar

- A quarter cup of olive oil

- One tablespoon of honey

- One teaspoon of Dijon mustard

- A quarter teaspoon of garlic powder

- A quarter teaspoon of salt, or more to taste

- Pinch freshly ground black pepper

Salad

- Four cups of chopped red leaf lettuce

- Half cup of cherry or grape tomatoes halved

- Half English cucumber, sliced in quarters lengthwise and then cut into bite-size pieces

- Any combination of fresh, torn herbs (parsley, oregano, basil, or chives)

- One tablespoon of roasted sunflower seeds

Instructions

Make the Dressing

- Combine the vinegar, olive oil, honey, mustard, garlic powder, salt, and pepper in a jar with a lid. Shake well.

Make the Salad

- In a bowl, combine the lettuce, tomatoes, cucumber, and herbs. Toss well.

- Pour all or as much dressing as desired over the tossed salad. Toss it again to coat the salad dressing.

- Top with the sunflower seeds before serving.

Mushroom and barley salad

Preparation time-10 minutes |Cook time-15 minutes |Servings-2 to 4 |Difficulty-Easy

Nutritional value: ~Calories-238 | Proteins-6g | Fat-16g | Carbohydrates-17g

Ingredients

- Half cup of extra-virgin olive oil, divided
- One and a half pounds assorted mushrooms, halved and divided
- Salt and freshly ground pepper to taste
- Two heads of Bibb lettuce leaves separated
- One and a half cups of cooked barley
- Half cup of toasted chopped hazelnuts
- Half cup of fresh flat-leaf parsley

For Dressing

- One shallot, minced
- Three tablespoons of sherry vinegar, divided
- Half cup of low-fat sour cream
- Three tablespoons of chopped fresh chives
- Three teaspoons of fresh thyme
- Salt and freshly ground pepper to taste

Instructions

- Heat one tablespoon of olive oil in a large skillet over medium heat. Add half of the mushrooms and sauté until golden brown, often stirring.
- Transfer to a large salad bowl. Repeat for the remainder of the mushrooms. Add salt and pepper to taste mushrooms in a bowl. In the same bowl, add lettuce, barley, hazelnuts, and parsley.
- Add dressing, tossing to coat, and while serving, occasionally toss to continue to coat.

Dressing

- Add one tablespoon of olive oil and shallots to a skillet (you can use the same skillet) and cook shallots on low heat until softened.
- Add two tablespoons of vinegar and let simmer until reduced by half. Remove from heat and whisk in sour cream and the rest of the vinegar.
- Add the balance of the olive oil and whisk to combine. Add chives, thyme, salt, and pepper to taste and allow the mixture to cool.

Oriental Slaw

Preparation time-15 minutes | Cook time-0 minutes | Servings-6 | Difficulty-Easy

Nutritional value- Calories-100 | Fat-1g | Carbohydrates-7g | Protein-3g

Ingredients

- Four tablespoons of cider vinegar
- One teaspoon of black pepper
- 3/4 teaspoon of salt
- One tablespoon of sesame oil
- Three tablespoons of sugar substitute
- A quarter cup of sliced almonds
- A quarter cup of unsalted sunflower seeds
- A quarter cup of julienne-cut red bell pepper
- A quarter cup of water chestnuts, drained and cut into thin strips
- One cup of shredded carrots
- Two cups of finely shredded cabbage
- A quarter cup of green onion, sliced

Instructions

- This salad is very simple to prepare. Just throw in everything and refrigerate before serving.

Orzo and Salmon Salad

Preparation time-10 minutes | Cook time-20 minutes | Servings-6 | Difficulty-Easy

Nutritional value- Calories-254 | Fat-12g | Carbohydrates-41g | Protein-20g

Ingredients

- Two tablespoons of fresh lemon juice
- One pound of salmon fillet, about 1 inch thick, cut into 6 pieces
- Half teaspoon of black pepper, divided
- 1/2-inch cubes of 4 plum tomatoes
- ¾ cup of dry orzo
- Half cup of diced red bell pepper
- ¾ teaspoon of salt, divided
- 1/3 cup of chopped fresh dill
- Three tablespoons plus two teaspoons of olive oil
- Half medium cucumber, peeled, halved, seeds removed, cut into 1/2-inch cubes
- Half cup of sliced mushrooms

Instructions

- Throw in the tomatoes, cucumber, and half a teaspoon of salt and drain for 15 minutes.
- Boil the pasta until done. Discard the hot water.
- Add Three tablespoons of olive oil over the pasta with red bell peppers, mushrooms, lemon juice, and dill, A quarter teaspoon of black pepper, tomatoes, and cucumbers.

- Preheat the broiler. Brush the salmon with Two teaspoons of oil, 1/4 teaspoon salt, and 1/4 teaspoon pepper.

- Broil the salmon on the top oven rack for 4 minutes. Flip it over and broil for 4 minutes again. When it's still translucent in the middle but golden-brown outside and the meat flakes easily with a fork, it's cooked.

- Serve pasta with salmon on top.

Parsley and Corn Salad

Preparation time-5 minutes |Cook time-0 minutes | Servings-2 to 4 | Difficulty-Easy

Nutritional value: ~Calories-121|Proteins-1.9g| Fat-9.5g|Carbohydrates-4.1g

Ingredients

- One and a half teaspoons of balsamic vinegar

- Two tablespoons of lime juice

- Two tablespoons of olive oil

- Black pepper and sea salt to taste

- Four cups of corn

- Half cup of parsley, chopped

- Two spring onions, chopped

Instructions

- In a salad bowl, combine the corn with the onions and the rest of the ingredients, toss, and serve cold.

Pasta and shrimp salad

Preparation time-10 minutes |Cook time-15 minutes | Servings-2 to 4 | Difficulty-Easy

Nutritional value: ~Calories-411|Proteins-32g| Fat-10g|Carbohydrates-57g

Ingredients

- Half pound whole-wheat fettuccine

- One pound of large pre-cooked shrimp

- Twelve pitted black olives, halved

- Six cherry tomatoes halved

- Half cup of diced roasted red peppers

- A quarter cup of chopped fresh parsley

- A quarter cup of chopped fresh basil

- Four scallions, trimmed and sliced

- A quarter-pound of feta cheese, crumbled

- Salt and freshly ground pepper to taste

- Extra-virgin olive oil to drizzle

Instructions

- Fill a large pot with water and heat to boiling, add pasta, and cook until al dente. When ready, drain pasta well and transfer to a large serving bowl.

- Add cooked shrimp, olives, tomatoes, peppers, parsley, basil, scallions, and feta cheese to the pasta. Toss to mix.

- Add salt and pepper and drizzle with olive oil to lightly moisten pasta; serve.

Pear and walnut salad

Preparation time-10 minutes |Cook time-20 minutes | Servings-2 to 4 | Difficulty-Easy

Nutritional value: ~Calories-244|Proteins-6g| Fat-13g|Carbohydrates-27g

Ingredients

- Two cups of low-sodium, fat-free chicken broth

- One cup of white grain quinoa

- Two tablespoons of canola oil

- One tablespoon of raspberry vinaigrette

- A quarter cup of snipped fresh chives

- Salt and freshly ground pepper to taste

- Two ripe-but-firm pears, cored and diced

- Half cup of toasted walnuts for garnish

Instructions

- In a large saucepan, heat broth to a boil. Stir in quinoa, cover and reduce to a simmer, and cook until liquid is absorbed about 15–20 minutes.

- While quinoa simmers, in a bowl, whisk together canola oil, vinaigrette, chives, and salt and pepper. Add pears and toss to coat.

- Drain any excess remaining liquid from quinoa and add quinoa to pears. Toss to mix well.

- Place pear-quinoa mixture in refrigerator and chill for about 15 minutes.

- Serve cold with a sprinkling of walnuts.

Peppers and Lentils Salad

Preparation time-10 minutes |Cook time-0 minutes | Servings-2 to 4 | Difficulty-Easy

Nutritional value: ~Calories-200|Proteins-5.6g| Fat-2.5g|Carbohydrates-11g

Ingredients

- Fourteen ounces of canned lentils, drained and rinsed

- Two spring onions, chopped

- One red bell pepper, chopped

- One green bell pepper, chopped

- One tablespoon of fresh lime juice

- 1/3 cup of coriander, chopped
- Two teaspoons of balsamic vinegar

Instructions

- In a salad bowl, combine the lentils with onions, bell peppers, and the rest of the ingredients. Toss and serve.

Peppery watercress salad

Preparation time-10 minutes |Cook time-0 minutes |Servings-2 to 4|Difficulty-Easy

Nutritional value: ~Calories-67|Proteins-4g| Fat-7g|Carbohydrates-1g

Ingredients

- Two bunches of watercress, rinsed and stems removed
- Two teaspoons of champagne vinegar
- Salt and freshly ground pepper to taste
- Two tablespoons of extra-virgin olive oil

Instructions

- Allow watercress to drain. In a small bowl, whisk together vinegar, salt and pepper, and olive oil.
- Place watercress in a salad bowl and toss well with olive oil mixture to coat evenly.
- Serve immediately.

Quinoa and kale protein power salad

Preparation time-5 minutes |Cook time-15 minutes |Servings-2 to 4|Difficulty-Easy

Nutritional value: ~Calories-107|Proteins-5g| Fat-3g|Carbohydrates-16g

Ingredients

- One sliced zucchini
- Half tablespoon of extra virgin olive oil
- A quarter teaspoon of turmeric
- A quarter teaspoon of cumin
- A quarter teaspoon of paprika
- Two teaspoons of minced garlic
- One pinch of red pepper flakes
- Half cup of cooked quinoa Salt to taste
- One cup of drained chickpeas
- One cup of chopped curly kale

Instructions

- In a bowl, whisk chili flakes, cumin, paprika, salt, olive oil, garlic, and turmeric. Keep it aside.
- Toast quinoa for one minute in olive oil.

- Cook toasted quinoa following the instructions given over the package. Set aside.
- Sauté garlic, kale, chickpeas, and zucchini in heated olive oil in the same skillet used to toast quinoa.
- Cook for a few minutes until the mixture starts to sweat. Sprinkle salt and remove skillet from flame.
- In a bowl, combine veggies mixture and quinoa and leave for 10 minutes.
- In a skillet, sauté spices in oil for two minutes and add in veggies mixture.
- Serve and enjoy.

Quinoa Arugula Salad

Preparation time- 5 minutes| Cook time-25 minutes| Servings-4 |Difficulty-Easy

Nutritional value- Calories-233| Fat-1.8g |Carbohydrates-35g| Protein-7.3g

Ingredients

- One and a half cups of quinoa
- Zest and juice of two oranges
- Zest and juice of one lime
- A quarter cup of brown rice vinegar
- Four cups of arugula
- One small red onion, peeled and thinly sliced
- One red bell pepper, seeded and cut into ½-inch cubes
- Two tablespoons of pine nuts, toasted
- Salt and freshly ground black pepper to taste

Instructions

- Rinse the quinoa under cold water and drain. Bring three cups of water to a boil in a pot. Add the quinoa and bring the pot back to a boil over high heat. Reduce the heat to medium, cover, and cook for 15 to 20 minutes, or until the quinoa is tender. Drain any excess water, spread the quinoa on a baking sheet, and refrigerate until cool.
- While the quinoa cools, combine the orange zest and juice, lime zest and juice, brown rice vinegar, arugula, onion, red pepper, pine nuts, and salt and pepper in a large bowl. Add the cooled quinoa and chill for 1 hour before serving.

Quinoa Tabbouleh

Preparation time-15 minutes| Cook time-0 minutes| Servings-4 |Difficulty-Easy

Nutritional value- Calories-226| Fat-1.8g |Carbohydrates-32g| Protein-9.3g

Ingredients

- Two and a half cups of quinoa, cooked and cooled to room temperature

- Zest of one lemon and juice of two lemons, or to taste

- Three Roma tomatoes, diced

- One cucumber, peeled, halved, seeded, and diced

- Two cups of cooked chickpeas or one 15-ounce can of chickpeas, drained and rinsed

- Eight green onions (white and green parts), thinly sliced

- One cup of chopped parsley

- Three tablespoons of chopped mint

- Salt and freshly ground black pepper to taste

Instructions

- Combine all ingredients in a large bowl. Chill for 1 hour before serving.

Quinoa, Corn and Black Bean Salad

Preparation time-5 minutes| Cook time-25 minutes| Servings-4 |Difficulty-Easy

Nutritional value- Calories-178| Fat-2.8g |Carbohydrates-26g| Protein-5.3g

Ingredients

- Two and a half cups of cooked quinoa

- Three ears corn, kernels removed

- One red bell pepper, roasted, seeded, and diced

- Half small red onion, peeled and diced

- Two cups of cooked black beans or one 15-ounce can drain and rinse

- One cup of finely chopped cilantro

- Six green onions (white and green parts), thinly sliced

- One jalapeño pepper, minced (for less heat, remove the seeds)

- Zest of one lime and juice of two limes

- One tablespoon of cumin seeds, toasted and ground

- Salt to taste

Instructions

- Combine all ingredients in a large bowl and mix well. Chill for 1 hour before serving.

Rice Salad with Fennel, Chickpeas and Orange

Preparation time-5 minutes| Cook time-25 minutes| Servings-4 |Difficulty-Easy

Nutritional value- Calories-222| Fat-1.8g |Carbohydrates-32g| Protein-2.3g

Ingredients

- Two cups of cooked chickpeas

- One orange, peeled, zested, and segmented

- Half teaspoon of crushed red pepper flakes

- One and a half cups of brown basmati rice

- One fennel bulb, diced and trimmed

- A quarter cup plus two tablespoons of white wine vinegar

- A quarter cup of finely chopped parsley

Instructions

- Combine the rice with three cups of cold water in a pot.

- Bring to a boil over high heat, then reduce the heat and cook for around 50 minutes.

- Mix the chickpeas, orange zest fennel, segments, crushed red pepper flakes, white wine vinegar, and parsley in a large mixing bowl while the rice boils. When the rice is done, pour it into the mixing dish and stir well.

Roasted Vegetable and Shrimp Salad

Preparation time-5 minutes| Cook time-20 minutes|Servings-4 |Difficulty-Easy

Nutritional value- Calories-71| Fat-3g |Carbohydrates-2g| Protein-10g

Ingredients

- Two tablespoons of nonfat plain Greek yogurt
- One and a half cups of canned baby shrimp
- A quarter cup of diced bell pepper
- Half teaspoon of garlic powder
- Two teaspoons of extra-virgin olive oil, divided
- Half teaspoon of ground cumin
- One teaspoon of apple cider vinegar
- A quarter cup of diced yellow or red onion
- Nonstick cooking spray

Instructions

- Preheat the oven to 400°F. Then with aluminum foil or parchment paper, line a baking sheet and coat with nonstick cooking spray.
- Place the pepper and onion on the baking sheet and then drizzle with one tablespoon of olive oil. Coat the veggies with olive oil and bake for about 20 minutes. Take the pan out.
- Mix the onion and pepper with yogurt, garlic powder, remaining oil, shrimp, vinegar, and cumin in a large mixing bowl.
- Serve warm or cold before serving.

Salmon and Cucumber Salad

Preparation time-10 minutes |Cook time-35 minutes |Servings-2 to 4 |Difficulty-Moderate

Nutritional value: ~Calories-380|Proteins-34g| Fat-4.8g|Carbohydrates-7g

Ingredients

Sauce

- A quarter teaspoon of kosher salt
- Two teaspoons of lemon juice
- Three teaspoons of pepper
- One tablespoon of olive oil
- One tablespoon of chopped dill
- One cup of yogurt

Cucumber salad

- Two teaspoons of olive oil
- Two teaspoons of chopped flat-leaf parsley
- Two teaspoons of chopped chives
- Three teaspoons of pepper
- Three teaspoons of kosher salt
- One and a half teaspoons of minced shallot

- ¾ teaspoons of lemon juice
- Half lb English cucumbers

Salmon and serving

- A quarter teaspoon of kosher salt
- A quarter teaspoon of pepper
- One tablespoon of olive oil
- Four salmon fillets
- Dill sprigs

Instructions

- Mix all the ingredients of the sauce list in a bowl. The sauce is ready.
- Combine all the items of salad in a bowl and set aside. The salad and dressing are ready.
- Place fish with skin placed downwards on a baking tray.
- Grill the fillets for 15 minutes.
- Place the grilled fillets on a plate and drizzle salad and dressing over it; serve.

Shrimp Louie

Preparation time-10 minutes| Cook time-0 minutes|Servings-2 |Difficulty-Easy

Nutritional value- Calories-260| Fat-15g |Carbohydrates-14g| Protein-20g

Ingredients

- One green onion, finely chopped
- Six ounces of the cooked bay (cold-water) shrimp
- A quarter avocado, peeled and chopped
- Two cups of mixed baby greens
- A quarter teaspoon of black pepper
- One and a half tablespoons of fresh lemon juice
- One and a half teaspoons of dry mustard
- One tablespoon of purchased chili sauce
- A quarter cup of light mayonnaise

Instructions

- For the salad dressing, just mix some mustard, lemon juice, mayonnaise, pepper, and chili sauce in a small bowl.
- Place greens on a dish and top with shrimp and avocado. Add the salad dressing and finish with green onions.

Simple Spanish salad

Preparation time-10 minutes |Cook time-0 minutes |Servings-2 to 4 |Difficulty-Easy

Nutritional value: ~Calories-107 | Proteins-2g | Fat-9g | Carbohydrates-7g

Ingredients

- One bag (2 bunches) cleaned and trimmed romaine lettuce, torn into bite-sized pieces

- Three medium ripe tomatoes, cut into 1/4-inch wedges

- One large sweet onion, thinly sliced

- One green bell pepper, seeded and thinly sliced

- One red bell pepper, seeded and thinly sliced

- A quarter cup of chopped and pitted marinated green olives

- A quarter cup of chopped and pitted black olives

- A quarter cup of extra-virgin olive oil

- Three tablespoons of balsamic vinegar

- Salt and freshly ground pepper to taste (optional)

Instructions

- Place a bed of romaine lettuce on chilled salad plates.

- Arrange tomatoes, onion, peppers, and olives on top of the lettuce on each plate. Mix olive oil and vinegar together; drizzle over salad.

- Add salt and pepper, if desired, and serve.

Smoked Salmon Lentil Salad

Preparation time-5 minutes | Cook time-25 minutes | Servings-2 to 4 | Difficulty-Easy

Nutritional value: ~Calories-233 | Proteins-18.7g | Fat-2g | Carbohydrates-35.5g

Ingredients

- One cup of green lentils, rinsed

- Two cups of vegetable stock

- Half cup of chopped parsley

- Two tablespoons of chopped cilantro

- One red pepper, chopped

- One red onion, chopped

- Salt and pepper to taste

- Four ounces of smoked salmon, shredded

- One lemon, juiced

Instructions

- Combine the stock and lentils in a saucepan. Cook on low heat for 20 minutes or until all the liquid has been absorbed completely.

- Transfer the lentils to a salad bowl and add the parsley, cilantro, red pepper, and onion. Season it with salt and pepper.

- Add the smoked salmon and lemon juice and mix well.

- Serve the salad fresh.

Spicy Asian Quinoa Salad

Preparation time-5 minutes | Cook time-25 minutes | Servings-4-6 | Difficulty-Easy

Nutritional value- Calories-223 | | Carbohydrates-32g | Protein-2.3g Fat-3.8g

Ingredients

- A quarter cup plus two tablespoons of brown rice vinegar

- Four cloves garlic, peeled and minced

- Zest and juice of two limes

- One and a half tablespoons of grated ginger

- One and a half teaspoons of crushed red pepper flakes

- Four cups of cooked quinoa

- Two cups of cooked adzuki beans or one 15-ounce can drain and rinse

- ¾ cup of mung bean sprouts

- Half cup of finely chopped cilantro

- Six green onions (white and green parts), thinly sliced

- Salt to taste

- Four cups of spinach

Instructions

- Combine the brown rice vinegar, ginger, lime zest and juice, garlic, and crushed red pepper flakes in a large bowl and mix well.

- Add the quinoa, green onions, mung bean sprouts, adzuki beans, cilantro, and salt and toss to coat. Refrigerate for 30 minutes before serving on top of the spinach.

Spring Asparagus Salad with Lemon Vinaigrette

Preparation time-35 minutes | Cook time-0 minutes | Servings-4 | Difficulty-Easy

Nutritional value- Calories-288 | | Carbohydrates-12g | Protein-11g Fat-23g

Ingredients

- Half lemon juiced & zested
- Two scallions chopped
- One and a half lb. of asparagus spears
- Three teaspoons of white wine vinegar
- Black pepper
- One and a half teaspoons of mint finely diced
- 1/3 cup of sliced almonds toasted
- One cup of grape tomatoes quartered
- Four tablespoons of olive oil
- Sea salt
- Half cup of shaved Parmesan/Manchego cheese

Instructions

- In a bowl, combine the lemon zest and scallions, vinegar, lemon zest & juice, and salt and pepper to taste. Stir and let sit for 15 minutes.
- In a frying pan, toast the sliced almonds over medium-low heat for 5 minutes, often stirring, until golden brown. Remove and cool from the stovetop.
- To thinly slice the asparagus into strips, use a vegetable peeler. Pace the sliced spears with the quartered tomatoes in a large bowl.
- Drizzle the oil in a thin and steady stream into the lemon-vinegar mixture, whisking constantly. Season with salt and pepper to taste.
- Toss half of the cheese, asparagus, almonds, mint, and tomatoes in the dressing. If desired, season with pepper and salt again. Allow the salad to sit before serving for 10 minutes, then top with the remaining cheese.

Steamed Broccoli Salad

Preparation time-10 minutes |Cook time-2 minutes |Servings-2 to 4|Difficulty-Easy

Nutritional value: ~Calories-118|Proteins-5g| Fat-17g|Carbohydrates-11g

Ingredients

- One tablespoon of red wine vinegar
- 1/3 cup of olive oil
- A quarter teaspoon of black pepper
- A quarter teaspoon of red pepper flakes
- Two teaspoons of cumin seeds
- Two teaspoons of sesame oil, roasted
- 3/4 teaspoons of salt
- Four minced garlic cloves
- One lb of broccoli florets

Instructions

- Cook raw broccoli: In the red wine vinegar, toss broccoli with salt and pepper. Set aside for 10 minutes, the broccoli will be pickled gently, almost ceviche.
- Garlic, seasoning, and oil mix: Melt the oil over medium heat in a small skillet. Cumin seeds, garlic, and flakes of red pepper are added. Cook until the garlic is bright golden, stirring.
- Broccoli toss: Dump the oil mix over the broccoli immediately. Using the rubber spatula to clean up the oil from all the bowl sides, throw very well.
- Marinate: Leave to marinate for at least 1 hour, or refrigerate for 48 hours (it gets better over time).
- For the best taste, serve at room temperature, not cold!

Sun-Dried Tomatoes Salad

Preparation time-15 minutes |Cook time-0 minutes |Servings-2 to 4|Difficulty-Easy

Nutritional value: ~Calories-120|Proteins-9g| Fat-7g|Carbohydrates-5g

Ingredients

- One cup of sun-dried tomatoes, chopped
- Four eggs, hard-boiled, peeled and chopped
- Half cup of olives, pitted, chopped
- One small red onion, finely chopped
- Half cup of Greek yogurt
- One teaspoon of lemon juice
- One teaspoon of Italian seasonings

Instructions

- In the salad bowl, mix up all the ingredients and shake well.

Sweet red cabbage salad

Preparation time-10 minutes |Cook time-15 minutes |Servings-2 to 4|Difficulty-Easy

Nutritional value: ~Calories-85|Proteins-1g| Fat-2g|Carbohydrates-16g

Ingredients

- One small head of red cabbage
- One tablespoon of balsamic vinegar
- Two tablespoons of olive oil
- Half cup of raisins
- 1/3 cup of water
- 3/4 teaspoon of freshly squeezed lemon juice
- Salt and freshly ground pepper to taste

Instructions

- Cut cabbage head in half and remove the stem. Slice cabbage halves into thin slices and place them in a large bowl.

- Add vinegar, olive oil, and raisins and toss to coat the cabbage.

- In a large saucepan, add cabbage mixture and water and cook over medium-high heat until tender, about 15 minutes.

- Stir occasionally. Add lemon juice and salt and pepper to taste, and serve.

Tabbouleh salad

Preparation time-20 minutes |Cook time-0 minutes |Servings-2 to 4 | Difficulty-Easy

Nutritional value: ~Calories-190 | Proteins-3.2g | Fat-10g | Carbohydrates-26g

Ingredients

- Half cup of bulgur wheat

- One chopped English cucumber

- Four chopped tomatoes

- Two chopped parsley

- Four chopped green onions

- Thirteen chopped mint leaves

- Salt to taste

- Four tablespoons of extra virgin olive oil

- Four tablespoons of lime juice

- Romaine lettuce leaves to garnishing

Instructions

- Soak bulgur for 10 minutes in water.

- Drain to remove all the excess water and keep it aside.

- Now, mix all the ingredients in a large salad bowl and place them for 30 minutes in the refrigerator to get the best results.

Tabouli salad

Preparation time-10 minutes |Cook time-8 minutes |Servings-2 to 4 |Difficulty-Easy

Nutritional value: ~Calories-112 | Proteins-3g | Fat-2g | Carbohydrates-9g

Ingredients

- Four Roma tomatoes

- One large cucumber

- One medium red onion, diced

- One cup of Cauliflower Couscous

For the dressing

- A quarter cup of chopped fresh mint

- Half cup of chopped fresh parsley

- Three tablespoons of lemon juice

- A quarter cup of extra-virgin olive oil

- Fine sea salt and ground black pepper

Instructions

- Cut the tomatoes in half, core them, remove the seeds, and dice them. Peel the cucumber, cut it in half lengthwise, remove the seeds, and dice it.

- Put the onion, cucumber, tomatoes, and cauliflower couscous in a large bowl.

- In a small bowl, whisk together the mint, parsley, lemon juice, olive oil, and a pinch of salt and pepper. Pour the dressing over the cauliflower mixture and toss well. Adjust the seasoning to taste.

- Chill for 30 minutes, if desired, before serving.

Tangy orange roasted asparagus salad

Preparation time-10 minutes |Cook time-15 minutes |Servings-2 to 4 | Difficulty-Easy

Nutritional value: ~Calories-124 | Proteins-4g | Fat-10g | Carbohydrates-6g

Ingredients

- Four tablespoons of extra-virgin olive oil

- Four tablespoons of fresh, sweet orange juice (no pulp)

- Two cloves finely minced garlic

- Six cups of chopped fresh romaine lettuce

- One tablespoon of minced fresh basil leaf

- One pound of fresh asparagus, trimmed and cut into Half-inch diagonal pieces

- Salt to taste

- One tablespoon of lime juice (freshly squeezed)

- Freshly grated Romano cheese (optional)

- Salt and freshly ground pepper to taste

- Three tablespoons of pine nuts (toasted)

Instructions

- Place the nuts on a non-stick baking sheet in a single layer. Bake at 375 degrees for 15-20 minutes, stirring periodically, until lightly browned. Remove from the oven and set aside to cool.

- With two tablespoons of olive oil, toss asparagus and season with salt and pepper to taste.

- Place it in a single layer in a baking dish and bake it. Roast for about ten minutes, or until soft and crispy. Set aside.

- Whisk together the orange juice, garlic, lime juice, and the remaining two tablespoons of olive oil in a mixing bowl until well combined; season with pepper and salt to taste.

- Divide lettuce into servings, lay on plates and top with asparagus when ready to serve.

- Pour the dressing over the asparagus and lettuce salad after whisking it briefly.

- Basil and pine nuts are sprinkled over the top. If preferred, top with a sprinkling of Romano cheese.

Tomato and Avocado Salad

Preparation time-10 minutes |Cook time-0 minutes |Servings-2 to 4|Difficulty-Easy

Nutritional value: ~Calories-148|Proteins-5.5g| Fat-7.8g|Carbohydrates-5.4g

Ingredients

- One pound of cherry tomatoes, cubed

- Two avocados, pitted, peeled, and cubed

- One sweet onion, chopped

- A pinch of sea salt

- Black pepper

- Two tablespoons of lemon juice

- One and a half tablespoons of olive oil Handful basil, chopped

Instructions

- Mix the tomatoes with the avocados and the rest of the ingredients in a serving bowl. Toss and serve right away.

Tomato, Basil, and Cucumber Salad

Preparation time-15 minutes| Cook time-0 minutes|Servings-4 |Difficulty-Easy

Nutritional value- Calories-72| Fat-4g |Carbohydrates-8g| Protein-1g

Ingredients

- Half teaspoon of freshly ground black pepper

- Half teaspoon of Dijon mustard

- One tablespoon of extra-virgin olive oil

- Three tablespoons of red wine vinegar

- Half cup of chopped fresh basil

- One medium red onion, thinly sliced

- Four medium tomatoes, quartered

- One large cucumber, seeded and sliced

Instructions

- Combine the red onion, tomatoes, cucumber, and basil in a mixing bowl.

- Then, beat together the mustard, olive oil, vinegar, and pepper in a small bowl.

- Pour the salad dressing on top of the veggies and combine well.

- Refrigerate for a minimum of 30 minutes and serve.

Tomato pasta salad

Preparation time-10 minutes |Cook time-0 minutes |Servings-2 to 4|Difficulty-Easy

Nutritional value: ~Calories-293|Proteins-14g| Fat-7g|Carbohydrates-45g

Ingredients

- Eight ounces of penne pasta, cooked

- One pint of grape tomatoes halved

- Six ounces of fresh mozzarella cheese

- One medium red bell pepper, coarsely chopped

- One small sweet onion, diced

- Two cloves fresh garlic, minced

- Half cup of fresh basil leaves, torn into pieces

For Dressing

- Two tablespoons of balsamic vinegar

- Two tablespoons of extra-virgin olive oil

- One teaspoon of Dijon mustard

- Salt and freshly ground pepper to taste

Instructions

- In a large salad bowl, combine cooked pasta, tomatoes, mozzarella cheese, red bell pepper, onion, garlic, and basil.

Dressing

- In a salad dressing carafe, combine vinegar, olive oil, mustard, salt and pepper, and shake well. Pour dressing over salad to coat and gently toss.

- Cover and chill overnight before serving.

Tossed Brussel Sprout Salad

Preparation time-20 minutes |Cook time-0 minutes |Servings-2| Difficulty-Easy

Nutritional value: ~Calories-107|Proteins-2g| Fat-9g|Carbohydrates-7g

Ingredients

- Six Brussels sprouts
- Half teaspoon of apple cider vinegar
- One teaspoon of olive/grapeseed oil
- A quarter teaspoon of salt
- A quarter teaspoon of pepper
- One tablespoon of freshly grated parmesan

Instructions

- Break and clean Brussels sprouts in half lengthwise, root on, then cut thin slices through them in the opposite direction.
- Cut the roots and remove them until chopped.
- Toss the apple cider, oil, pepper and salt together.
- Sprinkle, blend and eat with your parmesan cheese.

Tuna Salad

Preparation time-10 minutes |Cook time-0 minutes |Serving-4 |Difficulty- Easy

Nutritional value: ~Calories-185| Fat-3g| Protein-10g| Carbohydrates-9g

Ingredients

One tablespoon of pickle juice

One tablespoon of powdered eggs

One can (6 oz.) tuna packed in water, drained

One and a half tablespoons of mayonnaise

Instructions

Combine ingredients in a blender and puree until smooth.

Tunisian carrot salad

Preparation time-10 minutes |Cook time-10 minutes |Servings-2 to 4|Difficulty-Easy

Nutritional value: ~Calories-138|Proteins-7g| Fat-15g|Carbohydrates-13g

Ingredients

- Ten medium carrots, peeled and sliced into Half-inch-thick slices
- Five teaspoons of freshly minced garlic
- Salt to taste
- Two teaspoons of caraway seed
- One tablespoon of Harissa

- Six tablespoons of cider vinegar
- A quarter cup of extra-virgin olive oil
- One cup of crumbled feta cheese, divided
- Twenty pitted Kalamata olives, reserving some for garnish

Instructions

- In a medium saucepan filled with water, cook carrots until tender. Drain and cool under cold running water, then drain again and place in a bowl.
- Combine garlic, salt, and caraway seed in a mortar and grind until it forms a rough paste, then pulse the paste in a food processor.
- Add Harissa and vinegar to the bowl with the carrots and mix well. Mash the carrots.
- Add the garlic-caraway mixture to Harissa-carrot mixture, blend well, and mix in olive oil.
- Add 3/4 cup feta cheese and olives and toss again.
- Place salad in a shallow bowl and garnish with remaining feta cheese and olives.

Watercress Salad with Tarragon and Mint Leaves

Preparation time-5 minutes |Cook time-0 minutes |Serving-4 |Difficulty- Easy

Nutritional value: ~ Calories-43| Fat-3.6g| Protein-1g| Carbohydrates-4.9g

Ingredients

- One tablespoon of olive oil
- Three tablespoons of apple cider vinegar
- Two teaspoons of lemon juice
- A quarter teaspoon of salt
- A quarter teaspoon of black pepper
- Two cups of watercress
- A quarter cup of fresh spearmint leaves
- A quarter cup of fresh tarragon leaves

Instructions

- In a small bowl, combine the oil, vinegar, and lemon juice and whisk briefly until emulsified. Add the salt and pepper.
- In a serving bowl, place the watercress, mint, and tarragon.
- Pour the dressing on top and gently toss with salad tongs, just enough to ensure complete coverage.

Waldorf Salad

Preparation time-15 minutes| Cook time-0 minutes| Servings-6 |Difficulty-Easy

Nutritional value- Calories-218| Fat-13g |Carbohydrates-2g| Protein-21g

Ingredients

- 1/3 cup of nonfat plain Greek yogurt
- Two tablespoons of sugar substitute
- Two cups of peeled and chopped apples
- Three tablespoons of chopped walnuts
- Three tablespoons of light mayonnaise
- One tablespoon of lemon juice
- Half cup of halved grapes

Instructions

- Put all the ingredients and mix well. Refrigerate before serving.

Warm Chicken Pasta Salad

Preparation time-10 minutes |Cook time-18 minutes |Servings-2 to 3|Difficulty-Easy

Nutritional value: ~Calories-105|Proteins-47g| Fat-48g|Carbohydrates-85g

Ingredients

- ¾ cup of dried rigatoni pasta
- One cup of Lilydale Free Range Chicken Breast, trimmed
- One medium brown onion, thinly sliced
- One garlic clove, crushed
- Half cup of semi-dried tomatoes, drained, chopped
- ¾ cup of pure cream
- 1/8 cup of baby rocket
- Half teaspoon of dried chili flakes
- A quarter cup of olive oil

Instructions

- Take frypan and cook pasta until it becomes soft to follow the pasta packet's instructions and drain the remaining water.
- Along with that, heat one tablespoon of. Oil in a pan and add chicken to it.
- Cook every side until it is completely cooked. Remove frypan from the stove, cover it & set it aside for 6 minutes.
- Take the remaining oil in a frypan, heat it over medium heat, and then add the onion. Cook for 4 to 6 minutes, mix frequently, or till the onion has softened.
- Onions, Garlic, & chili are added. Cook for 1 minute or till the smell is floral.
- Now add cream, then cook for 4 to 6 minutes, or till the mixture thickens, stirring regularly.

- Put a bowl of spaghetti, chicken, and rocket. Add the onions mixture. To combine, toss. Just serve.

Warm Rice and Bean Salad

Preparation time-5 minutes |Cook time-25 minutes |Servings-4|Difficulty-Easy

Nutritional value: ~Calories-218|Proteins-5.3g| Fat-1.8g|Carbohydrates-27g

Ingredients

- One and a half cups of brown basmati rice, toasted in a dry skillet over low heat for 2 to 3 minutes
- Two cups of cooked navy beans or one 15-ounce can drained and rinsed
- A quarter cup plus two tablespoons of balsamic vinegar
- A quarter cup of brown rice syrup
- Zest and juice of one lemon
- One cup of thinly sliced green onion (white and green parts)
- Two tablespoons of minced tarragon
- A quarter cup of minced basil
- Salt and freshly ground black pepper to taste
- Four cups of packed baby spinach

Instructions

- Rinse the toasted rice under cold water and drain. Add it to a pot with 3 cups of cold water. Bring it to a boil over high heat, reduce the heat to medium, and cook, covered, for 45 to 50 minutes, or until the rice is tender.
- While the rice is cooking, add the beans, balsamic vinegar, brown rice syrup, lemon zest and juice, green onion, tarragon, basil, and salt and pepper to a large bowl and mix well. When the rice is finished cooking, drain off the excess water, add it to the bowl and mix well. Divide the spinach between four plates and spoon the salad on top.

Whole-Wheat Elbow Macaroni Salad

Preparation time-5 minutes |Cook time-20 minutes |Serving-8 |Difficulty- Easy

Nutritional value: ~ Calories-70| Fat-0.5g| Protein-2.5g| Carbohydrates-15g

Ingredients

- One cup of dry whole-wheat macaroni
- Half cup of nonfat mayonnaise
- One teaspoon of Dijon mustard
- One tablespoon of lemon juice
- One teaspoon of celery salt
- Half teaspoon of black pepper

- Half cup of finely chopped red onion

- 3/4 cup of finely chopped celery

- Half cup of finely chopped red bell pepper

- One tablespoon of sliced black olives

- One tablespoon of chopped fresh parsley

- Half teaspoon of finely chopped green onion

Instructions

- Cook the macaroni according to package instructions, omitting the salt and oil. Drain the macaroni and cool completely in the refrigerator.

- While the macaroni cools, place the mayonnaise, mustard, lemon juice, celery salt, and pepper in a small mixing bowl and stir to combine.

- When the pasta is completely cooled, place it in a large mixing bowl along with the onion, celery, bell pepper, olives, parsley, and green onion and pour the dressing over the top.

- Using a large spoon or rubber spatula, gently stir the pasta until it is completely covered with a dressing. Transfer to a serving bowl.

Winter Greens Salad with Pomegranate & Kumquats

Preparation time-5 minutes | Cook time-35 minutes | Servings-12 | Difficulty-Easy

Nutritional value: ~Calories-337 | Proteins-28g | Fat-13g | Carbohydrates-28g

Ingredients

- Six tablespoons of pomegranate juice

- One and a half teaspoons of cornstarch

- One and a half teaspoons of sugar

- ⅛ teaspoon of garlic salt

- One cup pomegranate arils/raspberries

- A quarter cup of extra-virgin olive oil

- One and a half tablespoons of orange juice

- Two heads of Belgian endive without

- A quarter cup of toasted walnuts

- Five cups of bitter baby greens

- Half cup of kumquats, thinly sliced/ orange segments

- One small head torn radicchio

- Half teaspoon of orange zest

- A quarter cup of toasted pepitas/pistachios

Instructions

- In a small saucepan, combine the orange zest, sugar, pomegranate juice, orange juice, cornstarch, and

garlic salt, and whisk well. Heat over medium-high heat, constantly stirring, before the mixture starts to boil, darkens, and becomes cooler, around 5 minutes. Remove from the heat and leave to cool for 20 minutes at room temperature. Whisk the oil in.

- On a plate, arrange radicchio, endive, and baby greens. Cover with oranges and raspberries and drizzle with the dressing. Sprinkle with pistachios and walnuts.

Zucchini and Avocado Salad with Garlic Herb Dressing

Preparation time-20 minutes | Cook time-25 minutes | Servings-4 | Difficulty-Moderate

Nutritional value: ~Calories-775 | Proteins-21g | Fat-49g | Carbohydrates-72g

Ingredients

Chickpeas

- Fifteen ounces of chickpeas

- Salt to taste

- One tablespoon of olive oil

- Black pepper to taste

Salad

- Four medium zucchinis

- One jicama

- Two large avocados

- Kale

- Arugula

- Basil

- Microgreens

- Chopped parsley

- Half cup of chopped green onion

Dressing

- Half cup of tahini

- Half cup of cilantro

- One lemon juiced

- One and a quarter cup of parsley without stem

- Pepper to taste

- One tablespoon of apple cider vinegar

- One tablespoon of honey

- Salt to taste

- Water

Instructions

Chickpeas

- Preheat the oven to 400 ° F. Toss the dried and rinsed chickpeas with salt, pepper, and olive oil in a medium bowl. Spread the chickpeas over the baking sheet evenly and roast for around 30 minutes, or until crispy. Remove from the oven and cool aside.

- Meanwhile, shave the zucchini thinly while the chickpeas are roasting. Slice the jicama and cube the avocado into thin matchsticks. Just set aside.

- Arrange the greens in a large salad bowl — arugula, kale, microgreens (if required), chopped green onions, and fresh herbs. To combine, toss. On top of the greens, arrange the zucchini ribbons, jicama, and avocado and top it with cooled roasted chickpeas.

Dressing

- In a blender, add all ingredients and process until creamy and smooth. Add water if required and any necessary seasoning.

- Drizzle and serve with your preferred amount of dressing garlic herb. The dressing will last up to 3-4 days in the refrigerator.

Chapter 11~Vegetable and Vegetarian Recipes

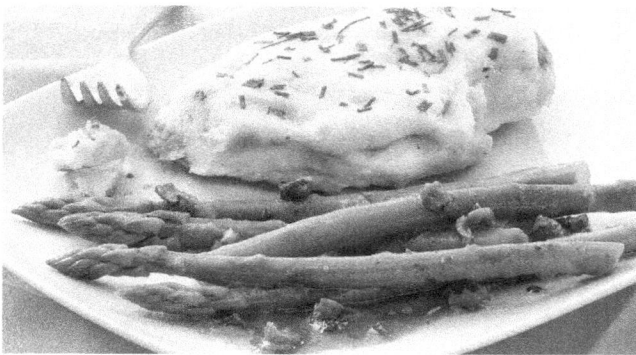

Asparagus with curried walnut butter

Preparation time~10 minutes |Cook time~16 minutes|Servings~3 |Difficulty~Easy

Nutritional value: ~189 Calories| Fat~19g|Protein~3g|Carbohydrates~5g

Ingredients

- One pound of asparagus
- A quarter cup of butter
- Two tablespoons of chopped walnuts
- One teaspoon of curry powder
- Half teaspoon of ground cumin
- Nine drops liquid stevia (English toffee)

Instructions

- Snap the ends off of the asparagus where they want to break naturally. Put in a microwavable container with a lid, or use a glass pie plate and plastic wrap. Either way, add a tablespoon or two (15 to 28 ml) of water and cover.

- Microwave on high for 5 minutes. Don't forget to uncover as soon as the microwave goes beep, or your asparagus will keep cooking.

- While that's cooking, put the butter in a medium skillet over medium heat. When it's melted, add the walnuts. Stir them around for 2 to 3 minutes until they're getting toasty.

- Now stir in the curry powder, cumin, and stevia, and stir for another 2 minutes or so.

- Your asparagus is done by now. Fish it out of the container with tongs, put it on your serving plates, and top with the curried walnut butter.

Asparagus with soy and sesame mayonnaise

Preparation time~10 minutes |Cook time~20 minutes|Servings~3 |Difficulty~Easy

Nutritional value: ~298 Calories| Fat~33g|Protein~3g|Carbohydrates~4g

Ingredients

- One pound of asparagus
- Half cup of mayonnaise
- Two teaspoons of soy sauce
- One teaspoon of dark sesame oil
- A quarter teaspoon of chili garlic sauce
- One scallion

Instructions

- Snap the ends off the asparagus where they want to break naturally. Put them in a microwave steamer or a glass pie plate.

- Add a couple of tablespoons (28 ml) of water, cover, and nuke on high for 5 minutes.

- In the meantime, combine everything else in your food processor with the S-blade in place and run until the scallion is pulverized.

- The standard way to serve this is to give everyone a puddle of sauce to dip their asparagus in.

- The fancy way is to spoon the sauce into a baggie, snip a teeny bit off the corner, and pipe artistic squiggles of sauce over your plates of asparagus.

Black Bean Noodles with Creamy Chipotle~Roasted Pepper Sauce

Preparation time~20 minutes |Cook time~20 minutes |Serving~4 |Difficulty~Moderate

Nutritional value: ~ Calories~260| Fat~8g| Protein~27g| Carbohydrates~28g

Ingredients

- Three chipotle peppers, canned in adobo sauce
- One red bell pepper
- One poblano pepper
- One garlic clove, peeled
- ⅓ cup of low-fat, plain Greek yogurt
- One tablespoon of extra-virgin olive oil
- One teaspoon of white vinegar
- One teaspoon of honey
- Juice of half lime
- A quarter teaspoon of salt
- A quarter teaspoon of freshly ground black pepper
- Eight ounces of black bean noodles

For Garnishes

- Fresh cilantro
- Avocado

- Grape tomatoes
- Lime slices

Instructions

- Preheat the oven to 400°F. Line a baking sheet with aluminum foil.
- Lay all of the peppers and the garlic clove on their sides on the prepared baking sheet. Roast for 20 minutes or until fork-tender.
- Using tongs, flip the peppers and garlic, and roast for another 20 minutes. Remove from the oven and let cool. Once cool, remove the stems and seeds from the peppers.
- In a blender, combine the roasted peppers and garlic with the yogurt, olive oil, vinegar, honey, lime juice, salt, and black pepper, and blend until smooth.
- Cook the black bean noodles according to package directions.
- In a separate small saucepan, gently heat the sauce until warm but not boiling.
- Plate the pasta, add the sauce, top with desired garnishes, and serve.

Black Bean Veggie Burger

Preparation time-10 minutes| Cook time-15 minutes| Servings-4 |Difficulty-Easy

Nutritional value- Calories-150| Fat-2g |Carbohydrates-27g| Protein-7g

Ingredients

- Half teaspoon of pepper
- Half teaspoon of chili powder
- Half teaspoon of dried thyme
- One teaspoon of onion powder
- One teaspoon of garlic powder
- Half cup of all-purpose flour
- One 14- to 15-ounce can of black beans
- Half cup of diced onion
- One teaspoon of canola oil

Instructions

- Preheat the oven to 350 degrees. Add oil and sauté the onion for 3 minutes.
- Mash the beans in a separate bowl until they become smooth. Throw in sautéed onion and other ingredients and combine.
- Then, make four ½ inch thick patties from the bean mixture. Now bake for 15 minutes. Enjoy.

Black beans and brown rice

Preparation time-10 minutes |Cook time-40 minutes |Servings-2 |Difficulty-Moderate

Nutritional value: ~Calories-350|Proteins-17g| Fat-6g|Carbohydrates-57g

Ingredients

- One and a half cups of dry black beans
- Five cups of water or canned low-sodium, fat-free chicken broth
- Two bay leaves
- One teaspoon of freshly ground black pepper
- Salt to taste
- Two cloves fresh garlic, chopped
- One medium onion, chopped
- One medium green bell pepper, chopped
- Half teaspoon of cayenne pepper
- Ten green Manzanilla olives pitted and halved
- One tablespoon of extra-virgin olive oil
- Half cup of Edmundo cooking wine or a dry white wine
- Three cups of cooked brown rice
- Raw chopped onion for garnish

Instructions

- Wash beans under cold running water. Place beans, water or broth, and bay leaves in a large heavy-bottomed pot and bring to a boil. Boil for about 2–3 minutes.
- Remove from heat, cover, and soak beans for 1 hour.
- Add black pepper, salt to taste, garlic, onion, and bell pepper bring to boil, then reduce heat to simmer, cover, and cook until beans are tender (about one to one and a half hours), adding extra water or broth if needed.
- When beans are tender, add cayenne, olives, olive oil, and wine. Cook on simmer for roughly 20–30 minutes to allow alcohol to evaporate and flavors to marry.
- Serve over brown rice and garnish with raw chopped onion.

Buffalo Seitan Bites

Preparation time-15 minutes |Cook time-15 minutes |Serving-4 |Difficulty- Easy

Nutritional value: ~Calories-87| Fat-4g| Protein-8g| Carbohydrates-5g

Ingredients

- Nonstick cooking spray
- One large egg

- Half cup of flaxseed meal

- One and a half tablespoons of garlic powder

- One and a half tablespoons of onion powder

- One (8-ounce) package seitan (cut into strips or small, 2-inch pieces if not already)

- Half cup of buffalo wing sauce

- Low-fat Greek yogurt mixed with ranch seasoning (optional)

Instructions

- Preheat the oven to 350°F. Coat a baking sheet with cooking spray.

- In a medium bowl, whisk the egg.

- In another medium bowl, mix together the flaxseed meal, garlic powder, and onion powder.

- One by one, coat each seitan piece in egg, allowing the excess egg to drip off, then lightly coat with the dry mixture.

- Gently transfer coated pieces to the prepared baking sheet. Bake for 12 to 15 minutes, or until crispy, flipping halfway through.

- Transfer to a large bowl and coat with the buffalo wing sauce.

- Serve with Greek yogurt mixed with ranch seasoning (if desired).

Butternut Squash and Black Bean Enchiladas

Preparation time-15 minutes| Cook time-40 minutes| Servings-8 |Difficulty-Moderate

Nutritional value- Calories-233| Fat-8g |Carbohydrates-27g| Protein-8g

Ingredients

- Two scallions, chopped

- Half cup of sliced black olives

- Eight small whole-wheat tortillas

- One (10-ounce) can diced tomatoes or 2 large fresh tomatoes, diced

- One small butternut squash

- One (10-ounce) can of red enchilada sauce, divided

- A quarter cup of water

- One teaspoon of low-sodium taco seasoning

- One teaspoon of ground cumin

- One red bell pepper, finely diced

- One jalapeño pepper, seeded and finely diced

- One can of black beans

- One onion, diced

- Two teaspoons of minced garlic

- One teaspoon of extra-virgin olive oil

Instructions

- Preheat the oven to 425°F.

- Heat up the olive oil. Now add garlic and sauté until the garlic is fragrant. Then add jalapeños, onion and bell pepper, and sauté for a few minutes.

- Add the taco seasoning, cumin, and squash. Now sauté until everything is well-mixed. Throw in some beans, water, and tomatoes. Cook for 30 minutes.

- In a 9x13" baking dish, spread A quarter cup of enchilada sauce.

- Now, put a half cup of squash on every single tortilla. Fold them over and arrange them in the baking pan.

- Put the leftover enchilada sauce on top. Seal with tin foil and bake for about 10 minutes.

- Garnish some scallions and olives. Enjoy.

Cannellini Bean Lettuce Wraps

Preparation time-10 minutes |Cook time-10 minutes |Servings-2 to 4 |Difficulty-Easy

Nutritional value: ~Calories-211|Proteins-10g| Fat-8g|Carbohydrates-28g

Ingredients

- One tablespoon of extra-virgin olive oil

- Half cup of diced red onion

- ¾ cup of chopped fresh tomatoes (about one medium tomato)

- A quarter teaspoon of freshly ground black pepper

- One can cannellini or great northern beans

- A quarter cup of finely chopped fresh curly parsley

- Half cup of Lemony Garlic Hummus or a half cup of prepared hummus

- Eight romaine lettuce leaves

Instructions

- In a large frypan over medium heat, warm the oil. Add the onion and cook for 3 minutes, occasionally stirring.

- Add the tomatoes and pepper and cook for three more minutes, occasionally stirring. Add the beans and cook for three more minutes, occasionally stirring. Take away from the heat, then mix in the parsley.

- Spread one tablespoon of hummus over each lettuce leaf. Evenly spread the warm bean mixture down the center of each leaf.

- Fold one side of the lettuce leaf over the filling lengthwise, then fold over the other side to make a wrap and serve.

Cauliflower and Broccoli

Preparation time-10 minutes |Cook time-35 minutes |Servings-2 to 4 |Difficulty-Moderate

Nutritional value: ~Calories-83|Proteins-1g| Fat-2g|Carbohydrates-12g

Ingredients

- Ten bubs of Cauliflower
- One Broccoli
- Three Carrots
- Two tablespoons of butter or margarine
- A quarter Chopped onion
- A quarter teaspoon of Garlic salt
- Half cup of Water

Instructions

- Cut veggies (carrots cauliflower, & broccoli) into bite-size slices & add garlic salt, butter/margarine, & onion in it.
- Bring water to a boil & steam vegetables until cooked, for around 30 minutes in a very large pot.

Cheesy Vegetarian Chili

Preparation time-25 minutes| Cook time-30 minutes| Servings-8 |Difficulty-Moderate

Nutritional value- Calories-195| Fat-3g |Carbohydrates-34g| Protein-13g

Ingredients

- 2 garlic cloves
- 1 large green bell pepper (diced)
- Two teaspoons of olive oil
- One cup of chopped onion
- 1/2 pound of sliced mushrooms
- 1 can of diced tomatoes, 14.5-ounce or Two cups of fresh tomatoes
- 2 tablespoon chili powder
- 8 ounces tomato sauce
- 2 cans red kidney beans, 15-ounce (rinsed)
- 1 10-ounce package of frozen corn
- 1 medium zucchini, thinly sliced
- One cup of low-fat cheddar cheese, shredded

Instructions

- In a large saucepan, heat the olive oil and garlic.
- Combine the green pepper, onions and mushrooms in a medium bowl. Cook until the vegetables are tender.

- Bring to a boil, then diced tomatoes, tomato sauce and chili powder.
- Reduce to low heat add kidney beans and zucchini and. Cook for 10–15 minutes.
- Combine frozen corn and a half cup of cheddar cheese in a medium bowl. Stir.
- Continue simmering on low heat for an additional 10-15 minutes.
- Garnish with cheddar cheese.

Chicken-almond rice

Preparation time-10 minutes |Cook time-18 minutes|Servings-5 |Difficulty-Easy

Nutritional value: ~104 Calories| Fat-9g|Protein-2g|Carbohydrates-4g

Ingredients

- Half head cauliflower
- Half medium onion, chopped
- Two tablespoons of butter, divided
- A quarter cup of dry white wine
- One tablespoon of chicken bouillon concentrate
- One teaspoon of poultry seasoning
- A quarter cup of sliced or slivered almonds

Instructions

- Turn your cauliflower into Cauli-Rice according to the instructions.
- While that's cooking, sauté the onion in one tablespoon of the butter in a large, heavy skillet over medium-high heat.
- When the cauliflower is done, pull it out of the microwave, drain it, and add it to the skillet with the onion.
- Add the wine, chicken bouillon concentrate, and poultry seasoning, and stir. Turn the heat down to low.
- Let that simmer for a minute or two while you sauté the almonds in the remaining tablespoon (14 g) of butter in a small, heavy skillet.
- When the almonds are golden, stir them into the "rice" and serve.

Chickpea and fresh spinach sandwich

Preparation time-10 minutes |Cook time-10 minutes |Servings-2 |Difficulty-Easy

Nutritional value: ~Calories-227|Proteins-15g| Fat-5g|Carbohydrates-40g

Ingredients

- One (15-ounce) can of chickpeas
- Two teaspoons of extra-virgin olive oil

- Two cloves fresh garlic, minced
- Half medium white onion, diced
- Salt and freshly ground pepper to taste
- Crushed red hot pepper flakes, if desired
- Four slices of whole wheat grain bread
- One clove of fresh garlic, cut in half
- Three ounces of fresh spinach leaves

Instructions

- Rinse and drain chickpeas thoroughly. Mash to a paste and set aside.
- In one teaspoon of olive oil, sauté garlic and onion until golden brown. Add chickpea paste, salt and pepper to taste, and hot pepper flakes, if desired.
- Drizzle pasta with the remaining teaspoon of olive oil and set aside. Toast whole wheat bread slices and rub one side of each piece with fresh garlic halves.
- Divide paste mixture and spinach leaves into two portions and make them into two sandwiches. Serve.

Cucumber Olive Rice

Preparation time-10 minutes |Cook time-14 minutes | Servings-2 to 4 | Difficulty-Easy

Nutritional value: ~Calories-229 | Proteins-5g | Fat-5g | Carbohydrates-40g

Ingredients

- Two cups of rice, rinsed
- Half cup of olives pitted
- One cup of cucumber, chopped
- One tablespoon of red wine vinegar
- One teaspoon of lemon zest, grated
- One tablespoon of fresh lemon juice
- Two tablespoons of olive oil
- Two cups of vegetable broth
- Half teaspoon of dried oregano
- One red bell pepper, chopped
- Half cup of onion, chopped
- One tablespoon of olive oil
- Pepper
- Salt

Instructions

- Add oil into the inner pot, then put the onion and sauté for 3 minutes.
- Add bell pepper and oregano and sauté for 1 minute. Add rice and broth and stir well.

- Cook on high for 6 minutes.
- Add the remaining ingredients and stir everything well to mix. Serve immediately and enjoy it.

Cumin mushrooms

Preparation time-10 minutes |Cook time-10 minutes | Servings-3 | Difficulty-Easy

Nutritional value: ~93 Calories | Fat-8g | Protein-2g | Carbohydrates-4g

Ingredients

- Eight ounces of sliced mushrooms
- One and a half tablespoons of butter
- One and a half tablespoons of olive oil
- One teaspoon of ground cumin
- A quarter teaspoon of ground black pepper
- Two tablespoons of sour cream

Instructions

- Start sautéing the mushrooms in the butter and oil in a skillet over medium-high heat.
- When they've gone limp and changed color, stir in the cumin and pepper.
- Let the mushrooms cook with the spices for a minute or two, then stir in the sour cream. Cook just long enough to heat through and serve.

Curried Eggplant and Chickpea Quinoa

Preparation time-15 minutes | Cook time-40 minutes | Servings-4 | Difficulty-Moderate

Nutritional value- Calories-131 | Fat-2g | Carbohydrates-23g | Protein-6g

Ingredients

- Low-fat plain Greek yogurt, for garnish
- One cup of vegetable broth
- Half cup of packaged quinoa
- Half cup of water
- Three tomatoes, diced
- One tablespoon of ground cumin
- One teaspoon of ground turmeric
- Two teaspoons of smoked paprika
- One medium eggplant, cut into ½-inch chunks
- A quarter teaspoon of cayenne pepper
- One red bell pepper, chopped
- One yellow summer squash, cut into ½-inch chunks
- One large onion, chopped

- One (15-ounce) can chickpeas, drained and rinsed

- One teaspoon of extra-virgin olive oil

- Four teaspoons of minced garlic

Instructions

- Sauté the garlic in olive oil. Add bell pepper, onion, and sauté again until tender.

- Then cook some turmeric, cumin, paprika, and cayenne pepper for a few minutes.

- Add the eggplant, tomatoes, water, chickpeas, and squash. Cook on medium-low for 15 minutes.

- Then, in a small saucepan, put the broth and quinoa over medium-high heat and boil. Cook for 15 minutes. Remove from the heat.

- Top the curried vegetables with yogurt and serve with quinoa.

Dragon's teeth

Preparation time-10 minutes |Cook time-15 minutes|Servings-4 |Difficulty-Easy

Nutritional value: ~175 Calories| Fat-9g|Protein-0g|Carbohydrates-3g

Ingredients

- One head napa cabbage

- A quarter cup of chili garlic paste

- Two tablespoons of soy sauce

- Two teaspoons of dark sesame oil

- One teaspoon of salt

- Twelve drops of liquid stevia (plain)

- Two tablespoons of peanut or canola oil

- Two teaspoons of rice vinegar

Instructions

- Cut the head of napa cabbage in half lengthwise, then lay it flat-side down on the cutting board and slice it about Half-inch (1 cm) thick. Cut it one more time, lengthwise down the middle, and then do the other half head.

- Mix together the chili garlic paste, soy sauce, sesame oil, salt, and stevia in a small dish, and set by the stove.

- In a wok or extra-large skillet, over the highest heat, heat the peanut or canola oil. Add the cabbage and start stir-frying.

- After about a minute, add the seasoning mixture and keep stir-frying until the cabbage is just starting to wilt—you want it still crispy in most places.

- Sprinkle in the rice vinegar, stir once more, and serve.

Easy baked eggplant parmesan

Preparation time-10 minutes |Cook time-20 minutes |Servings-2 |Difficulty-Easy

Nutritional value: ~Calories-196|Proteins-13g| Fat-5g|Carbohydrates-23g

Ingredients

- Half cup of liquid eggs

- A quarter cup of bread crumbs

- One large eggplant, with skin, on and sliced lengthwise into eight slices (about Half-inch thickness each)

- Olive oil cooking spray

- Garlic salt to sprinkle (optional)

- One cup of shredded low-fat mozzarella cheese

- One (14.5-ounce) can of diced tomatoes with basil, garlic, and oregano, drained

- One (8-ounce) can of tomato sauce with basil, garlic, and oregano

- Chopped fresh parsley for garnish

- Grated Parmesan cheese for garnish

Instructions

- Preheat oven to 425 degrees. Place eggs in a large, shallow dipping bowl. Place bread crumbs in another large, shallow bowl.

- Dip each slice of eggplant into eggs and then into bread crumbs, coating both sides of each piece.

- Place pieces on a lightly oil-sprayed baking sheet. If desired, lightly sprinkle each slice with garlic salt. Bake eggplant until slices are tender and lightly browned, roughly 5 minutes on each side.

- Sprinkle tops of one side of the eggplant with shredded mozzarella cheese and bake for 1-minute longer until cheese softens and browns slightly.

- While eggplant is baking, combine tomatoes and sauce in a saucepan and heat on medium-low heat to let simmer until slightly thickened, about 10 minutes.

- Divide tomato mixture into shallow serving plates and top each plate with two slices of eggplant. Sprinkle each serving with parsley and Parmesan cheese and serve.

Flavors Herb Risotto

Preparation time-10 minutes |Cook time-15 minutes |Servings-2 to 4 |Difficulty-Moderate

Nutritional value: ~Calories-514|Proteins-9g| Fat-17g|Carbohydrates-78g

Ingredients

- Two cups of rice

- Two tablespoons of parmesan cheese, grated

- Two ounces of heavy cream

- One tablespoon of fresh oregano, chopped

- One tablespoon of fresh basil, chopped

- Half tablespoon of sage, chopped

- One onion, chopped

- Two tablespoons of olive oil

- One teaspoon of garlic, minced

- Four cups of vegetable stock

- Pepper

- Salt

Instructions

- Sauté the garlic and onion within 2-3 minutes in a pot with olive oil.

- Put the rest of the ingredients except for parmesan cheese and heavy cream and stir well.

- Cook on high for 12 minutes. Stir in cream and cheese and serve.

Flavors Taco Rice Bowl

Preparation time-10 minutes | Cook time-15 minutes | Servings-2 to 4 | Difficulty-Easy

Nutritional value: ~Calories-468 | Proteins-32g | Fat-15g | Carbohydrates-45g

Ingredients

- One lb. of ground beef

- Eight ounces of cheddar cheese, shredded

- Fourteen ounces can of red beans

- Two ounces of taco seasoning

- Sixteen ounces of salsa

- Two cups of water

- Two cups of brown rice

- Pepper

- Salt

Instructions

- Set instant pot on sauté mode. Add meat to the pot and sauté until brown. Add water, beans, rice, taco seasoning, pepper, and salt and stir well.

- Top with salsa—cook on high for 14 minutes. Add cheddar cheese and stir until the cheese is melted. Serve and enjoy.

Garlic pasta

Preparation time-10 minutes | Cook time-20 minutes | Servings-2 | Difficulty-Easy

Nutritional value: ~Calories-247 | Proteins-8g | Fat-8g | Carbohydrates-33g

Ingredients

- Four ounces of thin whole grain pasta

- One tablespoon of extra-virgin olive oil

- Garlic powder to taste

- Salt and freshly ground pepper to taste

Instructions

- Cook and drain pasta according to package directions.

- Place well-drained hot pasta in a bowl and toss with olive oil, garlic powder, and salt and pepper to taste.

- Serve while hot.

Italian Baked Beans

Preparation time-10 minutes | Cook time-15 minutes | Servings-2 to 4 | Difficulty-Easy

Nutritional value: ~Calories-236 | Proteins-10g | Fat-4g | Carbohydrates-42g

Ingredients

- Two teaspoons of extra-virgin olive oil

- Half cup of minced onion

- One (12-ounce) can of low-sodium tomato paste

- A quarter cup of red wine vinegar

- Two tablespoons of honey

- A quarter teaspoon of ground cinnamon

- Half cup of water

- Two cans cannellini or great northern beans, undrained

Instructions

- In a medium saucepan over medium heat, heat the oil.

- Add the onion, then cook it for 5 minutes, frequently stirring. Add the tomato paste, vinegar, honey, cinnamon, and water, and mix well. Turn the heat to low.

- Trench and rinse one can of the beans in a colander and add to the saucepan. Pour the entire second can of beans (including the liquid) into the saucepan.

- Let it cook for 10 minutes, occasionally stirring, and serve.

Italian roasted vegetables

Preparation time-10 minutes | Cook time-30 minutes | Servings-2 to 4 | Difficulty-Moderate

Nutritional value: ~Calories-88 | Proteins-4g | Fat-1g | Carbohydrates-14.3g

Ingredients

- Eight ounces of mushrooms

- Twelve ounces of Campari tomatoes

- Extra virgin olive as required

- Two sliced zucchinis

- Twelve ounces of sliced baby potatoes

- Ten chopped garlic cloves

- One teaspoon of dried thyme

- Salt to taste

- Shredded Parmesan cheese

- Black pepper to taste

- Half tablespoon of dried oregano

- Red pepper flakes to taste

Instructions

- Add salt, mushrooms, olive oil, pepper, veggies, oregano, garlic, and thyme in a mixing bowl and toss well. Set aside.

- Roast potatoes in a preheated oven at 425 degrees for 10 minutes.

- Mix the mushroom mixture with baked potatoes and bake for another 20 minutes.

- Garnish with cheese and pepper flakes and serve.

Jambalaya with Vegetarian Sausage

Preparation time-10 minutes |Cook time-25 minutes |Serving-6 |Difficulty- Easy

Nutritional value: ~Calories-148| Fat-7g| Protein-7g| Carbohydrates-10g

Ingredients

- Two tablespoons of extra-virgin olive oil, divided

- Half package (7 ounces) vegetarian andouille sausage, sliced into quarter-inch-thick rounds

- One green bell pepper, diced

- Half small onion, diced

- One celery stalk, diced

- Three garlic cloves, minced

- One tablespoon of Cajun seasoning

- One (14.5-ounce) can of diced tomatoes

- Four ounces of jumbo shrimp, tails removed, peeled, and deveined

- One cup of cauliflower rice

Instructions

- In a large skillet over medium-high heat, heat one tablespoon of oil. Add the sliced sausage, and cook

until browned on both sides, about 10 minutes total. Transfer the sausage to a plate.

- Heat another tablespoon of oil in the pan, and add the bell pepper, onion, celery, and garlic. Sauté for 5 minutes. Add the Cajun seasoning, and stir well.

- Add the tomatoes, sausage, and shrimp. Cook for 2 to 3 minutes until the shrimp is opaque and cooked through, then add the cauliflower rice. Cook for another 5 to 7 minutes until the cauliflower is hot and soft, and serve.

Japanese fried rice

Preparation time-10 minutes |Cook time-15 minutes|Servings-5 |Difficulty-Easy

Nutritional value: ~91 Calories| Fat-6g|Protein-4g|Carbohydrates-5g

Ingredients

- Half head cauliflower

- Two eggs

- One cup of fresh snow pea pods

- Two tablespoons of butter

- Half cup of diced onion

- Two tablespoons of shredded carrot

- Three tablespoons of soy sauce

- Salt and ground black pepper, to taste

Instructions

- Turn your cauliflower into Cauli-Rice according to the instructions.

- While that's happening, whisk the eggs, pour them into a non-stick skillet (or one you've coated with non-stick cooking spray), and cook over medium-high heat. As you cook the eggs, use your spatula to break them up into pea-sized bits.

- Remove from the skillet and set aside.

- Remove the tips and strings from the snow peas and snip them into 1/4-inch (6 mm) lengths. (By now, the microwave has beep—take the lid off your cauliflower, or it will turn into a mush that bears not the slightest resemblance to rice!)

- Melt the butter in the skillet and sauté the pea pods, onion, and carrot for 2 to 3 minutes. Add the cauliflower and stir everything together well.

- Stir in the soy sauce and cook the whole thing, often stirring, for another 5 to 6 minutes. Add a little salt and pepper, and serve.

Lemon-herb zucchini

Preparation time-10 minutes |Cook time-15 minutes|Servings-4 |Difficulty-Easy

Nutritional value: ~78 Calories| Fat-7g|Protein-1g|Carbohydrates-4g

Ingredients

- Two medium zucchini
- Two tablespoons of olive oil
- Two tablespoons of lemon juice
- Half teaspoon of ground coriander
- A quarter teaspoon of dried thyme
- One clove of garlic, minced
- Two tablespoons of chopped fresh parsley

Instructions

- Cut your zukes in half lengthwise, then slice them 1/4 inch (6 mm) thick.
- Coat your large, heavy skillet with non-stick cooking spray, and put over medium-high heat.
- Add the olive oil. When it's hot, add your sliced zucchini, and sauté, frequently stirring, till it's just softening.
- Add the lemon juice, coriander, thyme, and garlic. Stir everything together, reduce the heat to medium-low, and let it simmer for another few minutes.
- Stir in the parsley just before serving.

Lentil Sloppy Joes

Preparation time-5 minutes |Cook time-35 minutes |Serving-6 |Difficulty- Easy

Nutritional value: -Calories-163| Fat-3g| Protein-10g| Carbohydrates-26g

Ingredients

- Two cups of vegetable broth
- One cup of green lentils, well rinsed
- One tablespoon of extra-virgin olive oil
- Half medium yellow onion, minced
- Half green bell pepper, minced
- Two garlic cloves, minced
- One (15-ounce) can of tomato sauce
- One to Two tablespoons of sugar substitute
- One tablespoon of Worcestershire sauce
- Two teaspoons of chili powder
- One teaspoon of ground cumin
- One teaspoon of paprika
- Lettuce leaves, sliced jalapeños and red onion for serving

Instructions

- In a small saucepan over medium-high heat, combine the broth and lentils. Bring to a boil, then reduce to a

simmer and cook uncovered for about 18 minutes, or until tender. Drain any excess liquid.

- In a large skillet over medium heat, heat the oil. Add the onion, bell pepper, and garlic, and cook for 4 to 5 minutes, until tender and onions are slightly brown.
- Add the tomato sauce, sugar substitute, Worcestershire, chili powder, cumin, paprika, and lentils. Stir to combine.
- Continue cooking for 5 to 10 minutes over medium heat until warmed through and thickened.
- Refrigerate leftovers in an airtight container. Reheat in the microwave or on the stovetop, adding extra water or broth if needed to soften.
- Serve in lettuce leaves with sliced jalapeños and red onion.

Lettuce-Wrapped Veggie Burgers

Preparation time-10 minutes| Cook time-10 minutes| Servings-4 |Difficulty-Easy

Nutritional value- Calories-466| Fat-34g |Carbohydrates-13g| Protein-26g

Ingredients

- One red onion, sliced
- Four tablespoons of Secret Burger Sauce
- Four slices of steak tomato
- Four veggie patties
- Eight Bibb lettuce leaves

For the Sauce

- Two tablespoons of dill pickle relish
- A quarter teaspoon of salt
- Half teaspoon of Worcestershire sauce
- One teaspoon of hot sauce
- A quarter teaspoon of freshly ground black pepper
- A quarter cup of low-sugar ketchup
- Half cup of olive oil mayonnaise

Instructions

- Make the vegan patties according to the package.
- Put one patty in each lettuce leaf. Pour one teaspoon of sauce, place 1 tomato slice, 1 slice of red onion. Finish with a lettuce leaf on top.
- Continue the same for all the patties. Serve hot.

For the Sauce

- Beat the relish well, hot sauce, salt ketchup, mayonnaise, Worcestershire sauce and pepper.
- Refrigerate for up to 5 days.

Mushroom Casserole

Preparation time-15 minutes |Cook time-One hour |Servings-2 to 4 |Difficulty-Hard

Nutritional value: ~Calories-156|Proteins-11.2g| Fat-9.7g|Carbohydrates-7g

Ingredients

- Two eggs, beaten
- One cup of mushrooms, sliced
- Two shallots, chopped
- One teaspoon of marjoram, dried
- Half cup of artichoke hearts, chopped
- Three ounces of Cheddar cheese, shredded
- Half cup of plain yogurt

Instructions

- Mix up all the ingredients in a casserole mold and cover it with foil.
- Bake the casserole for 60 minutes at 355°F.

Mushroom risotto

Preparation time-10 minutes |Cook time-20 minutes|Servings-5 |Difficulty-Easy

Nutritional value: ~139 Calories| Fat-11g|Protein-6g|Carbohydrates-4g

Ingredients

- Half head cauliflower
- Three tablespoons of butter
- One cup of sliced mushrooms
- Half medium onion, diced
- One teaspoon of minced garlic or two cloves of garlic, minced
- Two tablespoons of dry vermouth
- One tablespoon of chicken bouillon concentrate
- 3/4 cup of grated Parmesan cheese
- Guar or xanthan, as needed
- Two tablespoons of chopped fresh parsley

Instructions

- Turn your cauliflower into Cauli-Rice according to the instructions.
- While the cauliflower is cooking, melt the butter in a large skillet over medium-high heat.
- Add the mushrooms, onion, and garlic, and sauté them all together.
- When the cauliflower is done, pull it out of the microwave and drain it. When the mushrooms have changed color and are looking done, add the cauliflower to the skillet and stir everything together.
- Stir in the vermouth and bouillon, add the cheese, and let the whole thing cook for another 2 to 3 minutes.
- Sprinkle just a little guar or xanthan over the "risotto," stirring all the while to give it a creamy texture.
- Stir in the parsley just before serving.

Mushrooms with bacon, sun-dried tomatoes, and cheese

Preparation time-10 minutes |Cook time-12 minutes|Servings-4 |Difficulty-Easy

Nutritional value: ~113 Calories| Fat-8g|Protein-6g|Carbohydrates-5g

Ingredients

- Four slices of bacon
- Eight ounces of sliced mushrooms
- Half teaspoon of minced garlic or 1 clove fresh garlic, minced
- A quarter cup of diced sun-dried tomatoes—about 10 pieces before dicing
- Two tablespoons of heavy cream
- 1/3 cup of shredded Parmesan cheese

Instructions

- Chop up the bacon or snip it up with kitchen shears. Start cooking it in a large, heavy skillet over medium-high heat. As some grease starts to cook out of the bacon, stir in the mushrooms.
- Let the mushrooms cook until they start to change color and get soft. Stir in the garlic and cook for 4 to 5 more minutes.
- Stir in the tomatoes and cream and cook until the cream is absorbed.
- Scatter the cheese over the whole thing, stir it in, let it cook for just another minute, and serve.

Navy Bean Bake

Preparation time-15 minutes| Cook time-36 minutes| Servings-6 |Difficulty-Moderate

Nutritional value- Calories-180| Fat-3g |Carbohydrates-26g| Protein-13g

Ingredients

- One cup of diced tomato
- One cup of shredded low-fat cheddar cheese
- Half cup of low-sodium vegetable broth
- One 14.5-ounce canned low-sodium pinto beans, rinsed and drained
- One 14.5-ounce canned navy beans, rinsed and drained

- A quarter cup of diced green pepper

- One teaspoon of dried thyme

- Half cup of diced onion

- Two cloves of fresh garlic chopped fine

- One teaspoon of olive oil

Instructions

- Preheat the oven to 325 degrees. Coat an 8x8" pan with nonstick cooking spray.

- To a medium pan over medium-high heat, add olive oil. Then throw in the onion, tomato, green pepper, thyme, and garlic and sauté for 3 minutes. Then introduce the broth and beans and simmer them for 3 minutes.

- Put the bean blend in the baking pan. Bake for half an hour. Cool a bit and serve.

Pepperoncini spinach

Preparation time-10 minutes |Cook time-12 minutes|Servings-3 |Difficulty-Easy

Nutritional value: ~47 Calories| Fat-3g|Protein-5g|Carbohydrates-5g

Ingredients

- One package of (10 ounces) frozen chopped spinach, thawed

- One and a half teaspoons of olive oil

- Two pepperoncini peppers, drained and minced

- One clove of garlic

- One tablespoon of lemon juice

Instructions

- Put your thawed spinach in a strainer, and either press it with the back of a spoon or actually pick it up with clean hands and squeeze it—you want all the excess water out of it.

- Give your medium skillet a shot of non-stick cooking spray, put it over medium-high heat, and add the olive oil.

- When it's hot, add spinach, pepperoncini, and garlic.

- Sauté, often stirring, for about 5 minutes. Stir in the lemon juice, let it cook another minute, and serve.

Portobello Burger

Preparation time- 5 minutes| Cook time-10 minutes| Servings-4 |Difficulty-Easy

Nutritional value- Calories-240| Fat-8g |Carbohydrates-30g| Protein-13g

Ingredients

- Four romaine lettuce leaves

Four tomato slices

- One tablespoon of balsamic vinegar

- Four whole-wheat hamburger buns

- A quarter teaspoon of salt

- One teaspoon of onion powder

- One teaspoon of garlic powder

- One tablespoon of olive oil

- Four large portobello mushroom stems removed

Instructions

- Mix whole garlic powder, salt, mushrooms caps, onion powder, balsamic vinegar, olive oil and let it marinate for 20 minutes.

- Preheat the broiler on high. Arrange the marinated mushrooms on a dry cooking sheet and broil for 4 minutes. Flip the side midway and broil for another 4 minutes.

- Put each mushroom on a whole-wheat bun, place 1 tomato slice, 1 lettuce leaf, and serve.

Ratatouille

Preparation time-20 minutes |Cook time-40 minutes |Servings-2 to 4 |Difficulty-Hard

Nutritional value: ~Calories-230|Proteins-5g| Fat-11g|Carbohydrates-32g

Ingredients

Veggies

- Two zucchinis

- Two eggplants

- Two yellow squashes

- Six Roma tomatoes

Sauce

- One onion diced

- Four cloves minced garlic

- Two tablespoons of olive oil

- One diced red bell pepper

- One diced yellow bell pepper

- Twenty-eight ounces of crushed tomatoes

- Two tablespoons of chopped basil Herb seasoning

- Two tablespoons of chopped basil

- One teaspoon of garlic minced

- Two tablespoons of fresh parsley Chopped

- Two teaspoons of thyme

- Salt and pepper to taste

- Four tablespoons of olive oil

Instructions

- Preheat oven to 375°F.

- Heat olive oil in an oven-safe pan. Sauté onion, garlic, & bell peppers for about 10 minutes. Then season with salt & pepper, add the crushed tomatoes. Mix. Remove from heat, and then add basil. Stir until smooth.

- Arrange sliced veggies on top of the sauce and then season with salt & pepper.

- In a small bowl, mix the basil, parsley, thyme, garlic, salt, pepper, & olive oil. Spoon herb seasoning on vegetables.

- Cover pan with foil & bake for 40 minutes. Now, uncover, and bake for the next 20 minutes, till vegetables are softened.

- Serve.

Roasted cauliflower with lemon and cumin

Preparation time-15 minutes | Cook time-25 minutes | Servings-2 to 4 | Difficulty-Moderate

Nutritional value: ~Calories-213 | Proteins-3g | Fat-17g | Carbohydrates-10g

Ingredients

- Eleven ounces of cauliflower

- One tablespoon of lemon juice

- 1/3 cup of olive oil

- Salt to taste

- Zest of one lemon

- One tablespoon of ground sumac

- One tablespoon of ground cumin

- One teaspoon of garlic powder

- Black pepper to taste

Instructions

- Mix all the ingredients in a large mixing bowl.

- Transfer the cauliflower to a baking tray and bake in a preheated oven at 425 degrees for 25 minutes.

- Serve and enjoy it.

Sautéed mushrooms and spinach with pepperoni

Preparation time-10 minutes | Cook time-20 minutes | Servings-6 | Difficulty-Easy

Nutritional value: ~90 Calories | Fat-7g | Protein-3g | Carbohydrates-5g

Ingredients

- One ounce of sliced pepperoni

- Two tablespoons of olive oil, divided

- One pound of sliced mushrooms

- One bunch of scallions, sliced

- Two cloves of garlic, crushed

- One bag of (5 ounces) baby spinach

- Salt and ground black pepper, to taste

Instructions

- Slice your pepperoni into teeny strips.

- Heat one tablespoon of the olive oil in your large, heavy skillet, add the pepperoni and sauté it until it's crisp. Lift out with a slotted spoon, and drain on paper towels.

- Add the remaining one tablespoon of oil to the skillet, and let it heat over a medium-high burner.

- Add the mushrooms, and sauté them until they've softened and started to brown.

- Add the sliced scallions and sauté for another few minutes until they're starting to brown, too. Stir in the garlic, then add the spinach.

- Turn the whole thing over and over, just until the spinach wilts. Stir in the pepperoni bits, season with salt and pepper to taste, and serve.

Spaghetti Squash Chow Mein

Preparation time-10 minutes | Cook time-55 minutes | Serving-3 | Difficulty- Easy

Nutritional value: ~ Calories-252 | Fat-11g | Protein-6g | Carbohydrates-39g

Ingredients

- Nonstick cooking spray

- One small (3- to 4-pound) spaghetti squash

- A quarter cup of low-sodium soy sauce

- Three garlic cloves, minced

- One tablespoon of oyster sauce

- One inch ginger root, peeled and minced

- Two tablespoons of extra-virgin olive oil

- One small white onion, diced

- Three celery stalks, thinly sliced

- Two cups of shredded cabbage (or coleslaw mix)

Instructions

- Preheat the oven to 350°F. Coat a baking sheet with cooking spray.

- Halve the spaghetti squash, remove and discard the seeds, and place the halves cut-side down on the prepared baking sheet. Bake for 30 to 45 minutes, or until the flesh is tender and can be scraped with a fork.

- Remove from the oven, and let cool. Scrape out the flesh with a fork, creating small noodles. Set aside.

- In a small bowl, whisk together the soy sauce, garlic, oyster sauce, and ginger.

- In a large skillet over medium heat, heat the oil. Add the onion and celery and cook, stirring, until tender, 3 to 4 minutes. Add the cabbage and cook, stirring, until heated through, 1 to 2 minutes.

- Add the spaghetti squash and sauce mixture. Continue cooking for another 2 minutes.

- Serve immediately.

Spicy eggplant

Preparation time-10 minutes | Cook time-20 minutes | Servings-2 | Difficulty-Easy

Nutritional value: ~Calories-117 | Proteins-1g | Fat-10g | Carbohydrates-3g

Ingredients

- Four tablespoons of extra-virgin olive oil

- One (1-pound) eggplant, thinly sliced (about 1/8-inch thick)

- Half cup of liquid egg substitute

- A quarter cup of all-purpose flour

- Two tablespoons of finely minced fresh garlic

- Salt and freshly ground pepper to taste

- Cholula hot sauce or other spicy red hot sauce to taste

- One and a half cups of fresh marinara sauce

Instructions

- Heat one tablespoon of olive oil in a heavy-bottomed skillet over medium-high heat. Dip eggplant slices in egg and then lightly into flour.

- Sprinkle slices with garlic and salt and pepper to taste. Cook, adding only as much olive oil as needed, until golden brown, and transfer to a warmed plate.

- Repeat until all eggplant slices are cooked.

- Layer cooked eggplant in an oven-safe casserole dish and drizzle each layer with a small amount of hot sauce and fresh marinara sauce.

- Repeat layers until all eggplant is used. Do not overdo sauces! Keep in a 175-degree F oven until ready to serve.

Spinach fettuccine with baby artichokes

Preparation time-10 minutes | Cook time-20 minutes | Servings-2 | Difficulty-Easy

Nutritional value: ~Calories-437 | Proteins-17g | Fat-3g | Carbohydrates-51g

Ingredients

- Eight ounces of spinach fettuccine

- Nine-ounce package of baby artichokes, thawed

- Three tablespoons of extra-virgin olive oil

- Six cloves fresh garlic, finely chopped

- Sixteen large raw shrimp, peeled and deveined

- Half cup of dry vermouth

- Two large plum tomatoes, finely chopped

- One cup of canned low-sodium, fat-free chicken broth

- Twelve pitted black olives, halved

- One and a half tablespoons of trans fat-free canola/olive oil spread

- One teaspoon of fresh lemon peel, finely grated

- Salt to taste (optional)

- Half teaspoon of ground nutmeg

- One tablespoon of chopped fresh parsley

- Lemon wedges for garnish

Instructions

- Cook pasta per box directions, then remove from heat, drain pasta, and return to pot, drizzling with the scant amount of olive oil to keep the pasta from sticking together. Set aside.

- Cut artichokes lengthwise, remove outer leaves, cut off bases, and trim off tops about

- 1/3 way down. Remove fuzzy choke inside, discard, and cut remaining choke in half again.

- Repeat the procedure until all chokes are cleaned and quartered. In a large skillet, add Two tablespoons of olive oil and garlic and sauté for 1 minute; add artichokes and cook for another 1–2 minutes.

- Add shrimp and vermouth; continue cooking, often stirring, until shrimp are pink. Add tomatoes, broth, olives, canola/olive oil spread, lemon peel, salt, nutmeg, and pasta.

- Toss to coat pasta with sauce. Heat mixture until warmed through. Stir in parsley and drizzle with remaining olive oil. Garnish with lemon wedges.

Sweet-and-sour cabbage

Preparation time-10 minutes | Cook time-18 minutes | Servings-4 | Difficulty-Easy

Nutritional value: ~46 Calories | Fat-3g | Protein-2g | Carbohydrates-4g

Ingredients

- Three slices of bacon

- Four cups of shredded cabbage

- Two tablespoons of cider vinegar

- Twelve drops of liquid stevia (English toffee)

Instructions

- In a heavy skillet, cook the bacon until crisp. Remove and drain.

- Add the cabbage to the bacon grease and sauté it until tender-crisp about 10 minutes.

- Stir together the vinegar and stevia. Stir this into the cabbage. Crumble in the bacon just before serving, so it stays crisp.

Tabbouleh with Avocado

Preparation time-15 minutes| Cook time-20 minutes| Servings-4 |Difficulty-Easy

Nutritional value- Calories-149| Fat-7g |Carbohydrates-21g| Protein-4g

Ingredients

- Half teaspoon of salt

- A quarter cup of finely chopped yellow onion

- One tablespoon of olive oil

- Half avocado

- One cup of peeled, seeded, and diced cucumbers

- One cup of diced tomato

- One clove of garlic

- A quarter cup of mint leaves

- Half cup of parsley leaves

- Half cup of fine cracked wheat

- One tablespoon of lemon juice, or to taste

- Half cup of boiling water

Instructions

- Put some boiling water over the bulgur, cover the bowl and leave it for 20 minutes till it becomes tender.

- Add garlic, onion, chopped herbs, cucumber, tomato, and add to the bulgur.

- Mix the lemon juice, salt, and oil and put them in the wheat mixture.

- Chill for a few hours, throw avocado on top and serve.

Tempeh BLTA Lettuce Wrap

Preparation time-10 minutes |Cook time-30 minutes |Serving-4 |Difficulty- Easy

Nutritional value: ~Calories-129| Fat-7g| Protein-7g| Carbohydrates-10g

Ingredients

- One (8-ounce) package bacon-flavored tempeh

- A quarter cup of low-sodium soy sauce

- A quarter cup of apple cider vinegar

- One teaspoon of sugar substitute

- A quarter teaspoon of ground cumin

- One and a half teaspoons of liquid smoke

- Four romaine lettuce leaves

- Two teaspoons of mayonnaise

- Four tomato slices

- Half avocado, quartered

Instructions

- Preheat the oven to 350°F. Line a baking sheet with parchment paper.

- Slice the tempeh lengthwise into quarter-inch slices. You will get about 12 slices per package. It is easiest to cut the tempeh loaf in half lengthwise. Then cut each half into thirds, and then each third in half to make 12 total slices.

- To make the marinade, in a medium bowl, combine the soy sauce, vinegar, sugar substitute, cumin, and liquid smoke. Whisk well. Place the tempeh in a 9-by-13-inch dish, and cover with marinade. Cover and chill overnight, or at least for one hour. 5. Place the marinated tempeh strips on the prepared baking sheet.

- Bake for 15 minutes, or until lightly brown and crispy. Flip and bake for another 15 minutes.

- Serve 2 strips of tempeh in each lettuce leaf with mayo, a tomato slice, and an avocado quarter.

Tofu and Broccoli Quiche

Preparation time-10 minutes| Cook time-20 minutes| Servings-6 |Difficulty-Easy

Nutritional value- Calories-190| Fat-8g |Carbohydrates-8g| Protein-13g

Ingredients

- One tablespoon of pickled plum paste (umeboshi paste) or white miso

- One tablespoon of sesame oil

- Half pound of broccoli, chopped

- One and a half pounds of tofu

- Half cup of uncooked bulgur wheat

- Pinch of salt

- One yellow onion, chopped

- A quarter-pound of mushrooms, chopped

- Two tablespoons of sesame tahini

Instructions

- Preheat the oven to 350 degrees Fahrenheit (180 degrees Celsius).

- Bring one cup of water to a boil in a small saucepan. Bring the water back to a boil with the salt and bulgur.

- Cook for 16 minutes after lowering the heat to a low level and covering it.

- Bake for 13 minutes, or until the bulgur is crusty and dry, pressing it into an oiled nine-inch pie pan. Remove the item from the table.

- Heat the oil in a large skillet over medium-high heat.

- In a skillet, cook broccoli, onions, and mushrooms for a few minutes.

- Remove the skillet from the heat and cover it; set it away while you make the tofu mixture.

- Combine tahini, tofu, tamari, and umeboshi paste in a food processor and process until smooth.

- Place the mixture in a mixing bowl and add the cooked vegetables. Toss gently to blend.

- Bake for 32 minutes after filling the bulgur crust halfway with veggie mixture.

- Turn off the oven and leave it turned off for 10 minutes.

- Serve warm or cold, cut into 6 slices.

Tofu Stir-Fry

Preparation time-15 minutes | Cook time-40 minutes | Serving-4 | Difficulty-Moderate

Nutritional value: ~Calories-163 | Fat-8g | Protein-12g | Carbohydrates-11g

Ingredients

- One (14 ounces) block extra-firm tofu
- Nonstick cooking spray
- One tablespoon of sesame oil
- Three cups of frozen stir-fry vegetable blend
- Half cup of Stir-Fry Sauce

Instructions

- Preheat the oven to 400°F.
- Drain the tofu, and wrap in a kitchen towel. Place a plate on top of the tofu, and top with something heavy, such as a book or skillet. Let dry for 15 minutes, changing the towel if it gets too wet.
- Once dry, chop into 1-inch cubes or rectangles. Arrange the tofu on a lightly greased or parchment paper-covered baking sheet, and bake for 25 to 35 minutes, or until golden brown, flipping halfway through.
- Once golden brown, remove from the oven and let cool while you continue cooking.
- Heat a large skillet over medium-high heat. Add the sesame oil, and swirl to coat. Add the veggies, and stir-fry or toss to coat. Cook for 5 minutes.
- Add the stir-fry sauce, and stir to coat.
- Add the tofu, and stir. Cook for 3 to 5 minutes, gently stirring constantly.
- When the veggies reach the tenderness of your liking, remove from the heat and serve.

Tofu with mushrooms

Preparation time-25 minutes | Cook time-17 minutes | Servings-2 to 4 | Difficulty-Moderate

Nutritional value: ~Calories-235 | Proteins-16g | Fat-14g | Carbohydrates-11g

Ingredients

- Black pepper to taste
- One tablespoon of sweetener
- One tablespoon of Hoisin sauce
- Fourteen ounces of tofu
- Five tablespoons of soy sauce
- One lb of Cremini mushrooms
- One pinch of red color
- One tablespoon of rice vinegar
- Two teaspoons of peanut oil
- Three sliced ginger
- One teaspoon of sesame oil
- Three sliced garlic cloves
- Half cup of sliced green onions

Instructions

- Marinate tofu with a mixture of vinegar, pepper, soy sauce, and sesame oil in a bowl.
- Drain tofu after 30 minutes of marination. Add it to the marination mixture.
- Sauté ginger and garlic in heated oil over medium flame.
- Mix in tofu and cook for ten minutes. After seven minutes, take out tofu and set it aside.
- Pour oil add mushrooms, and cook for five more minutes.
- Again put tofu in the pan and cook. Pour in the sauce mixture, reduce the flame and cook for five minutes.
- Stir in onions and cook for two minutes.
- Serve and enjoy it.

Two-cheese cauliflower

Preparation time-10 minutes | Cook time-15 minutes | Servings-8 | Difficulty-Easy

Nutritional value: ~213 Calories | Fat-17g | Protein-13g | Carbohydrates-3g

Ingredients

- One head cauliflower, cut into florets One and a half pounds frozen cauliflower
- One large egg
- One cup of small-curd whole-milk cottage cheese
- One cup of sour cream
- Half teaspoon of salt
- 1/8 teaspoon of ground black pepper
- Eight ounces of sharp Cheddar cheese, shredded
- Two tablespoons of chopped fresh parsley (optional)

Instructions

- Preheat oven to 350°F,
- Lightly coat a 2-quart baking dish with non-stick cooking spray.
- Put the cauliflower florets in a microwavable casserole dish, add Two tablespoons of water (28 ml), and cover.
- Microwave it for 10 to 11 minutes, or until very tender.

- Stir two tablespoons of poppy seeds into the cauliflower before baking. This gives it a kind of polka-dot look and adds subtle sophistication to the flavor.

Veggie wrap

Preparation time-10 minutes |Cook time-40 minutes |Servings-2 to 4 |Difficulty-Moderate

Nutritional value: ~Calories-170|Proteins-9g| Fat-1g|Carbohydrates-36g

Ingredients

- Olive oil cooking spray

- Two medium tomatoes, cut into Half-inch thick slices

- Two small cucumbers, sliced lengthwise into Half-inch thick slices

- Two small onions, cut into Half-inch thick slices

- One green bell pepper, cut into strips

- Two medium zucchini, sliced lengthwise into Half-inch thick slices

- Extra-virgin olive oil to drizzle

- 3/4 tablespoon of crumbled dried oregano

- A quarter tablespoon of crumbled dried rosemary

- 3/4 teaspoon of dried thyme

Half (15-ounce) can chickpeas, rinsed and drained

- A quarter teaspoon of cumin (optional)

- Salt and freshly ground pepper to taste

- Six whole wheat flatbreads (8–10-inch), warmed

- Alfalfa sprouts (optional)

Instructions

- Spray a non-stick pan with cooking spray. Place tomatoes, cucumbers, onions, green bell pepper, and zucchini on the pan, and drizzle with olive oil.

- Sprinkle with oregano, rosemary, and thyme, and roast for 15–20 minutes at 425 degrees F.

- Add chickpeas and cumin, plus salt and pepper to taste, and cook an additional 15–20 minutes until tender.

- Fill warmed flatbread with bean and veggie mix, top with alfalfa sprouts, if desired, roll up, and serve.

Whopper Veggie Burger

Preparation time- 5 minutes| Cook time-5 minutes| Servings-1 |Difficulty-Easy

Nutritional value- Calories-260| Fat-5g |Carbohydrates-5g| Protein-19g

Ingredients

- One hamburger bun (whole-wheat)

- One tablespoon of ketchup

- One tablespoon of mustard

- One tablespoon of Miracle Whip Light

- One Boca-Burger (Mushroom Mozzarella flavor)

- Lettuce

- Onion

- Tomato

Instructions

- Prepare the Boca Burger according to the package directions.

- Spread tomato, ketchup, light miracle whip, lettuce, and onion on a bun.

Zucchini Enchilada Boats with Meatless Crumbles

Preparation time-10 minutes |Cook time-30 minutes |Serving-6 |Difficulty-Moderate

Nutritional value: ~Calories-145| Fat-4g| Protein-17g| Carbohydrates-16g

Ingredients

- Three cups of meatless crumbles, such as Tofurky brand

- Two tablespoons of Taco Seasoning

- Half cup of water

- Three large zucchini, as wide and uniform as possible

- One and a half cups of red enchilada sauce

- Half cup of shredded Cheddar cheese

Optional toppings

- Chopped fresh cilantro

- Diced tomatoes

- Diced scallions

- Diced avocado

- Low-fat, plain Greek yogurt

Instructions

- Preheat the oven to 425°F.

- In a large skillet, prepare the meatless crumbles per package directions. Add the taco seasoning and water, and mix well. Simmer until the liquid has evaporated.

- Halve the zucchini lengthwise, and scoop out the seeds to make a "boat," leaving quarter-inch-thick edges.

- In a 9-by-13-inch baking dish, place the zucchini boat's flesh side up.

- Fill the zucchini with meatless crumbles.

- Pour the enchilada sauce over the zucchini, then sprinkle with the cheese.

- Cover the dish with aluminum foil, and bake for 20 minutes. Remove the foil, and bake for another 5 to 10 minutes uncovered, or until the cheese is melted and the zucchini is cooked through.

- Add desired toppings, and serve.

Zucchini Lasagna Roll-Ups

Preparation time-30 minutes | Cook time-30 minutes | Serving-6 | Difficulty-Hard

Nutritional value: -Calories-240 | Fat-13g | Protein-18g | Carbohydrates-16g

Ingredients

- Three large zucchinis, trimmed and sliced lengthwise into -inch-thick strips

- One teaspoon of salt

- Nonstick cooking spray

- One (10-ounce) bag of fresh spinach

- One cup of part-skim ricotta

- Half cup of Parmesan cheese

- One large egg

- Two garlic cloves, minced

- Two teaspoons of Italian seasoning

- One and a half cups of marinara sauce, divided

- One cup of part-skim shredded mozzarella

Instructions

- Preheat the oven to 400°F.

- Lay the zucchini slices flat on a paper towel-lined baking sheet, and sprinkle with salt. Let's sit for 15 minutes.

- Meanwhile, spray a small skillet with nonstick cooking spray, and set over medium heat.

- Add the spinach and cook for 2 minutes, or until wilted. Remove from the heat.

- In a medium bowl, mix the ricotta, Parmesan, egg, garlic, and Italian seasoning until well combined.

- Pat the zucchini dry, removing excess salt.

- Spread one cup of marinara in the bottom of a 9-by-9-inch baking dish.

- Spread each zucchini slice with a spoonful of ricotta mixture, then gently roll up and place in the prepared baking dish, seam-side down. Repeat with the remaining zucchini and filling.

- Top with the remaining half cup of marinara, and sprinkle with the mozzarella cheese.

- Bake for 25 to 30 minutes, or until the lasagna rolls are heated through, and the cheese begins to brown.

- Serve immediately.

Chapter 12~Beverages Recipes

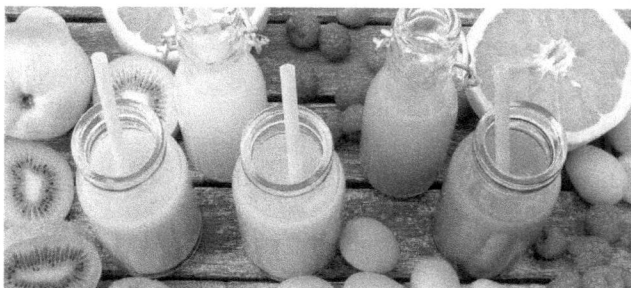

Apricot~orange smoothie

Preparation time~10 minutes |Cook time~0 minutes |Servings~2 |Difficulty~Easy

Nutritional value: ~Calories~119|Proteins~8g| Fat~2g|Carbohydrates~8g

Ingredients

- Two cups of full-fat, canned coconut milk
- Two medium apricots pitted
- One large navel orange, peeled
- One tablespoon of lemon juice
- One teaspoon of rose water
- Two cups of ice
- Two tablespoons of grass-fed beef gelatin

Instructions

- Combine the coconut milk, apricots, orange, lemon juice, rose water, if using, and ice in a blender and pulse until smooth.
- Add the gelatin and pulse again until smooth. Pour into two 8-ounce glasses and enjoy.

Avocado and Apple Smoothie

Preparation time~5 minutes |Cook time~0 minutes |Servings~2 |Difficulty~Easy

Nutritional value: ~Calories~168|Proteins~2.1g| Fat~10g|Carbohydrates~21g

Ingredients

- Three cups of spinach
- One green apple, cored and chopped
- One avocado, peeled, pitted, and chopped
- Three tablespoons chia seeds
- One teaspoon of honey
- One banana, frozen and peeled
- Two cups of coconut water

Instructions

- In your blender, blend the spinach with the apple and the rest of the ingredients.
- Pulse and divide into glasses and serve.

Banana caramel milkshake

Preparation time~15 minutes |Cook time~0 minutes |Serving~2 |Difficulty~ Easy

Nutritional value: ~ Calories~124| Fat~9g| Protein~4g| Carbohydrates~8g

Ingredients

- One cup of Vanilla ice cream
- Half cup of Milk
- Four tablespoons of Salted caramel sauce
- One large ripe banana

Instructions

- Process all ingredients until smooth, around 2-3 minutes, in a blender.
- Serve in separate glasses immediately and top with extra car mail sauce if needed.

Banana cream pie smoothie

Preparation time~5 minutes |Cook time~0 minutes |Serving~2 |Difficulty~ Easy

Nutritional value: ~ Calories~124| Fat~9g| Protein~4g| Carbohydrates~8g

Ingredients

- One cup of sliced ripe banana
- One cup of vanilla low-fat yogurt
- Half cup of low-fat milk
- Two tablespoons of whole wheat graham cracker crumbs
- One tablespoon of nonfat dry milk
- Half teaspoon of vanilla extract
- Three ice cubes
- Graham cracker crumbs

Instructions

- On a baking sheet, arrange the collar pieces on a single layer and leave them to stand until firm (about 1 hour).
- In a blender, place the frozen bananas and the remaining ingredients until a smooth process. Use graham cracker crumbs to sprinkle. Immediately serve.

Banana Cream Protein Shake

Preparation time~5 minutes |Cook time~0 minutes |Serving~2 |Difficulty~ Easy

Nutritional value: ~Calories-226 | Fat-4g | Protein-17g | Carbohydrates-30g

Ingredients

- One and a half cups of low-fat milk
- A quarter cup of low-fat, plain Greek yogurt
- One small banana
- One teaspoon of vanilla extract
- One scoop (¼ cup) vanilla protein powder
- One tablespoon of sugar-free instant banana pudding mix

Instructions

- In a blender, combine the milk, yogurt, banana, vanilla, protein powder, and pudding mix. Blend on high for 2 to 3 minutes, until the powder has dissolved and the mixture is smooth.
- Pour half of the shake into a glass, and enjoy.
- Store the remaining half in an airtight container in the refrigerator for up to a week, and re-blend prior to serving.

Banana peach vanilla soy milk smoothie

Preparation time-10 minutes | Cook time-0 minutes | Servings-2 | Difficulty-Easy

Nutritional value: ~Calories-204 | Proteins-5g | Fat-3g | Carbohydrates-19g

Ingredients

- One cup of light vanilla soy milk
- One medium banana
- One medium peach, pitted and sliced
- One cup of ice
- One teaspoon of vanilla extract
- Non-caloric sweetener

Instructions

- In a blender, combine soy milk, banana, peach, and ice. The process to desired consistency; with the machine running, add vanilla extract and sweetener.
- Serve immediately.

Banana, Orange, and Kiwi Smoothie

Preparation time-15 minutes | Cook time- 0 minutes | Servings-3 | Difficulty-Easy

Nutritional value- Calories- 231 | Fat- 6 g | Protein- 14 g | Carbohydrates- 33 g

Ingredients

- One cup of crushed ice

- One and a half banana
- ¾ cup of orange juice
- One kiwi
- A quarter cup of coconut milk
- One tablespoon of agave syrup
- Three tablespoons of protein powder

Instructions

- Add all the ingredients to a food processor and blend to get a smooth mixture.
- Serve and enjoy it.

Berry Blast Protein Shake

Preparation time- 5 minutes | Cook time-0 minutes | Servings-2 | Difficulty-Easy

Nutritional value- Calories-126 | Fat-3g | Carbohydrates-14g | Protein-15g

Ingredients

- Five ice cubes
- A quarter cup of vanilla or plain protein powder
- One cup of low-fat milk or unsweetened soy milk
- ¾ cup of mixed frozen berries

Instructions

- Mix the ice cubes, berries, milk, and protein powder and blend till all the powder is well incorporated.
- Pour and chill the leftover in an airtight container. Throw away any leftovers after a week.

Berry Bliss Protein Shake

Preparation time-5 minutes | Cook time-0 minutes | Serving-2 | Difficulty- Easy

Nutritional value: ~ Calories-206 | Fat-4g | Protein-18g | Carbohydrates-24g

Ingredients

- One cup of low-fat milk
- Half cup of low-fat, plain Greek yogurt
- One scoop (¼ cup) vanilla protein powder
- One cup of frozen mixed berries
- One small handful of spinach
- One teaspoon of vanilla extract
- One tablespoon of freshly squeezed lemon juice

Instructions

- In a blender, combine the milk, yogurt, protein powder, berries, spinach, vanilla, and lemon juice. Blend on high until smooth.

- Pour half of the shake into a glass, and enjoy.

- Store the remaining half in an airtight container in the refrigerator for up to a week, and re-blend prior to serving.

Berry breakfast smoothie

Preparation time-5 minutes |Cook time-5 minutes |Servings-2 |Difficulty-Easy

Nutritional value: ~Calories-117|Proteins-8g| Fat-1g|Carbohydrates-18g

Ingredients

- Two cups of milk

- Half cup of oats

- Two cups of berries

- Two teaspoons of chia seeds

Instructions

- Add milk with fruit and oats in a blender.

- Blend it smoothly, mix in chia seeds and serve instantly.

Berry-Mango Breakfast Shake

Preparation time-5 minutes |Cook time-0 minutes |Serving-4 |Difficulty- Easy

Nutritional value: ~ Calories-104| Fat-0.5g| Protein-4g| Carbohydrates-19g

Ingredients

- One and a half cups of frozen berries

- One cup of fresh or canned mango slices, chilled

- One cup of soft, silken, low-fat tofu

- One cup of diet cranberry juice cocktail

- Half teaspoon of vanilla extract

- Six teaspoons of sugar substitute

- Four sprigs mint

Instructions

- In a blender, process the berries, mango, tofu, juice, vanilla, and sugar substitute, until the consistency is smooth.

- Pour into glasses and top with the mint.

Blueberry brainpower smoothie

Preparation time-5 minutes |Cook time-0 minutes |Serving-3 |Difficulty- Easy

Nutritional value: ~ Calories-124| Fat-9g| Protein-4g| Carbohydrates-8g

Ingredients

- Six ounces of light vanilla soy milk (or your choice of milk)

- One scoop of natural vanilla protein powder

- ⅓ cup of frozen blueberries

- ⅓ cup of natural vanilla yogurt

- One tablespoon of ground flaxseed

- Sweetener of your choice

- Ice

Instructions

- Add all ingredients to the blender.

- Process until smooth, adding sweetener and ice as desired. Enjoy!

Blueberry burst whey smoothie

Preparation time-10 minutes |Cook time-0 minutes |Servings-2 |Difficulty-Easy

Nutritional value: ~Calories-124|Proteins-22g| Fat-1g|Carbohydrates-10g

Ingredients

- Half cup of cold water

- A quarter cup of fresh or unsweetened frozen blueberries

- Two packets of non-caloric sweetener

- A quarter cup of plain non-fat yogurt

- One scoop of natural-flavored whey protein powder

- Eight ice cubes

- Fat-free whipped cream

- Sprinkle of crushed almonds for garnish

Instructions

- In an ice-crushing blender, add water, berries, and sweetener and blend until smooth. Add yogurt and

whey and blend until smooth again.

- Add ice cubes and chop until crushed. Pour into glass and top with whipped cream and almonds.

Blueberry Vanilla Smoothie

Preparation time- 5 minutes| Cook time-0 minutes| Servings-1 |Difficulty-Easy

Nutritional value- Calories-185| Fat-0g |Carbohydrates-18g| Protein-29g

Ingredients

- One tablespoon of unsweetened vanilla whey protein powder

- Half cup of fresh or frozen blueberries

- ¾ cup of non-fat plain Greek yogurt

Instructions

- Put the blueberries, protein powder, stevia, and yogurt in the blender. Now blend for around 2 minutes or till everything is well-mixed.

- Serve and enjoy.

Body Pumping Smoothie

Preparation time-10 minutes| Cook time-0 minutes| Servings-2 |Difficulty-Easy

Nutritional value- Calories-185| Fat-0g |Carbohydrates-18g| Protein-29g

Ingredients

- One beetroot

- One Apple

- Three tablespoons of yogurt

- Handful of mint

- One thumb of a two-inch ginger

- Half teaspoon of black salt or rock salt

- One teaspoon of honey or sugar

- A quarter cup of water

Instructions

- Clean and remove the beet peel.

- Slice the medium-sized apple and remove the nuts.

- Add all the ingredients into the blender.

- Add ice, then proceed to mix into a paste that is smooth.

- Add juice from the lemon.

- Enjoy and serve.

Breakfast green smoothie

Preparation time-5 minutes |Cook time-0 minutes |Servings-2 |Difficulty-Easy

Nutritional value: ~Calories-229|Proteins-5g| Fat-5g|Carbohydrates-48g

Ingredients

- Two tablespoons of hemp hearts

- Two cups of spinach

- One medium banana

- Two cups of pineapple

- Half apple

- Two cups of water

Instructions

- Blend all the items in the blender and serve.

Bright Morning Smoothie

Preparation time-15 minutes |Cook time-0 minutes |Serving-2 |Difficulty- Easy

Nutritional value: ~ Calories-110| Fat-2g| Protein-11g| Carbohydrates-9.2g

Ingredients

- Two cups of Washed Spinach

- Two Large Strawberries

- A quarter cup of Lemon Juice or Fresh Squeezed Orange Juice

- Two tablespoons of Chia Seeds or Powder

- One cup of Green Tea

- One cup of Ice

- Four tablespoons of sweetener of choice

Instructions

- Place all of the ingredients in a mixer.

- Blend it all until smooth.

- Let it rest for about 5-10 minutes, then serve.

Café Mocha Protein Blend

Preparation time-5 minutes |Cook time-0 minutes |Serving-2 |Difficulty- Easy

Nutritional value: ~ Calories-95| Fat-2g| Protein-10g| Carbohydrates-9g

Ingredients

- Half cup of low-fat milk

- One cup of decaffeinated coffee, brewed and chilled

- One scoop (¼ cup) vanilla protein powder

- One teaspoon of unsweetened cocoa powder

- Half teaspoon of vanilla extract

- Four ice cubes

Instructions

In a blender, combine the milk, coffee, protein powder, cocoa powder, vanilla, and ice. Blend on high until smooth.

Pour half of the shake into a glass, and enjoy.

Store the remaining half in an airtight container in the refrigerator for up to a week, and re-blend prior to serving.

Chocolate mousse whey smoothie

Preparation time-10 minutes |Cook time-0 minutes |Servings-2 |Difficulty-Easy

Nutritional value: ~Calories-145|Proteins-24g| Fat-1g|Carbohydrates-11g

Ingredients

- Half cup of cold water

- Half cup of plain fat-free yogurt

- One scoop of natural-flavored whey protein powder

- Two packets of non-caloric sweetener

- One tablespoon of fat-free, sugar-free chocolate syrup

- One teaspoon of almond extract

- Eight ice cubes

- Fat-free whipped cream

- Fat-free, sugar-free chocolate syrup to drizzle

- Sprinkle of crushed almonds for garnish (optional)

Instructions

- In an ice-crushing blender, add water, yogurt, whey, sweetener, chocolate syrup, and almond extract, and blend until smooth. Add ice and chop until crushed.

- Pour into a glass and top with whipped cream, chocolate syrup, and almonds, if desired.

Chocolate raspberry soy milk smoothie

Preparation time-10 minutes | Cook time-0 minutes | Servings-2 | Difficulty-Easy

Nutritional value: ~Calories-317 | Proteins-8g | Fat-4g | Carbohydrates-66g

Ingredients

- One cup of light chocolate soy milk

- One medium banana

- One cup of frozen unsweetened raspberries

- One cup of ice

- One teaspoon of vanilla extract

- Non-caloric sweetener to taste

Instructions

- In a blender, combine soy milk, banana, raspberries, and ice. The process to desired consistency; with the machine running, add vanilla extract and sweetener.

- Serve immediately.

Chocolate-Mint Protein Shake

Preparation time-5 minutes | Cook time-0 minutes | Serving-2 | Difficulty- Easy

Nutritional value: ~ Calories-170 | Fat-3g | Protein-19g | Carbohydrates-15g

Ingredients

- One cup of low-fat milk

- Half cup of low-fat cottage cheese

- One scoop (¼ cup) chocolate protein powder

- One tablespoon of cocoa powder

- A quarter teaspoon of mint extract

- Four ice cubes

Instructions

- In a blender, combine the milk, cottage cheese, protein powder, cocoa powder, mint extract, and ice. Blend on high until smooth.

- Pour half of the shake into a glass, and enjoy.

- Store the remaining half in an airtight container in the refrigerator for up to a week, and re-blend prior to serving.

Chocolate-Raspberry Truffle Protein Shake

Preparation time-5 minutes | Cook time-0 minutes | Serving-1 | Difficulty- Easy

Nutritional value: ~ Calories-285 | Fat-5g | Protein-27g | Carbohydrates-33g

Ingredients

- One cup of low-fat milk

- One scoop (¼ cup) chocolate protein powder

- Two teaspoons of unsweetened cocoa powder

- One teaspoon of vanilla extract

- Half cup of frozen raspberries

Instructions

- In a blender, combine the milk, protein powder, cocoa powder, vanilla, and raspberries. Blend on high until smooth.

- Pour half of the shake into a glass, and enjoy.

- Store the remaining half in an airtight container in the refrigerator for up to a week, and re-blend prior to serving.

Chunky Monkey Smoothie

Preparation time- 5 minutes| Cook time-0 minutes| Servings-2 |Difficulty-Easy

Nutritional value- Calories-298| Fat-16g |Carbohydrates-2.8g| Protein-20.9g

Ingredients

- Half cup of Greek yogurt

- One cup of ice cubes

- Two tablespoons of powdered peanut butter

- One cup of unsweetened almond milk

- A quarter cup of chocolate protein powder

- 1 small banana, frozen

Instructions

- Mix the banana, milk, yogurt, protein powder, powdered peanut butter, and ice cubes, then puree until the consistency is smooth, there are no lumps, and the powder is well incorporated. You can add two to three tablespoons of water.

- Pour and chill the leftover in an airtight container. Throw away any leftovers after a week.

Cool-as-a-Cucumber Water

Preparation time-5 minutes |Cook time-0 minutes |Serving-8 cups |Difficulty- Easy

Nutritional value: ~ Calories-8| Fat-0g| Protein-0g| Carbohydrates-3g

Ingredients

- Eight cups of water

- One lemon, sliced

- One lime, sliced

- Half cucumber, sliced

- Two fresh mint sprigs

Instructions

- In a 2¼-quart pitcher, combine the water, lemon, lime, cucumber, and mint. Muddle, if desired.

- Chill for 30 minutes before drinking, or for best flavor, overnight.

Creamy Pumpkin Pie Smoothie

Preparation time- 5 minutes| Cook time-0 minutes| Servings-1 |Difficulty-Easy

Nutritional value- Calories-242| Fat-1g |Carbohydrates-25g| Protein-36g

Ingredients

- A pinch of salt (optional)

- One and a quarter teaspoon of ground cinnamon

- Half teaspoon of stevia (optional)

- ⅔ cup of unsweetened canned pumpkin

- One cup of non-fat plain Greek yogurt

- One tablespoon of unsweetened vanilla whey protein powder

Instructions

- Put the pumpkin, stevia (if preferred), salt (if preferred), cinnamon, protein powder, and yogurt in the blender.

- Now blend for around 2 minutes or till everything is well-mixed. Serve and enjoy.

Frosty Peppermint Shake

Preparation time-5 minutes |Cook time-0 minutes |Serving-3 |Difficulty- Easy

Nutritional value: ~ Calories-124| Fat-9g| Protein-4g| Carbohydrates-8g

Ingredients

- Eight ounces of milk, skim

- One scoop of chocolate protein powder

- One tablespoon of sugar-free, chocolate fudge instant pudding mix

- A quarter teaspoon of peppermint extract

- A handful of ice cubes

Instructions

- Add all ingredients to a blender. Let whirl until smooth, creamy, and frosty. Drink immediately.

Green Machine Protein Shake

Preparation time-5 minutes |Cook time-0 minutes |Serving-2 |Difficulty- Easy

Nutritional value: ~ Calories-133| Fat-5g| Protein-10g| Carbohydrates-16g

Ingredients

- One and a half cups of water

- Half medium banana

- Half small Granny Smith apple

- Two loose handfuls of spinach

- One small handful of fresh parsley

- A quarter avocado, peeled

- Juice of one lemon

- One scoop (¼ cup) unflavored protein powder

Instructions

- In a blender, combine the water, banana, apple, spinach, parsley, avocado, lemon juice, and protein powder. Blend on high until smooth.

- Pour half of the shake into a glass, and enjoy.

- Store the remaining half in an airtight container in the refrigerator for up to a week, and re-blend prior to serving.

High Protein Milk

Preparation time-5 minutes |Cook time-0 minutes |Serving-4 |Difficulty- Easy

Nutritional value: ~ Calories-127| Fat-3g| Protein-11g| Carbohydrates-15g

Ingredients

- Four cups of low-fat milk

- One and ⅓ cups of instant nonfat dry milk powder

Instructions

- In a large pitcher, mix the milk and milk powder well.

- Chill in the refrigerator for up to 5 days.

Iced Strawberry and Greens

Preparation time-5 minutes |Cook time-0 minutes |Serving-2 |Difficulty- Easy

Nutritional value: ~ Calories-127| Fat-3g| Protein-11g| Carbohydrates-15g

Ingredients

- Half cup coconut water

- One cup of ice

- One cup of washed spinach

- Three large strawberries

- Sweetener to taste

Instructions

- Blend all the ingredients together in a blender until smooth.

- Let it rest for 5 minutes and then serve chilled.

Kale Avocado Smoothie

Preparation time- 10 minutes| Cook time- 0 minutes| Servings-2 |Difficulty-Easy

Nutritional value- Calories-114| Fat-6.7g |Carbohydrates-5g| Protein-10.9g

Ingredients

- One cup of sliced new kale

- Half cup of avocado

- 3/4 cup of almond unsweetened milk

- A quarter cup of yogurt full-fat, simple

- Three to four cubes of ice

- One spoonful of fresh lemon juice

- Stevia powder in oil

Instructions

- In a mixer, add spinach, avocado, and almond milk.

- Pulse several times on the ingredients.

- Add remaining ingredients and blend together until smooth.

- Pour into a large bottle and instantly drink it.

Kiwi Dream Blender

Preparation time-5 minutes |Cook time-0 minutes |Serving-2 |Difficulty- Easy

Nutritional value: ~ Calories-127| Fat-3g| Protein-11g| Carbohydrates-15g

Ingredients

- A quarter average avocado

- One small wedge of Galia melon (or Honeydew, Cantaloupe)

- One scoop of vanilla whey protein powder (vanilla or plain)

- powdered gelatin

- Six drops liquid Stevia extract

- Ice as per the need

- A quarter cup of coconut milk (or coconut cream or full-fat cream)

- A quarter cup of kiwi berries or kiwi fruit

- One tablespoon of chia seeds (or psyllium)

- Half cups of water

Instructions

- Strip and peel the avocado and put it in a blender.

- Add the kiwi, melon and the remaining ingredients to the flesh.

- Blend until completely smooth.

- Serve.

Lemon Meringue Pie Smoothie

Preparation time- 5 minutes| Cook time-0 minutes| Servings-1 |Difficulty-Easy

Nutritional value- Calories-179| Fat-1g |Carbohydrates-14g| Protein-29g

Ingredients

- A quarter teaspoon of stevia

- One tablespoon of unsweetened vanilla whey protein powder

- One teaspoon of vanilla extract

- Half cup of unsweetened almond milk

- Two small lemons juice

- ¾ cup of non-fat plain Greek yogurt

Instructions

- Put the vanilla extract, lemon juice, yogurt, protein powder, stevia, and almond milk in the blender.

- Now blend for around 2 minutes or till everything is well-mixed. Serve and enjoy.

Lemon Pie Protein Shake

Preparation time-5 minutes |Cook time-0 minutes |Serving-2 |Difficulty- Easy

Nutritional value: ~ Calories-189| Fat-4g| Protein-18g| Carbohydrates-21g

Ingredients

- One cup of low-fat milk

- Half cup of low-fat, plain Greek yogurt

- Half medium banana

- One teaspoon of lemon zest

- Two teaspoons of freshly squeezed lemon juice

- ⅛ teaspoon of lemon extract

- A quarter teaspoon of vanilla extract

- One scoop (¼ cup) vanilla protein powder

- Two to four ice cubes

Instructions

- In a blender, combine the milk, yogurt, banana, lemon zest, lemon juice, lemon extract, vanilla, protein powder, and ice. Blend on high until smooth.

- Pour half of the shake into a glass, and enjoy.

- Store the remaining half in an airtight container in the refrigerator for up to a week, and re-blend prior to serving.

Low-Carb Caribbean Cream

Preparation time-10 minutes |Cook time-0 minutes |Serving-1 |Difficulty- Easy

Nutritional value: ~ Calories-127| Fat-3g| Protein-11g| Carbohydrates-15g

Ingredients

- Half cup of unsweetened coconut milk

- A quarter cup of coconut water or water (iced)

- One shot of dark or white rum

- One slice of fresh pineapple

- Five drops of liquid Stevia extract

Instructions

- In an ice cube tray, freeze the coconut water for 1-2 hours.

- Blend coconut milk and pineapple until creamy.

- Add the coconut water ice cubes and rum to the serving bottle.

- Add the combined solution.

- Use the pineapple to garnish.

- Serve and enjoy.

Melon madness whey smoothie

Preparation time-10 minutes |Cook time-0 minutes |Servings-2 |Difficulty-Easy

Nutritional value: ~Calories-204|Proteins-22g| Fat-2g|Carbohydrates-27g

Ingredients

- Half cup of cold water

- Half (5–6-inch) fresh cantaloupe

- Two packets of non-caloric sweetener

- A quarter cup of plain non-fat yogurt

- One scoop of natural-flavored whey protein powder

- Eight ice cubes

- Fat-free whipped cream

- Crushed almonds for garnish

Instructions

- In an ice-crushing blender, add water, cantaloupe, sweetener, yogurt, and whey, and blend until smooth. Add ice and chop until crushed.

- Pour into glass and top with whipped cream and almonds.

Mexican Comfort Cream

Preparation time-5 minutes | Cook time-15 minutes | Serving-2 | Difficulty- Easy

Nutritional value: ~ Calories-127| Fat-3g| Protein-11g| Carbohydrates-15g

Ingredients

- Two handfuls of almonds blanched
- One cup of almond milk (unsweetened)
- One large egg
- Two tablespoons of whole or ground chia seeds
- One tablespoon of lime zest
- One teaspoon of cinnamon powder or one whole cinnamon stick
- Three tablespoons of erythritol or another healthy low-carb sweetener
- Twenty drops of liquid Stevia extract (Clear / Cinnamon)
- Two cups of warm water

Instructions

- Put in a bowl lime zest, the blanched almonds and cinnamon stick and cover with two teaspoons of hot water.
- Let it rest for about eight hours or overnight.
- Remove the lime zest and cinnamon stick after the almonds have been softened and put them in a shallow saucepan.
- Mix almond milk. Purée until it's really smooth.
- Steam the mixture and mix cinnamon and sweeteners before it begins to sizzle.
- Whisk the egg when stirring constantly and pour it gently into the mixture.
- Stir for a minute or two over the heat.
- Remove from the heat and add in the seeds of chia.
- To thicken the remainder.
- Serve cold and pour in a bottle.

Minted Iced Berry Sparkler

Preparation time-5 minutes | Cook time-0 minutes | Serving-2 | Difficulty- Easy

Nutritional value: ~ Calories-127| Fat-3g| Protein-11g| Carbohydrates-15g

Ingredients

- One cup of mixed frozen berries
- One lime or lemon
- One cup of fresh mint

- Twenty drops liquid Stevia extract (Clear / Berry)
- One large bottle of water
- Ice

Instructions

- Wash the mint.
- Cut the lime into wedges that are thin.
- Use your option of sparkling or still water to put mint, frozen berries, lemon wedges or lime and leftover ingredients into all in a jar.
- Let yourself relax for 15 minutes or more. The longer you keep it, the taste gets bolder.
- Serve.

Neapolitan Smoothie

Preparation time- 5 minutes| Cook time-0 minutes| Servings-1 | Difficulty-Easy

Nutritional value- Calories-189| Fat-2g |Carbohydrates-20g| Protein-24g

Ingredients

- A quarter teaspoon of stevia (optional)
- Half tablespoon of unsweetened cocoa powder
- One teaspoon of vanilla extract
- A quarter cup of unsweetened almond milk
- Half cup of fresh or frozen strawberries
- One cup of non-fat plain Greek yogurt

Instructions

- Put strawberries, vanilla extract, cocoa powder, almond milk, stevia, and yogurt (if preferred) in the blender.
- Now blend for around 2 minutes or till everything is well-mixed. Serve and enjoy.

Peaches and Cream Smoothie

Preparation time-5 minutes| Cook time-0 minutes| Servings-1 | Difficulty-Easy

Nutritional value- Calories-110| Fat-0g |Carbohydrates-20g| Protein-8g

Ingredients

- One packet sugar substitute, or to taste
- A quarter cup of ice
- A quarter cup of plain nonfat yogurt
- A quarter teaspoon of vanilla extract
- Half cup of canned no-sugar-added peaches, drained
- Two tablespoons of nonfat dry powdered milk

- A quarter cup of nonfat milk

Instructions

- Mix the powdered milk and the nonfat milk and put them aside for 2 to 3 minutes. Then place all ingredients in a blender and blend well.

Peaches and Creamy Coconut Smoothie

Preparation time- 5 minutes| Cook time-0 minutes| Servings-1 |Difficulty-Easy

Nutritional value- Calories-162| Fat-4g |Carbohydrates-13g| Protein-19g

Ingredients

- A quarter teaspoon of stevia (optional)

- Two tablespoons of unsweetened vanilla whey protein powder

- A quarter cup of coconut cream

- ¾ cup of frozen peaches

- ¾ cup of non-fat plain Greek yogurt

Instructions

- Put the coconut cream, peaches, yogurt, stevia, and protein powder, in the blender.

- Now blend for around 2 minutes or till everything is well-mixed. Serve and enjoy.

Peanut Butter and Banana Power Smoothie

Preparation time- 5 minutes| Cook time-0 minutes| Servings-2 |Difficulty-Easy

Nutritional value- Calories-178| Fat-2g |Carbohydrates-20g| Protein-24g

Ingredients

- A quarter teaspoon of stevia (optional)

- One tablespoon of unsweetened vanilla whey protein powder

- One small banana

- A quarter cup of unsweetened dry peanut butter powder

- Half cup of ice

- One cup of non-fat plain Greek yogurt

Instructions

- Put the ice, protein powder, banana, yogurt, peanut butter powder, and stevia in the blender.

- Now blend for around 2 minutes or till everything is well-mixed. Serve and enjoy.

Peanut Butter and Chocolate Protein Shake

Preparation time-5 minutes |Cook time-0 minutes |Serving-2 |Difficulty- Easy

Nutritional value: ~ Calories-189| Fat-5g| Protein-21g| Carbohydrates-18g

Ingredients

- One cup of low-fat milk

- Half cup of low-fat, plain Greek yogurt

- One scoop (¼ cup) chocolate whey protein powder

- Two tablespoons of powdered peanut butter

- One tablespoon of unsweetened cocoa powder

- Three ice cubes

Instructions

- In a blender, combine the milk, yogurt, protein powder, peanut butter, cocoa powder, and ice. Blend on high until smooth.

- Pour half of the shake into a glass, and enjoy.

- Store the remaining half in an airtight container in the refrigerator for up to a week, and re-blend prior to serving.

Piña Colada Protein Shake

Preparation time-5 minutes |Cook time-0 minutes |Serving-2 |Difficulty- Easy

Nutritional value: ~ Calories-195| Fat-5g| Protein-14g| Carbohydrates-18g

Ingredients

- One and a half cups of unsweetened coconut milk

- Half cup of low-fat cottage cheese

- One cup of frozen pineapple chunks

- One teaspoon of coconut extract

- One scoop (¼ cup) vanilla protein powder

- Four to five ice cubes

- The sugar substitute for added sweetness (optional)

Instructions

In a blender, combine the coconut milk, cottage cheese, pineapple, coconut extract, protein powder, ice, and sugar substitute (if using). Blend on high until smooth.

Pour half of the shake into a glass, and enjoy.

Store the remaining half in an airtight container in the refrigerator for up to a week, and re-blend prior to serving.

Pineapple delight whey smoothie

Preparation time-10 minutes |Cook time-0 minutes |Servings-2 |Difficulty-Easy

Nutritional value: ~Calories-149|Proteins-20g| Fat-1g|Carbohydrates-16g

Ingredients

- Half cup of cold water

- Half cup of fresh pineapple, diced
- One teaspoon of pineapple extract
- Two packets of non-caloric sweetener
- A quarter cup of plain non-fat yogurt
- One scoop of natural-flavored whey protein powder
- Eight ice cubes
- Fat-free whipped cream
- Crushed walnuts for garnish

Instructions

- In an ice-crushing blender, add water, pineapple, pineapple extract, and sweetener, and blend until smooth. Add yogurt and whey and blend until smooth again.
- Add ice and chop until crushed. Pour into a glass and top with whipped cream and walnuts.

Pineapple Raspberry Smoothie

Preparation time-20 minutes | Cook time-15 minutes | Servings-2 | Difficulty-Easy

Nutritional value: ~Calories-50 | Proteins-8g | Fat-0.5g | Carbohydrates-8g

Ingredients

- One and a half lb. of pineapple
- Ten ounces of frozen raspberries
- One and a quarter cups of vanilla rice milk
- Three tablespoons of buckwheat flakes
- Mint to taste

Instructions

- A piece of pineapple peels and removes the core. Cut into medium pieces.
- Raspberries can be put frozen can be thawed overnight on the top shelf of the refrigerator.
- Take one cup of rice milk (in the absence of it, of course, you can replace it with non-fat milk), buckwheat flakes, slices of mandarin and pineapple, and beat at high speed in a blender.
- Let stand for about 10-15 minutes. During this time, buckwheat flakes will swell.
- Add another quarter cup of rice drink and punch in the blender again. If the smoothie is still thick, bring the water or rice drink to the desired concentration.
- Garnish with fresh mint leaves.

Pineapple Upside Down

Preparation time- 5 minutes | Cook time-0 minutes | Servings-2 | Difficulty-Easy

Nutritional value- Calories-110 | Fat-1g | Carbohydrates-21g | Protein-7g

Ingredients

- 1 packet sugar substitute, or to taste
- A quarter cup of plain nonfat yogurt
- 1/8 teaspoon lemon extract
- 1/8 teaspoon butter extract
- A quarter teaspoon of coconut extract
- A quarter cup of crushed pineapple, drained
- A quarter cup of plain calcium-enriched soy milk
- Two tablespoons of nonfat dry powdered milk
- A quarter cup of ice

Instructions

- Mix the powdered milk and the soy milk and put it aside for 2 to 3 minutes. Then place all ingredients in a blender and blend well.

Pomegranate-blueberry smoothie

Preparation time-10 minutes | Cook time-0 minutes | Servings-2 | Difficulty-Easy

Nutritional value: ~Calories-121 | Proteins-12g | Fat-8g | Carbohydrates-5g

Ingredients

- Two cups of full-fat, canned coconut milk
- One cup of pomegranate seeds
- One tablespoon of rose water or grated orange zest
- Two cups of frozen blueberries
- One tablespoon of honey
- Two tablespoons of grass-fed beef gelatin

Instructions

- Place the coconut milk and pomegranate seeds in a blender and blend until almost smooth (there will still be small bits of seed).
- Pour the mixture through a strainer(wire-mesh) set over a bowl, pressing against the seeds to extract as much liquid as possible. Discard the seeds.
- Rinse out the blender. Pour the strained coconut and pomegranate mixture back into the blender and add the rose water, blueberries, and honey.
- Pulse a few more seconds, add the gelatin, and pulse again until smooth. Pour into two 8-ounce glasses and enjoy.

Protein hot chocolate

Preparation time-5 minutes |Cook time-10 minutes |Serving-3 |Difficulty- Easy

Nutritional value: - Calories-124| Fat-9g| Protein-4g| Carbohydrates-8g

Ingredients

- One scoop of protein powder (unsweetened)
- Two tablespoons of unsweetened cocoa powder
- Two tablespoons of monk fruit sweetener
- One teaspoon of vanilla bean paste
- A quarter cup of hot water
- One tablespoon of hot coffee
- One cup of almond milk

Instructions

- In a small saucepan, measure all of the dry ingredients (including the honey). On low heat, put the saucepan. Then stir together until well blended with the dry ingredients.
- Gently stir in hot water (this will make your hot chocolate nice and creamy) until a creamy paste is formed.
- Turn the bottom of the pan to medium-high and shake gently over the non-dairy milk and coffee. (if you are using it)
- Shake the liquid until the mixture is hot and boiling over medium-high heat. It can take 3-5 minutes or so.

- Transfer the mixture carefully to a large mug and enjoy it!

Protein Hot Cocoa

Preparation time-5 minutes |Cook time-5 minutes |Serving-2 |Difficulty- Easy

Nutritional value: - Calories-254| Fat-5g| Protein-28g| Carbohydrates-23g

Ingredients

- One cup of low-fat milk
- One package sugar-free hot chocolate mix
- One scoop (¼ cup) unflavored protein powder

Instructions

- In a small saucepan over medium-low heat, whisk together the milk, hot chocolate mix, and protein powder.
- Whisk continuously just until warm. Do not boil.
- Pour into a heat-proof mug, and enjoy.

Protein-Packed Peanut Butter Cup Shake

Preparation time- 5 minutes| Cook time-0 minutes| Servings-2 |Difficulty-Easy

Nutritional value- Calories-215| Fat-3g |Carbohydrates-18g| Protein-27g

Ingredients

- A quarter cup of chocolate protein powder
- Two tablespoons of cocoa powder
- Half cup of Greek yogurt
- Two tablespoons of powdered peanut butter
- A quarter cup of nonfat ricotta cheese
- One cup of low-fat milk

Instructions

- Mix milk, powdered peanut butter, ricotta, cocoa powder, protein powder, yogurt, and blend at high speed for 3 to 4 minutes on high speed or until the consistency is smooth and the powder is well incorporated.
- Pour and chill the leftover in an airtight container. Throw away any leftovers after a week.

Pumpkin Pie Keto Spiced Latte

Preparation time- 5 minutes| Cook time-15 minutes| Servings-2 |Difficulty-Easy

Nutritional value- Calories-215| Fat-3g |Carbohydrates-18g| Protein-27g

Ingredients

- Two cups of strong and freshly brewed coffee
- One cup of Coconut Milk
- A quarter cup of Pumpkin Puree
- Half teaspoon of Cinnamon
- One teaspoon of Vanilla Extract
- Two teaspoons of Pumpkin Pie Spice Blend
- Fifteen drops of Liquid Stevia
- Two tablespoons of Butter
- Two tablespoons of Heavy Whipping Cream

Instructions

- Cook the pumpkin, butter, milk and spices over medium-low flame,
- Add two cups of solid coffee and blend together until bubbling.
- Remove from the stove, apply cream and stevia, and then whisk together with an electric mixer.
- Top with whipped cream and enjoy.

Pumpkin Spice Latte Protein Shake

Preparation time- 5 minutes| Cook time-5 minutes| Servings-2 |Difficulty-Easy

Nutritional value- Calories-125| Fat-0g |Carbohydrates-12g| Protein-15g

Ingredients

- One teaspoon of ground cinnamon
- ⅛ teaspoon of ground cloves
- A quarter teaspoon of ground nutmeg
- A quarter teaspoon of ground ginger
- ¾ cup of brewed decaf coffee
- A quarter cup of protein powder
- Half cup of pumpkin puree
- One cup of low-fat milk

Instructions

- Put the pumpkin puree, coffee, nutmeg, ginger, cloves, milk, cinnamon, and protein powder in a and then blend for about 3 minutes, until the consistency becomes smooth and the ingredients are well-incorporated.

- Pour it into a glass and enjoy.
- Place any leftovers in an airtight container for up to 7 days.

Raspberry strawberry smoothie

Preparation time-10 minutes |Cook time-10 minutes |Servings-2 |Difficulty-Easy

Nutritional value: ~Calories-317|Proteins-12g| Fat-5g|Carbohydrates-58g

Ingredients

- One tablespoon of honey
- One cup of hulled fresh strawberries
- Half cup of milk
- Half cup of raspberries
- Half cup of vanilla yogurt
- One teaspoon of vanilla extract

Instructions

- Put all the ingredients in a blender and blend until a smooth consistency is attained.

Refreshing Strawberry Smoothie

Preparation time- 5 minutes| Cook time-0 minutes| Servings-1 |Difficulty-Easy

Nutritional value- Calories-170| Fat-0g |Carbohydrates-20g| Protein-24g

Ingredients

- A quarter teaspoon of stevia
- One cup of frozen unsweetened strawberries
- One cup of non-fat plain Greek yogurt

Instructions

- Put the strawberries, stevia, and yogurt in the blender.
- Now blend for around 2 minutes or till everything is well-mixed. Serve and enjoy.

Smart Banana Blender

Preparation time-10 minutes| Cook time-0 minutes| Servings-2 |Difficulty-Easy

Nutritional value- Calories-170| Fat-0g |Carbohydrates-20g| Protein-24g

Ingredients

- One cup of Spinach
- One cup of Banana
- Half cup of water and yogurt
- Two tablespoons of Pomegranate
- Two tablespoons of Almond meal/Almonds

- One teaspoon of Cinnamon powder

- One teaspoon of Vanilla sugar or Honey or Sugar and vanilla extract

- Ice

Instructions

- Clean the spinach and chop it coarsely.

- Cut the Banana into medium-sized portions.

- To make a half-cup of milk, blend two to three tablespoons of yogurt with water.

- In a blender, mix all ingredients and process until smooth.

- If the ideal thickness is met, add ice when blending.

- Then serve.

Smoothie Bowl

Preparation time-5 minutes |Cook time-0 minutes |Servings-2 |Difficulty-Easy

Nutritional value: ~Calories-224|Proteins-2g| Fat-5g|Carbohydrates-51g

Ingredients

- One tablespoon of shredded coconut

- ¾ cup of blueberries

- One teaspoon of Honey

- Half sliced banana

- Three tablespoons of plain coconut milk

- One tablespoon of Blueberries

- Half cup of Organic and Frozen strawberries

- Half cup of Water

Instructions

- Combine all the smoothie bowl ingredients (except coconut and fresh berries) in a high-speed blender.

- Allow all the ingredients to be like a creamy sorbet; blend.

- Pour the mixture into a bowl.

- Garnish the smoothie with coconut and fresh berries.

Spiced Apple Pie Smoothie

Preparation time- 5 minutes| Cook time-0 minutes| Servings-1 |Difficulty-Easy

Nutritional value- Calories-100| Fat-0g |Carbohydrates-19g| Protein-7g

Ingredients

- Two packets of sugar substitute, or to taste

- A quarter cup of ice

- Half cup of plain nonfat yogurt

- 1/8 teaspoon of vanilla extract

- A quarter teaspoon of apple pie spice

- A quarter cup of unsweetened applesauce

- A quarter cup of nonfat milk

Instructions

- Blend everything well and serve.

Spinach Superfood Smoothie

Preparation time- 5 minutes| Cook time-0 minutes| Servings-1 |Difficulty-Easy

Nutritional value- Calories-148| Fat-4g |Carbohydrates-17g| Protein-13g

Ingredients

- One teaspoon of chia seeds

- Ten to twelve ice cubes

- One cup of spinach

- A quarter cup of unflavored or vanilla protein powder

- One tablespoon of ground flaxseed

- One cup of unsweetened almond milk or low-fat milk

- Half small banana

- Half medium cucumber, peeled

- One kiwi

Instructions

- Mix the spinach, kiwi, cucumber, banana, milk, flaxseed, chia seeds, protein powder, and ice cubes, then blend at high speed or until the consistency is smooth; there are no lumps, and the powder is well incorporated. You can add two to three tablespoons of water.

- Pour and chill the leftover in an airtight container. Throw away any leftovers after a week.

Strawberry-Banana Protein Smoothie

Preparation time-5 minutes| Cook time-0 minutes| Servings-2 |Difficulty-Easy

Nutritional value- Calories-131| Fat-1g |Carbohydrates-14g| Protein-16g

Ingredients

- ⅓ Ripe banana

- Five ice cubes

- Half cup of frozen strawberries

- A quarter cup of vanilla or unflavored protein powder

- One cup of low-fat milk

Instructions

- Mix the ice cubes, banana, frozen strawberries, milk, protein powder, and blend at high speed till the consistency is smooth, there are no lumps, and the powder is well incorporated.

- Pour and chill the leftover in an airtight container. Throw away any leftovers after a week.

Strawberry Lime Ginger Punch

Preparation time- 5 minutes| Cook time-0 minutes| Servings-2 |Difficulty-Easy

Nutritional value- Calories-132| Fat-4g |Carbohydrates-12g| Protein-7g

Ingredients

- Two cups of water

- Two tablespoons of raw apple cider vinegar

- Three packets of NuStevia or any other sweetener

- Juice of one lime

- Half teaspoon of ginger powder

- Five frozen strawberries

Instructions

- Blend all the ingredients together in a blender until smooth.

- Let it rest for 5 minutes and then serve chilled.

Strawberry Protein Smoothie

Preparation time- 5 minutes| Cook time-0 minutes| Servings-2 |Difficulty-Easy

Nutritional value- Calories-154| Fat-5g |Carbohydrates-17g| Protein-15g

Ingredients

- Half cup water

- One cup of ice

- One scoop of strawberry protein powder

- One egg

- Two tablespoons of cream

- Two strawberries

Instructions

- Blend ice cubes and water together.

- Apply the egg, powder and strawberries and start blending.

- Pour in the cream.

- Blend it again until smooth in a blender.

- Serve and enjoy.

Strawberry sundae whey smoothie

Preparation time-10 minutes |Cook time-0 minutes |Servings-2 |Difficulty-Easy

Nutritional value: ~Calories-134|Proteins-21g| Fat-2g|Carbohydrates-11g

Ingredients

- Half cup of cold water

- Half cup of fresh or unsweetened frozen strawberries

- A quarter teaspoon of vanilla extract

- Two packets of non-caloric sweetener

- A quarter cup of plain non-fat yogurt

- One scoop of natural-flavored whey protein powder

- Eight ice cubes

- Fat-free whipped cream

- Fat-free, sugar-free chocolate syrup to drizzle

Instructions

- In an ice-crushing blender, add water, strawberries, vanilla extract, and sweetener, and blend until smooth. Add yogurt and whey, and blend until smooth again.

- Add ice and chop until crushed. Pour into glass and top with whipped cream and chocolate syrup.

Summer rhubarb cooler

Preparation time-10 minutes |Cook time-10 minutes |Servings-2 |Difficulty-Easy

Nutritional value: ~Calories-35|Proteins-0g| Fat-2g|Carbohydrates-7g

Ingredients

- A quarter cup of low-calorie baking sweetener

- One cup of water

- Half pound of fresh rhubarb, trimmed and cut into 1-inch pieces

- One cup of sliced fresh strawberries plus extra for garnish

- Three tablespoons of freshly squeezed lemon juice

- Drinking glasses chilled in the freezer

Instructions

- Bring sweetener and water to a boil in a large saucepan over high heat. Cook, often stirring, to dissolve sugar, about 2 minutes.

- Reduce heat to medium and add rhubarb, then cook until tender. Add strawberries and lemon juice and cook for two additional minutes.

- Strain the mixture through a sieve to remove solids. Pour strained mixture into a 9x13-inch baking dish, cover with plastic wrap, and place in freezer. Every 30 minutes, stir the mixture with the tips of the fork to break up any forming ice chunks.

- Freeze mixture until slushy and frozen, about 3 hours. When frozen, scoop into chilled glasses and garnish with remaining sliced strawberries.

Tropical Mango Smoothie

Preparation time-5 minutes| Cook time-0 minutes| Servings-2 |Difficulty-Easy

Nutritional value- Calories-115| Fat-2.6g |Carbohydrates-9g| Protein-15g

Ingredients

- Five ice cubes

- A quarter cup of canned pineapple chunks in 100% natural juice or water, drained

- A quarter cup of frozen mango chunks

- One cup of low-fat milk

- A quarter cup of protein powder

- Half cup of Greek yogurt

Instructions

- Mix the ice cubes, pineapple, yogurt, protein powder, mango, milk and blend at high speed for up 4 to minutes till the consistency is smooth and the powder is well incorporated.

- Pour and chill the leftover in an airtight container. Throw away any leftovers after a week.

Vanilla Bean Protein Shake

Preparation time-5 minutes |Cook time-0 minutes |Serving-2 |Difficulty- Easy

Nutritional value: ~ Calories-153| Fat-2g| Protein-16g| Carbohydrates-14g

Ingredients

- One cup of low-fat milk

- Half cup of low-fat, vanilla Greek yogurt

- One teaspoon of vanilla extract

- One scoop (¼ cup) vanilla protein powder

- Four ice cubes

Instructions

- In a blender, combine the milk, yogurt, vanilla, protein powder, and ice. Blend on high for 2 to 3 minutes, until the protein powder has dissolved and the mixture is smooth.

- Pour half of the shake into a glass, and enjoy.

- Store the remaining half in an airtight container in the refrigerator for up to a week, and re-blend prior to serving.

Vanilla Probiotic Shake

Preparation time- 5 minutes| Cook time-0 minutes| Servings-2 |Difficulty-Easy

Nutritional value- Calories-153| Fat-2g |Carbohydrates-8g| Protein-22g

Ingredients

- One teaspoon of vanilla extract

- Five ice cubes

- A quarter cup of Greek yogurt

- Half cup of low-fat plain kefir

- A quarter cup of protein powder

- One cup of unsweetened vanilla soy milk or low-fat milk

Instructions

- Mix the protein powder, ice cubes, yogurt, kefir, vanilla, and milk and blend at high speed for 3 to 4 minutes on high speed or until the consistency is smooth and the powder is well incorporated.

- Pour and chill the leftover in an airtight container. Throw away any leftovers after a week.

Zero waste protein milk

Preparation time~12 hours | Cook time~10 minutes | Serving~3 | Difficulty~Hard

Nutritional value: ~ Calories~124 | Fat~9g | Protein~4g | Carbohydrates~8g

Ingredients

- One cup of almonds

- Four and a half cups of water

- A quarter teaspoon of salt

- Two tablespoons of Maple Syrup

- 3/4 cup of hemp hearts

Instructions

- Overnight, soak the nuts. Keep them in a cup that has enough space to cover them with water completely. In these ingredients, not the 4 cups of water listed.

- Wash them after the nuts are soaked overnight until the water is clear.

- Add the nuts to the high-speed blender container.

- Add four cups of water and for 30 seconds, blend higher.

- Pour milk into a bowl of nuts in a bowl or measuring cup. And for some more fun, save the nuts.

- Rinse the drained milk in a blender and pour it back into the bottle.

- Add salt, maple syrup and the heart of the horn. For a time of 45 seconds, blend.

- Put it in refrigerator containers and store.

Chapter 13~Desserts Recipes

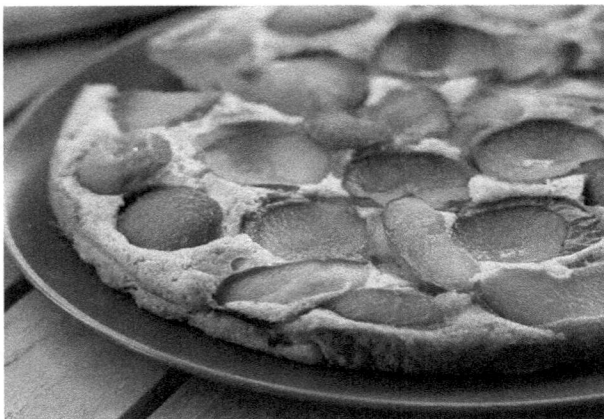

Apples and Plum Cake

Preparation time~10 minutes | Cook time~40 minutes | Servings~2 to 4 | Difficulty~Easy

Nutritional value: ~Calories~209 | Proteins~4g | Fat~7g | Carbohydrates~8g

Ingredients

- Seven ounces of almond flour
- One egg whisked
- Five tablespoons stevia
- One teaspoon of baking powder
- Three ounces of warm almond milk
- Two pounds of plums pitted and cut into quarters
- Two apples, cored and chopped
- Zest of one lemon, grated

Instructions

- In a bowl, blend the almond milk with the egg, stevia, and the rest of the ingredients except the cooking spray and whisk well.
- Grease a cake pan with the oil, pour the cake mix inside, introduce in the oven, then bake at 350 degrees F for 40 minutes.
- Cool down, slice, and serve.

Apple-walnut raisin wrap

Preparation time~10 minutes | Cook time~15 minutes | Servings~2 to 4 | Difficulty~Easy

Nutritional value: ~Calories~383 | Proteins~5g | Fat~24g | Carbohydrates~41g

Ingredients

- Four tablespoons of trans fat–free canola/olive oil spread, divided
- Two large apples (Granny Smith or Gala) to yield about three and a half cups of diced

- One (One and a half-ounce) box black raisins
- A quarter cup of maple syrup
- One teaspoon of ground cinnamon
- Pinch of salt
- Half cup of walnut pieces
- Four (8-inch) flour tortillas
- Low-fat vanilla yogurt or fat-free vanilla ice cream (optional)

Instructions

- In a large skillet, heat Two tablespoons of canola/olive oil spread over medium heat until melted. Add apples, raisins, maple syrup, cinnamon, and salt.
- Reduce heat to a simmer and cook, occasionally stirring, until apples are tender, about 8–10 minutes.
- Stir in walnut pieces and cook for an additional 2–3 minutes, until heated through.
- In a separate skillet, melt the remaining two tablespoons of canola/olive oil spread over low heat.
- Add tortillas, one at a time, and heat, turning once, until lightly browned.
- Place tortillas on a work surface and spoon apple mixture down the centers of the tortillas. Fold ends over filling and roll-up.
- Serve warm with an optional dollop of yogurt or ice cream on the side, if desired.

Apricot sorbet

Preparation time~10 minutes | Cook time~20 minutes | Servings~2 to 4 | Difficulty~Easy

Nutritional value: ~Calories~62 | Proteins~0g | Fat~0g | Carbohydrates~15g

Ingredients

- One cup of low-calorie baking sweetener
- One pound of very ripe apricots pitted and sliced plus three extra, ripe-but-firm apricots, pitted and thinly sliced
- 3/4 cup of sparkling champagne
- Two cups of water + extra as needed

Instructions

- Bring sweetener, one pound of apricots, champagne, and two cups of water to a boil in a medium saucepan.
- Reduce heat to a simmer and cook, often stirring, until apricots are very tender. Allow cooling.
- Transfer mixture to a blender and puree until smooth. Add extra water to the mixture as needed to make two to four cups.
- Transfer mixture to a large, shallow baking dish, gently mix in thin slices of apricots and freeze mixture until solid (at least 4–5 hours).

- Scoop into individual bowls when ready and serve.

Banana Cheesecake Chocolate Cookies

Preparation time-20 minutes | Cook time-25 minutes | Servings-2 to 4 | Difficulty-Easy

Nutritional value: ~Calories-351 | Proteins-4g | Fat-25g | Carbohydrates-31g

Ingredients

Crust

- Two tablespoons of butter
- Twelve cookies of Oreo

Cheesecakes

- One teaspoon of vanilla extract
- Two tablespoons of flour
- A quarter cup of cream
- Half cup of sugar
- Half cup of chocolate chips
- Two eight ounces cream cheese
- Half cup of banana
- One egg

Chocolate Whipped Cream

- One cup of heavy whipping cream
- A quarter cup of cocoa powder
- Two tablespoons of mini chocolate chips
- Half cup of powdered sugar
- Half teaspoon of rum extract
- One yellow banana, sliced

Instructions

- Blend all the mixture in the blender except eggs and bananas.
- Now whisk egg and banana and make a batter.
- Bake the batter in the oven at 350 degrees for twenty-five minutes. Top the cookies with cocoa, cream, vanilla, and sugar mixture.
- Serve and enjoy.

Banana Cinnamon Cupcakes

Preparation time-10 minutes | Cook time-20 minutes | Servings-2 to 4 | Difficulty-Easy

Nutritional value: ~Calories-142 | Proteins-2g | Fat-5.8g | Carbohydrates-5.6g

Ingredients

- Four tablespoons avocado oil

- Four eggs
- Half cup of orange juice
- Two teaspoons of cinnamon powder
- One teaspoon of vanilla extract
- Two bananas, peeled and chopped
- ¾ cup of almond flour
- Half teaspoon of baking powder
- Cooking spray

Instructions

- In a bowl, combine the oil with the eggs, orange juice, and the other ingredients except for the cooking spray.
- Whisk well, pour in a cupcake pan greased with the cooking spray, and introduce it in the oven 350 degrees F bake for 20 minutes.
- Cool the cupcakes down and serve.

Berry Delicious Cream of Wheat

Preparation time-5 minutes | Cook time-0 minutes | Serving-3 | Difficulty- Easy

Nutritional value: ~ Calories-219 | Fat-3g | Protein-24g | Carbohydrates-23g

Ingredients

- 3/4 cup of instant Cream of Wheat, no salt added
- Half teaspoon of vanilla extract
- Half cup of fresh raspberries
- Two tablespoons of protein powder supplement
- Two tablespoons of nonfat milk or low-fat, low-sugar soy milk
- Two sprigs of spearmint

Instructions

- Prepare Cream of Wheat per the package instruction for servings, adding the vanilla to the water before boiling. Just before removing the Cream of Wheat from the pan, stir in the raspberries.
- Add the protein powder just prior to serving.
- Serve in warmed bowls, topped with milk and garnished with fresh spearmint sprigs.

Blackberry and Apples Cobbler

Preparation time-10 minutes | Cook time-30 minutes | Servings-2 to 4 | Difficulty-Easy

Nutritional value: ~Calories-221 | Proteins-9g | Fat-6.3g | Carbohydrates-6g

Ingredients

- ¾ cup of stevia

- Six cups of blackberries

- A quarter cup of apples, cored and cubed

- A quarter teaspoon of baking powder

- One tablespoon of lime juice

- Half cup of almond flour

- Half cup of water

- Three and a half tablespoons of avocado oil

- Cooking spray

Instructions

- In a bowl, mix the berries with half of the stevia and lemon juice, sprinkle some flour

- all over, whisk and pour into a baking dish greased with cooking spray.

- In another bowl, mix flour with the rest of the sugar, baking powder, water, and oil, and stir the whole thing with your hands.

- Spread over the berries, introduce in the oven at 375 degrees F, and bake for 30 minutes. Serve warm.

Blueberry and Banana Protein Bread

Preparation time-10 minutes | Cook time-40 minutes | Servings-2 to 4 | Difficulty-Moderate

Nutritional value: ~Calories-139 | Proteins-10.2g | Fat-5.8g | Carbohydrates-14.2g

Ingredients

- One cup of Blueberries

- Two Egg

- One teaspoon of Cinnamon

- Two Bananas

- One teaspoon of Vanilla Extract

- Two teaspoons of Baking Powder

Instructions

- Preheat oven to 350 degrees F.

- In a mixing bowl, mix almond flour, baking powder, cinnamon, and protein powder.

- In a large bowl, mix applesauce, eggs, yogurt, and vanilla with mashed banana. Add it into dry ingredients with half of the blueberries.

- Put the other half of the blueberries into the lower layer; now put the bread on top.

- Bake at 350 degrees till the toothpick comes out clean from the center.

Blueberry Cake

Preparation time-10 minutes | Cook time-30 minutes | Servings-2 to 4 | Difficulty-Easy

Nutritional value: ~Calories-225 | Proteins-4.5g | Fat-9g | Carbohydrates-10.2g

Ingredients

- Two cups of almond flour

- Three cups of blueberries

- One cup of walnuts, chopped

- Three tablespoons of stevia

- One teaspoon of vanilla extract

- Two eggs whisked

- Two tablespoons of avocado oil

- One teaspoon of baking powder

- Cooking spray

Instructions

- Mix the flour with the blueberries, walnuts, and the other ingredients except for the cooking spray in a bowl, and stir well.

- Grease a cake pan with the cooking spray, pour the cake mix inside, introduce everything in the oven at 350 degrees F and bake for 30 minutes.

- Cool the cake down, slice, and serve.

Blueberry Pancakes

Preparation time-10 minutes | Cook time-15 minutes | Servings-2 to 4 | Difficulty-Easy

Nutritional value: ~Calories-117 | Proteins-3g | Fat-5.4g | Carbohydrates-16.2g

Ingredients

- Fifteen ounces of black beans

- A quarter teaspoon of salt

- Three flavorless oils

- Three eggs

- One teaspoon of vanilla

- 2/3 cup of sugar

- A quarter cup of cocoa powder

- Half teaspoon of baking powder

- Half cup of chocolate chips

Instructions

- In a bowl, mix all flour, salt, baking powder, and sugar.

- In another bowl, beat egg and milk. Add milk and egg into the flour mixture. Mix it and fold it with blueberries. Set down for one hour.

- Heat a pan over medium-high heat. Pour the batter onto the griddle. Turn its both sides brown to eat.

Blueberry Yogurt Mousse

Preparation time~30 minutes |Cook time~0 minutes |Servings~2 to 4 |Difficulty~Easy

Nutritional value: ~Calories~142 |Proteins~0.8g| Fat~4.8g |Carbohydrates~8.4g

Ingredients

- Two cups of Greek yogurt
- A quarter cup of stevia
- ¾ cup of heavy cream
- Two cups of blueberries

Instructions

- In a blender, combine the yogurt with the other ingredients, pulse well, divide into cups, and put it in the fridge for 30 minutes before serving.

Brownie Batter Fruit Dip

Preparation time~ 5 minutes| Cook time~0 minutes |Servings~8 |Difficulty~Easy

Nutritional value~ Calories~131 | Fat~5g |Carbohydrates~18g| Protein~5g

Ingredients

- Fresh fruit, for serving
- Four tablespoons of water, divided
- A quarter teaspoon of flaky sea salt
- One and a half teaspoons of vanilla extract
- Three tablespoons of maple syrup
- A quarter cup of unsweetened cocoa powder
- A quarter cup of tahini
- One (15-ounce) can chickpeas, drained and rinsed

Instructions

- Blend the chickpeas, maple syrup, vanilla, salt, cocoa powder, and tahini until smooth. Then add one tablespoon of water slowly until the dip has reached your desired thickness.
- Serve alongside fresh fruit.

Brownies

Preparation time~10 minutes |Cook time~35 minutes |Servings~20 brownies |Difficulty~Easy

Nutritional value: ~Calories~54 |Proteins~12g| Fat~3g |Carbohydrates~5g

Ingredients

- One and a quarter cup of cake flour (or substitute a combination of all-purpose flour and cornstarch as follows: Two and a half tablespoons of cornstarch plus enough flour to fill one and a quarter cups)
- Half teaspoon of sodium-free salt substitute

- ¾ teaspoon of baking powder
- Three tablespoons of unsweetened dark baking cocoa
- Two and a quarter cups of low-calorie baking sweetener
- One cup of liquid egg substitute
- Four tablespoons of canola oil
- One tablespoon of vanilla extract

Instructions

- Combine all dry ingredients in a large bowl and whisk to incorporate. In a separate bowl, combine egg, canola oil, and vanilla extract.
- Pour egg mixture into dry ingredients and mix until batter is smooth and blended. Pour batter into a nonstick 9x13-inch baking pan and spread the batter out evenly over the bottom. Place pan on the middle shelf in a 350-degree oven.
- Bake brownies for roughly 30 minutes; the center should spring back when touched with a finger, or you can insert a toothpick into the center.
- Brownies are done when the toothpick comes out with just a few moist crumbs on it. Do not overbake brownies, or they will be dry.
- Immediately remove the pan from the oven and allow brownies to cool on the cooling rack before cutting.

Caramelized pears

Preparation time~10 minutes |Cook time~25 minutes |Servings~2 to 4 |Difficulty~Easy

Nutritional value: ~Calories~102 |Proteins~2g| Fat~5g |Carbohydrates~14g

Ingredients

- Two ripe Bartlett pears, peeled, cut in half, and cored
- Three tablespoons of fresh lemon juice
- One tablespoon of vanilla extract
- Three tablespoons of trans fat–free canola/olive oil spread
- Half cup of low-calorie baking sweetener
- Four tablespoons of low-fat plain yogurt
- Four lemon slices for garnish (optional)

Instructions

- Preheat oven to 400 degrees F. Place pears in a large bowl; add vanilla extract and lemon juice.
- Gently toss ingredients to coat pears. Melt spread in an oven-safe skillet over medium-high heat. Add sweetener and stir to distribute sweetener evenly in the pan.
- Place pears cut side down in skillet and drizzle remaining lemon juice mixture from bowl over pears.

- Cook until sweetener begins to dissolve and mixture bubbles, shaking pan often to move the mixture around and under pears while cooking. Cook for about 5 minutes.

- Transfer skillet to oven and bake until pears are soft and juices are golden-colored (about 15–20 minutes).

- Serve pears warm, drizzled with mixture from pan; add a tablespoon of yogurt on the side and garnish with a lemon slice.

Caramelized pineapple and pistachios

Preparation time-10 minutes | Cook time-25 minutes | Servings-2 to 4 | Difficulty-Easy

Nutritional value: ~Calories-184 | Proteins-4g | Fat-4g | Carbohydrates-20g

Ingredients

- A quarter cup of dark brown, low-calorie baking sweetener (firmly packed)

- Half cup of no-pulp orange juice

- Three tablespoons of honey

- One medium ripe pineapple, cored, peeled, and cut lengthwise into eight wedges

- 1/3 cup of pistachios (unsalted), coarsely chopped

- A quarter cup of plain low-fat yogurt

Instructions

- Preheat oven to 450 degrees F.

- Line a parchment paper on a rimmed baking sheet. In a large bowl, combine sweetener, orange juice, and honey. Stir until sweetener dissolves.

- Add pineapple wedges and toss to coat. Allow marinating for 20–25 minutes, tossing occasionally.

- Place pineapple wedges flat side down on the baking sheet and reserve marinade.

- Roast pineapple for about 14-15 minutes, turn and brush on the marinade, and continue roasting until caramelized and tender.

- Remove from oven, drizzle the remaining marinade over pineapple, and allow to cool to room temperature.

- Divide among plates, sprinkle each with pistachios and add a spoonful of yogurt to the side of each plate.

Cardamom Almond Cream

Preparation time-30 minutes | Cook time-0 minutes | Servings-2 to 4 | Difficulty-Easy

Nutritional value: ~Calories-283 | Proteins-7g | Fat-12g | Carbohydrates-6g

Ingredients

- Juice of one lime

- Half cup of stevia

- One and a half cups of water

- Three cups of almond milk

- Half cup of honey

- Two teaspoons of cardamom, ground

- One teaspoon of rose water

- One teaspoon of vanilla extract

Instructions

- In a blender, blend the cardamon with almond milk and the rest of the ingredients.

- Pulse well, divide into cups and keep in the fridge for 30 minutes before serving.

Cheesecake Ice Cream

Preparation time-20 minutes | Cook time-20 minutes | Servings-2 to 4 | Difficulty-Moderate

Nutritional value: ~Calories-272 | Proteins-7g | Fat-16g | Carbohydrates-24g

Ingredients

- One cup of milk

- Two eggs

- Two and a half cups of cream

- One teaspoon of vanilla extract

- One and a quarter cups of sugar

- Twelve ounces of cream cheese

- One tablespoon of lemon juice

Instructions

- Melt sugar in cream and milk mixture.

- Whisk in egg and transfer in a pan. Cook over medium flame.

- Remove from flame and mix in cream cheese.

- Cool the mixture and stir in lemon juice and vanilla extract.

- Refrigerate it for 120 minutes and serve.

Chia Chocolate Pudding

Preparation time- 5 minutes | Cook time- 20 minutes | Servings-1 | Difficulty-Easy

Nutritional value- Calories-257 | Fat-12g | Carbohydrates-21g | Protein-25g

Ingredients

- Half teaspoon of stevia or no-calorie sweetener

- One teaspoon of unsweetened cocoa powder

- One tablespoon of vanilla whey protein

- Two tablespoons of chia seeds

- Half cup of nonfat plain Greek yogurt

- Half cup of unsweetened almond milk

Instructions

- Mix the almond milk with chia seeds, cocoa powder, stevia, yogurt, and whey protein in a canning jar.

- Close the lid and refrigerate it overnight.

- When it's done freezing, you can consume it right from the jar.

Chocolate and Strawberry Layered Pudding

Preparation time-15 minutes| Cook time- 20 minutes|Servings-4 |Difficulty-Easy

Nutritional value- Calories-118| Fat-2g |Carbohydrates-18g| Protein-5g

Ingredients

- One teaspoon of almond extract

- One cup of light whipped topping

- Eight whole strawberries stem removed, rinsed, and cut in half

- Instant chocolate pudding mix

- One 1-ounce package sugar-free, fat-free

- Two cups of nonfat milk

Instructions

- In a large bowl, add milk with almond extract and the instant pudding mix. Now whisk for 2 minutes. Leave it there for just 5 minutes.

- Take an 8-ounce glass and simply add one layer of a quarter cup of pudding. Then put 2 strawberry halves. Make 2 layers and finish with a quarter cup of whipped cream. Make 3 such glasses. Refrigerate, take out and enjoy.

Chocolate Bombs

Preparation time-10 minutes| Cook time- 10 minutes|Servings-12 |Difficulty-Easy

Nutritional value- Calories-118| Fat-2g |Carbohydrates-18g| Protein-5g

Ingredients

- Ten tablespoons of coconut oil

- Three tablespoons of chopped macadamia nuts

- Two packets of stevia

- Five tablespoons of unsweetened coconut powder

- A pinch of salt

Instructions

- Place coconut oil in a casserole dish and melt over medium heat.

- Apply stevia, salt and cocoa powder, mix well and remove from the heat.

- Spoon this into a tray of candy and store it for a while in the freezer.

- Sprinkle the macadamia nuts on top and hold them in the refrigerator until served.

Chocolate Covered Strawberries

Preparation time-15 minutes |Cook time-10 minutes |Servings-2 to 4|Difficulty-Easy

Nutritional value: ~Calories-115|Proteins-1.4g| Fat-7.3g|Carbohydrates-12.7g

Ingredients

- Sixteen ounces of milk chocolate chips

- Two tablespoons of shortening

- One pound of fresh strawberries with leaves

Instructions

- In a bain-marie, melt chocolate and shortening, occasionally stirring until smooth.

- Pierce the tops of the strawberries with toothpicks and immerse them in the chocolate mixture.

- Turn the strawberries and put the toothpick in Styrofoam so that the chocolate cools.

Chocolate Cups

Preparation time-Two hours |Cook time-0 minutes |Servings-2 to 4|Difficulty-Easy

Nutritional value: -Calories-174|Proteins-2.8g| Fat-9.1g|Carbohydrates-3.9g

Ingredients

- Half cup of avocado oil

- One cup of chocolate, melted

- One teaspoon of matcha powder

- Three tablespoons of stevia

Instructions

- In a bowl, mix the chocolate, avocado oil, and the rest of the ingredients.

- Divide into cups and keep in the freezer for 2 hours before serving.

Chocolate Ganache

Preparation time-15 minutes |Cook time-10 minutes |Servings-2 to 4|Difficulty-Easy

Nutritional value: -Calories-142|Proteins-1.4g| Fat-10.8g|Carbohydrates-9.4g

Ingredients

- Nine ounces of bittersweet chocolate, chopped

- One cup of heavy cream

- One tablespoon of dark rum (optional)

Instructions

- Place the chocolate in a medium bowl. Warm up the cream in a small saucepan on medium heat.

- Bring to a boil. When the cream has reached a boiling point, pour the chopped chocolate over it and beat until smooth. Stir the rum if desired.

- Allow the ganache to cool slightly before you pour it on a cake. For a fluffy icing or chocolate filling, let it cool until thick and beat with a whisk until light and fluffy.

Chocolate ice cream with toasted almonds

Preparation time-5 minutes |Cook time-0 minutes |Serving-3 |Difficulty- Easy

Nutritional value: - Calories-124| Fat-9g| Protein-4g| Carbohydrates-8g

Ingredients

- One frozen banana

- Two teaspoons of natural almond butter

- Two teaspoons of cocoa powder

- One to three tablespoons of almond milk

- One teaspoon of sliced almonds toasted sweetener, to taste

Instructions

- In a food processor or blender, combine banana, almond butter, and cocoa powder. Process it with 3-4 pulses.

- Add almond milk, a tablespoon at a time, and process until the mixture clumps up and resembles ice cream.

- Add sweetener as needed. Spoon mixture into a cup and top with toasted almonds.

- Makes a smooth and creamy treat that tastes just like ice cream!

Chocolate Pie

Preparation time-3 hours| Cook time-15 minutes|Servings-10 |Difficulty-Hard

Nutritional value- Calories-118| Fat-2g |Carbohydrates-18g| Protein-5g

Ingredients

For the filling

- One tablespoon vanilla extract

- Four tablespoons of sour cream

- One teaspoon of vanilla extract

- Four tablespoons of butter

- Sixteen ounces of cream cheese

- Half cup of cut stevia

- Two teaspoons of granulated stevia

- Half cup of cocoa powder

- One cup of whipping cream

For crust

- Half teaspoons of baking powder

- One and a half cups of the almond crust

- A quarter cup of stevia

- A pinch of salt

- One egg

- One and a half teaspoons of vanilla extract

- Three tablespoons of butter

- One teaspoon of butter for the pan

Instructions

- With one teaspoon of butter, oil a springform pan and leave aside for now.

- Mix the baking powder with a quarter cup of stevia, almond flour and a pinch of salt in a bowl and stir.

- Add three tablespoons of butter, one teaspoon of egg, and one and a half teaspoons of vanilla extract, then mix till the time the dough is ready.

- Press it well into the springform pan, place it at 375 degrees F in the oven and cook it for 11 minutes.

- Take the pie crust out of the oven, cover it with tin foil and cook for another 8 minutes.

- Take it out of the oven again and set it aside to cool down.

- Meanwhile, add sour cream, four tablespoons of butter, one tablespoon of vanilla extract, half a cup of cocoa powder and stevia to the cream cheese in a bowl and mix it well.

- Mix two teaspoons of stevia and one teaspoon of vanilla extract with the whipping cream in another bowl and stir using your mixer.

- Combine two mixtures, pour into the pie crust, spread well, place for 3 hours in the refrigerator and serve.

Chocolate Protein Pudding Pops

Preparation time-Four hours | Cook time-0 minutes | Serving-4 | Difficulty- Hard

Nutritional value: ~ Calories-215 | Fat-2g | Protein-12g | Carbohydrates-36g

Ingredients

- One (3.9-ounce) package chocolate-flavored instant pudding

- Two cups of cold low-fat milk

- Two scoops of chocolate protein powder

Instructions

- In a medium bowl, whisk the pudding mix, milk, and protein powder for at least 2 minutes.

- Spoon into ice pop molds or paper cups. Insert an ice pop stick into the center of each mold or cup.

- Freeze for 4 hours, or until firm. Remove from the molds or cups before serving.

Chocolate Quinoa Crisps

Preparation time-15 minutes | Cook time-10 minutes | Serving-16 | Difficulty- Easy

Nutritional value: ~ Calories-92 | Fat-5g | Protein-2g | Carbohydrates-10g

Ingredients

- Five tablespoons of coconut oil, melted, divided

- One cup of dry quinoa

- Two tablespoons of maple syrup

- Two tablespoons of unsweetened cocoa powder

- One teaspoon of vanilla extract

- Sea salt

Instructions

- In a wide, heavy-bottomed saucepan (at least 6 inches deep with a lid) over medium heat, heat one tablespoon of coconut oil.

- Add a few dried quinoa seeds. Once the pan is hot enough, the quinoa should pop. It will not expand as much as a popcorn kernel, but it will brown and jump in the air.

- Cover the base of the pot with the remaining quinoa.

- Gently shake the pot constantly to prevent sticking or burning of seeds. Remove from the heat once the popping starts to slow, usually after 1 to 5 minutes. Be sure not to let the quinoa burn.

- Once the quinoa has stopped popping, pour it onto a baking sheet to cool.

- In a medium bowl, whisk together the remaining four tablespoons of coconut oil with maple syrup, cocoa powder, and vanilla until smooth. Add salt to taste.

- Fold in the puffed quinoa.

- Scoop 1-tablespoon mounds of the mixture onto a lined baking sheet, and gently press to flatten.

- Chill in the refrigerator or freezer for 30 to 60 minutes, until hardened.

- Transfer to a large bag or airtight container, and keep refrigerated.

Chocolate Truffles

Preparation time-10 minutes | Cook time- 20 minutes | Servings-22 pieces | Difficulty-Easy

Nutritional value- Calories- 201 | Carbohydrates- 8.3g | Fat-15.6g | Protein-9.8g

Ingredients

- One cup of sugar-free chocolate chips
- Two tablespoons of butter
- 2/3 cups of heavy cream
- Two teaspoons of brandy
- Two tablespoons of swerving
- A quarter teaspoon of vanilla extract
- Cocoa powder

Instructions

- In a fire-proof mug, add heavy cream, swerve, chocolate chips and butter, stir, put in the microwave and heat for 1 minute.
- Leave for 5 minutes, blend well, and combine with the vanilla and the brandy.
- Stir again. Set aside for a few hours in the fridge.
- Shape the truffles using a melon baller, cover them in cocoa powder and then serve them.

Chocolate-Orange Pudding

Preparation time-10 minutes |Cook time-0 minutes |Serving-4 |Difficulty- Easy

Nutritional value: ~ Calories-111| Fat-2g| Protein-10g| Carbohydrates-15g

Ingredients

- One package sugar-free instant chocolate pudding mix
- One scoop (¼ cup) unflavored or chocolate protein powder
- Two cups of low-fat milk
- One tablespoon of cocoa powder
- One teaspoon of orange extract

Instructions

- In a small bowl, whisk the pudding and protein powders together with the milk for 2 minutes.
- Add the cocoa powder and orange extract, and mix for 3 more minutes before serving. The pudding will continue to firm after you've finished mixing.

Cinnamon Chickpeas Cookies

Preparation time-10 minutes |Cook time-20 minutes |Servings-2 to 4 |Difficulty-Easy

Nutritional value: ~Calories-200|Proteins-2.4g| Fat-4.5g|Carbohydrates-10g

Ingredients

- One cup of canned chickpeas, drained, rinsed, and mashed

- Two cups of almond flour
- One teaspoon of cinnamon powder
- One teaspoon of baking powder
- One cup of avocado oil
- Half cup of stevia
- One egg whisked
- Two teaspoons of almond extract
- One cup of raisins
- One cup of coconut, unsweetened and shredded

Instructions

- In a bowl, combine the chickpeas with the flour, cinnamon, and the other ingredients, and whisk well until you obtain a dough.
- Scoop tablespoons of dough on a baking sheet lined with parchment paper, put them in the oven at 350 degrees F, and bake for 20 minutes.
- Leave it cool for a few minutes and serve.

Cinnamon-Apple Walnut Crumble

Preparation time-15 minutes| Cook time-40 minutes|Servings-8 |Difficulty-Hard

Nutritional value- Calories-206| Fat-13g |Carbohydrates-22g| Protein-3g

Ingredients

- A quarter cup of walnuts, chopped
- A quarter cup of melted coconut oil
- Half cup of old-fashioned rolled oats
- Half cup of almond flour
- A quarter teaspoon of salt
- One teaspoon of vanilla extract
- One teaspoon of ground cinnamon
- Two tablespoons of maple syrup
- Six cups of diced apple (about 3 apples)

Instructions

- Preheat the oven to 375°F.
- Put the apples in a 9x9" baking dish. Mix them with cinnamon, salt, vanilla, and maple syrup.
- Then mix the melted oil, oats, and almond flour.

Crumble this mixture with your hands and add the walnuts.

- Sprinkle it on top of the apples, and close the bowl with tin foil. Bake for 25 to 30 minutes. Now take the foil off and bake again for 10 minutes. Enjoy.

Cocoa and Pears Cream

Preparation time-10 minutes | Cook time-0 minutes | Servings-2 to 4 | Difficulty-Easy

Nutritional value: ~Calories-172 | Proteins-1g | Fat-5.6g | Carbohydrates-7.6g

Ingredients

- Two cups of heavy creamy
- 1/3 cup of stevia
- ¾ cup of cocoa powder
- Six ounces of dark chocolate, chopped
- Zest of one lemon
- Two pears, chopped

Instructions

- Pulse the cream, stevia, and the rest of the ingredients in a blender.
- Divide into cups and serve cold.

Cocoa Brownies

Preparation time-10 minutes | Cook time-20 minutes | Servings-2 to 4 | Difficulty-Easy

Nutritional value: ~Calories-200 | Proteins-4.3g | Fat-4.5g | Carbohydrates-8.7g

Ingredients

- Thirty ounces of canned lentils, rinsed and drained
- One tablespoon of honey
- One banana, peeled and chopped
- Half teaspoon of baking soda
- Four tablespoons almond butter
- Two tablespoons of cocoa powder
- Cooking spray

Instructions

- In a food processor, combine the lentils with the honey and the other ingredients except for the cooking spray and pulse well.
- Pour this into a pan greased with cooking spray, spread evenly, introduce in the oven at 375 degrees F, then bake for around 20 minutes.
- Cut the brownies and serve cold.

Corn Pudding

Preparation time-15 minutes | Cook time-40 minutes | Servings-2 to 4 | Difficulty-Moderate

Nutritional value: ~Calories-180 | Proteins-5g | Fat-10g | Carbohydrates-21g

Ingredients

- Butter
- Two tablespoons of all-purpose flour
- Half teaspoon of baking soda
- Three eggs
- ¾ cup of rice milk
- Three tablespoons of melted butter
- Two tablespoons of light sour cream
- Two tablespoons of granulated sugar
- Two cups corn kernels

Instructions

- Heat the oven before 350°F.
- Lightly lubricate with butter an eight by an eight-inch baking dish, and put it aside.
- Take a small bowl, mix flour and baking soda substitute, and put it aside.
- Take a medium-sized bowl and beat together sugar, butter, sour cream, eggs, and rice milk.
- Blend the egg mixture into the flour mixture until even.
- Mix the corn to the mixture and stir until even.
- Spoon this mixture in the baking dish and bake until the pudding is set, for almost forty minutes.
- Let it cool for fifteen minutes and serve warm.

Cottage Cheese Bake

Preparation time-8 minutes | Cook time-30 minutes | Servings-8 | Difficulty-Easy

Nutritional value- Calories-78 | Fat-3g | Carbohydrates-3g | Protein-2g

Ingredients

- One pack of frozen spinach, 10-ounce (thawed and drained)
- Two whole eggs
- Half cup of Parmesan cheese
- Two cups of low-fat cottage cheese

Instructions

- Preheat the oven to 350 degrees Fahrenheit.

- In a large mixing bowl, combine all ingredients thoroughly.

- Distribute evenly into an 8x8 pan.

- Bake for 20–30 minutes, or until the outside of the cheese bubbles.

- Set aside for 5 minutes before serving.

- Season with pepper, salt and garlic powder to taste.

Cottage Cheese Fluff

Preparation time-3 minutes| Cook time-0 minutes|Servings-8 |Difficulty-Easy

Nutritional value- Calories-170| Fat-12g |Carbohydrates-4g| Protein-15g

Ingredients

- One sugar-free whipped topping 8-ounce

- Two containers fat-free cottage cheese, 24-ounce

- Two packages sugar-free gelatin, the flavor of choice, 3-ounce

Instructions

- In a large mixing bowl, combine all ingredients.

- Add your favorite fruit as an option.

Creamy Coconut Fruit Delight

Preparation time-10 minutes| Cook time- 0 minutes|Servings-2 |Difficulty-Easy

Nutritional value- Calories-80| Fat-0g |Carbohydrates-14g| Protein-6g

Ingredients

- Half cup of blueberries

- One cup of sliced strawberries

- One medium banana, sliced

- One teaspoon of vanilla extract

- One tablespoon of stevia

- One teaspoon of coconut extract

- 1/3 cup of fat-free sour cream

- 1/3 cup of nonfat dry powdered milk

- One cup of plain nonfat Greek yogurt

Instructions

- Mix the Yogurt with vanilla, sour cream, coconut extract, powdered milk, and stevia in a bowl.

- Now add the banana, blueberries, and strawberries, and then slowly fold them in. Refrigerate for 2 hours before serving.

Dark double chocolate pudding

Preparation time-10 minutes |Cook time-10 minutes |Servings-2 |Difficulty-Easy

Nutritional value: ~Calories-92|Proteins-4g| Fat-2g|Carbohydrates-13g

Ingredients

- A quarter cup of egg substitute

- Three cups of skim milk

- 2/3 cup of low-calorie baking sweetener

- A quarter cup of cornstarch

- Three tablespoons of unsweetened dark cocoa powder

- 1/8 teaspoon of low-sodium salt

- Half teaspoon of pure vanilla extract

- Two ounces of dark chocolate chips

- Fat-free whipped cream for garnish (optional)

Instructions

- Beat egg substitute lightly and set aside. Gradually heat milk over low heat until it begins to bubble. Remove from heat and add sweetener, cornstarch, cocoa, and salt. Bring mixture to a boil over medium heat while constantly whisking.

- When the mixture thickens slightly, remove it from heat. Slowly add egg substitute to one cup of milk mixture (do this, so that egg substitute does not immediately cook) and whisk. Pour egg mixture into remaining milk mixture and return to a boil, constantly whisking.

- When the mixture thickens to pudding consistency, remove from heat and add vanilla extract and chocolate chips. Stir to incorporate, then pour into a bowl and cover with plastic wrap.

- Push wrap down into the bowl, so it touches the top of the pudding; this keeps pudding from developing skin on the top.

- Refrigerate until ready to serve and garnish with whipped cream, if desired.

Easy peach cobbler

Preparation time-10 minutes |Cook time-10 minutes |Servings-2 |Difficulty-Easy

Nutritional value: ~Calories-76|Proteins-1g| Fat-1g|Carbohydrates-12g

Ingredients

- Half cup of low-calorie baking sweetener
- One tablespoon of cornstarch
- One (10-ounce) can sliced peaches, drained, liquid reserved
- Half tablespoon of ground cinnamon
- One tablespoon of trans fat–free canola/olive oil spread
- Half cup of self-rising flour
- Half tablespoon of trans fat–free shortening
- A quarter cup of almond milk

Instructions

- Preheat oven to 400 degrees. In a saucepan, combine a half cup of sweetener and cornstarch, gradually stirring in reserved peach juice and bringing to a boil for 1 minute, stirring constantly.
- Add peaches, pour the mixture into a 9x13-inch baking dish, sprinkle with cinnamon, dot with canola/olive oil spread, and set aside.
- Mix flour and remaining sweetener, cut with shortening, then add milk and stir until ingredients are well blended. Spoon dough onto fruit and bake for 25–30 minutes. Serve warm.

Fruited nutty pastry rolls

Preparation time-10 minutes |Cook time-20 minutes |Servings-2 to 4 |Difficulty-Easy

Nutritional value: ~Calories-78|Proteins-4g| Fat-6g|Carbohydrates-5g

Ingredients

- Canola oil cooking spray
- Four tablespoons of trans fat–free canola/olive oil spread
- A quarter cup of low-calorie baking sweetener
- One egg
- One teaspoon of almond extract
- 2/3 cup of all-purpose unbleached flour, sifted
- Four tablespoons of natural chunky peanut butter
- Four tablespoons of low-sugar fruit jam
- 1/8 cup of finely chopped walnuts

Instructions

- Lightly coat a baking sheet with cooking spray. In a bowl, beat together canola/olive oil spread and sweetener until soft and fluffy.
- Crack the egg and separate the yolk from the white; reserve white. Beat the egg yolk and almond extract into the spread and sweetener mixture. Add in flour. Stir to mix all ingredients and form a firm dough ball.

- Add in a small amount of extra flour if the dough is too soft. Divide the dough in half and roll each half into a log about 10 inches long.
- Place both logs on the baking sheet. Lightly spray the handle of a dinner knife with cooking spray.
- Starting about 1/8 inch from the beginning of each log, use the knife handle to make a channel down the center, stopping about 1/8 inch before the end of the log.
- Whisk the egg white gently and brush it over each log.
- Fill the channel with peanut butter and top with jam. Sprinkle with walnut pieces. Chill logs for about 30–45 minutes.
- Heat oven to 350 degrees and bake chilled logs until they are a light golden brown (about 10–12 minutes).
- Remove from oven and allow logs to cool until jam sets. Slice each roll diagonally into ten slices before serving.

Grilled Stone Fruit with Greek Yogurt

Preparation time-5 minutes |Cook time-5 minutes |Serving-6 |Difficulty- Easy

Nutritional value: ~ Calories-78| Fat-3g| Protein-4g| Carbohydrates-11g

Ingredients

Nonstick cooking spray

- Three large fresh peaches halved and pitted
- One teaspoon of extra-virgin olive oil
- Six ounces of low-fat, honey-flavored Greek yogurt
- A quarter cup of sliced almonds
- Ground cinnamon for garnishing

Instructions

- Spray your grill (or a grill pan on the stovetop) with cooking spray. Heat the grill or grill pan to high heat, about 500°F.
- Brush each peach half with olive oil.
- Place the cut fruit on the grill flesh-side down, and grill for two minutes. Using tongs, turn the fruit over and cook for another 2 minutes. Transfer to a serving dish.
- Serve the fruit with Greek yogurt, and garnish with almonds and cinnamon.

Hazelnut Pudding

Preparation time-10 minutes |Cook time-40 minutes |Servings-2 to 4|Difficulty-Moderate

Nutritional value: ~Calories-178|Proteins-1.4g| Fat-8g|Carbohydrates-11g

Ingredients

- Two and a quarter cups of almond flour

- Three tablespoons of hazelnuts, chopped
- Five eggs whisked
- One cup of stevia
- One and 1/3 cups of Greek yogurt
- One teaspoon of baking powder
- One teaspoon of vanilla extract

Instructions

- Mix the flour with the hazelnuts plus the other ingredients in a bowl, and pour into a cake pan lined with parchment paper.
- Introduce in the oven at 350 degrees F, bake for 30 minutes, cool down, slice, and serve.

Healthy banana-nut muffins

Preparation time-10 minutes | Cook time-30 minutes | Servings-2 to 4 | Difficulty-Easy

Nutritional value: ~Calories-100 | Proteins-5g | Fat-6g | Carbohydrates-9g

Ingredients

- One cup (8 ounces) of soy flour
- Two teaspoons of baking powder
- Two tablespoons of low-calorie baking sweetener
- A quarter cup of finely chopped walnuts
- Two medium-sized ripe bananas, mashed
- One teaspoon of vanilla extract
- One and a quarter cup of s vanilla soy milk
- A quarter cup of egg substitute
- Two tablespoons of canola oil
- Two tablespoons of dry oatmeal

Instructions

- Line a 12-cup muffin pan with paper muffin cups. Sift soy flour and baking powder together into a mixing bowl.
- Add sweetener and walnuts and stir to mix ingredients. Make a well in the center of the mix and add bananas, vanilla extract, soy milk, egg substitute, and canola oil.
- Pour batter into muffin cups, sprinkle tops with oatmeal, and bake in a 350-degree oven for 20–25 minutes or until muffins are firm and a toothpick inserted into the center of a muffin comes back dry.
- Remove from oven and allow to cool.

Healthy chocolate cupcakes

Preparation time-10 minutes | Cook time-20 minutes | Servings-2 to 4 | Difficulty-Easy

Nutritional value: ~Calories-135 | Proteins-7g | Fat-6g | Carbohydrates-17g

Ingredients

- One and a quarter cup of s pastry flour
- Three tablespoons of ground flaxseed
- One cup of low-calorie baking sweetener
- Half cup of unsweetened dark cocoa
- Half teaspoon of baking soda
- Half teaspoon of baking powder
- Half teaspoon of sodium-free salt substitute
- Half cup of concentrated pomegranate juice or other clear concentrated juice
- 3/4 cup of vanilla soy milk
- Three tablespoons of canola oil
- 1/3 cup of chopped walnuts

Instructions

- Mix together flour, flaxseed, sweetener, cocoa, baking soda, baking powder, and salt substitute. Blend all ingredients well with a whisk. Make a well in the center of the mixture. In a separate bowl, add juice, soy milk, canola oil, and 2/3 of the walnuts (reserve 1/3 for garnish).
- Stir ingredients well and pour the mixture into the well of the flour mixture. With a spatula, blend all ingredients until well mixed. Line a 12-cup cupcake pan with paper cupcake liners and fill each liner until almost full.
- Sprinkle a small amount of the reserved chopped walnuts on top of each cupcake. Place pan in a 350-degree oven on center rack and bake for 18–20 minutes or until a toothpick inserted in the center of a cupcake comes out clean. Do not overbake. Allow cooling for 10–15 minutes before serving.

Honey mousse delight

Preparation time-10 minutes |Cook time-10 minutes |Servings-2 to 4 |Difficulty-Easy

Nutritional value: ~Calories-196|Proteins-7g| Fat-6g|Carbohydrates-29g

Ingredients

- 1/3 cup of honey
- Two teaspoons of freshly grated orange rind
- Twelve ounces of part-skim ricotta cheese
- Two and a half cups of halved fresh strawberries
- Two and a half cups of fresh blackberries
- A quarter cup of fresh orange juice
- Three tablespoons of non-caloric sweetener
- Two tablespoons of finely chopped walnuts

Instructions

- Mix honey, orange rind, and ricotta cheese in a medium bowl; cover and refrigerate to chill. Combine berries, juice, and sweetener, gently toss, and let stand for 5 minutes before covering and re-chilling.
- When well chilled, spoon 1/3 berry mixture (divided equally) into serving bowls and top each with about a quarter cup of ricotta mixture.
- Divide the remaining fruit mixture and add on top of the cheese.
- Sprinkle with walnuts and serve.

Keto Cheesecakes

Preparation time-10 minutes |Cook time-20 minutes |Servings-9 |Difficulty-Easy

Nutritional value: ~Calories-78|Proteins-2g| Fat-2g|Carbohydrates-5g

Ingredients

For the cheesecakes

- Two tablespoons of butter
- Eight ounces of cream cheese
- Three tablespoons of coffee
- Three eggs
- 1/3 cup of swerve
- One tablespoon of sugar-free caramel syrup

For the frosting

- Three tablespoons of sugar-free caramel syrup
- Three tablespoons of butter
- Eight ounces of soft mascarpone cheese
- Two tablespoons of swerving

Instructions

- Combine eggs with cream cheese, two tablespoons of butter, one tablespoon caramel syrup, coffee, and 1/3 cup of swerving in your blender and pulse very well.
- Spoon this into a pan of cupcakes, place it at 350 degrees F in the oven and cook for 15 minutes.
- To cool down, leave aside and then keep in the freezer for three hours.
- Meanwhile, mix three tablespoons butter with three tablespoons caramel syrup, two tablespoons swerve and mascarpone cheese in a bowl and mix well.
- Spoon the cheesecakes over and serve them.

Keto Doughnuts

Preparation time-10 minutes |Cook time-20 minutes |Servings-24 |Difficulty-Easy

Nutritional value: ~Calories-135|Proteins-7g| Fat-6g|Carbohydrates-17g

Ingredients

- A quarter cup of erythritol
- A quarter cup of flaxseed meal
- 3/4 cups of almond flour
- One teaspoon of baking powder
- One teaspoon of vanilla extract
- Two eggs
- Three tablespoons of coconut oil
- A quarter cup of coconut milk
- Twenty drops of red food coloring
- A pinch of salt
- One tablespoon of cocoa powder

Instructions

- Mix together the almond flour, cocoa powder, baking powder, erythritol and salt in a bowl and stir.
- Mix the coconut oil with vanilla, coconut milk, food coloring and eggs in another bowl and stir.
- Mix mixtures, use a hand mixer to stir, move to a bag, cut a hole in the bag and shape a baking sheet with 12 doughnuts.
- Place it in the oven at 350 degrees F and cook for 15 minutes.
- On a tray, place them and eat them.

Lemon cakes

Preparation time-10 minutes |Cook time-35 minutes |Servings-2 to 4 |Difficulty-Easy

Nutritional value: ~Calories-78|Proteins-2g| Fat-2g|Carbohydrates-5g

Ingredients

- Two tablespoons of trans fat–free canola/olive oil spread plus more, softened, to coat ramekins
- 1/3 cup of all-purpose flour, spooned and leveled
- Half teaspoon of baking powder
- A quarter teaspoon of salt
- Three large eggs, separated
- A quarter cup plus 1/8 cup of low-calorie baking sweetener
- One teaspoon of finely grated lemon zest
- 1/3 cup of freshly squeezed lemon juice
- One and a quarter cups of almond milk
- Confectioners' sugar for dusting, the scant amount

Instructions

- Preheat oven to 325 degrees F. Brush the sides and bottoms of 2 to 4 (6-ounce) ramekins with softened canola/olive oil spread. Place ramekins in a shallow baking casserole.
- In a bowl, combine flour, baking powder, and salt. In a separate larger bowl, whisk together egg yolks with a quarter cup of sweetener until the mixture is pale and smooth. Whisk in Two tablespoons of canola/olive oil spread, lemon zest, lemon juice, milk, and flour mixture. Cover and refrigerate the mixture for 3 hours.
- In another large bowl, using an electric mixer, beat egg whites with 1/8 cup of sweetener until mixture peaks, about minutes, and fold into chilled batter. With a ladle, divide batter among ramekins, wiping any dripped excess from edges.
- Add enough water to the casserole to come halfway up the sides of the ramekins. Place casserole with ramekins in the oven and bake until cakes puff and are slightly golden on top, about 30 minutes.
- Dust with confectioners' sugar and serve while hot.

Lemon Mousse

Preparation time-15 minutes| Cook time-5 minutes|Servings-4 |Difficulty-Easy

Nutritional value- Calories-85| Fat-6g |Carbohydrates-6g| Protein-1g

Ingredients

- One and a half cups of whipped topping
- Two cups of ice cubes
- One (6-ounce) package sugar-free lemon-flavored gelatin
- One and a half cups of boiling water

Instructions

- Mix the gelatin with boiling water until the gelatin is completely dissolved.
- Put in the ice cubes, and mix until melted. Put it in the refrigerator for about 5 to 10 minutes.
- Now add in the whipped cream on top.
- Make four portions out of it and refrigerate until it thickens; it'll take 4 hours.
- Top with fresh fruit (optional) and serve.

Lime Vanilla Fudge

Preparation time-Three hours |Cook time-0 minutes |Servings-2 to 4|Difficulty-Easy

Nutritional value: ~Calories-200|Proteins-5g| Fat-4.5g|Carbohydrates-13.5g

Ingredients

- 1/3 cup of cashew butter
- Five tablespoons of lime juice
- Half teaspoon of lime zest, grated
- One tablespoon of stevia

Instructions

- In a bowl, mix the cashew butter with the other ingredients and whisk well.
- Line a muffin tray with parchment paper, scoop one tablespoon of lime fudge, mix in each of the muffin tins and keep in the freezer for 3 hours before serving.

Mango Bowls

Preparation time-30 minutes |Cook time-0 minutes |Servings-2 to 4|Difficulty-Easy

Nutritional value: ~Calories-122|Proteins-4.5g| Fat-4g|Carbohydrates-6.6g

Ingredients

- Three cups of mango, cut into medium chunks
- Half cup of coconut water
- A quarter cup of stevia
- One teaspoon of vanilla extract

Instructions

- Mix the mango with the rest of the ingredients in a blender.
- Pulse well, divide into bowls and serve cold.

Mango Cream

Preparation time- 5 minutes| Cook time-0 minutes|Servings-4 |Difficulty-Easy

Nutritional value- Calories-60| Fat-0g |Carbohydrates-17g| Protein-1g

Ingredients

- Two tablespoons of fresh lime juice

- Two cups of peeled and cubed mango

Instructions

- Put the mango cubes into an airtight plastic bag and freeze it for 2 hours.

- Now, take the bag out, put the frozen cubed mango with lime juice in a blender, and pulse until the consistency becomes creamy.

Meringue cookies

Preparation time-10 minutes | Cook time-One hour 10 minutes | Servings-20 cookies | Difficulty-Easy

Nutritional value: ~Calories-5 | Proteins-1g | Fat-0g | Carbohydrates-0.5g

Ingredients

- One cup of liquid egg whites

- Pinch of cream of tartar

- A quarter cup of low-calorie baking sweetener

- One teaspoon of white wine vinegar

- One teaspoon of vanilla extract

Instructions

- Preheat oven to 275 degrees. Line 2 cookie trays with parchment paper. Place egg whites in a mixing bowl and slowly whisk on low speed with an electric beater until they begin to bubble.

- Add cream of tartar and increase speed slightly; whisk until the mixture begins to peak. Increase speed to medium and slowly add sweetener, vinegar, and vanilla extract. Continue whisking until the mixture is satiny and firmly holds a peak.

- Ladle a soup spoon–sized portion of the mixture onto parchment-lined trays to make 20–24 cookies. Put trays of meringues in the oven and bake for about 1 hour.

- Turn off the oven and allow cookies to stand in a closed oven for an additional hour to dry. When meringues are pierced with a toothpick that comes back dry, they are ready.

- Transfer cookies to cooling racks to continue to cool.

Mini Cheesecake Bites

Preparation time-10 minutes | Cook time-30 minutes | Serving-6 | Difficulty-Moderate

Nutritional value: ~Calories-196 | Fat-19g | Protein-5g | Carbohydrates-3g

Ingredients

- One tablespoon of butter, melted

- A quarter cup of almond flour

- Eight ounces of low-fat cream cheese softened

- Two tablespoons of erythritol

- One large egg

- One teaspoon of vanilla extract

- One and a half tablespoons of low-fat sour cream

- Two tablespoons of freshly squeezed lemon juice

- ⅛ teaspoon of salt

- Fresh fruit, for serving (optional)

Instructions

- Preheat the oven to 325°F.

- Line a 6-compartment muffin tin with muffin liners.

- In a small bowl, combine the butter and almond flour until almost doughy. Divide the mixture evenly among the 6 muffin liners. Using your fingers, press the crust into an even layer. Bake for 10 minutes, remove from the oven and set aside.

- In a medium mixing bowl with a hand mixer, beat the cream cheese until fluffy. Add the erythritol slowly, and continue mixing.

- Add the egg, vanilla, sour cream, lemon juice, and salt; beat until combined.

- Pour Two tablespoons of cheesecake mixture on top of each almond meal crust. Tap the muffin tin on the counter to bring any air bubbles to the top, then pop them.

- Bake for 18 to 22 minutes, or until no longer jiggly. Remove from the oven and allow to cool for 15 minutes. Transfer to a wire rack to cool completely. Chill in the refrigerator for 2 to 4 hours or overnight.

- Serve topped with fresh fruit (if desired).

Mixed Berries Stew

Preparation time-10 minutes | Cook time-15 minutes | Servings-2 to 4 | Difficulty-Easy

Nutritional value: ~Calories-172 | Proteins-2.3g | Fat-7g | Carbohydrates-8g

Ingredients

- Zest of one lemon, grated
- Juice of one lemon
- Half-pint of blueberries
- One pint of strawberries halved
- Two cups of water
- Two tablespoons of stevia

Instructions

- Mix the berries with the water, stevia, and the other ingredients in a pan.
- Bring to a simmer, cook over medium heat for 15 minutes, divide into bowls and serve cold.

No-Bake Blueberry Cheesecake Bars

Preparation time- 5 minutes | Cook time- 20 minutes | Servings-10-12 | Difficulty-Easy

Nutritional value- Calories-264 | Fat-20g | Carbohydrates-2.1g | Protein-18.9g

Ingredients

For the shortbread crust

- Two (8-ounce) packages of cream cheese, softened
- Half cup of powdered erythritol-based sweetener
- One teaspoon grated lemon zest
- A quarter cup of heavy whipping cream, room temperature

For the blueberry topping

- One cup of frozen blueberries
- A quarter cup of water
- A quarter cup of powdered erythritol-based sweetener
- One tablespoon fresh lemon juice
- A quarter teaspoon of xanthan gum Fresh mint, for garnish (optional)

Instructions

For the bars

- Firmly and uniformly push the shortbread crust mixture into the bottom of a 9-inch square baking pan. Freeze the crust when cooking filling for the cheesecake. (Freezing the crust will allow it to stay together as the filling is poured over the top.)

- Use an electric mixer in a wide bowl to pound the cream cheese up until creamy with the sweetener and lemon zest. Beat in the milk until it mixes properly.
- Spread the crust over the filling. Refrigerate for at least 2 hours until strong.

For the topping and assembly

- Bring the blueberries, sugar, and sweetener to a boil in a medium saucepan over medium heat, then simmer for 5 minutes.
- Remove from oil, and whisk in the juice of a lemon. Sprinkle quickly with the xanthan gum, then whisk off. Before use, let cool.
- Pour over the cheesecake the blueberry topping-either the whole pan or individual servings. When needed, garnish with fresh mint.

Orange and Apricots Cake

Preparation time-10 minutes | Cook time-20 minutes | Servings-2 to 4 | Difficulty-Easy

Nutritional value: ~Calories-221 | Proteins-5g | Fat-8.3g | Carbohydrates-14.5g

Ingredients

- ¾ cup of stevia
- Two cups of almond flour
- A quarter cup of olive oil
- Half cup of almond milk
- One teaspoon of baking powder
- Two eggs
- Half teaspoon of vanilla extract
- Juice and zest of two oranges
- Two cups of apricots, chopped

Instructions

- Mix the stevia with the flour and the rest of the ingredients in a bowl. Whisk and pour into a cake pan lined with parchment paper.
- Introduce in the oven at 375 degrees F, bake for 20 minutes, cool down, slice, and serve.

Peanut Butter Balls

Preparation time-10 minutes | Cook time-0 minutes | Servings-24 | Difficulty-Easy

Nutritional value- Calories-49 | Fat-3g | Carbohydrates-5g | Protein-1g

Ingredients

- One teaspoon of vanilla extract
- Two tablespoons of chocolate whey protein powder
- A quarter cup of mini dark chocolate chips
- Two tablespoons of flaxseed meal
- A quarter cup of natural peanut butter
- Two tablespoons of honey
- ⅓ cup coconut shreds
- ⅓ cup old-fashioned rolled oats

Instructions

- Mix the coconut, flaxseed, peanut butter, oats, chocolate chips, protein powder, honey, and vanilla.
- Refrigerate for 30 minutes.
- Make 2-inch balls and serve.

Peanut Butter Fudge

Preparation time-15 minutes| Cook time-0 minutes|Servings-12 |Difficulty-Easy

Nutritional value- Calories-49| Fat-3g |Carbohydrates-5g| Protein-1g

Ingredients

- One cup of unsweetened peanut butter
- A quarter cup of almond milk
- Two teaspoons of vanilla stevia
- One cup of coconut oil
- A pinch of salt

For the topping

- Two tablespoons of swerving
- Two tablespoons of melted coconut oil
- A quarter cup of cocoa powder

Instructions

- Combine peanut butter with one cup of coconut oil in a heat-proof bowl, stir and heat in your microwave until it melts.
- Add stevia, a pinch of salt and almond milk, mix it well and pour into a lined loaf pan.
- Keep it for 2 hours in the refrigerator and then slice it.
- Mix two tablespoons of cocoa powder and melted coconut in a bowl and swirl and stir well.
- Drizzle over your peanut butter fudge with the sauce and serve.

Plum sorbet

Preparation time-10 minutes |Cook time-40 minutes |Servings-2 to 4 |Difficulty-Moderate

Nutritional value: ~Calories-56|Proteins-0.6g| Fat-2g|Carbohydrates-11g

Ingredients

- One pound of (about 14) red plums, halved and pitted
- Six ounces of sweet red sherry
- 3/4 cup of water
- One and a half cups of non-caloric sweetener
- One cinnamon stick
- One teaspoon of vanilla extract
- Zest from half a lemon

Instructions

- Place the freezer canister of an ice cream maker in the freezer. Combine plums, sherry, water, sweetener, cinnamon stick, vanilla extract, and zest in a heavy saucepan and cook, covered, over medium heat, occasionally stirring, until plums fall apart (about 20–30 minutes). Remove cinnamon stick.
- Place plum mixture in a blender or food processor and process until smooth. Strain pureed mixture through a mesh strainer to separate any remaining large pieces.
- Allow to cool, then transfer mixture to cold ice cream canister and return to freezer uncovered for about 2 hours. When the sorbet is cold, transfer it to an airtight freezer container for at least one more hour before serving.

Pumpkin pudding

Preparation time-10 minutes |Cook time-0 minutes |Servings-2 to 4 |Difficulty-Easy

Nutritional value: ~Calories-55|Proteins-5g| Fat-0g|Carbohydrates-9g

Ingredients

- One and 3/Four cups of skim milk
- One (1-ounce) package sugar-free instant vanilla pudding mix
- Half cup of canned pumpkin
- Half teaspoon of pumpkin spice

Instructions

- Combine cold milk and pudding mix in a chilled bowl and stir until smooth.
- Blend in pumpkin and spice and refrigerate to chill before serving.

Raspberry and Coconut Dessert

Preparation time-5 minutes| Cook time- 20 minutes| Servings-12 |Difficulty-Easy

Nutritional value- Calories- 198 | Carbohydrates- 8.3g | Fat-18.6g | Protein-8.8g

Ingredients

- Half cup of coconut butter
- Half cup of coconut oil
- Half cup of dried raspberries
- A quarter cup of swerve
- Half cup of shredded coconut

Instructions

- Mix the dried berries in your food processor very well.
- Heat a pan over medium heat with the butter.
- Stir in the coconut oil and swerve, stir and cook for 5 minutes.
- Pour half of this and spread well into a lined baking pan.
- Add raspberry powder and also spread.
- Spread the rest of the butter mix on top and keep it in the fridge for a while.
- Cut and serve into pieces.

Raspberry meringues

Preparation time-10 minutes | Cook time-35 minutes | Servings-30 cookies | Difficulty-Easy

Nutritional value: ~Calories-51 | Proteins-6g | Fat-0.7g | Carbohydrates-8g

Ingredients

- 3/4 cup of liquid egg whites
- Half cup of sliced raw almonds
- Two tablespoons of low-calorie baking sweetener
- A quarter teaspoon of almond extract
- 1/8 teaspoon of sodium-free salt substitute
- 1/3 cup of non-caloric sweetener
- 1/3 cup of low-calorie raspberry jam

Instructions

- Egg whites need to be at room temperature for 30 minutes before use. Preheat oven to 275 degrees. Line cookie sheets with parchment paper.
- Combine sliced almonds and two tablespoons of sweetener in a food processor or blender, and process until finely ground.
- In a large bowl, add egg whites, almond extract, and salt substitute, and whip on medium speed until mixture begins to bubble. Gradually add 1/3 cup of sweetener a little at a time, increasing speed to high, and whip until mixture forms stiff peaks. Gently fold in almond mixture.

- Ladle soup spoon–sized portions of mixture onto parchment paper, making about 30–40 cookies. Bake for 20–25 minutes. Turn the oven off and allow cookies to stand in the closed oven for an additional hour to dry.
- Transfer cookies to cooling racks to continue to cool. When completely cooled, spoon a small amount of raspberry jam into the center of each cookie.

Raspberry muffins

Preparation time-15 minutes | Cook time-15 minutes | Serving-3 | Difficulty- Easy

Nutritional value: ~ Calories-124 | Fat-9g | Protein-4g | Carbohydrates-8g

Ingredients

- Two cups of all-purpose flour
- Two eggs
- Half cup of granulated sugar
- One cup of dairy-free milk
- A quarter cup of softened dairy-free butter
- Half teaspoon of salt
- One tablespoon of baking powder
- One teaspoon of pure vanilla extract
- One pint of raspberries

Instructions

- Preheat the oven to 425 degrees F. Place a muffin tin 12 cups. About 12-15 large muffins will be made.
- Blend together the flour, granulated sugar, salt and baking powder in a big bowl.
- Add the eggs, milk, butter and pure vanilla extract. Just stir well.
- Into the batter, fold the raspberries
- Fill the baffle with the muffin tin so that it is nearly finished.
- For about 15 minutes, bake the muffins.

Ricotta Lemon Curd

Preparation time-5 minutes | Cook time-0 minutes | Servings-4 | Difficulty-Easy

Nutritional value- Calories-140 | Fat-7g | Carbohydrates-8g | Protein-11g

Ingredients

- One teaspoon of lemon zest
- A quarter cup of sugar substitute
- Half teaspoon of butter extract
- A quarter cup of lemon juice
- Half cup of plain nonfat Greek Yogurt
- One and a half cups of part-skim ricotta cheese

Instructions

- Add all the ingredients. Then beat with a beater on medium speed for 2 minutes.
- Freeze for 2 hours before serving.

Sautéed peaches or nectarines with maple syrup

Preparation time-10 minutes | Cook time-10 minutes | Servings-2 | Difficulty-Easy

Nutritional value: ~Calories-130 | Proteins-1g | Fat-0g | Carbohydrates-31g

Ingredients

- Two teaspoons of canola oil
- Two ripe peaches or nectarines, pitted, skinned, and sliced
- Two tablespoons of pure maple syrup
- Dash of ground cinnamon
- A dollop of plain yogurt per serving

Instructions

- Heat canola oil in a skillet over medium-high heat and sauté peaches or nectarines until golden, roughly 1–2 minutes.
- When golden, stir in maple syrup and allow syrup to thicken slightly.
- Serve warm with a sprinkling of ground cinnamon and a dollop of yogurt.

Simple and Delicious Mousse

Preparation time-10 minutes | Cook time-0 minutes | Servings-12 | Difficulty-Easy

Nutritional value: ~Calories-130 | Proteins-1g | Fat-0g | Carbohydrates-31g

Ingredients
- Eight ounces of mascarpone cheese
- 3/4 teaspoons of vanilla stevia

- One cup of whipping cream
- Half-pint of blueberries
- Half-pint of strawberries

Instructions

- Combine the whipped cream with mascarpone and stevia in a cup and blend well with your mixer.
- Assemble twelve glasses with a coating of strawberries and blueberries, then a layer of milk, and so on.
- Serve cool.

Sour cream and walnut cookies

Preparation time-10 minutes | Cook time-10 minutes | Servings-2 | Difficulty-Easy

Nutritional value: ~Calories-82 | Proteins-3g | Fat-1g | Carbohydrates-5g

Ingredients

- Canola oil cooking spray
- Half cup of trans fat–free canola/olive oil spread
- 2/3 cup of low-calorie baking sweetener
- 2/3 cup of low-fat sour cream
- One and a half cups of all-purpose unbleached flour
- One teaspoon of baking soda
- Half cup of chopped walnuts

Instructions

- Lightly coat two cookie sheets with cooking spray. In a bowl, combine canola/olive oil spread and sweetener. Use an electric beater on very low to whip the mixture into a soft consistency. Add sour cream and whip again for a few seconds to blend. Sift flour and baking soda into sour cream mixture.
- With a wooden spatula, fold the flour and baking soda into the mixture until well blended. Add walnuts to the dough mixture. Drop one tablespoon of dough on the cookie sheet for each cookie. Allow room between cookies.
- Press cookies flat with a wooden spatula and bake at 350 degrees, until golden brown (about 10–15 minutes).
- Remove from the oven and allow cookies to cool before serving.

Squash Apple Bake

Preparation time-15 minutes | Cook time-One hour | Servings-6 | Difficulty-Hard

Nutritional value- Calories-133 | Fat-8g | Carbohydrates-17g | Protein-1g

Ingredients

- One tablespoon of all-purpose flour

- 1/3 teaspoon of salt

- One medium peeled butternut squash, cut into ¾" cubes

- One tablespoon of Splenda

- Two teaspoons of ground cinnamon

- A quarter cup of melted butter

- Two medium peeled & cored apples, cut into thin wedges

Instructions

- In a casserole dish, combine the squash and apples.

- Combine remaining ingredients in a mixing bowl and spoon over squash and apples.

- Bake at 350 degrees for 50–60 minutes, covered, or until tender.

- If you prefer a crispier topping, remove the lid from the casserole dish during the final 10 minutes of cooking.

Strawberries Cream

Preparation time-10 minutes | Cook time-20 minutes | Servings-2 to 4 | Difficulty-Easy

Nutritional value: ~Calories-152 | Proteins-1g | Fat-5g | Carbohydrates-6g

Ingredients

- Half cup of stevia

- Two pounds of strawberries, chopped

- One cup of almond milk

- Zest of one lemon, grated

- Half cup of heavy cream

- Three egg yolks whisked

Instructions

- Heat a pan with the milk over medium-high heat, add the stevia and the rest of the ingredients.

- Whisk well, simmer for 20 minutes, divide into cups and serve cold.

Strawberry and poached pears

Preparation time-10 minutes | Cook time-30 minutes | Servings-2 | Difficulty-Easy

Nutritional value: ~Calories-120 | Proteins-1g | Fat-2g | Carbohydrates-5g

Ingredients

- Four large ripe Anjou or Bartlett pears, peeled and cored

- Two tablespoons of fresh lemon juice

- Half cup of red wine (not cooking wine)

- One and a half cups of water

- Two tablespoons of low-calorie baking sweetener

- One cinnamon stick

- One teaspoon of freshly grated orange rind

- Half teaspoon of freshly grated lemon rind

- A quarter teaspoon of cloves, ground

- Fresh mint leaves for garnish

For Strawberry Sauce

- One pint of fresh strawberries, cleaned and sliced

- Three tablespoons of non-caloric sweetener

- One teaspoon of Grand Marnier liqueur

Instructions

- Slice off the bottom of pears to allow them to sit flat in a pan. Brush body of pears with lemon juice.

- In a saucepan, combine wine, water, sweetener, cinnamon, orange rind, lemon rind, and cloves.

- Bring to a boil over medium heat, reduce heat, and simmer for 5 minutes. Add pears, cover, and poach for 20 minutes until tender. Let pears stand in liquid until cool.

- Refrigerate until ready to serve.

- When serving, place pears on dessert plates and drizzle with a small amount of strawberry sauce. Garnish with a mint leaf.

Sauce

- Put strawberries in a bowl and sprinkle with sweetener and Grand Marnier.

- Let stand at room temperature for 1 hour.

- Blend or process until puréed, then refrigerate sauce to chill.

Strawberry Frozen Yogurt

Preparation time-5 minutes | Cook time-0 minutes | Servings-4 | Difficulty-Easy

Nutritional value- Calories-135 | Fat-1g | Carbohydrates-25g | Protein-6g

Ingredients

- Two tablespoons of honey

- One teaspoon of freshly squeezed lemon juice

- Two teaspoons of vanilla extract

- Four cups of frozen strawberries

- One cup of low-fat, plain Greek Yogurt

Instructions

- Mix the Yogurt with vanilla, honey, lemon juice, and strawberries in the blender. Then pulse until everything becomes creamy.

- Pour it into a loaf pan and freeze for 2 hours. It should still be soft enough to scoop by the end. Enjoy!

Strawberry Pie

Preparation time-20 minutes | Cook time-15 minutes | Servings-4 | Difficulty-Easy

Nutritional value- Calories-135 | Fat-1g | Carbohydrates-25g | Protein-6g

Ingredients

For the filling

- One teaspoon of gelatin

- Eight ounces of cream cheese

- Four ounces of strawberries

- Two tablespoons of water

- Half tablespoon of lemon juice

- A quarter teaspoon of stevia

- Half cups of heavy cream

- Eight ounces of chopped strawberries for serving

- Sixteen ounces of heavy cream for serving

For the crust

- One cup of shredded coconut

- One cup of sunflower seeds

- A quarter cup of butter

- A pinch of salt

Instructions

- Mix the sunflower seeds with coconut, butter and a pinch of salt in your food processor and stir well.

- Place this in a greased springform pan and push the bottom well.

- Heat a skillet over medium heat with the water, add gelatin, mix until it dissolves, remove the heat and leave to cool off.

- Add it to your food processor, mix and blend well with 4 ounces of cream cheese, lemon juice, strawberries and stevia.

- Stir well, pour half a cup of heavy cream and scatter over the crust.

- Before slicing and serving, top with 8 ounces of strawberries and 16 ounces of heavy cream and keep in the refrigerator for 2 hours.

Strawberry-rhubarb quinoa pudding

Preparation time-10 minutes | Cook time-40 minutes | Servings-2 to 4 | Difficulty-Easy

Nutritional value: ~Calories-106 | Proteins-5g | Fat-1g | Carbohydrates-18g

Ingredients

- Three cups of water, divided

- One and a half cups of chopped rhubarb, fresh or frozen

- One cup of chopped strawberries, fresh or frozen, plus more for garnish

- Half cup of quinoa

- Half teaspoon of ground cinnamon

- Dash of salt

- A quarter cup plus one and a half teaspoons of low-calorie baking sweetener

- Half teaspoon of freshly grated lemon zest

- One tablespoon of cornstarch

- One cup of plain non-fat yogurt

- One teaspoon of pure vanilla extract

Instructions

- In a saucepan, combine two and 2/3 cups of water, rhubarb, strawberries, quinoa, cinnamon, and salt. Bring to a boil and reduce heat to a simmer.

- Cover and cook for about 25 minutes or until quinoa is tender. Stir in a quarter cup of sweetener and lemon zest.

- In a small bowl, combine the remaining quarter cup of water with cornstarch and whisk until smooth, then add to quinoa mixture and continue to let simmer, constantly stirring for 1 minute.

- Remove from heat, divide among serving bowls, and refrigerate to cool for 1 hour.

- Meanwhile, combine yogurt, vanilla extract, and the remaining one and a half teaspoon of sweetener in a small bowl.

- Top each serving with a generous dollop of yogurt mixture and sliced fresh strawberries.

Strawberry-walnut trifle

Preparation time-10 minutes | Cook time-15 minutes | Servings-2 | Difficulty-Easy

Nutritional value: ~Calories-72 | Proteins-1g | Fat-0g | Carbohydrates-17g

Ingredients

- One small, no-sugar-added angel food cake

- Three ounces of sugar-free strawberry gelatin

- Ten ounces of frozen, unsweetened strawberries, thawed and halved (reserve one cup for garnish)

- Two bananas, sliced

- One (One and a half-ounce) package sugar-free instant vanilla pudding mix

- Three cups of almond milk

- Fat-free whipped cream

- Chopped walnut pieces to sprinkle

Instructions

- Tear cake into bite-sized pieces and place in the bottom of a glass trifle bowl. Dissolve gelatin in one cup of boiling hot water and add to strawberries.

- Spoon strawberry mixture evenly over cake pieces. Add banana slices to the top of strawberries and refrigerate while preparing pudding.

- Combine pudding mix with almond milk and whisk for roughly 2 minutes until it begins to set. Refrigerate pudding for an additional 5 minutes to set more firmly before adding it to the trifle bowl, spooning evenly over bananas and strawberries. Refrigerate trifle bowl mixture for at least 2 hours before serving.

- Top each serving with reserved strawberries, a dollop of whipped cream, and a sprinkle of chopped walnuts.

Stuffed dates

Preparation time-10 minutes |Cook time-0 minutes |Servings-2 |Difficulty-Easy

Nutritional value: ~Calories-152 |Proteins-9g| Fat-14g |Carbohydrates-9g

Ingredients

- Eight pitted dates

- Eight whole almonds

- Three tablespoons of almond paste

Instructions

- Slice dates open on one side.

- Pull back skin from the meat of the date and stuff each date with one almond and one teaspoon of almond paste. Serve.

Sweet Potato Blueberry Protein Muffins

Preparation time-25 minutes| Cook time-30 minutes |Servings-3 |Difficulty-Moderate

Nutritional value- Calories-130| Fat-3g |Carbohydrates-18g| Protein-7g

Ingredients

- One and a half cups of old-fashioned rolled oats

- One small sweet potato, peeled, cooked and mashed

- One cup of plain low-fat yogurt

- Two large eggs

- Half teaspoon of baking soda

- Two scoops of vanilla protein powder

- One teaspoon of baking powder

- Pinch of salt

- One tablespoon of cinnamon

- One and a half cups of blueberries (fresh or frozen)

Instructions

For Sweet Potato

- Peel and cut cubes of sweet potato in a glass bowl.

- Microwave on high power for 5 minutes.

- Stir well and microwave for an additional 2:32 minutes, or until soft.

- In the glass bowl, mash with a fork.

For Muffins

- Preheat the oven to 350 degrees Fahrenheit. Coat 12 muffin cups in cooking spray or arrange with paper cups.

- Add oats to blender and process for about 30 seconds, or until flour forms.

- Combine the sweet potato, yogurt, baking soda, eggs, protein powder, baking powder, salt and cinnamon in a large mixing bowl. Blend until smooth (or whisk in a bowl). The batter will be extremely thick.

- Spoon into a bowl and stir in blueberries.

- Scoop batter into prepared muffin cups.

- Bake in the oven for 25-30 minutes.

- Remove from heat and then allow to cool for 5 minutes. Enjoy!

Vanilla Custard

Preparation time-10 minutes |Cook time-20 minutes |Servings-2 to 4 |Difficulty-Easy

Nutritional value: ~Calories-272 |Proteins-6g| Fat-16g |Carbohydrates-24g

Ingredients

- One tablespoon of corn-flour

- 1/3 cup of sugar

- One Vanilla Bean

- One cup of milk

- Four yolks of egg

- One cup of cream

Instructions

- Cook vanilla, milk, and cream in a saucepan with continuous stirring.

- Pour cream mixture over the egg, sugar, and cornflour mixture in a bowl.

- Cook until the required thickness is achieved.

- Cool and serve.

Vanilla Ice Cream

Preparation time-20 minutes| Cook time-0 minutes|Servings-6|Difficulty-Easy

Nutritional value- Calories-130| Fat-3g |Carbohydrates-18g| Protein-7g

Ingredients

- Four eggs, yolks and whites separated

- A quarter teaspoon of cream of tartar

- Half cups of swerving

- One tablespoon of vanilla extract

- One and a quarter cups of heavy whipping cream

Instructions

- Mix the egg whites with the tartar cream in a bowl and swerve and swirl using your mixer.

- Whisk the cream with the vanilla extract in another bowl and mix thoroughly.

- Combine and gently whisk the two mixtures.

- Whisk the egg yolks very well in another bowl and then apply the combination of two egg whites.

- Gently stir, put it into a container and leave it in the refrigerator for 3 hours until the ice cream is eaten.

Walnuts Cake

Preparation time-10 minutes |Cook time-40 minutes |Servings-2 to 4|Difficulty-Moderate

Nutritional value: ~Calories-205|Proteins-3.4g| Fat-14.8g|Carbohydrates-9.4g

Ingredients

- Half pound of walnuts, minced

- Zest of one orange, grated

- One and a quarter cups of stevia

- Eggs whisked

- One teaspoon of almond extract

- One and a half cups of almond flour

- One teaspoon of baking soda

Instructions

- In a bowl, combine the walnuts with the orange zest and the other ingredients. Put into a cake pan lined with parchment paper.

- Introduce in the oven at 350 degrees F, bake for 40 minutes, cool down, slice, and serve.

Watermelon-Basil Granita

Preparation time-10 minutes |Cook time-0 minutes |Serving-8-10 |Difficulty- Easy

Nutritional value: ~ Calories-76| Fat-0g| Protein-1g| Carbohydrates-20g

Ingredients

- Half medium watermelon, peel removed, roughly chopped (about 8 to 9 cups)

- Juice of two limes

- A quarter cup of sugar (or sugar substitute)

- One cup of fresh basil leaves, finely chopped

Instructions

- In a blender, combine the watermelon chunks, lime juice, and sugar (if using). Blend on high until smooth.

- Pour the watermelon mixture into a 9-by-13-inch baking dish, and stir in the basil leaves. Freeze for 1 hour.

- Remove from the freezer, and using a fork, scrape the frozen areas until broken apart. Return the dish to the freezer, and continue this process every half hour for at least 2 to 3 hours, or until the granita resembles coarse crystals.

- Before serving, scrape the frozen mixture again with a fork.

Chapter 14-Dips, Dressings and Sauces Recipes

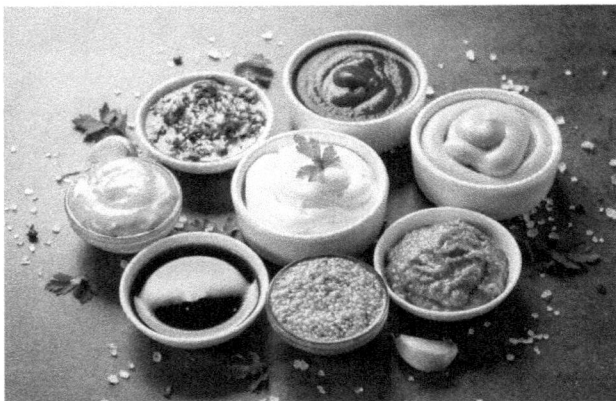

Asian-Inspired Dipping Sauce

Preparation time-15 minutes |Cook time-0 minutes |Serving-2 |Difficulty- Easy

Nutritional value: ~ Calories-51| Fat-2g| Protein-0.3g| Carbohydrates-8g

Ingredients

- Two tablespoons of minced or grated ginger
- Two tablespoons of minced or pressed garlic
- Two teaspoons of chili-garlic sauce (or more to taste)
- Six tablespoons of soy sauce
- Half cup of rice vinegar
- Half cup of hoisin sauce
- Half cup of low-sodium vegetable stock

Instructions

- Merge together all the ingredients in a small bowl, or place in a jar with a tight-fitting lid and shake until well mixed.
- Use immediately.

Avocado Cream

Preparation time-5 minutes |Cook time-0 minutes |Serving-3 |Difficulty- Easy

Nutritional value: ~ Calories-124| Fat-9g| Protein-4g| Carbohydrates-8g

Ingredients

- Two avocados
- Two garlic cloves
- Half jalapeño
- Six ounces of low-fat, plain Greek yogurt
- A quarter teaspoon of salt

- Juice of one lime

Instructions

- In a food processor, combine the avocado, garlic, jalapeño, yogurt, salt, and lime, and pulse until well combined.
- Refrigerate in an airtight container for up to 5 days.
- Serve with eggs, meats, soups, salads, and more for a tasty garnish that packs a nutritional punch.

Béchamel sauce

Preparation time-5 minutes |Cook time-15 minutes |Serving-2 |Difficulty- Easy

Nutritional value: ~ Calories-73| Fat-1.8g| Protein-2.3g| Carbohydrates-12g

Ingredients

- A quarter cup of grapeseed oil
- Three tablespoons of all-purpose flour
- Two and a half cups of unflavored non-dairy milk, preferably soy or rice
- A quarter small yellow onion, studded with one whole clove
- One bay leaf
- A quarter teaspoon of kosher salt
- Pinch of freshly ground black pepper
- Pinch of freshly grated nutmeg

Instructions

- In a small saucepan over medium-high heat, heat grapeseed oil. Add all-purpose flour all at once, and stir vigorously with a whisk.
- When flour mixture is golden and begins to smell nutty (but before it browns about 2 minutes), add non-dairy milk, continuing to whisk vigorously to prevent lumps.
- Add clove-studded yellow onion and bay leaf, reduce heat to low, and cook, frequently stirring, for about 10 minutes or until sauce is thickened.
- Remove from heat, and stir in kosher salt, black pepper, and nutmeg. Taste and adjust seasonings.
- Strain sauce through a fine-mesh strainer to remove solids, and use immediately.

Blue Cheese Dressing

Preparation time-5 minutes |Cook time-0 minutes |Serving-10 |Difficulty- Easy

Nutritional value: ~ Calories-24| Fat-0.29g| Protein-3.23g| Carbohydrates-1.7g

Ingredients

- One cup of nonfat cottage cheese
- 1/3 cup of nonfat buttermilk
- Two tablespoons of blue cheese crumbles
- Half teaspoon of Worcestershire sauce
- Half teaspoon of fresh lemon juice
- One teaspoon of finely chopped fresh parsley
- Half teaspoon of black pepper

Instructions

- Place all of the ingredients in a blender or food processor and blend until smooth.

Carrot-Tomato Sauce

Preparation time-5 minutes |Cook time-15 minutes |Serving-3 |Difficulty- Easy

Nutritional value: ~ Calories-284| Fat-14g| Protein-10g| Carbohydrates-35g

Ingredients

- Ten medium-sized, quartered tomatoes
- Eight medium-sized, diced carrots
- Eight minced garlic cloves
- Half chopped white onion
- Half cup of soaked cashews
- A quarter cup of water
- One tablespoon of olive oil

Instructions

- Heat oil in a deep-bottomed saucepan and add garlic.
- When fragrant, add onions and stir for 1-2 minutes. Add carrots and tomatoes. Cook for another few minutes. Pour in water and stir.
- Close and seal the lid.
- Cook on low pressure for 15 minutes.
- Turn down the heat and let it stand for some time.
- Move to a blender and puree.
- Pour the sauce back into the saucepan, leaving one cup in the blender.
- Add your soaked cashews to the blender and puree.

- Pour back into the pot and simmer without the lid for 10 minutes, until thickened.
- Season to taste.

Cashew ricotta

Preparation time-15 minutes |Cook time-0 minutes |Serving-2 |Difficulty- Easy

Nutritional value: ~ Calories-51| Fat-2g| Protein-0.3g| Carbohydrates-8g

Ingredients

- Two cups of raw cashews
- A quarter cup of extra-virgin olive oil
- A quarter cup of warm water
- Juice of one and a half medium lemons
- Two tablespoons of nutritional yeast
- One tablespoon of finely chopped fresh parsley
- One tablespoon of finely chopped chives
- One teaspoon of white (Shiro) miso
- Half teaspoon of dried marjoram
- Half teaspoon of kosher salt
- Half teaspoon of freshly ground black pepper

Instructions

- Soak cashews in water overnight.
- Discard soaking water, rinse cashews well, and drain.
- In a food processor fitted with a metal blade, process cashews, extra-virgin olive oil, warm water, lemon juice, nutritional yeast, parsley, chives, white (Shiro) miso, marjoram, kosher salt, and black pepper until smooth, scraping down the bowl several times with a spatula.
- Use immediately, or store in the refrigerator for up to 5 days.

Cinnamon peanut butter dip

Preparation time-5 minutes |Cook time-0 minutes |Serving-3 |Difficulty- Easy

Nutritional value: ~ Calories-124| Fat-9g| Protein-4g| Carbohydrates-8g

Ingredients

- Half cup of peanut butter
- One (6 ounces) container of light vanilla yogurt
- Half teaspoon of ground cinnamon

Instructions

- Place peanut butter into a small bowl or container. Add half of the vanilla yogurt, mixing with a spatula to combine.

- Add the rest of the yogurt and cinnamon and mix until a smooth texture is reached. Serve with carrots, celery, bell peppers, apples, bananas, pears, or any product that you can think of.

Creamy Italian Dressing

Preparation time-5 minutes |Cook time-0 minutes |Serving-10 |Difficulty- Easy

Nutritional value: - Calories-20.3| Fat-0.08g| Protein-2.9g| Carbohydrates-1.8g

Ingredients

- One cup of nonfat cottage cheese
- 1/3 cup of low-fat buttermilk
- One teaspoon of fresh lemon juice
- Half teaspoon of dried basil
- Half teaspoon of dried oregano
- Half teaspoon of dried thyme
- Half teaspoon of garlic powder

Instructions

- Place all of the ingredients in a blender or food processor and blend until smooth.

Creamy Lemon-Herb Dressing

Preparation time-5 minutes |Cook time-0 minutes |Serving-10 |Difficulty- Easy

Nutritional value: - Calories-20| Fat-0.08g| Protein-2.9g| Carbohydrates-1.7g

Ingredients

- One cup of nonfat cottage cheese
- 1/3 cup of low-fat buttermilk
- Two teaspoons of fresh lemon juice
- Half teaspoon of lemon zest
- One teaspoon of chopped fresh tarragon leaves
- One teaspoon of chopped fresh parsley
- One teaspoon of chopped fresh green onion (white and green parts)

Instructions

- Place all of the ingredients in a blender or food processor and blend until smooth.

Cucumber and Ranch Dressing

Preparation time-5 minutes |Cook time-0 minutes |Servings-2 |Difficulty-Easy

Nutritional value: ~Calories-232|Proteins-2g| Fat-21g|Carbohydrates-12g

Ingredients

- Half chopped onion
- A quarter teaspoon of pepper and salt each
- Two sliced cucumbers
- Half teaspoon of dill
- Half cup of ranch dressing

Instructions

- Whisk all the ingredients in a large bowl and set aside. Serve.

Cucumber salsa

Preparation time-10 minutes |Cook time-0 minutes |Servings-2 |Difficulty-Easy

Nutritional value: ~Calories-152|Proteins-1g| Fat-15g|Carbohydrates-6g

Ingredients

- Two cups of finely diced cucumber, peeled and deseeded
- Half cup of finely diced red onion
- Half cup of chopped fresh cilantro
- One clove of fresh garlic, minced
- One finely diced jalapeño pepper
- Three tablespoons of fresh lime juice
- One tablespoon of extra-virgin olive oil
- Salt and freshly ground pepper to taste

Instructions

- In a medium bowl, combine cucumber, onion, cilantro, garlic, and jalapeño. Toss to mix, then add in lime juice, olive oil, and salt and pepper to taste.
- Toss again and refrigerate for 15 minutes to allow flavors to blend. Let cool to room temperature before serving. Serve as a great addition over grilled fish, like tuna or swordfish.

Dill Dressing

Preparation time-5 minutes |Cook time-0 minutes |Serving-10 |Difficulty- Easy

Nutritional value: - Calories-19.8| Fat-0.09g| Protein-2.9g| Carbohydrates-1.7g

Ingredients

- One cup of nonfat cottage cheese
- 1/3 cup of low-fat buttermilk
- One teaspoon of fresh lemon juice
- Half tablespoon of chopped fresh dill
- A quarter teaspoon of black pepper
- A quarter teaspoon of ground celery seed

Instructions

- Place all of the ingredients in a blender or food processor and blend until smooth.

Easy basil pesto

Preparation time-10 minutes |Cook time-0 minutes |Servings-2 |Difficulty-Easy

Nutritional value: ~Calories-1464|Proteins-24g| Fat-176g|Carbohydrates-6g

Ingredients

- Two cups of packed fresh basil leaves
- Three cloves of fresh garlic
- 1/3 cup of walnuts
- 2/3 cup of extra-virgin olive oil, divided
- Half cup of freshly grated Pecorino cheese
- Salt and freshly ground pepper to taste

Instructions

- Combine basil, garlic, and walnuts in a food processor and pulse until coarsely chopped. Add half a cup of oil and process until smooth.
- Add in Pecorino cheese, salt and pepper, and remaining olive oil and pulse again until blended.

Easy pizza sauce

Preparation time-15 minutes |Cook time-20 minutes |Servings-2 |Difficulty-Easy

Nutritional value: ~Calories-19|Proteins-0.5g| Fat-1g|Carbohydrates-2g

Ingredients

- One teaspoon of crumbled dried basil
- Half teaspoon of crumbled dried oregano
- A quarter teaspoon of crumbled dried marjoram
- A quarter cup of dry white wine
- Two cloves of fresh garlic, finely chopped
- One tablespoon of extra-virgin olive oil
- One and a half cups of chopped, crushed plum tomato
- Two tablespoons of tomato paste
- Salt and freshly ground pepper to taste

Instructions

- Add herbs to wine and marinate for 15 minutes. Meanwhile, over medium heat, sauté garlic in olive oil until soft but not brown. Add tomato, tomato paste, and herb/wine mixture. Cover and simmer for about 20 minutes.
- Remove from stove, put into a blender, and puree until smooth. Return to skillet uncovered and continue to simmer until sauce thickens slightly. Add salt and pepper to taste.

Eggplant dip (baba ghanoush)

Preparation time-5 minutes |Cook time-35 minutes |Servings-2 |Difficulty-Moderate

Nutritional value: ~Calories-216|Proteins-8g| Fat-19g|Carbohydrates-21g

Ingredients

- Two large purple eggplants
- Four cloves of garlic
- Fine sea salt and ground black pepper
- One teaspoon of ground cumin
- Two tablespoons of lemon juice
- Four tablespoons of tahini (sesame seed paste)
- Two tablespoons of chopped fresh cilantro for garnish
- Two tablespoons of extra-virgin olive oil for garnish

Instructions

- Preheat the oven to 350°F. Line a baking sheet with parchment paper.
- Place the whole eggplants on the baking sheet. In each eggplant, hollow out two holes large enough for a garlic clove. Stick a clove of garlic in each hole. Bake the eggplants for about 30 minutes, until soft.
- Let the eggplants cool for 5 minutes. Cut the stems off the eggplants and put them in a food processor, skin on. Add a pinch of salt and pepper, cumin, and lemon juice to the food processor. Pulse the mixture a few times until all of the ingredients are combined. Add the tahini and pulse for 10 seconds. Taste the dip and adjust the seasoning to your taste.
- Transfer the dip to a bowl and top with the cilantro and olive oil. Serve warm.

Fava Bean Dip

Preparation time-5 minutes |Cook time-15 minutes |Serving-2|Difficulty- Easy

Nutritional value: ~ Calories-415| Fat-26g| Protein-15g| Carbohydrates-31g

Ingredients

- Three cups of water
- Two cups of soaked split fava beans
- Two crushed garlic cloves
- Two tablespoons of vegetable oil
- One tablespoon of olive oil
- One zested and juiced lemon
- Two teaspoons of tahini

- Two teaspoons of cumin
- One teaspoon of harissa
- One teaspoon of paprika
- Salt to taste

Instructions

- The night before, soak the fava beans and drain the fava beans before beginning the recipe.
- Heat oil in a deep-bottomed pot.
- Add garlic when hot and cook until they become golden.
- Add beans, veggie oil, and three cups of water.
- Close and seal the lid.
- Cook on high pressure for 12 minutes.
- Turn down the heat and wait 10 minutes.
- Drain the cooking liquid from the pot, leaving about one cup.
- Toss in the tahini, cumin, harissa, and lemon zest.
- Puree until smooth. Add the salt and blend again.
- Serve with a drizzle of olive oil and a dash of paprika.

French Dressing

Preparation time-5 minutes |Cook time-0 minutes |Serving-10 |Difficulty- Easy

Nutritional value: ~ Calories-21| Fat-9g| Protein-3g| Carbohydrates-2g

Ingredients

- One cup of nonfat cottage cheese
- 1/3 cup of low-fat buttermilk
- Half teaspoon of paprika
- Half teaspoon of Worcestershire sauce
- Two teaspoons of unsalted tomato juice
- One teaspoon of onion powder
- Half teaspoon of dry mustard

Instruction

- Place all of the ingredients in a blender or food processor and blend until smooth.

Garden Goddess Dressing

Preparation time-5 minutes |Cook time-0 minutes |Serving-10 |Difficulty- Easy

Nutritional value: ~ Calories-21.9| Fat-0.25g| Protein-4g| Carbohydrates-1.7g

Ingredients

- One cup of nonfat cottage cheese
- 1/3 cup of low-fat buttermilk
- One teaspoon of fresh lemon juice
- Two teaspoons of anchovy paste
- One tablespoon of chopped fresh parsley
- Two teaspoons of chopped green onion
- One teaspoon of chopped fresh oregano leaves (stems removed)

Instructions

- Place all of the ingredients in a blender or food processor and blend until smooth.

Herb cucumber yogurt dip

Preparation time-10 minutes |Cook time-10 minutes |Servings-2 |Difficulty-Easy

Nutritional value: ~Calories-16|Proteins-0.5g| Fat-1g|Carbohydrates-1g

Ingredients

- One English cucumber
- Salt to taste
- Two cloves fresh garlic, chopped
- Two teaspoons of white wine vinegar
- Two tablespoons of extra-virgin olive oil
- Two cups of plain low-fat yogurt
- Two teaspoons of fresh dill
- Two teaspoons of dried mint
- Freshly ground pepper to taste
- Two tablespoons of chopped fresh mint for garnish

Instructions

- Peel and slice cucumber (if very seedy, remove seeds). Place in a bowl and sprinkle with a little salt; let sit for about 15 minutes to draw out water.
- In a separate bowl, mash garlic into a paste; add a pinch of salt, vinegar, and olive oil, and stir. Add yogurt, dill, and dried mint, and mix well.
- Rinse salt from cucumber slices and pat dry, removing any excess water. Combine cucumber with yogurt mixture; add salt and freshly ground pepper to taste.
- Garnish with fresh chopped mint and serve.

Homemade Ketchup

Preparation time-5 minutes |Cook time-15 minutes |Serving-3|Difficulty- Easy

Nutritional value: ~ Calories-20| Fat-0.3g| Protein-6g| Carbohydrates-1.7g

Ingredients

- Two pounds of quartered plum tomatoes
- One tablespoon of paprika
- One tablespoon of agave syrup
- One teaspoon of salt
- Six tablespoons of apple cider vinegar
- ⅓ cup of raisins
- ⅛ wedged onion
- Half teaspoon of Dijon mustard
- A quarter teaspoon of celery seeds
- ⅛ teaspoon of garlic powder
- ⅛ teaspoon of ground clove
- ⅛ teaspoon of cinnamon

Instructions

- Put everything in a deep-bottomed pot.
- Mash down, so the tomatoes release their juice, making sure you hit the one and a half cups minimum for the pot.
- Close and seal the lid.
- Cook for 5 minutes on high pressure.
- Turn down the heat and let it stand for some time.
- Take the lid off and simmer for 10 minutes to reduce.
- Puree in a blender before storing in a jar.
- Wait until it's cooled down before putting it in the fridge.

Honey mustard sauce

Preparation time-10 minutes | Cook time-0 minutes | Servings-2 | Difficulty-Easy

Nutritional value: ~Calories-372 | Proteins-3g | Fat-22g | Carbohydrates-46g

Ingredients

- Four tablespoons of Dijon mustard
- Four tablespoons of light mayonnaise
- Two tablespoons of honey
- Two tablespoons of red wine vinegar

Instructions

- Combine all ingredients in a covered container and chill in the refrigerator to blend flavors for 30 minutes.
- Serve room temperature with chicken, crab, or shrimp.

Horseradish Dressing

Preparation time-5 minutes | Cook time-0 minutes | Serving-10 | Difficulty- Easy

Nutritional value: ~ Calories-19.72 | Fat-0.79g | Protein-2.89g | Carbohydrates-1.6g

Ingredients

- One cup of nonfat cottage cheese
- 1/3 cup of low-fat buttermilk
- One teaspoon fresh lemon juice
- One tablespoon of freshly grated horseradish
- One teaspoon of chopped fresh parsley
- One teaspoon of chopped fresh green onion (white parts only)

Instructions

- Place all of the ingredients in a blender or food processor and blend until smooth.

Hot Artichoke Dip

Preparation time-5 minutes | Cook time-20 minutes | Serving-10 | Difficulty- Easy

Nutritional value: ~ Calories-74 | Fat-3g | Protein-5g | Carbohydrates-8g

Ingredients

- Two cans (14 ounces each) artichoke hearts, drained and cut into quarters
- One cup of shredded low-moisture, part-skim mozzarella cheese
- 3/4 cup of nonfat mayonnaise
- A quarter cup of shredded Parmesan cheese
- Half teaspoon of salt
- A quarter teaspoon of black pepper

Instructions

- Preheat the oven to 375°F.
- In a 1-quart (1-L) casserole oven-safe dish, place the artichoke hearts.
- Add the mozzarella cheese, mayonnaise, Parmesan cheese, salt, and pepper. Mix thoroughly with a large spoon, ensuring even distribution.
- Bake the dip for 15 minutes and serve immediately. (Avoid overheating to ensure the mayonnaise does not separate.)

Hummus with tahini dip

Preparation time-10 minutes | Cook time-0 minutes | Servings-2 | Difficulty-Easy

Nutritional value: ~Calories-84 | Proteins-3g | Fat-5g | Carbohydrates-8g

Ingredients

- Four cups of canned chickpeas, rinsed and drained
- Three tablespoons of tahini paste
- Three tablespoons of freshly squeezed lemon juice
- Four cloves of fresh garlic, crushed into a paste
- Salt to taste
- One tablespoon of chopped fresh cilantro for garnish
- Four tablespoons of extra-virgin olive oil

Instructions

- Puree chickpeas in a food processor or blender. Blend together the tahini, lemon juice, garlic, and salt. Combine this with the chickpeas and blend until it becomes a smooth paste.
- Serve garnished with cilantro and drizzled with olive oil.

Lemon and Thyme Sauce

Preparation time-5 minutes |Cook time-0 minutes |Servings-2 |Difficulty-Easy

Nutritional value: ~Calories-26|Proteins-3g| Fat-0.2g|Carbohydrates-1.8g

Ingredients

- One cup of low-sodium vegetable broth
- Half cup of freshly squeezed lemon juice
- A quarter cup of cooking oil
- A quarter cup of water
- One tablespoon of finely minced fresh chives
- One tablespoon of fresh thyme
- One tablespoon of finely minced garlic

Instructions

- Put ingredients in a medium bowl and whisk until combined. Use immediately or store refrigerated for up to 10 days.

Lemon dressing

Preparation time-10 minutes |Cook time-0 minutes |Servings-2 |Difficulty-Easy

Nutritional value: ~Calories-61|Proteins-0.2g| Fat-7g|Carbohydrates-1g

Ingredients

- A quarter cup of extra-virgin olive oil
- A quarter cup of fresh-squeezed lemon juice
- One medium clove of fresh garlic, crushed to a paste
- Scant pinch of salt
- Freshly ground pepper to taste

Instructions

- Combine all ingredients in a bowl and mix well.

Lemon-pepper salad dressing

Preparation time-10 minutes |Cook time-0 minutes |Servings-2 |Difficulty-Easy

Nutritional value: ~Calories-720|Proteins-0g| Fat-84g|Carbohydrates-2g

Ingredients

- Half cup of extra-virgin olive oil
- Two tablespoons of vinegar
- One tablespoon of non-caloric sweetener
- Two teaspoons of lemon pepper seasoning

Instructions

- Combine all ingredients in a salad dressing shaker and shake well to blend.
- Drizzle on salad.

Lentil Bolognese

Preparation time-5 minutes |Cook time-15 minutes |Servings-4-6 |Difficulty-Easy

Nutritional value: ~Calories-208|Proteins-12g| Fat-0g|Carbohydrates-39g

Ingredients

- Four cups of water
- One cup of washed black lentils
- One 28-ounce can of fire-roasted tomatoes
- Four minced garlic cloves
- Three diced carrots
- One diced yellow onion
- One can of tomato paste
- A quarter cup of balsamic vinegar
- Two tablespoons of Italian seasoning
- Red pepper flakes
- Salt and pepper

Instructions

- Add all your ingredients except the balsamic vinegar in a deep-bottomed saucepan. Stir. Close and seal the lid.
- Cook for 15 minutes on high pressure.
- Turn down the heat and wait 10 minutes.
- Add the balsamic vinegar, salt, and pepper and stir.
- Serve or pour in a jar that you let cool before storing in the fridge.

Light Alfredo Sauce

Preparation time- 5 minutes | Cook time-15 minutes | Servings-7 | Difficulty-Easy

Nutritional value- Calories-71 | Fat-4g | Carbohydrates-5g | Protein-5g

Ingredients

- Four cloves garlic, minced
- One cup of chicken warmed broth
- Half teaspoon of salt
- One tablespoon of extra-virgin olive oil
- Two cups of skim milk
- Three tablespoons of all-purpose flour
- A quarter teaspoon of black pepper
- Half cup of grated Parmesan cheese

Instructions

- In a medium saucepan over medium heat, heat olive oil.
- Add garlic and sauté until fragrant, about 30 seconds.
- Stir in flour until thick paste forms.
- Whisk in warmed chicken broth in a slow, steady stream.
- Stir in the milk, pepper and salt.
- Cook over low heat, constantly stirring until smooth and thick.
- To finish, stir in the Parmesan cheese.

Mango chutney

Preparation time-10 minutes | Cook time-0 minutes | Servings-2 | Difficulty-Easy

Nutritional value: ~Calories-82 | Proteins-0g | Fat-8g | Carbohydrates-6g

Ingredients

- One ripe mango, peeled, pitted, and diced into small cubes
- One bunch cilantro, finely chopped
- Half teaspoon of crushed red hot pepper flakes
- A quarter cup of extra-virgin olive oil
- Two tablespoons of freshly squeezed lime juice
- Salt and freshly ground pepper to taste

Instructions

- In a bowl, combine mango, cilantro, hot pepper flakes, olive oil, and lime juice. Stir to blend, then add salt and pepper to taste.
- Serve with fish or chicken.

Mixed-Veggie Sauce

Preparation time-10 minutes | Cook time-7 minutes | Servings-3 | Difficulty-Easy

Nutritional value: ~Calories-126 | Proteins-3g | Fat-3g | Carbohydrates-22g

Ingredients

- Four chopped tomatoes
- Five cubes of pumpkin
- Four minced garlic cloves
- Two chopped green chilies
- Two chopped celery stalks
- One sliced leek
- One chopped onion
- One chopped red bell pepper
- One chopped carrot
- One tablespoon of sugar
- Two teaspoons of olive oil
- One teaspoon of red chili flakes
- Splash of vinegar
- Salt to taste

Instructions

Prepare the vegetables.

- Heat your oil in a pot
- Add onion and garlic, and cook until the onion is clear.
- Add pumpkin, carrots, green chilies, and bell pepper.
- Stir before adding the leek, celery, and tomatoes.
- After a minute or so, toss in salt and red chili flakes. Close and seal the lid of the pot.
- Cook for 6 minutes with the lid on.
- Turn down the heat and let the pressure come down on its own. The veggies should be very soft.
- Let the mixture cool a little before moving to a blender.
- Puree until smooth.
- Pour back into the pot and add vinegar and sugar.
- Simmer on low for a few minutes before serving.

Orange ginger sauce

Preparation time-10 minutes | Cook time-5 minutes | Servings-2 | Difficulty-Easy

Nutritional value: ~Calories-60 | Proteins-0g | Fat-5g | Carbohydrates-5g

Ingredients

- Juice from three fresh oranges

- A quarter cup of light mayonnaise

- Two tablespoons of prepared fresh horseradish

- A quarter teaspoon of honey

- A quarter teaspoon of ground ginger

- One tablespoon of extra-virgin olive oil

- Salt and freshly ground pepper to taste

- Generous pinch of all-purpose flour

Instructions

- Combine orange juice, mayonnaise, horseradish, honey, ginger, olive oil, and salt and pepper in a small saucepan. Whisk to blend on low heat.

- When sauce begins to simmer, whisk in flour. Cook for 1–2 minutes, constantly whisking, until sauce is smooth.

Raspberry vinaigrette

Preparation time-10 minutes | Cook time-8 minutes | Servings-2 | Difficulty-Easy

Nutritional value: ~Calories-121 | Proteins-0.2g | Fat-14g | Carbohydrates-1g

Ingredients

- Half shallot

- Half teaspoon of Dijon mustard

- A quarter cup of raspberry vinegar

- Six drops of liquid stevia (plain)

- Half cup of olive oil

- Salt and ground black pepper, to taste

Instructions

- Put the shallot and mustard in your food processor, and turn it on. As the shallots are reaching the minced stage, add the raspberry vinegar and liquid stevia. Now slowly pour in the olive oil. When it's well incorporated, turn off the processor.

- Taste, add salt and pepper, then pulse just another second or two to mix, and it's ready to use.

Roasted garlic cauliflower hummus

Preparation time-10 minutes | Cook time-45 minutes | Servings-2 | Difficulty-Moderate

Nutritional value: ~Calories-146 | Proteins-6g | Fat-12g | Carbohydrates-24g

Ingredients

- One head of garlic

- Six tablespoons of extra-virgin olive oil, divided

- Six cups of cauliflower florets

- Two tablespoons of tahini (sesame seed paste)

- One tablespoon of lemon juice

- One teaspoon of ground cumin

- One teaspoon of paprika

- Fine sea salt and ground black pepper

Instructions

- Preheat the oven to 350°F.

- Chop the top off of the head of garlic and coat the head with Two tablespoons of olive oil. Place it in a small glass baking dish and roast it in the oven for 35 minutes.

- Place the cauliflower florets in a steamer pot with several inches of water over medium-high heat. Steam the cauliflower

- until it's cooked and fork-tender but not mushy, about 10 minutes. Drain the cauliflower and place it in a food processor.

- Squeeze 4 to 6 of the roasted garlic cloves out of their skins and into the food processor. Save the rest of the roasted garlic for another use, such as a pizza topping.

- Add the tahini, lemon juice, remaining Four tablespoons of olive oil, cumin, paprika, and a pinch of salt and pepper to the food processor. Pulse the mixture until smooth. Adjust seasonings to taste and chill before serving if desired.

Roasted pepper dip

Preparation time-10 minutes | Cook time-20 minutes | Servings-2 | Difficulty-Easy

Nutritional value: ~Calories-22 | Proteins-0.2g | Fat-2g | Carbohydrates-2g

Ingredients

- Four large red bell peppers

- One tablespoon of red wine vinegar

- Three tablespoons of extra-virgin olive oil

- Two cloves fresh garlic, peeled and minced

- Salt and freshly ground pepper to taste

Instructions

- Wash red bell peppers and pat dry. Place on a moderately hot grill, often turning until skin is charred and blistered (about 15–20 minutes). Remove from grill and let peppers cool.

- Rub off blackened skins. Cut each bell pepper in half, remove stalks and seeds, and cut into Half-inch strips. In a food processor, add vinegar and bell peppers and pulse, adding olive oil slowly until bell peppers are smooth.

- Transfer pepper mixture from processor to a bowl. Mash garlic and stir into pepper mixture; add salt and pepper to taste.

Sage~Butternut Squash Sauce

Preparation time-10 minutes | Cook time-10 minutes | Servings-4 | Difficulty-Easy

Nutritional value: ~Calories-179 | Proteins-3g | Fat-7g | Carbohydrates-30g

Ingredients

- Two pounds of chopped butternut squash
- One cup of veggie broth
- One chopped yellow onion
- Two chopped garlic cloves
- Two tablespoons of olive oil
- One tablespoon of chopped sage
- ⅛ teaspoon of red pepper flakes
- Salt and black pepper to taste

Instructions

- Preheat your saucepan with oil.
- Once the oil is hot, add the sage and stir so it becomes coated in oil.
- When the sage crisps up, move it to a plate.
- Add the onion to your cooker and cook until it begins to turn clear.
- Add garlic and cook until fragrant.
- Pour in one cup of broth and deglaze before adding squash.
- Close and seal the lid.
- Cook for straight 10 minutes.
- Turn down the heat and wait for 10 minutes.
- When a little cooler, add the pot's contents (and the sage) to a blender and puree till smooth.
- If it's too thick, add a little more veggie broth.
- Serve right away or store in the fridge no longer than 3-4 days.

Secret Burger Sauce

Preparation time-5 minutes | Cook time-0 minutes | Serving-2 | Difficulty- Easy

Nutritional value: - Calories-76 | Fat-6g | Protein-0g | Carbohydrates-3g

Ingredients

- Half cup of olive oil mayonnaise
- A quarter cup of low-sugar ketchup
- One teaspoon of hot sauce
- Two tablespoons of dill pickle relish
- Half teaspoon of Worcestershire sauce
- A quarter teaspoon of salt
- A quarter teaspoon of freshly ground black pepper

Instructions

- In a small bowl, whisk the mayonnaise, ketchup, hot sauce, relish, Worcestershire sauce, salt, and pepper until well combined.
- Refrigerate in an airtight container for up to 5 days.

Simply great marinara sauce

Preparation time-10 minutes | Cook time-One hour | Servings-2 | Difficulty-Hard

Nutritional value: ~Calories-74 | Proteins-17g | Fat-2g | Carbohydrates-13g

Ingredients

- Half cup of yellow onion, finely chopped
- Six cloves of fresh garlic, finely minced
- Three tablespoons of extra-virgin olive oil
- Two (28-ounce) cans of tomato puree with no salt added
- One (28-ounce) can of crushed tomatoes
- One tablespoon of tomato paste
- Half teaspoon of dried basil
- Two and a half cups of water
- One cup of canned low-sodium, fat-free chicken broth
- One teaspoon of low-calorie baking sweetener
- A quarter teaspoon of crushed red hot pepper flakes
- Salt and freshly ground pepper to taste

Instructions

- Sauté onion and garlic in olive oil over medium heat until soft; do not brown. Add tomato puree, crushed tomatoes, tomato paste, and basil. Stir to blend flavors.
- Add water, broth, sweetener, hot pepper flakes, and salt and pepper, then bring mixture to a boil, cover, reduce heat to low, and simmer for 1 hour.
- Store unused sauce (in a sealed container) in the freezer for up to 3–4 months.

Spicy and Cheesy Turkey Dip

Preparation time-15 minutes | Cook time-25 minutes | Servings-2 | Difficulty-Easy

Nutritional value: ~Calories-284 | Proteins-26g | Fat-19g | Carbohydrates-3.2g

Ingredients

- One Fresno chili pepper, deveined and minced

- One and a half cups of Ricotta cheese, creamed, 4% fat, softened

- A quarter cup of sour cream

- One tablespoon of butter, room temperature

- One shallot, chopped

- One teaspoon of garlic, pressed

- One pound of ground turkey

- Half cup of goat cheese, shredded

- Salt and black pepper, to taste

- One and a half cups of Gruyere, shredded

Instructions

- Dissolve the butter in a frying pan over a moderately high flame. Now, sauté the onion and garlic until they have softened.

- Stir in the ground turkey and continue to cook until it is no longer pink.

- Transfer the sautéed mixture to a lightly greased baking dish. Add in Ricotta, sour cream, goat cheese, salt, pepper, and chili pepper.

- Top with the shredded Gruyere cheese. Bake at 350 degrees F within 20 minutes in the preheated oven or until hot and bubbly on top.

Spicy Peanut Dressing

Preparation time-10 minutes | Cook time-0 minutes | Serving-2 | Difficulty- Easy

Nutritional value: ~Calories-76| Fat-4g| Protein-6g| Carbohydrates-6g

Ingredients

- A quarter cup of powdered peanut butter

- Two tablespoons of water

- Two tablespoons of rice vinegar

- Two tablespoons of low-sodium soy sauce

- One teaspoon of sesame oil

- One teaspoon of fresh ginger, minced

- Half teaspoon of sriracha (optional)

- Half teaspoon of fish sauce (optional)

Instructions

- In a medium bowl, whisk the powdered peanut butter, water, vinegar, soy sauce, sesame oil, ginger, sriracha, and fish sauce until well combined.

- Refrigerate in an airtight jar for up to one week.

Stir-Fry Sauce

Preparation time-10 minutes | Cook time-0 minutes | Serving-2 | Difficulty- Easy

Nutritional value: ~Calories-42| Fat-0g| Protein-1g| Carbohydrates-11g

Ingredients

- A quarter cup of low-sodium soy sauce

- One tablespoon of freshly grated ginger

- Two garlic cloves, minced

- Two tablespoons of brown sugar (or sugar substitute)

- A quarter cup of water

- One teaspoon of sriracha

- Two tablespoons of rice vinegar

Instructions

- In a medium bowl, whisk to combine the soy sauce, ginger, garlic, sugar, water, sriracha, and vinegar.

- Refrigerate in an airtight container for up to one week.

Sweet Lemon Poppy Seed Dressing

Preparation time-5 minutes | Cook time-0 minutes | Serving-10 | Difficulty- Easy

Nutritional value: ~ Calories-25| Fat-0.06g| Protein-2.93g| Carbohydrates-2.8g

Ingredients

- One cup of nonfat cottage cheese

- 1/3 cup of low-fat buttermilk

- Two teaspoons of fresh lemon juice

- Half teaspoon of lemon zest

- Two teaspoons of honey

- One teaspoon of poppy seeds

Instructions

- Place all of the ingredients in a blender or food processor and blend until smooth.

Taco Seasoning

Preparation time-10 minutes | Cook time-0 minutes | Serving-2 | Difficulty- Easy

Nutritional value: ~Calories-26| Fat-1g| Protein-1g| Carbohydrates-4g

Ingredients

- Two tablespoons of chili powder

- Three teaspoons of ground cumin

- One teaspoon of garlic powder

- Half teaspoon of onion powder

- One teaspoon of dried oregano

- Two teaspoons of ground paprika

- Half teaspoon of salt

- Half teaspoon of freshly ground black pepper

Instructions

- In a resealable container, combine the chili powder, cumin, garlic powder, onion powder, oregano, paprika, salt, and pepper, and mix well.

- Store in an airtight container for up to 3 months.

Tangy honey mustard dressing

Preparation time-10 minutes | Cook time-0 minutes | Serving-2 | Difficulty- Easy

Nutritional value: ~Calories-7 | Fat-0.1g | Protein-0.1g | Carbohydrates-1g

Ingredients

- Half cup of light olive oil

- A quarter cup of cider vinegar

- A quarter cup of brown mustard

- 1/8 teaspoon of liquid stevia (plain)

- A quarter teaspoon of ground black pepper

- A quarter teaspoon of salt

Instructions

- Just assemble everything in a clean jar, lid it tightly, and shake like mad. Store in the fridge, right in the jar, and shake again before using.

Teriyaki Sauce

Preparation time-15 minutes | Cook time-0 minutes | Servings-4 | Difficulty-Easy

Nutritional value- Calories-51 | Fat-2g | Carbohydrates-8g | Protein-0.2g

Ingredients

- Half cup of soy sauce

- Three tablespoons of honey

- One tablespoon of rice wine or dry sherry

- One tablespoon of rice vinegar

- Two teaspoons of minced fresh ginger

- Two smashed garlic cloves

Instructions

- Merge together all the ingredients in a small bowl.

- Use immediately.

Tofabulous crab dip

Preparation time-5 minutes | Cook time-20 minutes | Serving-4 | Difficulty- Easy

Nutritional value: ~ Calories-124 | Fat-9g | Protein-4g | Carbohydrates-8g

Ingredients

- ¾ cup of finely chopped soft tofu

- Half to ⅔ cup of fresh grated Parmesan cheese

- Two tablespoons of Dijon mustard

- Two teaspoons of dried oregano

- Half teaspoon of black pepper

- Half cup of fat-free or reduced-fat sour cream

- A quarter cup of 0% fat Greek yogurt

- Six ounces of lump crab meat (freshly cooked or canned)

- One cup of artichoke hearts (jarred in water, not oil!), chopped roughly paprika

Instructions

- Preheat oven to 350 F.

- Combine all ingredients except paprika into a medium bowl, mixing gently.

- Spoon mixture into a baking dish, and sprinkle with paprika. Bake for 20 minutes or until browned.

Tomato-basil sauce

Preparation time-10 minutes | Cook time-15 minutes | Servings-2 | Difficulty-Easy

Nutritional value: ~Calories-66 | Proteins-2g | Fat-3g | Carbohydrates-6g

Ingredients

- One tablespoon of olive oil

- Four cloves of fresh garlic, minced

- One shallot, finely chopped

- One (14.5-ounce) can diced tomatoes with chilies, well-drained

- Salt and freshly ground pepper to taste

- Four sprigs of basil, chopped

Instructions

- In a skillet over medium-high heat, combine olive oil, garlic, and shallot. Sauté garlic and shallot until soft and fragrant. Reduce heat to low.

- Add tomatoes, salt and pepper, and basil, and cook uncovered until heated through and liquid absorbed.

- Serve as a chunky sauce over fish or chicken.

Tzatziki Greek Yogurt and Cucumber Sauce

Preparation time-15 minutes | Cook time-30 minutes | Servings-9 | Difficulty-Moderate

Nutritional value- Calories-53| Fat-0g |Carbohydrates-8g| Protein-6g

Ingredients

- One chopped garlic clove

- One tablespoon of salt

- Salt to taste

- One tablespoon of finely chopped dill

- Three tablespoons of lemon juice

- Two medium cucumbers (seeded, peeled & diced)

- Three cups of plain Greek yogurt (fat-free)

- Pepper to taste

Instructions

- Cucumbers should be peeled and cut in half lengthwise. Scrape out and throw away the seeds with a small spoon.

- Cucumbers should be diced and placed in a colander with one tablespoon of salt. Allow standing for 30 minutes to allow the water to evaporate. Drain thoroughly and dry cucumber slices with a paper towel.

- Combine garlic, cucumbers, dill, lemon juice, and a few grinds of black pepper in a food processor fitted with a steel blade.

- Process until smooth.

- Add the mixture to the yogurt and stir well.

- Taste before adding any additional salt, then season with additional salt if necessary.

- Refrigerate for at least two hours before serving to allow flavors to meld (do not skimp on the resting time).

- Before serving, drain any excess water and stir.

Tzatziki Sauce

Preparation time-10 minutes |Cook time-0 minutes |Serving-4 |Difficulty- Easy

Nutritional value: ~Calories-40| Fat-2g| Protein-3g| Carbohydrates-2g

Ingredients

- One cup of shredded cucumber, seeded and grated

- One cup of low-fat, plain Greek yogurt

- One tablespoon of extra-virgin olive oil

- One tablespoon of fresh dill

- One tablespoon of freshly squeezed lemon juice

- One garlic clove, minced

- Salt

- Freshly ground black pepper

Instructions

- Using paper towels, pat dry the cucumber shreds, removing as much liquid as you can.

- In a large bowl, mix the cucumber, yogurt, olive oil, dill, lemon juice, garlic, and salt and pepper to taste.

- Serve immediately, or refrigerate in an airtight container for up to 5 days.

Vegan "Cheese" Sauce

Preparation time-10 minutes |Cook time-5 minutes |Serving-4 |Difficulty- Easy

Nutritional value: ~Calories-216| Fat-9g| Protein-13g| Carbohydrates-26g

Ingredients

- Two cups of peeled and chopped white potatoes

- Two cups of water

- One cup of chopped carrots

- Three peeled, whole garlic cloves

- Half cup of chopped onion

- Half cup of nutritional yeast

- Half cup of raw cashews

- One teaspoon of turmeric

- One teaspoon of salt

Instructions

- Put everything in a deep saucepan with a lid.

- Close and seal the lid.

- Cook for 5 minutes on high pressure.

- Turn down the heat and open the lid.

- Let the sauce cool for 10-15 minutes.

- Blend until smooth and creamy.

- Serve or store!

Vegan Alfredo Sauce

Preparation time-10 minutes |Cook time-0 minutes |Serving-4 |Difficulty- Easy

Nutritional value: ~Calories-20| Fat-1g| Protein-1g| Carbohydrates-2g

Ingredients

- Twelve ounces of cauliflower florets

- Two minced garlic cloves

- Half cup of water

- One teaspoon of coconut oil

- Half teaspoon of sea salt

- Black pepper to taste

Instructions

- Heat the oil in a deep-bottomed saucepan and add garlic.

- When the garlic has become fragrant, pour half a cup of water into the pan.

- Pour cauliflower in a steamer basket, and lower into the pot.

- Close and seal the lid.

- Cook for 3 minutes on high pressure.

- Turn down the heat and wait for the pressure to come down on its own.

- The cauliflower should be very soft. When a little cooler, add cauliflower and cooking liquid to a blender and process until smooth.

- Season with salt and pepper before serving with pasta.

Vinaigrette

Preparation time-10 minutes |Cook time-8 minutes |Serving-4 |Difficulty- Easy

Nutritional value: ~Calories-121| Fat-14g| Protein-0.3g| Carbohydrates-1g

Ingredients

- 3/4 cup of extra-virgin olive oil

- 1/3 cup of wine vinegar

- One teaspoon of Dijon mustard

- One clove of garlic, crushed

- Half teaspoon of salt

- A quarter teaspoon of ground black pepper

Instructions

- Just put everything in a clean jar, lid it tightly, and shake vigorously. You can store it in the jar and just shake it up again before use.

Vinegar Honey Sauce

Preparation time-10 minutes |Cook time-0 minutes |Serving-4 |Difficulty- Easy

Nutritional value: ~Calories-19| Fat-0.3g| Protein-0.2g| Carbohydrates-0.3g

Ingredients

- One and a quarter cup of balsamic vinegar
- Half cup of water
- A quarter cup of honey
- A quarter cup of cooking oil
- One tablespoon of Italian seasoning
- One teaspoon of salt
- One teaspoon of white pepper

Instructions

- Put ingredients in a medium bowl and whisk until combined. Use immediately or store refrigerated for up to 10 days.

White Albacore Tuna Dip

Preparation time-5 minutes| Cook time-0 minutes|Servings-6 |Difficulty-Easy

Nutritional value- Calories-90| Fat-20g |Carbohydrates-2g| Protein-8g

Ingredients

- Half cup of light mayonnaise
- Half cup of light sour cream
- Two tablespoons of fresh lemon juice
- Two teaspoons of minced garlic
- Two teaspoons of hot sauce
- Four tablespoons of chopped fresh dill weed
- Two 6-ounce pouches of white albacore tuna

Instructions

- In a blender, just put some garlic, dill, tuna, lemon juice, and hot sauce until pureed. Then add mayonnaise and sour cream, and purée again for 30 seconds. Enjoy.

White Wine Sherry Sauce

Preparation time-10 minutes |Cook time-0 minutes |Serving-4 |Difficulty- Easy

Nutritional value: ~Calories-32| Fat-2g| Protein-1g| Carbohydrates-2.3g

Ingredients

- One cup of dry white wine
- Half cup of water
- A quarter cup of cooking sherry
- A quarter cup of cooking oil
- Two tablespoons of finely minced shallots
- One tablespoon of dried parsley
- One tablespoon of finely minced garlic
- One tablespoon of finely minced capers
- One teaspoon of salt
- One teaspoon of pepper

Instructions

- Put ingredients in a medium bowl and whisk until combined. Use immediately or store refrigerated for up to 10 days.

Yogurt dressing

Preparation time-10 minutes |Cook time-0 minutes |Servings-2 |Difficulty-Easy

Nutritional value: ~Calories-160|Proteins-9g| Fat-8g|Carbohydrates-13g

Ingredients

- Crushed garlic or spearmint to taste
- One cup of plain yogurt

Instructions

- Mix garlic or spearmint into yogurt to taste.

Conclusion

The gastric bypass diet is a common method of losing weight in a short period of time. Unfortunately, the gastric bypass diet also necessitates significant modifications in one's way of life. The eating habits and cooking techniques you use must be changed totally if you want to lose weight using this method. When it comes to dietary limitations and food preparation procedures, you may find that your access to cooking devices is limited.

Finally, allow me to bring up an important point. You can only eat so much food at a time, no matter what type of weight-loss surgery you have undertaken. This is true regardless of the type of weight-loss procedure you have undergone. The size of your stomach before the operation was approximately the same as that of a tennis ball, with the ability to expand and grow. When you recover from surgery, your pouch shrinks dramatically in size and can only hold a few tablespoons of food. If you have a gastric bypass procedure, your pouch will be about the size of an egg when finished. In comparison to your previous stomach, this one will be smaller in size.

You've been through surgery and have taken in all of the information included in the book. What are your alternatives at this point? Listed below is a phrase to support you in your climb up the wellness ladder. To start, keep a food diary or journal of your eating habits to track your progress. In addition to aiding in weight reduction, keeping a diet record can be good for weight maintenance as well. It will be easier to keep track of your food intake and when you stray from your healthy eating plan with the help of a food journal. Additionally, keeping a food diary will assist you in becoming more conscious of when you are eating. By keeping a journal of your feelings when you assume you are hungry, it is possible to find that you are actually thirsty, fatigued, or agitated.

For the second time, good health starts in the kitchen. As a result, the first step toward becoming structured is to take stock of what you have, cut it down to what you absolutely require, and restructure it effectively with the goal of increasing efficiency. By planning your meals, you will be better able to maintain your diet regimen, keep within your financial constraints, and make the most of what you have. Spend some time each week preparing your weekly menus to prevent any guesswork and to give yourself a little extra time each day to get things done. You can design a shopping list based on your culinary preferences and make all of your weekly purchases in one trip, reducing the need to make frantic trips to the supermarket to pick up things that you may have forgotten about. If you were more organized, you might find it more fun to prepare healthy meals.

In this book, you'll find a full meal plan for each stage of your gastric post-op diet, as well as recipes for each of the food selections on the meal plan. There's also a wealth of additional information. Keep in mind that you are in command and that you can, with enough work, make significant improvements in your life.